PRINCIPLES AND MANAGEMENT OF SURGICAL INFECTIONS

PRINCIPLES AND MANAGEMENT OF SURGICAL INFECTIONS

Edited By:

John Mihran Davis, M.D.

Associate Professor, Department of Surgery, Cornell University Medical College,
Associate Attending Surgeon, The New York Hospital, New York, New York

G. Tom Shires, M.D.

Lewis Atterbury Stimson Professor and Chairman, Department of Surgery,
Cornell University Medical College,
Surgeon-in-Chief, The New York Hospital, New York, New York

WITH 42 CONTRIBUTORS

J. B. LIPPINCOTT COMPANY
Philadelphia

New York • St. Louis • London • Sydney • Tokyo

Acquisitions Editor: Lisa McAllister
Sponsoring Editor: Paula Callaghan
Project Editor: Tracy Resnik
Indexer: Julia Figures
Designer: Doug Smock
Production Manager: Helen Ewan
Production Coordinator: Kathryn Rule
Compositor: Circle Graphics
Printer/Binder: R.R. Donnelley & Sons Company

6 5 4 3 2 1

Library of Congress Cataloging in Publication Data

Principles and management of surgical infections / editors,
   John Mihran Davis and G. Tom Shires; with 42 contribu-
   tors.
      p.   cm.
   ISBN 0-397-50735-6
   1. Surgical wound infections. 2. Bacterial diseases.
I. Davis, John Mihran, 1946–   . II. Shires, G. Tom
(George Tom), 1925–   .
   [DNLM: 1. Bacterial Infections—prevention and con-
trol. 2. Surgical Wound Infection—prevention and con-
trol. WO 185 P957]
RD98.3.P75   1991
617′.01—dc20
DNLM/DLC
for Library of Congress   89-14281
                                            CIP

The authors and publisher have exerted every effort to ensure that drug selection and dosage set forth in this text
are in accord with current recommendations and practice at
the time of publication. However, in view of ongoing research, changes in government regulations, and the constant
flow of information relating to drug therapy and drug reactions, the reader is urged to check the package insert for
each drug for any change in indications and dosage and for
added warnings and precautions. This is particularly important when the recommended agent is a new or infrequently
employed drug.

CONTRIBUTORS

Anthony C. Antonacci, M.D.

Associate Professor of Surgery, Cornell University Medical College, Associate Attending Surgeon, The New York Hospital, New York, New York

Philip S. Barie, M.D.

Associate Professor of Surgery, Cornell University Medical College, Associate Attending Surgeon, Director, Surgical Intensive Care Unit, The New York Hospital, New York, New York

Arthur E. Brown, M.D.

Associate Professor Clinical Medicine and Clinical Pediatrics, Cornell University Medical College, Associate Attending Physician, Memorial Sloan–Kettering Cancer Center, Associate Attending Pediatrician, The New York Hospital, Chairman, Hospital Infection Committee, Memorial Sloan–Kettering Cancer Center, New York, New York

Eric J. Brown, M.D.

Associate Professor of Medicine, Washington University School of Medicine, St. Louis, Missouri

C. James Carrico, M.D.

Professor and Chairman, Department of Surgery, The University of Texas Southwestern Medical School, Dallas, Texas

Robert E. Condon, M.D., M.S.

Ausman Foundation Professor and Chairman, Department of Surgery, Medical College of Wisconsin, Director of Surgery, Milwaukee County Medical Complex, Chief of Surgery, Froedtert Memorial Lutheran Hospital, Milwaukee, Wisconsin

Paul P. Cook, M.D.

Assistant Professor of Medicine, Physician, Department of Medicine, East Carolina University School of Medicine, Greenville, North Carolina

Jerome J. DeCosse, M.D., Ph.D.

Professor of Surgery, Cornell University Medical College, Attending Surgeon, The New York Hospital, New York, New York

E. Patchen Dellinger, M.D.

Associate Professor of Surgery, University of Washington School of Medicine, Attending Surgeon, University of Washington Medical Center, Harborview Medical Center, Department of Surgery, University of Washington Medical Center, Seattle, Washington

R. Gordon Douglas, Jr., M.D.

Chairman, Department of Medicine, Cornell University Medical College, Physician-in-Chief, The New York Hospital, New York, New York

David L. Dunn, M.D., Ph.D.

Associate Professor of Surgery, Head, Surgical Infectious Diseases, Department of Surgery, University of Minnesota Medical School, University of Minnesota Hospitals and Clinics, Minneapolis, Minnesota

Richard L. Gamelli, M.D.

Professor and Vice Chairman, Department of Surgery, University of Vermont College of Medicine, Associate Surgeon-in-Chief, Medical Center Hospital of Vermont, Burlington, Vermont

Jeffrey P. Gold, M.D.

Assistant Professor of Surgery (Cardiothoracic Surgery), Assistant Professor of Surgery in Pediatrics, Cornell University Medical College, New York, New York

Leon D. Goldman, M.D.

Assistant Professor of Surgery, Harvard Medical School, Beth Israel Hospital, Boston, Massachusetts

Cleon W. Goodwin, M.D.

Associate Professor of Surgery, Cornell University Medical College, Director, The New York Hospital Burn Center, New York, New York

Barry Jay Hartman, M.D.

Associate Professor of Clinical Medicine, Cornell University Medical Center, Associate Attending Physician, The New York Hospital, New York, New York

Clifford M. Herman, M.D.

Professor of Surgery, University of Washington School of Medicine, Attending and Associate Surgeon-in-Chief, Harborview Medical Center, Seattle, Washington

O. Wayne Isom, M.D.

Professor of Surgery, Cornell University Medical College, Chairman, Division of Cardiothoracic Surgery, The New York Hospital, New York, New York

William G. Jones, M.D.

Resident, Department of Surgery, Cornell University Medical College, New York, New York

Mark S. Klempner, M.D.

Professor of Medicine, Tufts University School of Medicine, Physician, Department of Medicine, Division of Geographic and Infectious Diseases, New England Medical Center, Boston, Massachusetts

John N. Krieger, M.D.

Associate Professor, Department of Urology, University of Washington School of Medicine, Attending Surgeon, University of Washington Medical Center, Harborview Medical Center, Children's Hospital, Seattle V.A. Medical Center, Seattle, Washington

William J. Ledger, M.D.

Given Professor of Obstetrics and Gynecology, Cornell University Medical College, Obstetrician–Gynecologist-in-Chief, The New York Hospital, New York, New York

Stephen F. Lowry, M.D.

Associate Professor of Surgery, Director, Laboratory of Surgical Metabolism, Cornell University Medical College, Associate Attending Surgeon, The New York Hospital, New York, New York

Janet A. McGarr, M.D.

Department of Surgery, Washington University School of Medicine, St. Louis, Missouri

Albert T. McManus, M.D.

Chief, Microbiology Branch, U.S. Army Institute of Surgical Research, Brooke Army Medical Center, Fort Sam Houston, Texas

William F. McManus, M.D.

U.S. Army Institute of Surgical Research, Brooke Army Medical Center, Fort Sam Houston, Texas

J. Wayne Meredith, M.D.

Assistant Professor of Surgery, Bowman Gray School of Medicine, Wake Forest University Medical Center, Winston–Salem, North Carolina

John D. Meyer, M.D.

Department of Surgery, Harvard Medical School, Boston, Massachusetts

John S. Najarian, M.D.

Regents' Professor, Jay Phillips Chair in Surgery, University of Minnesota Medical School, Minneapolis, Minnesota

Claude H. Organ, Jr., M.D.

Professor and Vice Chair, Department of Surgery, University of California at Davis School of Medicine, Davis, California, Director, Residency Program, East Bay Hospital, Oakland, California

Paul M. Pellicci, M.D.

Associate Professor of Surgery (Orthopaedics), Assistant Professor of Anatomy, Cornell University Medical College, Associate Attending Orthopaedic Surgeon, Hospital for Special Surgery and The New York Hospital, New York, New York

Malcolm O. Perry, M.D.

The H. William Scott, Jr., Professor of Surgery, Chief, Division of Vascular Surgery, Vanderbilt University Medical Center, Nashville, Tennessee

Susan E. Pories, M.D.

Surgical Oncology Fellow, Harvard Medical School, New England Deaconess Hospital, Boston, Massachusetts

S. Frank Redo, M.D.

Professor of Surgery, Cornell University Medical College, Attending Surgeon, Chief of Pediatric Surgery, The New York Hospital, New York, New York

Craig D. Rhyne, M.D.

Assistant Professor, Department of Surgery, Texas Tech University, Lubbock, Texas

Eduardo A. Salvati, M.D.

Professor of Clinical Surgery (Orthopaedics), Cornell University Medical College, Attending Orthopaedic Surgeon, The Hospital for Special Surgery, The New York Hospital, New York, New York

William A. Silen, M.D.

Johnson & Johnson Professor of Surgery, Harvard Medical School, Surgeon-in-Chief, Beth Israel Hospital, Boston, Massachusetts

Michael L. Steer, M.D.

Professor of Surgery, Harvard Medical School, Associate Surgeon-in-Chief, Beth Israel Hospital, Boston, Massachusetts

Kevin J. Tracey, M.D.

Assistant Surgeon, Division of Neurosurgery, The New York Hospital, Cornell University Medical Center, Guest Investigator, Laboratory of Medical Biochemistry, Rockefeller University, New York, New York

Donald D. Trunkey, M.D.

Professor and Chairman, Department of Surgery, Oregon Health Sciences University, Portland, Oregon

Philip D. Wilson, Jr., M.D.

Professor of Surgery (Orthopaedics), Cornell University Medical Center, Attending Surgeon and Surgeon-in-Chief Emeritus, The Hospital for Special Surgery, New York, New York

Roger W. Yurt, M.D.

Associate Professor of Surgery, Vice Chairman, Department of Surgery, Cornell University Medical College, Associate Attending Surgeon, The New York Hospital, New York, New York

PREFACE

In the past two decades we have seen the emergence of two unrecognized pathogens, *Legionella pneumophila* (Legionnaire's disease) and *Borrelia burgdorferi* (Lyme disease), as the causes of serious infectious processes. Similarly, bacteria such as *Serratia marcescens* and *Acinetobacter calcoaceticus,* which were not believed to be pathogenic, have emerged as the causative agents in serious surgical infections. Certain pathogens not clinically evident for many years have reappeared. The causative agent of toxic shock syndrome, *Staphylococcus aureus,* is similar to the virulent strains of this microbe that plagued clinicians in the 1950s. A *Streptococcus pyogenes* has been identified that produces an exotoxin associated with shock, renal failure, and adult respiratory distress syndrome. This lethal pathogen is similar to the causative agent of scarlet fever seen in the 1930s and 1940s.

These clinical entities emphasize the continuing importance of infections in surgical practice. As the field of surgery moves into a new decade, surgeons are performing more complicated operations on sicker patients. Although we are armed with many new and potent antibiotics, the patients being treated are less resistant to infection. We feel justified in this setting to introduce a new text on surgical infections. This text is directed toward the clinical surgeon, who in this era should understand basic immunology, host resistance, and microbiology, as well as the major complications in the surgical specialties. With this in mind, we have attracted active clinicians who contribute regularly to their fields to address infectious topics of current importance.

John Mihran Davis, M.D.

CONTENTS

PRINCIPLES AND MANAGEMENT OF SURGICAL INFECTIONS

1

○   ○   ○   •   •   •

THE LYMPHOCYTE AND MONOCYTE RESPONSE

Craig D. Rhyne
Anthony C. Antonacci

The lymphocyte and monocyte response to pathogens commonly found in surgical infections involves a complex orchestrated interaction among serum proteins, cellular elements, and properties inherent to the invading microorganisms. It would be futile to attempt to cover in detail the entire immunologic chain of events that constitute the response to infection in the space of a single chapter. However, a description of the broader concepts involved in the body's resistance to infecting organisms as well as an overview of the humoral and cellular events that enable the body to kill and eliminate microbes will be presented.

GENERAL CONCEPTS

Invasion of Pathogens

The route by which pathogens gain entry in the host varies perhaps more extensively with surgical patients than with any other group. In addition to the usual portals of entry such as inhalation, ingestion, and cutaneous wounds, surgical patients are at risk from pathogens or opportunistic bacteria that gain access to tissue due to trauma, vascular accidents, burns, and surgically created wounds.

The normal host is remarkably well protected from all but the most inherently virulent microbial species. Patients with surgical disease frequently have disturbed physiologic homeostasis, which makes them susceptible to infection from otherwise harmless resident bacterial or fungal flora. These derangements vary and may result from injuries to protective structures such as the skin with penetrating wounds or burns. Loss of epithelial integrity due to vascular insult to the bowel or increased intraluminal pressure from obstruction may result in transudation of bacterial into the circulation or regional lymphatics even in the presence of intact mucosa. There is also substantial evidence that transudation of intestinal bacteria may occur during severe homeostatic disturbances such as trauma, burns, hypotension, and sepsis.[10,44] Blunt or penetrating trauma often results in rupture or perforation of hollow viscera with spill of contaminated bowel contents into the peritoneal, mediastinal, or retroperitoneal areas. Surgical wounds themselves provide an avenue of infection not usually encountered by other patients.

Although surgical patients are susceptible to the entire spectrum of pathogens from viral to parasitic, the majority of infections in surgical patients are bacterial or fungal. The emphasis of this chapter will concentrate, therefore, on these most common pathogens and attempt to provide an overview of the spectrum of host defenses that are called into play when these infections occur.

Mechanical and Chemical Defenses

The skin is a remarkably effective barrier to microorganisms of all types. Injuries to the skin that cause loss of integrity include abrasions, lacerations, crush injuries, and burns. Burns represent the most severe challenge to the host and provide an avenue for recurrent life-threatening infections. With the progress in recent years in resuscitation of burn patients, the fatal outcomes in any burn unit are usually related to infectious complications.[32]

Other normally active mechanisms that protect the host from infection are the production of mucus in the respiratory and gastrointestinal tract, and the bathing of tissues with secretions rich in immunoglobulins, such as tears or saliva. The ciliary action of the bronchial mucosa constantly cleanses the airways of inhaled bacteria and fungal spores trapped in the protective mucus. The explosive movement of air in both coughing and sneezing removes pathogens from the host (although paradoxically spreading infections in the population). The flow of intestinal contents and the act of defecation remove large numbers of bacteria from the body and maintain a protective balance in the microbial flora of the bowel.

The upper gastrointestinal tract is protected from ingested organisms by the acidic pH of the stomach. In patients with normal acid production in the stomach, the upper GI tract is essentially sterile. By contrast, achlorhydric patients may well have significant amounts of microbial species present in the stomach and proximal small intestine.

Finally, the unidirectional flow of some biologic fluids, such as urine or bile, provides protection against the encroachment of pathogens. Partial or complete obstruction of the normal flow of these fluids by stones, hypertrophic tissue, or tumors can produce potentially severe or fatal infectious complications.

Immune Defenses

The goal of the immune response may be simply stated. Once a pathogen gains access to the host's tissues, the body generates an elaborately orchestrated effort to control the further spread of infection and to identify, destroy, and eliminate the invading microbes. The basic elements that participate in this effort are the serum complement proteins, immunoglobulins produced by B lymphocytes, T-lymphocyte-mediated cellular responses, phagocytic cells such as neutrophils, and monocytic cells, which function both as phagocytes and as antigen-processing cells. These components are intimately interrelated, and each functions optimally only in the presence of an intact performance by the others. Congenital defects in these systems, such as agammaglobulinemia, selective immunoglobulin deficiencies, absent complement proteins, deficient intracellular killing, and deficient T-cell production, exist and are associated with recurrent or persistent infections, usually of a particular type.

Each of these systems will be reviewed individually in the context of its participation in the stated goal of containment, destruction, and elimination of pathogens. Additionally, an attempt will be made to emphasize the interrelationships of these systems in the immune response.

COMPLEMENT PROTEINS

The complement system represents a preformed defense against invading pathogens that does not require previous exposure or "immunity" in the usual sense. The system consists of at least 18 serum proteins, which constitute approximately 15% of the plasma globulin fraction. The function of these proteins is twofold: direct and indirect lysis of cells, which activate the proteolytic cascades, and the production of inflammatory mediators, which recruit leukocytes to areas of inflammation. There are two pathways by which the complement system is activated, the classical pathway and the alternate (or properdin system) pathway (Fig. 1-1).

The Classical Pathway

Activation of the classical pathway in the setting of infection requires the presence of antibodies to the invading microbes. This entails a requisite prior exposure to these organisms, and appreciable levels of antibody present at the time of subsequent infection. In this regard, the classical pathway is of less importance during first-time infections than the alternate pathway, which requires no antibody.

Not all antibodies will function in this regard. Only antibodies of the IgM, IgG_1, IgG_2, or IgG_3 classes or subclasses will effectively fix complement to initiate the cascade. These so-called complement-fixing antibodies are able to bind the C1

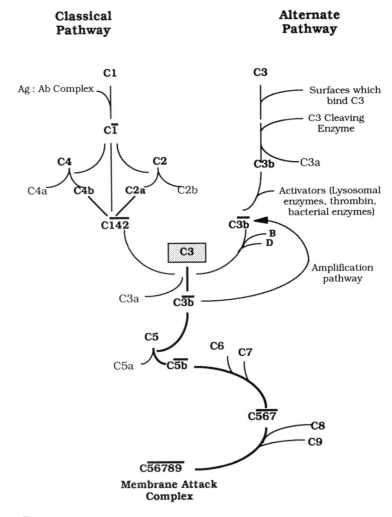

Figure 1–1.
The classical and alternate pathways of complement activation. The heavy bar
over the component numbers indicates the enzymatically activated complexes.

fragment to the Fc portion of the antibody molecule. This attachment protects the C1
from inactivation, perpetuating the cascade sequence. Additionally, not only do antigen–antibody complexes work in this regard, but aggregated immunoglobulin, C
reactive protein, DNA, staphylococcal protein A, and trypsinlike enzymes will also
trigger the classical pathway proteins.

The Alternate Pathway

Once thought to be a separate serologically active defense mechanism, the
alternate pathway has greater significance in the initial stages of infection than does

the classical pathway.[14] Originally named the properdin system,[31] the alternate pathway can be directly initiated by bacterial cell wall components without the need for specific antibody. Not only do certain bacterial polysaccharides trigger the alternate pathway, but the absence of other polysaccharides, such as sialic acid, seem to do so as well. Evidence indicates that sialic acid residues, which are absent from the cell walls of most bacteria, increase the affinity for cell-bound C3b for an inhibitory protein beta 1 H (factor I). This inhibitor protein can arrest the cascade. Conversely, the lack of sialic acid allows the activation of the C3b with protein B, which encourages and amplifies the cascade. Strong evidence that this is the case comes from two sources. First, those few bacteria that are known to have sialic acid residues in their walls, such as K1 *E. coli,* type III group B *Streptococci,* and groups B and C *Neisseria meningitidis,* are highly pathogenic in humans. Secondly, foreign cells such as sheep erythrocytes, which normally do not activate complement, will do so readily if sialic acid residues are cleaved from their membranes.[14]

Although the alternate pathway does not absolutely require antibody, some classes of antibody will activate complement proteins by way of the alternate pathway, including IgA and some IgG subclasses. Other activators include bacterial lipopolysaccharide, trypsinlike enzymes, and several types of bacterial and plant polysaccharides. Interestingly, cobra venom contains a very specific activator of the alternate pathway, which has provided a powerful experimental tool to study this system.

Shared Pathway

Despite differences in the two initial phases of complement activation, once having reached the activation of C3 to C3b, the terminal stages proceed rapidly in an identical fashion. The formation of C5–C9 complexes form an ionic pore in the membrane of the cell under attack, which leads to disruption and death of the cell.[27]

Control of Complement Activation

A complete review of the mechanisms that control this powerful biologic response system cannot be provided in this manuscript. However, it should be noted that multiple steps in both the classical and alternate pathways are susceptible to positive and negative influences. These control mechanisms include time-dependent associations of molecules, pH requirements, relative concentrations and availability of inhibitor proteins such as C1 inhibitor or factor I, and rates of formation of the activated complement proteins. (See Stites et al, *Basic and Clinical Immunology,* Chap. 11, "The Complement System," for a complete review.)

Defects in both the principal proteins of the complement system as well as the inhibitor proteins are associated with human disease states.[23] It is important to note that while congenital deficiencies of the components of the classical pathway are associated with autoimmune diseases such as systemic lupus erythematosus, deficiencies of the alternate or shared pathway (*i.e.,* C3 or C3b inactivator deficiencies) predispose a person to recurrent, severe infectious complications. Notably, those persons who have a genetic deficiency of the shared membrane attack sequence

(C5–C6–C7–C8–C9) often are susceptible to recurrent *Neisseria* infections of both gonococcal and meningococcal types.

Interaction with Other Immune System Components

In addition to autonomous activity against invading pathogens, the complement system also participates to a great degree in the function of the other immune mechanisms. It has been mentioned that complement proteins attach to specific sites on the Fc portions of IgM and three IgG subclasses. The C1 molecule has six binding sites for these immunoglobulin Fc receptors. Attachment of this complement protein to an antibody complexed with antigen initiates the classical pathway eventuating in disruption of the cell. Complement proteins also contribute to a phenomenon known as "immune adherence." This phenomenon (which is similar to opsonization with antibodies) is predominantly mediated by way of the attachment of the C3b component. The attachment of this complement protein allows for direct recognition of foreign cell surfaces through complement receptors on the surfaces of many cells of the immune system, including neutrophils, monocytes, tissue macrophages, and B lymphocytes.[13] While the function of complement receptors on B lymphocytes remains uncertain, the presence of complement protein fragments on bacterial surfaces promotes adherence of the microbes to the remainder of these cells and promotes eventual phagocytosis.[15]

Finally, components of the complement sequences, most notably C5A, are powerful chemoattractants for the cells of the immune system. The presence of C5A has been shown to promote granulocyte aggregation, to stimulate oxidative metabolism, and to promote release of monokines such as interleukin-1.

In summary, the complement system represents a tightly regulated, highly lethal, and nonspecific defense against invading pathogens that requires no prior immunologic exposure to be effective. It is, therefore, the first line of immunologic defense against infection once the body's physical barriers have been penetrated by an invading organism.

B LYMPHOCYTES— ANTIBODY PRODUCTION

Perhaps the most specific defense generated against an invading pathogen by the host is the production of antibody molecules. Antibodies are (usually) exquisitely precise in their affinity for non-self molecules on the surfaces of foreign cells or organisms. The ability to generate so elaborate a response has been a subject of intensive study for many decades. Recently, exciting new investigations have begun to define the exact molecular and genetic mechanisms by which the B lymphocytes are able to respond to a foreign antigen, to refine the response, and to "remember" the event, which enables an even more vigorous response should the same antigen be reencountered at a later date.

A given lymphocyte and its progeny, once stimulated by antigen, will produce antibodies with a single specificity. This cell can, however, switch the class of antibody produced from IgM, for example, to a more versatile antibody such as IgG. It has been estimated that the lymphocyte population in humans ranges from 1 million to 100 million clones of cells. The number of cells in each clone is highly variable, from a single cell to greater than one million cells directing a unified response against a given antigen. These lymphocytes possess an enormous capacity to produce immuno-globulins. Mathematical models predict that over one million different specificities can be produced by combining the various heavy and light chains encoded in the DNA. Also, a single stimulated plasma cell can release an estimated 10,000 antibody molecules per second.[8]

Antibody production, collectively called the humoral response, is most effective against extracellular pathogens. Antibodies probably have no effect against pathogens that have gained a foothold inside the cells of the host organism. As we have seen with certain complement proteins, the antibodies will attach to the surface of foreign cells and greatly magnify the phagocytic response of host leukocytes, a process known as opsonization. While antibodies are superior to the complement proteins in promoting phagocytosis, they are at a slight disadvantage in that several days are often required for the antibodies to become available after initial exposure to the antigen.

B Lymphocytes

The body's contingent of B lymphocytes is generated in the bone marrow and requires no further processing or "education" in another milieu. Approximately 10^9 B cells are released into the circulation daily, and, if unstimulated, the majority will die within a few days. The appropriate clone of B lymphocytes responds to cognate antigen by way of membrane-bound immunoglobulin molecules. The surface immu-noglobulin of the B lymphocyte, usually monomeric IgM or IgD, reflects the precise antigen specificity that subsequently released immunoglobulin from that expanding clone will manifest. It is now recognized that each B-cell progenitor develops antigenic specificity completely independent of exposure to that antigen.

Typically, B cells first encounter microbial antigens in the spleen or in the lymph nodes draining the portal of entry of the offending microbes. Once the B lymphocyte recognizes its antigenic "opponent," several events occur. B cells undergo rapid proliferation and subsequent differentiation into plasma cells, which are the mature antibody-secreting cells (Fig. 1-2). These plasma cells remain localized in the lym-phoid tissue and do not appear to reenter the circulation. Despite remaining in the spleen or regional nodes, these plasma cells secrete enormous amounts of antibody, which does recirculate freely in body. A small population of B-cell progeny will become memory cells, which do reenter the circulation. These memory cells continue to circulate and are available to promote a brisk secondary antibody response if they encounter the same antigen in the future.

Immunoglobulin Classes

When an antigen is identified and bound by immunoglobulin molecules, the net effect or response to that event depends to a large extent on the immunoglobulin class

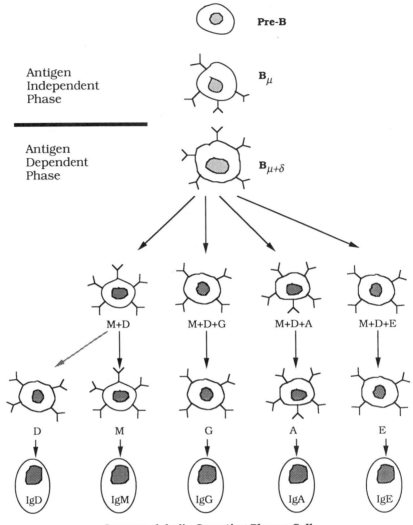

Immunoglobulin Secreting Plasma Cells

Figure 1–2.
B lymphocyte maturation and specialization. Pre-B cells develop into immature B cells with surface-bound monomeric IgM (B_μ) without antigenic exposure. Differentiation into mature B cells with both surface IgM and IgD ($B_{\mu+\delta}$) is thought to require antigenic exposure. Further stimulation with antigen and cytokines results in an intermediate stage of B-cell activation with both surface IgM and IgD, as well as surface immunoglobulin of the class that will ultimately be secreted. Loss of surface IgM and IgD occurs first, followed by loss of the class-specific surface immunoglobulin. Plasma cells bear no surface-bound immunoglobulins.

that is predominantly involved. Antibodies that recognize the same antigenic determinants may produce far different results based on the type of Fc portion (class) of the antibody. For example, the IgA class, which is secreted through mucous membranes into body fluids such as tears, sweat, saliva, bile, and intestinal fluids, may work primarily to block the sites on the microorganisms that would otherwise enable them to attach to epithelial surfaces. These microbes are not destroyed by this antibody "coating," only prevented from adhering to the epithelial cells of the host. By contrast, microbes that are bound to IgM or IgG antibodies in the blood or extracellular spaces may be directly lysed by complement proteins or phagocytosed by neutrophils or macrophages, which attach the Fc portions of those antibodies by way of their own Fc cell surface receptors.

The humoral system also undergoes a gradual maturation through the early years of life. Although human infants have intact production of B lymphocytes, the ability to produce the different classes of immunoglobulin varies as the person matures. This may, in part, be reflected in the different types of pathogens that typically affect infants and children as opposed to adults. A brief review of the different immunoglobulin subclasses and their properties follows (see Fig. 1-3).

IgM

IgM is the first antibody produced when a person is challenged by a hitherto unrecognized antigen. The molecule is extremely large with a molecular weight of 900,000 to 1 million. Because of its size the vast majority of IgM produced remains in the circulation and does not penetrate the extravascular spaces. Serum levels of IgM are usually 1.0 mg/ml, and its serum half-life is 5 to 6 days. It is a pentameric molecule composed of five immunoglobulin subunits linked by a J chain. The total number of combining sites for antigen is ten, making IgM extremely efficient at generating antigen–antibody networks, which are rapidly removed from the circulation. Complement is bound quite efficiently to the Fc portion of the IgM molecule, allowing activation of the full cascade and effecting eventual perforation and death of the microbe involved. IgM is also proficient at promoting phagocytosis of foreign cells through opsonization. The ability to synthesize IgM is attained early in life, with adult levels of IgM present in the circulation by 1 year of age.[8]

IgG

IgG antibodies exhibit several important functional differences from IgM. While still a relatively large molecule (molecular weight approximately 150,000), it is estimated that 50% of the total body pool of IgG resides in the extravascular spaces and lymphatics. Far more abundant in terms of total amount, approximately 12 mg/ml of IgG is measurable in normal serum. This makes IgG by far the most abundant antibody available. The half-life of IgG is considerably longer than IgM at 21 to 25 days. While some subclasses of IgG can fix and activate complement proteins, a more important function appears to be the opsonization of foreign cells. Four subclasses of IgG have been described, and each subclass appears to possess a slightly different functional

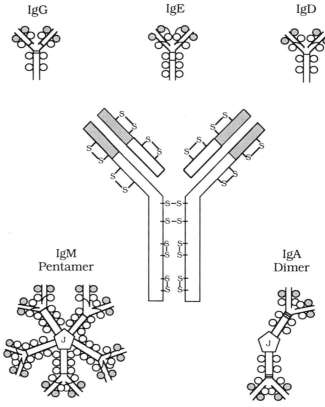

IgG   IgE   IgD

IgM
Pentamer

IgA
Dimer

Figure 1–3.
Immunoglobulin classes. The central figure schematically depicts the
monomeric immunoglobulin molecule. The shaded portions of both the
heavy and light chains represent the highly variable antigen combining
sites. The remaining domains are the constant regions of both light and
heavy chains, which are bounded by the indicated disulfide bonds. The
major classes of immunoglobulin are seen at the periphery. IgG subclasses (4) and IgA (2) are not shown.

repertoire. Maturation of the IgG system takes slightly longer than that of IgM, and
adult levels are not attained until about the fifth year of life.[8]

IgA

As mentioned in the overview, IgA is a unique immunoglobulin secreted through
epithelial cell surfaces. It is present in normal persons on external surfaces in sweat
and tears, and in the lumen of the biliary tree and the intestine. It is also secreted in
high quantities in maternal breast milk, conferring some degree of protection from
intestinal pathogens to infants. Normally accounting for 1.8 mg/ml of serum proteins,
it has a half-life of about 6 days. The major function of this immunoglobulin is not to

modulate killing of microbes; rather, it functions to augment local host resistance by coating the attachment surfaces of microbes and blocking their ability to adhere to the host epithelial cell surfaces. Despite the seeming importance of this function, persons have been identified who are deficient in IgA production. These persons do not seem to manifest a significantly increased susceptibility to infection, a paradox that may be explained by their compensatory secretion of IgM into the areas in which IgA is absent. Even in normal persons, adult levels of IgA are not reached until adolescence.

IgE

IgE is present in minute amounts in the serum, estimated at approximately 0.003 to 0.0003 mg/ml with a very short half-life of 2 days. Its function appears to be the mediation of allergic responses by way of the release of vasoactive substances, such as histamine from the cytoplasmic granules of basophils and mast cells. These local vasoactive phenomena may assist defenses in infectious processes by increasing availability of complement components and soluble immunoglobulins in extravascular tissue spaces. There is also evidence that IgE participates in the recruitment of cytotoxic eosinophils in some parasitic infections.[4]

IgD

Although the exact function of IgD remains speculative, it is present in the serum in minute quantities, about 0.03 mg/ml, and has a half-life of 2 to 3 days. It appears to be the second class of immunoglobulin produced in the differentiation of B lymphocytes, following IgM. Surface-bound IgD is present on a large percentage of circulating B cells. These surface IgD+ resting B cells will, when stimulated with antigen, differentiate into plasma cells that secrete predominantly IgG, not IgD. Thus, the presence of IgD on the surface of these B lymphocytes represents a developmental stage in their maturation to immunoglobulin-secreting effector cells.

The Antibody Response

During exposure to a novel infectious agent, the strongly antigenic portions are recognized by the appropriate clone of B lymphocytes, and these cells enter and remain localized to lymphoid tissue in the nodes or spleen. There they undergo differentiation and proliferate into plasma cells that eventually secrete immuno-globulin specific for the foreign antigen. Approximately 5 days after exposure, IgM directed against these antigenic foci is detectable in the serum. This is followed in 2 to 3 days by the appearance of IgG with the same specificity. As seen in Figure 1-4, the relative amounts of IgM and IgG are roughly equivalent following the primary expo-sure. Should the host encounter the same antigen at a later date, the IgM response is more rapid and is concomitantly associated with a markedly elevated IgG response. This "secondary response" demonstrates the capacity of the immune system to "remember" prior infectious challenges and to protect the host from these recurrent exposures.

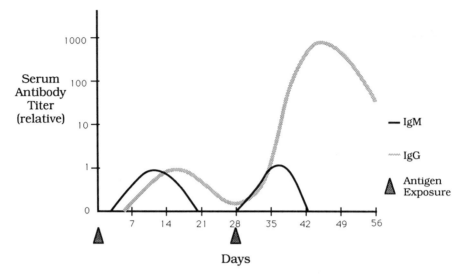

Figure 1–4.
The humoral response to antigen. After an antigenic challenge, detectable IgM appears in the serum in 4 to 5 days, followed in 2 or 3 more days by an equivalent amount of IgG. Subsequent exposure to the same antigen results in a slightly more brisk IgM response and a simultaneous and markedly heightened IgG response. (After Hood LE, ed., Immunology. 2nd ed. Menlo Park: Benjamin/Cummings 1984:288)

Lymphokines and T-Cell Help

The B lymphocytes cannot act alone in the production of immunoglobulin. Although the B cells are solely responsible for the production and release of the immunoglobulin molecules, both cytokines and T lymphocytes are necessary for the full humoral response. The B lymphocytes are able to recognize certain antigens with repeating determinants and to produce IgM without accessory T lymphocytes. In the vast majority of instances, however, T helper cells are required not only for IgM production, but also to affect immunoglobulin class switches to the production of IgG. Cell-to-cell contact between the T and B lymphocytes is required in these interactions, and intracytoplasmic events, such as microtubule orientation directed toward the opposite cell, appear to be involved.[21,34]

Recent evidence confirms that B cells participate in the induction of T-cell "help." In addition to recognizing antigen by surface-bound immunoglobulin, the B cell also internalizes and partially denatures the antigen. Following this, the partially denatured antigen is presented to T cells in a manner indistinguishable from antigen presentation by macrophages.[6] There is also evidence that B cells produce the membrane-bound form (only) of interleukin-1, which is a product required by T cells for activation. This cytokine was previously thought to be solely a monocyte/macrophage product.[22]

Additionally, soluble lymphokines (or cytokines) have been described that are requisite to the maturation of the B lymphocytes. They include interleukin-4 (formerly called B-cell-stimulating factor 1),[30] B-cell-stimulating factor 2, and gamma-interferon.[12]

The first of these factors, interleukin-4 (IL-4), is produced by activated T cells. B lymphocytes that have recognized an antigen through binding with their surface immunoglobulin are stimulated by this cytokine to proliferate and to express MHC class II molecules on their surface. These class II molecules (discussed more thoroughly in the sections entitled "T Cells" and "Monocytes") are crucial in allowing continued communication between the B lymphocytes and helper T lymphocytes. Interleukin-4 also exerts an influence on resting T cells to promote growth.[30]

Subsequent to the initial antigenic stimulation and IL-4 induced proliferation, the second of these cytokines, interleukin-6 (formerly, B-cell-stimulating factor 2), promotes differentiation of the expanding B-cell clone into immunoglobulin-secreting plasma cells. This factor may be identical with beta 2 interferon, plasmacytoma growth factor, and hepatocyte-stimulating factor.[12]

Other cytokines also appear to influence the B-cell clone, such as interleukin-1, interleukin-2, and gamma-interferon, which have been shown experimentally to augment the effects of the other cytokines. Figure 1-5 shows the principal steps in the activation of a resting B cell into a mature immunoglobulin-secreting plasma cell.

T LYMPHOCYTES

Overview

Classically and correctly regarded as mediators of the delayed type hypersensitivity reaction, it is now recognized that T lymphocytes play several crucial roles in many aspects of the immune response. While they do perform a surveillance function to attack and kill not only foreign tissue and certain tumors, T lymphocytes play a central role in the identification and destruction of autologous cells that harbor intracellular pathogens, either viral, fungal, or bacterial. Great diversity in the T-cell population exists and enables them to perform these effector functions and also to participate heavily in the control of other immune responses. It is increasingly apparent that the perception widely held as recently as 10 years ago of T lymphocytes divided into two large categories of "helpers" or "suppressors" is simplistic at best. The T cells that bear the CD4 surface markers and are collectively called "helpers" also contain a small group of cells that "help" to induce the activity of suppressor T lymphocytes. The "suppressor" T cells, recognized by their CD8 surface markers, not only control deleterious immune responses, but also have been shown to perform direct cytotoxic effector functions. These cytotoxic CD8 + T cells play an important role in destroying virally infected autologous tissue.

It is likely that other functions of these two groups remain to be discovered. It is important to note that T lymphocytes in both the CD4 + and CD8 + groups are "restricted" in their activity by gene products of the host major histocompatibility complex (MHC).[35] It is increasingly apparent that products of the MHC are involved in a majority of intercellular communications. Historically regarded as important in transplantation, it is clear that these gene products regulate the interactions between

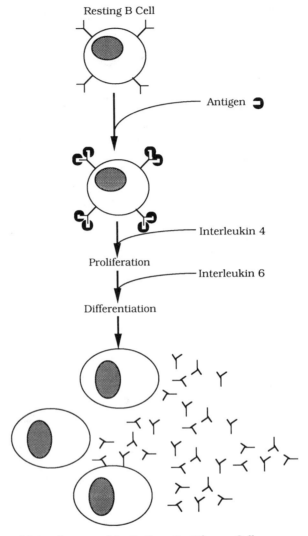

Resting B Cell

Antigen

Interleukin 4

Proliferation

Interleukin 6

Differentiation

Mature Immunoglobulin Secreting Plasma Cells

Figure 1–5.
B-cell activation. Following antigenic triggering of a responsive B-cell clone, both interleukin-4 and interleukin-6 are required to potentiate the production of immunoglobulin-secreting plasma cells.

the cells of the immune system. The class I markers are the molecules that discriminate "self" from "non-self" in the classical sense. The class II markers are now unquestionably involved in the initiation of T-cell responses. For a CD4 + T cell to initiate activity in response to an antigen, it must simultaneously recognize an autologous MHC class II molecule on the surface of an accessory cell.[43] Similarly, the CD8 + T cells require corecognition of a class I product to initiate their function.[16]

Class I   **Class II**   **Antibody**

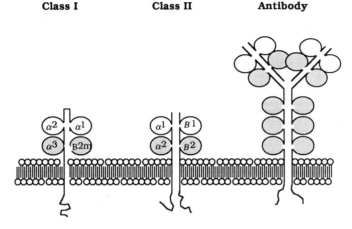

Figure 1–6.
The major histocompatibility complex/immunoglobulin gene family products. Shaded domains indicate considerable amino acid sequence homology, suggesting a common evolutionary ancestry for these structures. (Note that beta 2 microglobulin in the class I protein is not anchored to the membrane but is associated with the three domains of the membrane bound class I protein.) (After Hood LE, ed. Immunology. 2nd ed. Menlo Park: Benjamin/Cummings, 1984:204)

In recent years, advances in the field of molecular genetics have shown that many of the molecules involved in the immune responses share striking similarities despite their divergent functions. Amino acid sequence homologies in portions of the class I, class II, and the antibody molecules strongly suggest that these genes evolved from a common ancestral gene, which has been conserved and amplified to perform these specialized functions[39] (Fig. 1-6).

Thymic Processing

Unlike B lymphocytes, T cells require additional processing or "education" outside the bone marrow. Immature T lymphocytes released by the marrow are localized to the thymus where they undergo maturation or elimination. It has been estimated that 98% of all T lymphocytes that enter the thymus are destroyed there, and that only the remaining 2% are released into the peripheral circulation. It is likely that all T-cell clones that have the potential for recognizing self-antigens are selectively deleted in this way. Although the thymus undergoes involution at puberty, it remains active throughout life in the process of providing mature T cells to the body.

Investigators are beginning to understand how the thymus performs this educational and selection process. Briefly, the T cells may be allowed to recognize both MHC class I markers and class II markers in different regions of the thymus. This recognition, depending on the context in which it occurs, results in either maturation or elimination of the T cell in question.

Antigen Recognition—The T-Cell Receptor

T lymphocytes, unlike B lymphocytes, do not usually recognize antigen in its native form.[7,20,36] Additionally, it has been shown conclusively that the antigens recognized by T cells must be presented to the T cell by another cell bearing MHC. Class II proteins.[2] This introduces the intervention of another cell type, collectively called accessory cells. The primary accessory cells include monocytes, tissue macrophages, dendritic reticular cells, and Langerhans cells. Functions of these accessory cells include phagocytosis of antigens, partial degradation of the antigens by combining the phagosome with intracellular lysosomes containing proteolytic enzymes, and allowing the fragments of the original antigens to interact with class II molecules available on the internal membrane surface of the phagolysosome. Certain portions of the digested antigens may have the ability to combine with these molecules, probably through hydrogen bonding and hydrophobic/hydrophillic interactions.[11,17] The processed antigen and its phagolysosome are then exocytosed to the cell membrane, which, when everted, exposes the processed antigen and the associated class II molecule on the external surface of the accessory cell. T lymphocytes are then able to recognize the antigen fragment associated with this class II molecule, and clonal proliferation of the appropriate T-cell clone or clones will occur. This process results in a marked increase in the number of T cells bearing specific reactivity for the determinants of the infecting agent. It must be noted that antigen/MHC recognition is only one of the two known obligatory signals for the activation of T-cell responses. The second required signal is a cytokine, interleukin-1, which is available in either a membrane-bound form or as a soluble macrophage product.[28]

Extensive investigation has been performed in recent years searching for the identity of the T-cell antigen receptor. It now appears certain that the T-cell receptor is the T3/Ti complex consisting of five membrane-associated proteins present on all T cells following thymic processing (Fig. 1-7). The Ti portion of the complex, consisting of alpha and beta subunits, forms an antigen/MHC receptor "pocket," which is analogous to the surface immunoglobulin-binding site on B lymphocytes. This dimeric molecule, in all likelihood, evolved from the same primordial gene from which the immunoglobulin family arose as evidenced by the presence of variable, joining, diversity, and constant portions of these subunits.[40] When the receptor is occupied by a recognized antigen/MHC molecule, the associated T3 proteins (gamma, delta, and epsilon) act as transmembrane messengers that will activate the internal T-cell milieu by increasing intracytosolic free calcium and cleavage of phosphoinositol biphosphate

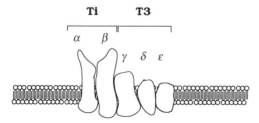

Figure 1–7.
Schematic representation of the T-cell receptor complex. The Ti portion is probably responsible for recognition of both the processed antigen and the class II MHC protein on the surface of an accessory cell. The T3 portion is likely involved in transmitting message signals to the cell interior (see text).

into putative second messengers, inositol triphosphate and diacylglycerol. Other activation messengers, such as kinases, may also be involved in these intracellular events.[33]

Lymphokines

In addition to direct clonal expansion of T cells to effect immunologic responses, the reactive T cells will manufacture and secrete numerous products that serve to amplify the immune response.[12] As previously discussed, T cells and their elaborated products, such as IL-4 and B-cell-stimulating factor 2, are required by B lymphocytes to generate the production of almost all antibodies. It is also now well documented that T cells exert autocrine regulation of their own function by making and releasing a lymphokine, interleukin-2 (IL-2), which is subsequently bound back to specialized receptors on their own cell membranes. When a T-cell clone is stimulated with processed antigen and IL-1, both the lymphokine and the IL-2 surface receptors are produced by the cell. If either the IL-2 or its receptor molecule are not produced in sufficient quantities, the T-cell response is impeded. Tight control of this response is possible, therefore, due to required threshold amounts of both interleukin-2 and the number of IL-2 cell surface receptors.

While these two examples are of prime importance in demonstrating the level of control that T cells exert on the overall response to infection, they are far from a complete list of immunomodulating T-cell products. The recruitment of other cells involved in the host response includes the elaboration of macrophage chemotactic factor, macrophage migration inhibition factor, and macrophage aggregation factor; all of which serve to promote the ingress and localization of phagocytic/accessory cells to areas of infection.

T cells also elaborate a broad-spectrum stimulator of bone marrow stem cells known as interleukin-3 (IL-3) whose exact role in immunologic responses remains to be defined. Preliminary evidence suggests that IL-3 is capable of stimulating the proliferation of blood monocytes and tissue macrophages.[5] Gamma-interferon, a potent immunomodulating T-cell product, performs multiple functions: (1) inducing both class I and class II MHC products, (2) augmenting the cytotoxic activity of natural killer (NK) cells and macrophages, and (3) amplifying (or inhibiting) the effects of other lymphokines.[1,12] Other lymphokines have been described, but their role in modifying the immune response in the setting of acute and chronic infections remains to be elucidated.

Other Possible T-Lymphocyte Functions

The elaborately complex set of T-lymphocyte responses to infection already described may not represent a completed picture. There is new evidence that T cells may participate in the direct killing of extracellular bacteria by way of elaboration of a soluble product, which as yet remains unidentified.[25,26] It appears experimentally that this is a primary T-cell function with the T lymphocyte as the final effector cell. Classically, the T-cell system has been thought to be involved only in the identification and cooperative killing (along with macrophages as the final effector cell) of tissue infected with either viruses or intracellular bacteria. Thus far, this newly described T-cell function does not seem to involve restriction by the class II MHC products. Although this represents a potentially exciting T-cell function, the clinical significance of this new experimental data remains to be clarified.

MONOCYTES

Overview

One of the first immune responses described was that of phagocytosis of foreign material by cells specialized for this purpose. The preservation of this function through the evolution from invertebrates to the vertebrates attests to the efficiency and efficacy of this system as a protective mechanism for the host. By contrast, the development of specialized immune response cells such as B and T lymphocytes is a relatively recent evolutionary occurrence and exists in only the "higher" vertebrate species.[9]

Origins and Differentiation

The cells of the human host that perform this function are principally the granulocytic and the monocytic leukocytes. This includes the tissue macrophages that represent the differentiation and unique tissue specialization of the circulating monocyte pool.

The granulocytes in the peripheral blood are the primary cells involved in the direct phagocytic attack against invading microbes. The importance of the granulocytes in localizing and eliminating an infective source is well appreciated.

The other lineage of bone-marrow-derived phagocytic cells, the monocytes, comprises only 3% to 7% of the normal number of circulating leukocytes. The vast majority of the total pool of mononuclear phagocytes resides in the tissues as macrophages. These tissue macrophages can be relatively quiescent physiologically until acted upon by inflammatory products that induce different states of priming or activation, allowing the macrophages to perform accessory or effector functions.[1]

The tissue macrophages share with the neutrophil the ability to phagocytose and kill microbes intracellularly. Additionally, however, macrophages play a pivotal role in the control of T lymphocytes. Not only do these mononuclear cells engage in intracellular killing of microbes, but they, unlike neutrophils, can use digested microbial fragments for antigen presentation if they constituitively or inductively express the class II MHC markers. The ability of the macrophages to elaborate monokines is also a major factor in the host response to infection. Tissue macrophages reside in both lymphoid and nonlymphoid tissues and are situated ideally to perform this dual role.

Monocyte Effector Functions

The repertoire of the macrophage is incredibly diverse and includes the direct attack of invasive organisms without other intervening cells. This is accomplished in part by either release of cellular products such as lysozyme or proteases, which can directly attack bacterial cell walls, or the phagocytosis and intracellular killing of microbes with lysosomal hydrolases or reactive oxygen intermediates.

The ability of the macrophage to ingest and kill microbes seems to depend in large part on the availability of specific cell surface receptors for either components of complement (C1 or C3), receptors for the Fc portion of immunoglobulins, or receptors for various polysaccharides such as a mannose–fructose receptor. The last of these may enable the macrophage to ingest bacteria directly if these sugar residues are available on the bacterial cell wall.

Accessory Functions of Macrophages

As discussed in the section on T-cell responses, the macrophages fulfill the T lymphocytes' unique requirement for stimulation by processed denatured antigen. This accessory function depends on several linked processing events. The macrophage must be able to phagocytose the native antigen and combine the phagosome with an intracellular lysosome containing acid hydrolases. The partially denatured antigen is then allowed to combine with the class II MHC protein on the inner surface of the phagolysosome. When an antigen is successfully combined with this molecule, it is protected from further degradation and, when exocytosed to the plasma membrane, is available for recognition by the T lymphocytes in conjunction with the obligatory class II marker. While this scheme seems complex, it enables the immune system to control tightly immune reactivity and explains one method by which the awesome power of the immune system is held in check against autoreactivity.[42,43]

Monokines and Serum Proteins

Monocytes and macrophages contribute to the overall immune response by the secretion of numerous cellular products (>75 different molecules). The most important of these regarding the response to infection are monokines that help to stimulate the immune response and those that contribute directly to kill or opsonize invading microbes.

In the first category are products such as interleukin-1 (IL-1), which has been conclusively shown to exert numerous physiologic effects that we associate with the acute response to infections such as fever, leukocytosis, and hypotension. It also appears responsible for the induction of hepatic acute phase proteins, increased insulin levels, release of ACTH and adrenal corticosteroids, induction of slow wave sleep, and muscle proteolysis. Immunologically, it is a potent chemotactic agent; an inducer of natural killer-cell activity; and, through its effect on T-cell activation and IL-2 production, an augmentor of B-cell production of immunoglobulin.[12,29,37]

Interleukin-1 is required for the clonal expansion of antigen responsive CD4 + T cells and the expression of IL-2 receptors by this "helper" T-cell clone.[18,28] Two forms of interleukin-1 have been identified and, despite being quite dissimilar in their primary amino acid sequences, have apparently identical immunologic effects.[19,24,43]

Another macrophage product that has received considerable attention is tumor necrosis factor (TNF, also known as cachectin). This macrophage product is released in large quantities following exposure to endotoxin. It has been shown to induce anorexia, wasting, acidosis, diarrhea, hypotension, and possibly diffuse intravascular coagulation. It also enhances the production of IL-1 and has been shown to generate a direct pyrogenic response of its own. There is little evidence that TNF modulates lymphocyte function, but it is a promoter of neutrophil adherence, activation, and degranulation. In short, this product is released in response to endotoxemia and may indeed be responsible for some of the consequences of severe gram-negative infections.[3]

Other potent compounds released by activated macrophages include several of the complement proteins, including some of both the classical and alternate pathways. As discussed in the earlier portion of this chapter, these proteins can exert direct toxic effects on invasive organisms as well as promote complement-mediated opsonization and subsequent phagocytosis by the granulocytes and macrophages themselves.

Finally, the control of monocyte/macrophage functions appears to be regulated tightly by their intrinsic production of arachidonic acid products such as the prostaglandins.[38,41] The level of autogenous prostaglandin production seems to vary inversely with the activation state of the macrophage in most tissues.

IMMUNOMODULATION— THE PAST AND FUTURE

The most significant advances in the manipulation of the immune system occurred before the nature of the system was even known. Immunization to prevent human disease was first documented in 1721 with the advent of variolation by Lady Montagu in Turkey. This little-known practice of interhuman vaccination against smallpox was superceded in 1798 by Edward Jenner's widely publicized discovery of the effectiveness of vaccination, again a successful attempt to prevent smallpox in humans. Pasteur expanded the techniques of immunization, first with attenuated cholera bacillus in 1880 and subsequently with a vaccine for rabies in 1885. In 1884 Metchnikoff provided the first understanding of the role of phagocytosis in immunity. In the past century, immunomodulation has become commonplace in the form of vaccines for numerous diseases such as tetanus, diptheria, pertussis, influenza, polio, measles, rubella, mumps, and hepatitis B.

The last 50 years has witnessed the greatest strides in the understanding of the associations of the cells and molecular elements of the immune response. It is possible that we are now at the threshold of learning how to control the individual elements of the immune system, to augment specific responses in the case of infections that already threaten a life, or to constrain unwanted responses such as the so-called autoimmune diseases.

Currently, nutritional support, especially in surgical patients, has been shown to increase markedly the patient's ability to recover successfully from an infectious challenge. The ability to produce monoclonal antibodies in unlimited quantities may someday be useful in treating established infections, with the potential impact on these infections that antibiotics have had in the past. The induction of selective classes of phagocytes or lymphocytes may also soon be possible, which could shift the course of septic complications. In short, we may be soon be able to alter radically the course of clinical infections, based on the knowledge of the various elements of the immune system and by selectively manipulating those elements.

SUMMARY

The physiologic events encompassing the lymphocyte and monocyte response to clinical infections are exceedingly complex. A comprehensive dissertation of these events is certainly beyond the scope of a single chapter in a clinical text. However, we hope to have provided some insight into the interrelationships at the cellular level that enable the host to combat and eliminate invasive microorganisms when normal anatomical barriers to infection have been overcome.

REFERENCES

1. Adams DO, Hamilton TA. Molecular transduction mechanisms by which IFN-gamma and other signals regulate macrophage development. Immunol Rev 1987;97:5.
2. Ashwell JD, Schwartz RH. T-cell recognition of antigen and the Ia molecule as a ternary complex. Nature 1986;320:176.
3. Beutler B, Cerami A. Cachectin and tumour necrosis factor as two sides of the same biological coin. Nature 1986;320:584.
4. Capron M, Bozin H, Joseph M, et al. Evidence for IgE-dependent cytotoxicity by rat eosinophils. J Immunol 1981;126:1764.
5. Chen BD, Clark CR. Interleukin 3 (IL-3) regulates the in vitro proliferation of both blood monocytes and peritoneal exudate macrophages: synergism between a macrophage lineage-specific colony-stimulating factor (CSF-1) and IL-3. J Immunol 1986;137:563.
6. Chesnut RW, Colon SM, Grey HM. Requirements for the processing of antigens by antigen-presenting B cells. I. Functional comparison of B cell tumors and macrophages. J Immunol 1982;129:2382.
7. Chesnut RW, Endrer RO, Grey HM. Antigen recognition of cross-reactivity between native and denatured forms of globular antigens. Clin Immunol Immunopathol 1980;15:397.
8. Cooper MD. B lymphocytes—Normal development and function. N Engl J Med 1987;317:1452.
9. Cramer DV, Gill TJ, III. Biology of disease: genetic aspects of cellular interactions in the immune response. Lab Invest 1986;55:126.
10. Deitch E, Winterton J, Li M, et al. The gut as a portal of entry for bacteremia—Role of protein malnutrition. Ann Surg 1987;205:681.
11. DeLisi C, Berzofsky JA. T-cell antigenic sites tend to be amphipathic structures. Proc Natl Acad Sci USA 1985;82:7048.
12. Dinarello CA, Meir JW. Lymphokines. N Engl J Med 1987;317:940.
13. Fearon DT. Cellular receptors for fragments of the third component of complement. Immunology Today 1984;5:105.
14. Fearon DT, Austen KF. The alternative pathway of complement—A system for host resistance to microbial infection. N Engl J Med 1980;303:259.
15. Fearon DT, Wong WW. Complement ligand–receptor interactions that mediate biological responses. Annu Rev Immunol 1983;1:243.
16. Goodman JW, Sercarz EE. The complexity of structures involved in T-cell activation. Annu Rev Immunol 1983;1:465.
17. Guillet JG, Lai MZ, Briner TJ, et al. Interactions of peptide antigens and class II major histocompatibility complex antigens. Nature 1986;324:260.

22

18. Kaye J, Gillis S, Mizel SB, et al. Growth of a cloned helper T-cell line induced by a monoclonal antibody specific for the antigen receptor: interleukin 1 is required for the expression of receptors for interleukin 2. J Immunol 1984;133:1339.
19. Kilian PL, Kaffka KL, Stern AS, et al. Interleukin 1a and interleukin 1b bind to the same receptor on T cells. J Immunol 1986;136:4509.
20. Kovak Z, Schwartz RH. The molecular basis of the requirement for antigen processing of pigeon cytochrome c prior to T cell activation. J Immunol 1985;134:3233.
21. Kupfer A, Swain SL, Janeway CA, et al. The specific direct interaction of helper T cells and antigen-presenting B cells. Proc Natl Acad Sci USA 1986;83:6080.
22. Kurt-Jones EA, Kiely JM, Unanue ER. Conditions required for expression of membrane IL-1 on B cells. J Immunol 1985;135:1548.
23. Lachmann PJ, Rosen FS. Genetic defects of complement in man. Springer Semin Immunopathol 1978;1:339.
24. March CJ, Mosley B, Larsen A, et al. Cloning, sequence and expression of two distinct human interleukin-1 complementary DNAs. Nature 1985;315:641.
25. Markham RB, Goellner J, Pier GB. In vitro T cell-mediated killing of *Pseudomonas aeruginosa*. I. Evidence that a lymphokine mediates killing. J Immunol 1984;133:962.
26. Markham RB, Pier GB, Goellner JJ, et al. In vitro T cell-mediated killing of *Pseudomonas aeruginosa*. II. The role of macrophages and T cell subsets in T cell killing. J Immunol 1985;134:4112.
27. Mayer M. The complement system. Sci Am 1973;229(5):54.
28. Mizel SB. Interleukin 1 and T cell activation, Immunol Rev 1982;63:51.
29. Oppenheim JJ, Gery I. Interleukin 1 is more than an interleukin. Immunology Today 1982;3:113.
30. Paul WE. Interleukin 4/B cell stimulatory factor 1: one lymphokine, many functions. FASEB Journal 1987;1:456.
31. Pillemer L, Blum L, Lepow IH, et al. The properdin system and immunity. I. Demonstration of isolation of a new serum protein and its role in immune phenomenon. Science 1954;120:279.
32. Pruitt BA. Host opportunist interaction in surgical infection. Arch Surg 1986;121:13.
33. Royer HD, Reinherz EL. T lymphocytes: ontogeny, function, and relevance to clinical disorders. N Engl J Med 1987;317:1136.
34. Sanders VM, Snyder JM, Uhr JW, et al. Characterization of the physical interaction between antigen-specific B cells and T cells. J Immunol 1986;137:2395.
35. Schwartz RH. T lymphocyte recognition of antigen in association with gene products of the major histocompatibility complex. Annu Rev Immunol 1985;3:237.
36. Shimonkevitz R, Kappler J, Marrack P, et al. Antigen recognition by H-2 restricted T cells. I. Cell free antigen processing. J Exp Med 1983;158:303.
37. Smith KA, Lachman LB, Oppenheim JJ, et al. The functional relationship of the interleukins. J Exp Med 1980;151:1551.
38. Snyder DS, Beller DI, Unanue ER. Prostaglandins modulate macrophage Ia expression. Nature 1982;299:163.
39. Steinmetz M, Hood L. Genes of the major histocompatibility complex in mouse and man. Science 1983;222:727.
40. Sui G, Clark SP, Yoshikai Y, et al. The human T cell antigen receptor is encoded by variable, diversity, and joining gene segments that rearrange to generate a complete V gene. Cell 1984;37:393.
41. Tripp CS, Wyche A, Unanue ER, et al. The functional significance of the regulation of macrophage Ia expression by endogenous arachidonate metabolites in vitro. J Immunol 1986;137:3915.
42. Unanue ER. Antigen-presenting function of the macrophage. Annu Rev Immunol 1984;2:395.
43. Unanue ER, Allen PM. The basis for the immunoregulatory role of macrophages and other accessory cells. Science 1987;236:551.
44. Woodruff PW, O'Carroll DE, Koizumi S, et al. Role of the intestinal flora in major trauma. J Infect Dis 1973;128:S290.

BIBLIOGRAPHY

Hood LE, Weissman IL, Wood WB, et al. Immunology. Menlo Park, CA: Benjamin/Cummings, 1984.
Meakins JL. The physiologic defense against infection. In: Burke JF, ed. Surgical physiology. Philadelphia: WB Saunders, 1983.
Stites DP, Stobo JD, Fudenberg HH, et al, eds. Basic and clinical immunology. Los Altos: Lange Medical Publications, 1982.

2

NECROTIZING SOFT-TISSUE INFECTIONS

E. Patchen Dellinger

Necrotizing soft-tissue infections constitute a small but very important portion of a surgeon's experience with soft-tissue infections. The presence of advancing tissue destruction signifies a process that is potentially life-threatening and that will not resolve without surgical intervention. On the other hand, the initial presentation of these conditions is often deceptive, leading to delay in diagnosis and definitive treatment. Unfortunately, the literature that refers to these infections is complex and confusing, identifying many separate syndromes and specific gangrenous infections when, in fact, the great majority of them fall on a continuous spectrum of signs and symptoms and relative severity.[15,30] One distinction that is often made and has some utility is that between histotoxic clostridial myonecrosis and all other necrotizing soft-tissue infections, both clostridial and nonclostridial.

Clostridial Infections

"Gas gangrene," or histotoxic clostridial myonecrosis is the most commonly discussed form of clostridial infection, but it is not the most common clostridial infection. Indeed, clostridial infections as a group are not the most common necrotizing soft-tissue infections. *Clostridium* are often found in "untidy" wounds that are not infected but merely need local care,[41] and in this setting they do not elicit much systemic response. *Clostridium* may be recovered with or without other bacteria in ordinary wound infections, which can be adequately treated with simple incision and drainage. They commonly appear as part of a mixed flora in cases of necrotizing fasciitis (see below). Clostridial myonecrosis is the most serious, rapidly progressive, potentially fatal clostridial infection. Although there are differences from the non-clostridial necrotizing infections in presentation and management, there are more similarities. These will be discussed below.

Nonclostridial Infections

Nonclostridial infections are more common than clostridial infections and are also life-threatening and potentially disfiguring. Many names have been used for these infections depending on the organisms isolated, the depth of tissue involvement, or the anatomical location of infection, but the similarities in clinical presentation and management outweigh these differences. Table 2-1 lists some specific terms for nonclostridial soft-tissue infections that have been described as separate syndromes in the medical literature but that are more usefully considered as different manifestations of the same clinical process.[15,30] The process may be relatively superficial, in which case the most commonly applied term is necrotizing fasciitis. This label is not ideal, because in the majority of cases the deep muscular fascia is not involved at all. The most common location of the infectious process is in the subcutaneous tissue with

Table 2–1
Terms Applied to Similar Necrotizing Soft-Tissue Infections in the Medical Literature

Gangrenous erysipelas
Necrotizing erysipelas
Hemolytic streptococcal gangrene
Nonclostridial crepitant cellulitis
Nonclostridial gas gangrene
Synergistic necrotizing cellulitis
Bacterial synergistic gangrene
Necrotizing fasciitis
Necrotizing cellulitis
Fournier's gangrene

relatively normal skin above and normal muscular fascia below most of the affected area (Fig. 2-1). The actual layer of tissue involved is usually the slight collagenous condensation in the subcutaneous tissue or superficial fascia. If the infection is caused by *Streptococcus pyogenes* alone, it has been called hemolytic streptococcal gangrene.[3,46] However, the clinical presentation and course are indistinguishable from cases caused by a polymicrobic flora of aerobic and anaerobic, gram-positive and gram-negative bacteria. High fever and other systemic signs occurring within the first 12 to 36 hours after an operative procedure, especially a clean procedure, should immediately raise the suspicion of an overwhelming, necrotizing streptococcal infection. This can progress to an irreversible stage with very minimal findings around the incision.[53,55]

When the infectious process involves tissues deep to the muscular fascia, it has been called necrotizing cellulitis to distinguish it from necrotizing fasciitis.[65] Individual muscle bundles may be infiltrated and in some cases rendered ischemic as the inflammatory process causes thrombosis of the blood supply. In most cases, however,

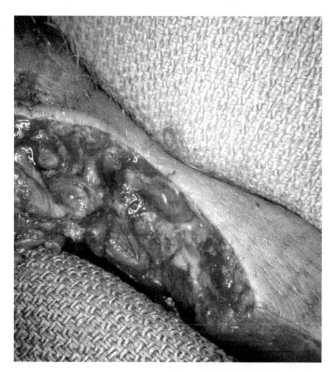

Figure 2–1.
Initial operative debridement of abdominal wall necrotizing fasciitis that originated in the scrotum. Note layer of necrotic, infected tissue with normal skin and subcutaneous tissue above and normal subcutaneous tissue below. The towel lies over normal, uninvolved, deep muscular fascia.

the involved muscle is viable and contracts on stimulation. Another muscle infection that may mimic this condition is pyomyositis. This is, in effect, multiple abscesses throughout a muscle group, usually caused by *Streptococcus pyogenes* or by *Staphylococcus aureus.*[1,22] The clinical presentation of this process, however, is similar to the other syndromes discussed. That is, the external evidence of infection is very slight compared with the extent of infection at deeper levels. Streptococcal myositis is much less common than the more superficial infections usually called necrotizing fasciitis. It has a tendency to progress more rapidly and is more likely to develop without a known portal of entry. Anyone treating soft-tissue infections should be aware of this syndrome because if initial surgical exploration of a patient with symptoms suggestive of necrotizing infection does not reveal infection superficial to the muscular fascia, then exploration below the fascia is necessary to locate and treat this infection. All of these syndromes contrast with clostridial myonecrosis in which the muscle is killed by toxins despite an intact blood supply and in advance of the actual bacterial infection.

When necrotizing fasciitis begins on the penis, scrotum, or vulva it has been called Fournier's gangrene. Only the anatomical location distinguishes this from other examples of the same infectious process. While the original descriptions of Fournier's gangrene emphasized the idiopathic nature of this infectious gangrene,[19,20] modern series recognize an underlying etiology (trauma, surgery, urinary tract infection, vulvar or anorectal pathology) in the majority of cases.[25,29,35,58] Even the distinction between clostridial myonecrosis and other necrotizing soft-tissue infections is less important than is often regarded in determining the clinician's initial response to infection. The most important issue is to recognize a necrotizing infection, whether or not *Clostridium* are involved. The subsequent steps in diagnosis and treatment will reveal the nature of the infection and allow the physician to make as precise a diagnosis as possible.

Diagnosis

The presence of diffuse tissue necrosis caused by infection is the most important distinguishing characteristic that must be recognized by the treating physician. A simple subcutaneous abscess has a central necrotic portion but is distinguished from the infections discussed here by being localized. The necrotizing soft-tissue infections are marked by the absence of localization or limitation. This accounts for their severity and for many of the delays encountered in recognition and treatment. In all cases the external evidence of infection and of gangrene is much less extensive than that found in deeper tissues. Both clostridial and nonclostridial infections appear rather unimpressive at their inception. Table 2-2 highlights the similarities and differences between clostridial myonecrosis and the nonclostridial infections in presentation, diagnosis, and management.

Clostridial infections are characterized by severe pain out of proportion to the local evidence of infection. There is often some local swelling but little evidence of an inflammatory reaction. By contrast, the nonclostridial infections exhibit a more marked inflammatory response, with redness, swelling, and tenderness at the site of infection. In either case there is little or no initial evidence of tissue death. As the

Table 2–2
Comparison of Clostridial and Nonclostridial Necrotizing Infections

	CLOSTRIDIAL MYONECROSIS	NONCLOSTRIDIAL NECROTIZING INFECTIONS
Erythema	Usually absent	Present, often mild
Swelling/edema	Mild to moderate	Moderate
Exudate	Thin	"Dishwater" to purulent
White cells	Usually absent	Present
Bacteria	GPR* ± others	Mixed ± GPR May be GPC† alone
Advanced signs	Hypesthesia Bronze discoloration Hemorrhagic bullae Dermal gangrene Crepitus	Hypesthesia Ecchymoses Bullae Dermal gangrene Crepitus
Deep involvement	Muscle much greater than skin	Subcutaneous tissue ± fascia ± muscle (uncommon) much greater than skin
Histology	Minimal or no inflammation Muscle necrosis	Acute inflammation Microabscesses Viable muscle
Physiology	Rapid onset of tachycardia, hypotension, volume deficit ± intravascular hemolysis	Variable—minimal to tachycardia, hypotension, and volume deficit
Treatment		
General	Aggressive cardiopulmonary resuscitation	Aggressive cardiopulmonary resuscitation
Antibiotics	Penicillin G‡ plus broad spectrum	Cefotaxime + metronidazole‡
Hyperbaric O₂	If it does not delay other treatment	No
Surgery	Aggressive removal of infected tissue; amputation of extremity often required	Debridement and exposure; not much removal required; usually no amputation
Antitoxin	No	No

* GPR—Gram-positive rods.
† GPC—Gram-positive cocci.
‡ See text for doses and alternate choices.
Adapted from Dellinger EP. Crepitus and Gangrene. In: Platt R and Kass EH, eds. *Current Therapy in Infectious Disease*. 3rd ed, 1979. Reprinted with permission of B.C. Decker, Inc.

infection advances, the skin above clostridial myonecrosis may develop a bronzed discoloration. Later hemorrhagic bullae may develop (Fig. 2-2). Gram's smear of the contents of these bullae may reveal gram-positive rods. Dermal gangrene and crepitus are late signs of infection.

Nonclostridial infections initially look no different from simple cellulitis without tissue necrosis. Erythema and swelling are usually present, but there is not an obvious

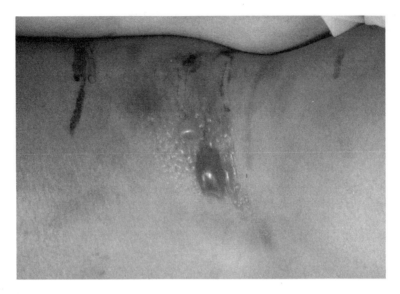

Figure 2–2.
Bullae adjacent to a traumatic wound of the antecubital fossa that developed clostridial myonecrosis. No organisms were present on Gram's stain or culture of the fluid.

border or clear transition between infected and uninvolved tissues. Rapid progression, a marked systemic hemodynamic response to infection, or failure to respond to conventional nonoperative therapy may be the earliest signs of the true nature of the process. Subtle bruising or ecchymoses (Fig. 2-3) probably reflect early dermal ischemia and almost invariably indicate underlying tissue necrosis. Bullae in an area of infection have the same significance. The bullous fluid may or may not contain bacteria. As the infection advances, there is an intense inflammatory process characterized by microabscesses in the superficial fascial layer while immediately adjacent tissues show little or no inflammatory changes. As the inflammatory process surrounds the nutrient blood vessels to the skin, thrombosis results. Veins are affected before arteries, and it is common to find thrombosed veins and patent arteries at operative exploration. The venous thrombosis may be the cause of the typical ecchymotic changes recorded in many cases of necrotizing fasciitis. Dermal gangrene and/ or crepitus, as in the case of clostridial myonecrosis, are very advanced signs and are unequivocal evidence of underlying necrosis, which demands operative intervention. While nonclostridial necrotizing infections usually progress rapidly, some cases, similar in other respects, advance slowly over many days with a correspondingly less severe systemic response.[71]

Crepitus refers to the crackling sensation detected by the palpation of gas in tissue, however, roentgenography, especially computerized tomography,[57] is a more sensitive technique than palpation for detecting gas. Soft-tissue gas is uncommon but always significant when found in conjunction with infection. It is more commonly

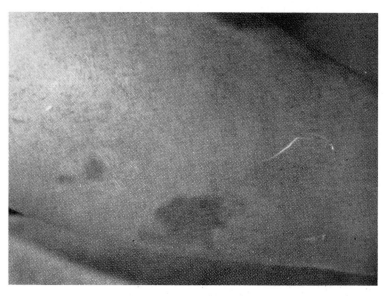

Figure 2–3.
Ecchymoses on the calf of a patient with necrotizing fasciitis that originated in a
deep heel ulcer. The underlying infection extended up to the buttocks.

associated with nonclostridial than with clostridial infections.[18,49] Most facultative
bacteria produce insoluble gases during anaerobic but not aerobic metabolism[68] (Figs.
2-4, 2-5, and 2-6). The presence of gas with infection, therefore, indicates an anaerobic
environment, incompatible with living human tissue (*i.e.,* gangrenous infection). For
gas to be clinically detectable, there must be a sufficient quantity and duration of
anaerobic bacterial metabolism, and this may explain the observation that, in general,
gas-producing infections are more serious than similar non-gas-producing infections.[14] Gas may also be present in tissue as a result of trauma or surgery or as a result
of a respiratory leak, either in association with severe obstructive pulmonary disease
or positive pressure ventilation. In either case, the source of gas should be evident
from the history, and the local signs of soft-tissue infection should be absent.

In both clostridial and nonclostridial necrotizing infections the initial local
exudate is usually unimpressive, being described as thin or like "dishwater." Nonclostridial infections may progress to display typical "purulent" discharge. Gram's stain of
drainage will often reveal multiple organisms and morphologic forms in both
clostridial and nonclostridial infections. In some cases of clostridial myonecrosis,
however, very few organisms are evident on Gram's smear and positive cultures may
not be obtained. *Clostridium* do not form spores in soft-tissue infections and, thus,
the absence of spores does not rule out *Clostridium* as the infectious agent.

White cells are usually absent or infrequent in Gram's smears or histologic
sections from cases of histotoxic clostridial infections.[41] This accounts for the thin
nature of the exudate and the absence of external signs of an inflammatory reaction.

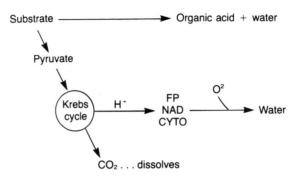

Figure 2-4.
Metabolic scheme normally used under aerobic conditions.

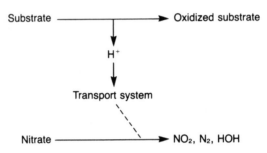

Figure 2-5.
Denitrification scheme of anaerobic metabolism.

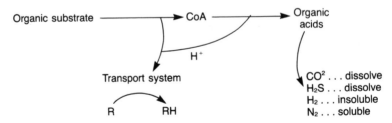

Figure 2-6.
Fermentation and deamination anaerobic metabolic pathways.

Culture of a clostridial infection may recover multiple species of clostridia and often includes other anaerobic and facultative bacteria. The presumed responsible *Clostridium* specie in cases of myonecrosis is *C. perfringens* in 60% to 80%, *C. novyi* in 30% to 60%, and *C. septicum* in 5% to 20% of reported cases.[41,70] *Clostridium histolyticum, C. bifermentans, C. sordelii,* and *C. falax* are rarely responsible for clostridial myonecrosis, but have all been reported in individual cases.[41] *Clostridium septicum,* in particular, has been reported as causing spontaneous myonecrosis in association with colonic malignancies.[32,50,61] In cases of clostridial myonecrosis, other, nonclostridial bacteria are usually recovered in addition.[9,41,62]

Only *Streptococcus pyogenes* is regularly reported as a solitary pathogen in cases of necrotizing fasciitis. Otherwise, nonclostridial necrotizing infections usually show multiple species. The bacterial spectrum mirrors that seen in cases of intra-abdominal infection (Table 2-3)[2,4,8,23,29,30,51,65] Cases of necrotizing fasciitis apparently due solely to *Streptococcus pneumoniae,*[38] to Group B streptococci,[44] *Staphylococcus aureus,*[45] *Hemophilus aphrophilus,*[10] and to marine vibrios[27,28] have also been described, but less commonly. *Clostridium* may be recovered as the predominant pathogen from infections that are not classic "gas gangrene" (histotoxic clostridial myonecrosis).[15,30,48,64] *Clostridium* are found more commonly in infections that are not myonecrosis, so this diagnosis and the subsequent therapeutic decisions must be made on clinical grounds, operative findings, and response to therapy, not simply on the presence of gram-positive rods on stain or recovery of *Clostridium* in culture. A Gram's smear that reveals many gram-positive rods and few or no white blood cells in the appropriate clinical setting, however, is most likely to represent clostridial myonecrosis. The presence of many white blood cells on smear suggests another process (Figs. 2-7, 2-8, 2-9, and 2-10).

When an infection begins in an open wound, one must take special care in obtaining specimens and interpreting culture results. Open wounds often contain a great variety of organisms, many of which are contaminants and not pathogenic in the infectious process. The most accurate cultures are obtained in the operating room after antiseptic preparation, through intact skin at a distance from any open wound. A

(text continued on page 34)

Table 2–3

Organisms Commonly Recovered from Cases of Necrotizing Soft-Tissue Infections

Aerobes and Facultative Anaerobes	Anaerobes
Escherichia coli	*Bacteroides fragilis*
Proteus mirabilis	*Bacteroides* spp
Proteus vulgaris	*Peptococcus* spp
Beta-hemolytic streptococci, group A and non-group A	*Peptostreptococcus* spp
Enterococcus	*Fusobacterium* spp
Streptococcus spp	*Clostridium* spp
Klebsiella spp	
Enterobacter spp	
Pseudomonas aeruginosa	
Staphylococcus aureus	
Serratia marsescens	
Morganella morgagni	

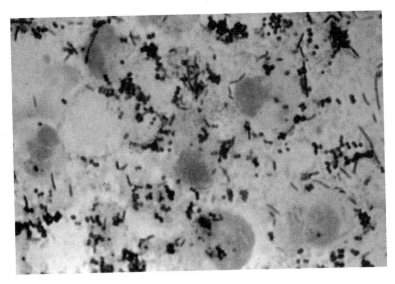

Figure 2–7.
Gram's smear from a case of necrotizing fasciitis that shows multiple morphologic forms of bacteria and many white blood cells.

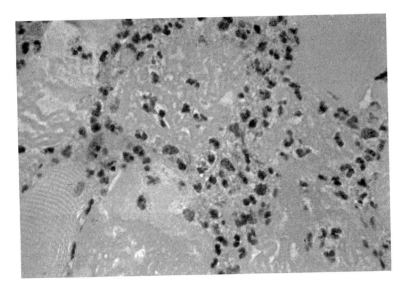

Figure 2–8.
Tissue section from a case of clostridial soft-tissue infection without myonecrosis or gangrene, showing intact muscle fibers and white blood cells. No bacteria are visible in this section.

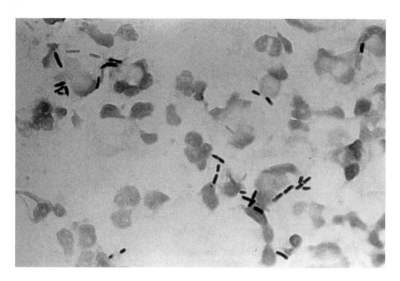

Figure 2–9.
Gram's smear of wound fluid from same infection as Fig. 2-8 showing multiple white blood cells and gram-positive rods.

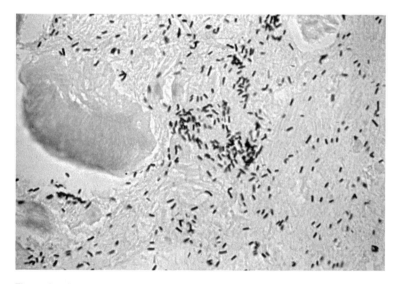

Figure 2–10.
Tissue section from a case of clostridial myonecrosis showing gram-positive rods, necrotic muscle, and no white blood cells.

needle aspirate of tissues at a distance from the open wound is an alternate approach.[37,67] If sufficient material is obtained in this manner, then the sample is reliable. If no material is obtained, however, this is not reliable evidence of the absence of a necrotizing infection. The location and extent of underlying involvement is unpredictable, and a needle aspirate may be unproductive despite an overwhelming infection.

The most common soft-tissue infections with crepitus and/or gangrene are not clostridial. They may involve subcutaneous tissue only, subcutaneous tissue and muscular fascia, or both and muscle. One rarely sees a deep infection that does not also involve subcutaneous tissue. The most common initiating event for necrotizing infections is a prior injury or operation, although for some cases no portal of entry can be discerned. Even the most trivial injuries such as mosquito bites or very minor operations can lead to these infections. Case reports document necrotizing infection after mucosal biopsy of the rectum,[13] Thiersch's operation,[59] hip repair,[40] episiotomy,[60] liposuction,[6] omphalitis,[34] tube thoracostomy,[52] percutaneous endoscopic gastrostomy,[42] intramuscular injection,[66] penile implant,[69] vasectomy,[54] and following an episode of dental infection,[43] and of porphyria cutanea tarda.[33] Essentially every site on the body has been reported involved, including the eyes.[11,17,39] The depth of tissue involvement is most commonly determined by the depth of the original wound of entry. Infections that follow very superficial wounds are more likely to be due to *Streptococcus pyogenes.* Wounds that have communicated with the bowel lumen or perineum are at higher risk for polymicrobic necrotizing infections, and any wound closed under tension is at higher risk. Necrotizing fasciitis of the abdominal wall often follows coeliotomy for treatment of intra-abdominal infection. If a necrotizing infection of the abdominal wall follows a prior bowel procedure, it may indicate a deeper intra-abdominal infection such as peritonitis or intra-abdominal abscess. Apparently, spontaneous episodes occur more commonly in the perineum and may be related to perirectal abscesses,[2,8,36,65] Bartholin cysts,[56] or other minor skin defects.[12] This condition occasionally serves as the presenting symptom of primary disease of the bowel.[21,31] These infections are usually polymicrobial with several anaerobic and facultative species present.

A source of difficulty with the necrotizing soft-tissue infections is that they are neither rare nor common. Thus, nearly every surgeon will see several over a lifetime of practice, but most see them quite infrequently and have little experience in their diagnosis or treatment. The primary physician must suspect the diagnosis, and the surgeon must have the courage to act aggressively once the diagnosis has been suspected to confirm or refute the diagnosis and institute treatment.[23,30,51,63] Essentially, this can be done only in the operating room where the infected, necrotic tissue can be exposed and the extent of involvement can be confirmed. Recently, some have suggested biopsy and frozen section tissue stains to confirm the diagnosis.[63] In fact, if the diagnosis is under serious enough consideration to warrant biopsy, the most important step has been taken. The incision made to obtain biopsy material will allow the diagnosis to be made by direct inspection, and definitive therapy can be initiated at once.[5,15,71] Improved outcome is related to early aggressive diagnosis and treatment.[23,30,51,63]

Treatment

Necrotizing soft-tissue infections result in significant fluid sequestration and a marked hemodynamic response. Clinical features among the nonclostridial infections range widely, from a minimal response to profound septic shock.[4,5,71] The spectrum parallels that seen with intra-abdominal infection. Clostridial myonecrosis is noted for a more rapid and severe hemodynamic picture. Cardiovascular collapse may occur with minimal evidence of infection.[41,70] This constitutes a major difference between the histotoxic clostridial infections and most others. In every case, the potential for profound cardiovascular compromise exists, and careful cardiorespiratory evaluation, monitoring, and support are mandatory. The other organism that occasionally presents with this type of early cardiovascular response in advance of obvious signs of infection is *Streptococcus pyogenes.*[55]

Empiric antibiotic selection must be directed against a range of potential pathogens similar to those found in intra-abdominal infections. Cefotaxime, 2 g, IV, every 8 hours, and metronidazole, 500 mg, IV, every 8 hours is a good initial choice. Another third-generation cephalosporin or an aminoglycoside can be substituted for cefotaxime. If an aminoglycoside is used, then penicillin should be added to ensure coverage of streptococcal species. Clindamycin, 900 mg, IV, every 8 hours can be given as a substitute for metronidazole and will also cover streptococci. Imipenem/cilastatin alone, 500 mg, IV, every 6 hours also provides appropriate coverage. If the initial Gram's stain shows a predominance of gram-positive rods and few or no white blood cells, penicillin G, 20 million units per day should be given. Because many cases of clostridial myonecrosis also involve other mixed bacterial flora, one should include cefotaxime and metronidazole as indicated above until the details of culture and clinical response are clear. For penicillin-allergic patients, chloramphenicol, 1 g, IV, every 6 hours initially, then 500 mg, IV, every 6 hours or cefotaxime and metronidazole are acceptable alternatives.

Hyperbaric oxygen prevents clostridial organisms from producing new toxins but does not inactivate toxins already present in tissue.[16,70] Hyperbaric oxygen may result in a transient improvement in the hemodynamic status of a patient with clostridial myonecrosis but is inadequate as a sole treatment.[16,24] No adequate clinical trials of its use in this condition have been or are likely to be done. If a hyperbaric chamber is readily available, it is prudent to add this treatment according to the protocol of the local chamber, but only after adequate hemodynamic resuscitation, antibiotic administration, and operative treatment have been instituted. It is contraindicated to delay resuscitation and initial debridement in order to transport a patient with clostridial myonecrosis for hyperbaric oxygen treatment before other measures have been instituted.[62] Many medical centers with hyperbaric chambers have acquired an interest and a large experience generated by patient referrals and thus provide excellent care for this condition.[9,62] There is no accepted role for antitoxins in the treatment of clostridial myonecrosis.

The extent of surgical excision and debridement is determined by the gross findings in the operating room. With clostridial myonecrosis, all infected tissue must be excised.[41] The excision margins in muscle must contract on stimulation and bleed freely. With extremity infections, amputation is often required. Complete excision is more difficult for truncal infections, and this may account for the higher mortality of these infections.[9,26] For nonclostridial infection, usually less excision of tissue is required. The critical task is to expose and debride all infected tissue, and the challenge is to find all extensions of the process.[5,15,71] Large areas of infection may communicate by narrow tracts. The intra-operative exploration is most efficiently done with blunt dissection using either a finger or blunt clamp. The infected tissues separate easily, admitting the probe, and a subsequent incision can be made over it. The incision must be carried beyond any evidence of infection into unaffected tissue.[15,71] After the infection has been completely exposed, all margins should be carefully inspected for signs of extension. Once all areas have been exposed and debrided, the infection usually resolves. The extensive unroofing required by some infections may result in interruption of the blood supply to superficial tissues and loss for that reason. Careful planning and placement of incisions can minimize such tissue loss.[7,71]

In all cases of diffuse necrotizing infection, either clostridial myonecrosis or nonclostridial gangrenous infections, a minimum of two operative procedures is required. The infectious process infiltrates widely beneath skin, and an extension may easily be overlooked at the first procedure or inadequately debrided in hopes of saving tissue. The second procedure should be scheduled within 24 to 48 hours of the time of the first. If significant infection is discovered at the second operation, a third must be scheduled and so on. When an operative inspection reveals no further infection, the surgical phase of treatment is completed.

The surgical management of these infections leaves large soft-tissue defects in most cases. The management and closure of these wounds is a significant problem. Topical agents such as mafenide and other techniques used in the management of large open burn wounds are useful in these circumstances. Indeed, mafenide may be a useful therapeutic agent, used topically, beginning at the time of the initial operative procedure, especially for cases of clostridial myonecrosis.[47] Often a consultation with a plastic surgeon or burn surgeon will be helpful in resolving these problems and achieving expeditious wound closure.

SUMMARY

Necrotizing soft-tissue infections involve a broad spectrum of clinical presentations, bacteriologic agents, and outcomes, but they require a unified initial approach to recognition and treatment. These infections have engendered an array of terms that focus on the anatomical location, antecedent events, or responsible bacterial species for categorization. All of the infections are potentially mutilating and life-threatening. Systemic reaction is often severe, and destruction of deep tissues is out of proportion to the external findings.

Infections caused both by *Clostridium* and by nonclostridial organisms can present with or without tissue gas, with or without muscular involvement, and vary widely in severity and speed of progression. The essential ingredient for successful management of these infections is timely recognition of the underlying necrotizing process and a systematic, aggressive approach to diagnosis and treatment. This does not depend on the initial bacterial isolates or on the specific label applied to the process. No specific bacterial species in the wound mandate operative intervention. No specific combination of bacteria is diagnostic of any particular variety of severe necrotizing infection. Clinical evidence of soft-tissue infection combined with any of the following should lead to early operative exploration: marked edema beyond the apparent limits of infection, blisters or bulla formation in the infected area, ecchymoses, crepitus or radiologic evidence of gas in tissues, rapidly advancing infection, especially with a severe systemic response, and failure to improve with nonoperative treatment. The findings at exploration will dictate subsequent management.

REFERENCES

1. Adams EM, Gudmundsson S, Yocum DE, et al. Streptococcal myositis. Arch Intern Med 1985;145:1020.
2. Adinolfi MF, Voros DC, Moustoukas NM, et al. Severe systemic sepsis resulting from neglected perineal infections. South Med J 1983;76:746.
3. Aitken DR, Mackett MCT, Smith LL. The changing pattern of hemolytic streptococcal gangrene. Arch Surg 1982;117:561.
4. Altemeier WA, Culbertson WR. Acute non-clostridial crepitant cellulitis. Surg Gynecol Obstet 1948;87:206.
5. Baxter CR. Surgical management of soft tissue infections. Surg Clin North Am 1972;52:1483.
6. Bello EF, Posalski l, Pitchon H, et al. Fasciitis and abscesses complicating liposuction. West J Med 1988;148:703.
7. Bongard FS, Elings VB, Markinson RE. New uses of fluorescence in the surgical management of necrotizing soft tissue infection. Am J Surg 1985;150:281.
8. Brightmore T. Perianal gas-producing infection of non-clostridial origin. Br J Surg 1972;59:109.
9. Caplan ES, Kluge RM. Gas gangrene. Arch Intern Med 1976;136:788.
10. Crawford SA, Evans JA, Crawford GE. Necrotizing fasciitis associated with *Haemophilus aphrophilus.* Arch Intern Med 1978;138:1714.
11. Crock GW, Heriot WJ, Janakiraman P, et al. Gas gangrene infection of the eyes and orbits. Br J Ophthalmol 1985;69:143.
12. Cruikshank SH, McLauchlan L. A *de novo* case of vulvar synergistic necrotizing fasciitis. Obstet Gynecol 1987;69:516.
13. Cunningham BL, Nivatvongs S, Shons AR. Fournier's syndrome following anorectal examination and mucosal biopsy. Dis Colon Rectum 1979;22:51.
14. Darke SG, King AM, Slack WK. Gas gangrene and related infection: classification, clinical features and aetiology, management and mortality. A report of 88 cases. Br J Surg 1977;64:104.
15. Dellinger EP. Severe necrotizing soft-tissue infections: multiple disease entities requiring a common approach. JAMA 1981;246:1717.
16. Demello FJ, Haglin JJ, Hitchcock CR. Comparative study of experimental *Clostridium perfringens* infection in dogs treated with antibiotics, surgery, and hyperbaric oxygen. Surgery 1973;73:936.
17. Einarsson OJ, Pers M. Streptococcal gangrene of the eyelids. Scand J Plast Reconstr Surg 1986;20:331.
18. Fisher JR, Conway MJ, Takeshita RT, et al. Necrotizing fasciitis. Importance of roentgenographic studies for soft-tissue gas. JAMA 1979;241:803.
19. Fournier AJ. Clinical study of fulminating gangrene of the penis. La Semaine Medicale 1884;4:69 (translated by J Hirschmann).
20. Fournier AJ. Fulminating gangrene of the penis. La Semaine Medicale, 1883;3:345 (translated by J Hirschmann).
21. Galbut DL, Gerber DL, Belgraier AH. Spontaneous necrotizing fasciitis: occurrence secondary to occult diverticulitis. JAMA 1977;238:2302

22. Gibson RK, Rosenthal SJ, Lukert BP. Pyomyositis: increasing recognition in temperate climates. Am J Med 1984;77:768.
23. Gozal D, Ziser A, Shupak A, et al. Necrotizing fasciitis. Arch Surg 1986;121:233.
24. Hart GB, O'Reilly RR, Cave RH, et al. The treatment of clostridial myonecrosis with hyperbaric oxygen. J Trauma 1974;14:712.
25. Himal HS, McLean APH, Duff JH. Gas gangrene of the scrotum and perineum. Surg Gynecol Obstet 1974;139:176.
26. Holland JA, Hill GB, Wolfe WG, et al. Experimental and clinical experience with hyperbaric oxygen in the treatment of clostridial myonecrosis. Surgery 1975;77:75.
27. Howard RJ, Pessa ME, Brennaman BH, et al. Necrotizing soft-tissue infections caused by marine vibrios. Surgery 1985;98:126.
28. Jenkins RD, Johnston JM. Inland presentation of *Vibrio vulnificus* primary septicemia and necrotizing fasciitis. West J Med 1986;144:78.
29. Jones RB, Hirschmann JV, Brown GS, et al. Fournier's syndrome: necrotizing subcutaneous infection of the male genitalia. J Urol 1979;122:279.
30. Kaiser RE, Cerra FB. Progressive necrotizing surgical infections—a unified approach. J Trauma 1981;21:349.
31. Klutke CG, Miles BJ, Obeid F. Unusual presentation of sigmoid diverticulitis as an acute scrotum. J Urol 1988;139:380.
32. Koranshy JR, Stargel MD, Dowel VR Jr. *Clostridium septicum* bacteremia: its clinical significance. Am J Med 1979;66:63.
33. Kranz KR, Reed OM, Grimwood RE. Necrotizing fasciitis associated with porphyria cutanea tarda. J Am Acad Dermatol 1986;14:361.
34. Lally KP, Atkinson JB, Wolley MM, et al. Necrotizing fasciitis: a serious sequela of omphalitis in the newborn. Ann Surg 1984;199:101.
35. Lamb RC, Juler GL. Fournier's gangrene of the scrotum: a poorly defined syndrome or a misnomer? Arch Surg 1983;118:38.
36. Ledingham IMcA, Tehrani MA. Diagnosis, clinical course and treatment of acute dermal gangrene. Br J Surg 1975;62:364.
37. Lee PC, Turnidge J, McDonald PJ. Fine-needle aspiration biopsy in diagnosis of soft tissue infections. J Clin Microbiol 1985;22:80.
38. Lewis RJ, Richmond AS, McGrory JP. *Diplococcus pneumoniae* cellulitis in drug addicts. JAMA 1975;232:54.
39. Lloyd RE. Necrotising fasciitis of the orbit. Br J Oral Maxillofac Surg 1987;25:323.
40. Mabie KN, Kulund DN, Whitehill R. Nonclostridial gas gangrene: late infection after hip pinning. South Med J 1983;76:269.
41. MacLennan JD. The histotoxic clostridial infections of man. Bacteriological Reviews 1962;26:176.
42. Martindale R, Witte M, Hodges G, et al. Necrotizing fasciitis as a complication of percutaneous endoscopic gastrostomy. JPEN J Parenter Enteral Nutr 1987;11:583.
43. McAndrew PG, Davies SJ, Griffiths RW. Necrotising fasciitis caused by dental infection. Br J Oral Maxillofac Surg 1987;25:314.
44. McCarty JM, Haber J. Group B streptococcal soft tissue infections beyond the neonatal period. West J Med 1987;147:558.
45. McCloskey RV. Scarlet fever and necrotizing fasciitis caused by coagulase-positive hemolytic *Staphylococcus aureus*, phage type 85. Ann Intern Med 1973;78:85.
46. Meleney FL. Hemolytic streptococcus gangrene. Arch Surg 1924;9:317.
47. Mendelson JA, Lindsey D. Sulfamylon® (mafenide) and penicillin as expedient treatment of experimental massive open wounds with *C. perfringens* infection. J Trauma 1962;2:239.
48. Moustoukas NM, Nichols RL, Voros D. Clostridial sepsis: unusual clinical presentations. South Med J 1985;78:440.
49. Nichols RL, Smith JW. Gas in the wound: what does it mean? Surg Clin North Am 1975;55:1289.
50. Pelfrey TM, Turk RP, Peoples JB, et al. Surgical aspects of *Clostridium septicum* septicemia. Arch Surg 1984;119:546.
51. Pessa ME, Howard RJ. Necrotizing fasciitis. Surg Gynecol Obstet 1985;161:357.
52. Pingleton SK, Jeter J. Necrotizing fasciitis as a complication of tube thoracostomy. Chest 1983;83:925.
53. Pollack MM, Schisgall RM. Overwhelming postoperative streptococcal infection. J Pediatr Surg 1978;13:527.
54. Pryor JP, Yates-Bell AJ, Pacham DA. Scrotal gangrene after male sterilization. Br Med J 1971;1:272.
55. Quintiliani R, Engh GA. Overwhelming sepsis associated with group A beta hemolytic streptococci. J Bone Joint Surg 1971;53-A:1391.

56. Roberts DB, Hester LI, Jr. Progressive synergistic bacterial gangrene arising from abscesses of the vulva and Bartholin's gland duct. Am J Obstet Gynecol 1972;114:285.

57. Rogers JM, Gibson JV, Farrar WE, et al. Usefulness of computerized tomography in evaluating necrotizing fasciitis. South Med J 1984;77:782.

58. Rudolph R, Soloway M, DePalma RG, et al. Fournier's syndrome: synergistic gangrene of the scrotum. Am J Surg 1975;129:591.

59. Rye BAO, Seidelin C, Dueholm S. Perineal progressive myonecrosis following Thiersch's operation for rectal prolapse. Ann Chir Gynaecol 1987;76:136.

60. Shy KK, Eschenbach DA. Fatal perineal cellulitis from episiotomy site. Obstet Gynecol 1979;54:292.

61. Sjølin SU, Andersen JC. Adenocarcinoma of the colon presenting as lower extremity gas gangrene (metastatic myonecrosis). Acta Chir Scand 1986;152:715.

62. Skiles MS, Covert GK, Fletcher HS. Gas-producing clostridial and nonclostridial infections. Surg Gynecol Obstet 1978;147:65.

63. Stamenkovic I, Lew PD. Early recognition of potentially fatal necrotizing fasciitis: the use of frozen-section biopsy. N Engl J Med 1984;310:1689.

64. Sterling JA, Ong TG, Klaus IG, et al. Gas gangrene of the perineum. Am J Surg 1954;87:874.

65. Stone HH, Martin JD. Synergistic necrotizing cellulitis. Ann Surg 1972;175:702.

66. Teo WS, Balasubramaniam P. Gas gangrene after intramuscular injection of adrenaline. Clin Orthop 1983;174:206.

67. Uman SJ, Kunin CM. Needle aspiration in the diagnosis of soft tissue infections. Arch Intern Med 1975;135:959.

68. VanBeek A, Zook E, Yaw P, et al. Nonclostridial gas-forming infections. Arch Surg 1974;108:552.

69. Walther PJ, Andriani RT, Maggio MI, et al. Fournier's gangrene: a complication of penile prosthetic implantation in a renal transplant patient. J Urol 1987;137:299.

70. Weinstein L, Barza M. Gas gangrene. N Engl J Med 1973;289:1129.

71. Wilson B. Necrotizing fasciitis. Am Surg 1952;18:416.

3

○   ○   ○   ●   ●   ●

THE ROLE OF THE SPLEEN IN HOST IMMUNITY

Eric J. Brown
Janet A. McGarr

Recognition of the importance of the spleen for host defense has grown over the past two or three decades. The syndrome of overwhelming postsplenectomy infection (OPSI) has had major impact on the development of our understanding of the role of the spleen in normal host defense. As splenectomy became a more common diagnostic and therapeutic procedure, particularly in patients with underlying medical abnormalities, such as Hodgkin's disease, Wiskott-Aldrich syndrome or autoimmune hemolytic anemia, it became increasingly clear that splenectomized patients were at increased risk for bacteremic infections. This observation led to renewed experimental interest in the role of the spleen in host defense against bacterial infections. In this chapter we will summarize recent experimental data that suggest that the spleen actually plays multiple essential roles in host immunity. We will also summarize clinical data on the susceptibility of asplenic individuals to bacterial infections, and, finally, we will attempt to outline a rationale for the prophylaxis and treatment of infections in these patients.

ANATOMY

The spleen is a major organ of the reticuloendothelial system (RES), which is also called the mononuclear phagocyte system (MPS). Each name emphasizes certain aspects of this grouping of cells that occur throughout the body, especially in liver, spleen, lymph nodes, lung, adrenal glands, bone marrow, and brain. The cells are perivascular and often in contact with blood elements through fenestrated endothelium, and they are cells of the monocyte–macrophage lineage. The RES was originally defined by Ludwig Aschoff as those cells that internalized intravenously injected analine dyes. These experiments emphasized the two most important features of the MPS, its phagocytic nature and its role in removing foreign material from the bloodstream. Thus, much of the interest in the role of the spleen in host defense has centered around its phagocytic potential and its role in removing particulate material, especially bacteria, from the blood.

The spleen is located in the left upper quadrant of the abdomen and weighs, on the average, 150 g with a range of 50 to 400 g.[84] At any given time, it is the residence of approximately 25% of the exchangeable T lymphocytes and 10% to 15% of the exchangeable B lymphocytes in the body.[28] The spleen receives up to 6% of the cardiac output at a rate of 300 ml per minute. It is surrounded by two coats: an external or serous coat formed by the peritoneum; and a fibroelastic capsule that sends out trabeculae that pass into the parenchyma and form the framework of the organ (Fig. 3-1).

At the hilus, the capsule is turned inward upon the blood vessels as a sheath. The splenic artery divides into five or more branches that enter the hilus and follow the trabeculae into the parenchyma of the spleen. Small arteriolar branches leave the course of the trabeculae and pass through both the white and red pulp. This architecture allows for efficient removal of particulate matter from the blood (*e.g.,* microorganisms and their products), which is important in the function of the spleen in host immunity. In the red pulp, the arterioles divide into a number of smaller vessels called penicilli. After a short distance, the penicilli develop a slight thickening of their coat due to the presence of macrophages and reticular cells. These macrophage-rich vessels are called ellipsoids. The ellipsoids continue as arterial capillaries that are continuous with the venous cords and sinuses within the red pulp. Blood that passes into the venous cords exists into the splenic veins along the trabeculae and leaves the organ at the hilus. Flow into the splenic cords and sinuses is highly regulated. The proportion of blood that bypasses the cords can be altered by physiologic and pharmacologic stimuli, such as epinephrine, blood loss, and hemolysis.[4,27] This decreases the efficiency of the spleen as a bloodstream filter because the shunted blood bypasses many of the splenic macrophages. This certainly affects the function of the spleen as an organ of host defense, but the significance of these various routes of blood flow through the spleen in various disease states has not been systematically investigated.

After the small arterioles leave the trabeculae and branch as capillaries, they are surrounded by a sheath of lymphatic tissue made up mostly of T lymphocytes. Along these periarterial lymphatic sheaths, the sheaths enlarge to form follicles made up of a

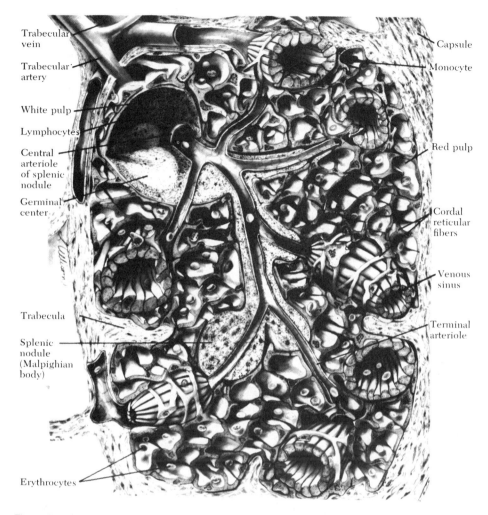

Trabecular vein

Trabecular artery

White pulp

Lymphocytes

Central arteriole of splenic nodule

Germinal center

Trabecula

Splenic nodule (Malpighian body)

Erythrocytes

Capsule

Monocyte

Red pulp

Cordal reticular fibers

Venous sinus

Terminal arteriole

Figure 3–1.
Diagrammatic representation of a splenic lobule. (Leeson CR, Leeson TS, Paparo AA. Atlas of histology. Philadelphia: WB Saunders, 1985: 135)

germinal center and a mantle layer. The germinal center contains B lymphocytes and macrophages while the mantle layer contains mostly small lymphocytes. Thus, the white pulp is quite similar in organization to a lymph node and probably serves a similar function. It is here that the immune system is first exposed to blood-borne foreign antigens.

The marginal zone intervenes between the white and red pulp. It contains macrophages, lymphocytes, and plasmablasts as well as mature plasma cells. The outer margin blends with the red pulp and merges with the splenic cords and sinuses.

The red pulp contains the splenic sinuses and a network of cells, the splenic cords. The basement membrane of the sinuses is fenestrated and allows communication between particulate matter of the blood and the cells of the splenic cords. These cells include erythrocytes, granulocytes, lymphocytes and numerous macrophages, either free or fixed in the pulp reticulum. Because of the large number of macrophages, the red pulp plays a major role in removing particulate and other foreign matter from the bloodstream.

FUNCTION

The spleen plays an important role in host defense both because of its own phagocytic capacity and because of its ability to produce soluble factors, particularly antibodies and the tetrapeptide tuftsin, which enhance phagocytosis throughout the body. We will review each of these facets of splenic function in detail.

Phagocytosis

The phagocytic cells of the spleen are the macrophages, present in large numbers in the splenic cords and lining the sinuses. The initial event in phagocytosis by these cells is recognition of circulating bacteria as foreign to the host. This occurs because of specific receptors on the macrophage plasma membrane (Fig. 3-2). Some of these receptors are cell surface lectins, which can recognize bacteria directly because of carbohydrates on the bacterial surface. For example, macrophages apparently have receptors capable of recognizing mannose[136] or beta-glucan.[35] However, most pathogenic bacteria have evolved mechanisms to evade this simple, direct recognition by macrophages. For these organisms, recognition as foreign by macrophages requires an intermediate step in which host plasma proteins bind to the bacteria. This process is termed *opsonization*. The most potent opsonins are antibodies and complement proteins, particularly C3, the third component of complement. In some circumstances, the plasma protein fibronectin may act as an opsonin, as may the acute phase reactant, C-reactive protein. Splenic macrophages have membrane receptors that can recognize these plasma proteins; in this manner, macrophages bind to the opsonized bacteria to begin the process of phagocytosis. The interaction of macrophage receptors with opsonized and unopsonized bacteria is aided by the slow blood flow through the splenic cords and the direct contact of blood elements with the lining macrophages. Thus, the architecture of the spleen allows for close contact of foreign particles with phagocytic cells, making it an ideal phagocytic organ.

Opsonins

Antibody. Type-specific IgG antibodies are major signals for phagocytosis of the organisms to which they are bound (Fig. 3-2). When IgG binds to its antigen, it then can bind to specific IgG receptors on the macrophage. Binding of IgG to these receptors is a sufficient signal for ingestion of the organism to which the IgG is bound.

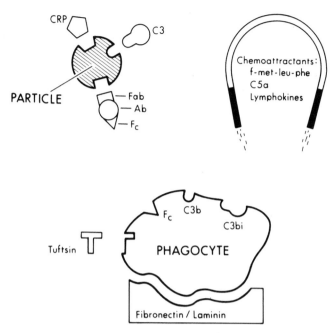

Figure 3–2.
Schematic representation of agents that affect the phagocyte (CRP = C-reactive protein; C3 = third component of complement; Ab = antibody; Fab = antigen-binding fragment of antibody molecule; Fc = crystallizable fragment of antibody molecule; T = tuftsin; C3b, C3bi = receptors for complement proteins C3b and C3bi). (See text for details.)

In humans, there is variation among the IgG subclasses with respect to their affinity for IgG receptors. IgG1 and IgG3 are bound more avidly than IgG2 or IgG4.[54] Thus, anticarbohydrate antibodies, which may be predominantly of the IgG2 subclass, interact rather inefficiently with IgG receptors. Because much of the immune response against bacteria is directed against their cell surface or capsular carbohydrates, opsonization with IgG alone might not be an efficient phagocytic signal. This may account, in part, for the necessity of complement for efficient antibacterial host defense. There are no cell surface receptors for IgM. Thus, IgM is not directly opsonic, and its efficacy in host defense clearly depends on its very efficient activation of complement. Receptors for IgA on macrophages have been described, but the role of IgA in host protection against bacteremia is unclear. In fact, there is evidence that IgA can actually inhibit complement activation by IgG when both are bound to *Neisseria meningitidis.*[64]

Complement. Complement activation is a less specific and evolutionarily older mechanism of opsonization than specific antibodies.[20] Complement activation may occur in the absence of antibodies, by either of two pathways, referred to as the classical and alternative pathways of complement activation. Although the alternative pathway is generally considered to be the mechanism of activation in the absence of antibody, certain bacteria, both gram-negative and gram-positive, can also activate the classical pathway in the absence of antibody. Complement activation leads to the deposition of a specific fragment of the component C3 on the activating surface. This fragment, called C3b, is recognized by a specific receptor on the macrophage surface, termed complement receptor type 1, or CR1 (Fig. 3-2). During the process of complement activation, C3b may be cleaved by the serum enzyme known as C3b inactivator (factor I). When this occurs, the majority of the C3b molecule remains bound to the bacterial surface, in a form known as iC3b. There is a separate receptor for iC3b on the macrophage surface, distinct from CR1. This receptor, which is absent in certain children with a congenital predisposition to bacterial infections,[135] is called complement receptor type 3, or CR3. Further action of the C3b inactivator leads to another cleavage in the C3 molecule, causing the release of the majority of iC3b from the bacterial surface. The piece of C3 that remains bound to the bacteria is known as C3dg. Although there is a receptor on some B lymphocytes for C3dg, the existence of a separate receptor for C3dg on macrophages is controversial.[76, 143, 150] The central role of C3 in the process of opsonization of bacteria for uptake by macrophages is underlined by the existence of at least two, and possibly three distinct receptors on the macrophage surface for products of C3 activation that can bind to invading bacteria.

Given the importance of C3 in the process of opsonization of bacteria for recognition and ingestion by macrophages, it is interesting that particle-bound C3b, iC3b, or C3dg may not be a sufficient signal for phagocytosis on its own. Instead, it appears that in many circumstances C3 interaction with its receptors provides a signal for binding of a foreign particle to a macrophage, but not for its ingestion.[91] Small amounts of a second signal are necessary for efficient ingestion. For example, C3 greatly augments the phagocytic efficiency of suboptimal amounts of IgG when both are bound to a model phagocytic target.[41]

Many macrophage functions, such as killing of tumors and the production of superoxide in response to certain stimuli, are latent. This means that, although resting macrophages are not able to perform these functions, macrophages can achieve a new state in which they are capable of these activities. The cell with increased effector capabilities is called an activated macrophage. Recent work has shown that C3 receptors can be phagocytic under certain circumstances, and that macrophage activation is in part reflected by this change in the function of its complement receptors. The ability of the host to control macrophage phagocytic function is most likely a very important element of host defense. Much of that control is exerted on the function of CR1 and CR3, because phagocytic function is greatly enhanced by conversion of complement receptors to their phagocytic state.

Fibronectin. The extracellular matrix proteins play more than one role in phagocytosis, because they can act as opsonins and also can exert a regulatory influence on the phagocytic function of macrophages. Fibronectin acts as a direct opsonin when it can bind to both the phagocytic target and the macrophage. The most studied examples of this directly opsonic effect of fibronectin involve its ability to mediate the ingestion of gelatin-coated particles and to enhance ingestion of rabbit erythrocytes.[37,66,144] Fibronectin will promote the ingestion of gelatinized particles *in vivo* as well, so it has been proposed that a major function of plasma fibronectin is to aid in removal of tissue debris from the circulation. Clinically, this would be most important in situations like massive traumatic injury, in which the body is faced with the removal of large amounts of devitalized tissue. Indeed, levels of plasma fibronectin have been reported to be reduced in cases of trauma, and the propensity of traumatized patients to infection has been inversely correlated with plasma fibronectin levels.[85,100,121,122] Clinical trials using fibronectin replacement in these patients have been undertaken. There has been no consistent effect of fibronectin therapy noted in these trials, so indications for the clinical use of fibronectin remain uncertain.

Fibronectin has also been shown to bind to certain bacteria. Most pathogenic *Staphylococcus aureus* bind fibronectin,[112] as do some streptococci[104] and certain mycobacteria (unpublished observations). However, the importance of this association for host defense is not clear. Studies of the effects of fibronectin on phagocytosis of bacteria have given variable results, but the best done studies suggest that fibronectin will enhance binding of bacteria to phagocytes but will not lead to phagocytosis.[113,140] In this respect, fibronectin is analagous to C3 as an opsonin for host defense. Unlike the case for the C3 receptors, regulation of the phagocytic potential of fibronectin receptors has not been studied.

Studies of the effects of fibronectin on the phagocytosis of rabbit erythrocytes suggest that intact fibronectin has no effect in this model system, but that a 180 kd fibronectin fragment augments phagocytosis by binding to both the erythrocyte and the macrophage.[36] While the physiologic significance of these studies is not entirely clear, the rabbit erythrocyte shares the property of activating the alternative pathway of complement with many bacteria. Thus, it is possible that this fibronectin fragment could be a significant opsonin for those bacteria that activate complement directly by way of the alternative pathway.

C-Reactive Protein (CRP). CRP is a pentameric protein of 105 kd that is present at extremely low levels in the uninfected host, but that appears rapidly in the blood in response to infection or inflammation. Because its synthesis is directly tied to the inflammatory stimulus, its regulation is currently of great interest to molecular biologists. However, its role in host defense is obscure. CRP will bind to phosphatidyl choline, which is present in the cell wall of some bacteria, particularly *Streptococcus pneumoniae*.[145] Moreover, there is evidence for CRP receptors on phagocytes, so that CRP may act as an opsonin like IgG or complement under certain circumstances. In fact, CRP-mediated ingestion of phosphatidyl choline-coated particles has been demonstrated, and there seems to be a close physical association between the CRP receptor and the IgG Fc receptor.[81] However, CRP will not act as an opsonin for encapsulated pneumococci that do not have phosphatidyl choline in their capsules, because the capsule sterically hinders the interaction of the cell-wall-bound CRP with the phagocyte plasma membrane. Thus, it is difficult to envision a direct opsonic role for CRP *in vivo*. CRP also activates the classical pathway of complement[80] and, thus, might play a role in the deposition of opsonic C3. However, because this C3 is also subcapsular, it is, like the CRP itself, poorly opsonic, and experimental evidence suggests that CRP does not aid phagocytosis of pneumococci by this mechanism either.[70]

Phagocytosis Enhancement

It is now clear that phagocytic function is a carefully regulated process of macrophages. At least three different types of potentially physiologic signals have been shown to enhance the rate and extent of macrophage phagocytosis. These signals act not as opsonins, which interact with both the macrophage and the phagocytic target, but as direct activators of macrophages. They do not require any interaction with the pathogen to exert their effect on phagocytosis. On the other hand, they do not stimulate macrophage recognition of the invader; this task is performed solely by conventional opsonins.

Extracellular Matrix Proteins. Fibronectin has been discussed above as a classic opsonin. However, fibronectin has another role in phagocytosis as well, perhaps more important than its directly opsonic function. Fibronectin can act as an enhancer of the phagocytic function of macrophages (Fig. 3-3). This has been demonstrated

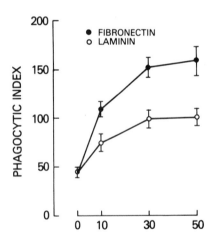

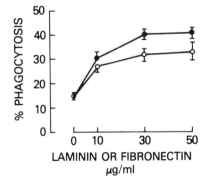

Figure 3–3.
Extracellular matrix proteins enhance macrophage phagocytosis of opsonized particles. Macrophages were exposed to varying concentrations of fibronectin (●) or laminin (○) and phagocytosis recorded as the number of IgG-coated targets eaten/100 macrophages (*top panel*) or the percentage of macrophages ingesting opsonized targets (*lower panel*). Both fibronectin and laminin enhance phagocytosis; fibronectin appears somewhat more stimulating than laminin. (Bohnsack JF, Kleinman HK, Takahashi T, et al. Connective tissue proteins and phagocytic cell function. J Exp Med 1985; 161:912)

using model sheep erythrocyte targets. Fibronectin enhances the phagocytosis of group B streptococci[69] *in vitro* as well. Because fibronectin is a ubiquitous component of the extracellular matrix, tissue macrophages are in contact with fibronectin (Fig. 3-2). Thus, splenic macrophages may be constantly under the influence of the phagocytosis-enhancing effects of fibronectin. Interestingly, other connective tissue components may have similar effects on macrophage phagocytosis. Both laminin[16] and serum amyloid P component[149] (a constituent of basement membranes) enhance macrophage receptor-mediated phagocytosis. For both laminin and fibronectin stimulation of macrophages, phagocytosis enhancement is not specific for a single opsonin receptor. IgG-dependent phagocytosis and complement-mediated phagocytosis are both increased by exposure of the phagocyte to these extracellular matrix proteins. Phagocytosis enhancement does not require interaction of the phagocytic target with extracellular matrix proteins. Thus, fibronectin and laminin might best be considered co-opsonins, because they increase the rate of phagocytosis of material that the phagocyte can already recognize. Their most important role is to regulate the phagocytic potency of the macrophage, rather than to enhance particle recognition by the phagocytic cell.

Lymphokines. A variety of lymphokines have been shown *in vitro* to be capable of regulating the phagocytic process. The earliest descriptions of such lymphokines came from Griffin and Griffin.[61,63] They showed that when T cells were present while macrophages ingested immune complexes, the T cells produced a lymphokine that could alter the phagocytic function of other macrophages. This lymphokine changed C3 receptors on resting macrophages from their nonphagocytic state to a state of phagocytic competence. The mechanism of activation of C3 receptors by this lymphokine seemed to depend on its ability to increase the rate of receptor diffusion in the plasma membrane. While extracellular matrix proteins seem to enhance phagocytosis by way of many receptors, lymphokine apparently enhances only complement receptor-mediated phagocytosis. In fact, in studies with human cells, this as yet uncharacterized lymphokine affects only CR1 function.[60] Recent work has shown that this lymphokine may also affect phagocyte function *in vivo.*[62]

Interferons may also affect phagocytic function. Gamma interferon increases the number of IgG Fc receptors on monocytes and macrophages.[146,147] This increases the rate and extent of IgG-mediated phagocytosis.

Tuftsin. In 1967, Fidalgo and Najjar[47] described leukokinin, a gamma globulin that bound to leukocytes and enhanced phagocytosis. Further studies[12,48,102,106,107] revealed that a tetrapeptide (l-threonyl-l-lysyl-l-prolyl-l-arginine) which they named tuftsin, was responsible for this enhancement. Tuftsin is a peptide within the Fc fragment of the leukokinin molecule. There are two enzymes involved in the cleavage of tuftsin from leukokinin that are necessary for the activity of the tetrapeptide. The first enzyme, which cleaves the heavy chain of the antibody, is located in the spleen. The second enzyme is named leukokininase and is found on the surface of the membrane of phagocytic cells (Fig. 3-2). Once the leukokinin has bound to the phagocyte membrane receptor, leukokininase can liberate the tetrapeptide. In addition to enhancing phagocytosis, tuftsin enhances chemotaxis of monocytes,[72] increases the reduction of nitroblue tetrazolium,[134] and enhances delivery of antigenic information to mouse spleen cells by mouse peritoneal macrophages.[139]

The importance of the spleen in the generation of tuftsin has been shown in the asplenic host. The tetrapeptide is not liberated in the absence of a functioning spleen, because one of the enzymes required for its release from IgG exists only in the spleen. Tuftsin levels are decreased in persons with sickle cell disease,[101] patients with Hodgkin's disease who have undergone staging splenectomy,[133] and patients splenectomized for other reasons.[32, 132] In patients who underwent splenectomy because of trauma, there is a correlation between tuftsin levels and the quantity of remaining splenic tissue, as measured by methyl-^{99}Tc scan. These patients have splenic tissue in nonstandard locations (splenosis) as the result of implantation of small islets of splenic tissue in the peritoneum at the time of trauma. Thus splenic tissue need not be in its anatomically correct location to bring about the synthesis and secretion of tuftsin. Because tuftsin levels are low in splenectomized patients, it has been postulated that tuftsin plays a part in the role of the spleen in host defense against bacterial pathogens.[29] A function for tuftsin in host defense also is suggested by the increased susceptibility to infection of persons with congenital tuftsin deficiency.[31, 101] The fact that bacteremia is rare in these persons suggests that tuftsin deficiency is not the sole cause for the serious infections that can occur in the splenectomized patient.

Splenic Phagocytic Function in Vivo

Most of the studies mentioned to this point were performed as *in vitro* experiments. However, much work has been done *in vivo* in experimental animals to examine the importance of the clearance and phagocytic functions of the MPS, and particular attention has been paid to the spleen. These studies suggest that the spleen plays an especially critical role in the clearance of poorly opsonized bacteria, or more virulent bacteria which have mechanisms for avoiding efficient opsonization by IgG and complement. Because ability of the liver to clear bacteria increases dramatically in the presence of antibacterial antibodies,[19] the spleen has its most important function as a phagocytic organ in the nonimmune host, during first exposure to the invading organism. Studies of the clearance of bacteria from the bloodstream in a variety of animals have shown that the bacteria are cleared less efficiently in splenectomized hosts.[15, 18, 126, 148] Our own studies[18] have examined the clearance of *Streptococcus pneumoniae* injected intravenously into guinea pigs (Fig. 3-4). These studies showed that the lethality of pneumococci for the guinea pigs depended on the capsular type used, and that lethality was markedly decreased in immune animals. Further investigation showed that the vast majority of the injected pneumococci were cleared by the RES of the liver and the spleen; importantly, the more lethal pneumococcal types were cleared to a greater extent by the spleen than the less lethal types. For example, approximately five times as many organisms were phagocytosed by the spleen when a virulent type 12 pneumococcus was injected as when an avirulent unencapsulated pneumococcus was injected. As would be expected from this finding, the consequences of splenectomy for the guinea pig were far worse when infected with the type 12 organisms than with the unencapsulated organisms. While type 12 bacteremia went unchecked in the splenectomized, nonimmune animal,

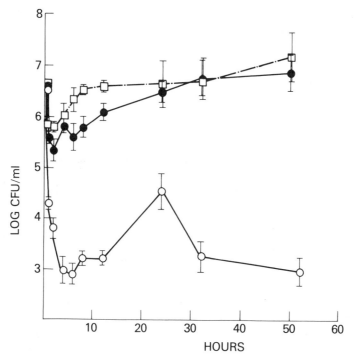

Figure 3–4.
Clearance of pneumococci in splenectomized guinea pigs. Normal guinea pigs (○), asplenic guinea pigs (●), and splenectomized guinea pigs with intraperitoneal splenosis (□) were injected with 100 million pneumococci at time 0. Splenectomy caused a major defect in removal of bacteria from the bloodstream, which was not corrected by splenosis. (Brown EJ, Hosea SW, Frank MM. The role of the spleen in experimental pneumococcal bacteremia. J Clin Invest 1981; 67:975)

bacteremia with unencapsulated organisms was cleared as rapidly in splenectomized as normal guinea pigs. Immunizing the guinea pigs against type 12 before splenectomy abrogated the clearance defect. The reason that immunization protected the splenectomized animals was that antibody binding to the pneumococci shifted clearance from the spleen to the liver. From the perspective of the RES, antibody converted a virulent encapsulated organism into an avirulent one.

This suggested that a major function of the spleen was to remove poorly opsonized organisms. Because of its unique architecture, the spleen provides more opportunity for the interaction of a lightly opsonized organism with the opsonin receptors of the macrophages in the cords and sinuses than does the liver. Further confirmation of this concept that the spleen is uniquely able to recognize and phagocytose poorly opsonized bacteria has come from work that showed that when animals are depleted of complement before injection of bacteria, more bacteria are cleared by the spleen and fewer by the liver.[19] Other work has shown that splenectomy and complement depletion are synergistic in their contribution to an animal's susceptibility to death from bacteremia.[141]

Studies of the clearance of IgG opsonized autologous erythrocytes have emphasized the role of the spleen in clearance of lightly opsonized particles. In these studies, the spleen was the site of erythrocyte clearance as long as the amount of IgG used for sensitization was low; as the amount of red cell bound IgG increased, the liver began to have a more and more predominant role in the removal of these cells from the circulation.[124] Taken together, these studies suggest a fundamental difference between the MPS in the liver and the spleen. Hepatic macrophages require more opsonization of the phagocytic target than do splenic phagocytes to achieve equivalent levels of binding and ingestion. Whether this simply reflects the difference in blood flow through the two organs, or whether it represents a fundamental biologic difference between the two populations of macrophages is not known.

All these *in vivo* studies suggest that the slow blood flow through the cords and sinuses of the spleen is critical for its clearance function. It is clear that the amount of splenic blood that actually arrives at the sinuses and cords can be affected by a variety of physiologic stimuli. For example, early in the course of malaria infection, blood is shunted away from the sinuses, to the closed circulation. This would be expected to decrease the effectiveness of the spleen as a clearance organ; this postulate has been tested experimentally to some extent.[109, 114, 152] The clearance of IgG-sensitized erythrocytes by the spleen decreases early in malaria infection, and then is restored to normal or supernormal levels as the parasitemia decreases. Increased clearance correlates with the return of normal blood flow through the splenic cords and sinuses. In phenylhydrazine-induced anemia, there is decreased blood flow to the splenic cords; this has been associated with increased mortality from *Hemophilus influenzae* bacteremia.[27] In fact, one of the major questions that remains unanswered about the role of the spleen as a clearance organ is how splenic blood flow is partitioned between the open and the closed circulations. Nothing is known about the mechanism of control of blood flow between the open and closed circulations or about the mediators that regulate this partitioning. Until these basic physiologic parameters are better understood, it will be difficult to examine how this basic variable affects host defense.

Reticuloendothelial Blockade

The fact that splenic clearance depends, in most cases, on specific opsonization and recognition of the opsonins by receptors on macrophages has been used for therapeutic advantage in idiopathic thrombocytopenic purpura (ITP).[22, 23, 45, 105] In this disease, platelets are trapped in the spleen and destroyed because they are sensitized with IgG, which binds the platelets to the splenic macrophages. A recent advance in therapy of ITP has been to treat patients with massive amounts of IgG intravenously, which blocks IgG receptor function in the spleen and inhibits the removal of platelets by the spleen. This is an example of a receptor-specific blockade of the MPS. In theory, this therapy might decrease the effectiveness of the spleen as a clearance organ in host defense. However, an increased incidence of bacteremia or sepsis has not been reported in these patients. Perhaps this is because the therapeutic blockade is receptor-specific and does not affect the function of complement receptors or lectins on the macrophage plasma membrane. Reticuloendothelial blockade in animals is generally receptor-specific as well. There are very few examples of blockade in which the total phagocytic function of the splenic macrophages is destroyed by experimental MPS blockaders such as carbon, zymosan, or sheep red blood cells. Only further clearance of the blockading particle is inhibited.[17] In fact, even in animals dying of overwhelming pneumococcal bacteremia, clearance of *Staphylococcus aureus* is normal.[93] However, at least two agents can destroy splenic macrophage function totally. Thorium dioxide is a radioactive compound taken up specifically by the MPS but never lost from the ingesting macrophages. It produces a total RES blockade.[94] Thorium dioxide is also radiopaque and was at one time used as a contrast agent for arteriography. Patients injected with thorium dioxide (Thorotrast) have been noted to have hepatic and splenic collections of the dye as long as 30 years after the contrast study. The mechanism by which thorium dioxide causes MPS blockade is not known, but is probably related to its long radioactive half-life and slow radiation-induced damage to the macrophages. Experimental animals injected with thorotrast have major clearance defects; an increased incidence of tumors and the occurrence of overwhelming pneumococcal sepsis have been reported in patients who received thorotrast for diagnostic purposes.

A recent report[128] suggests that ricin A chains may also be a specific macrophage toxin *in vivo.* Although intact ricin is a toxin for all cells, the A chain is taken up selectively by macrophages by way of their mannose receptors. This leads to selective ricin-mediated macrophage death. This induces a clearance defect in the experimental animals, which is associated with an acute depletion of macrophages from tissue.

The Spleen as Antibody-Producing Organ

Phagocytosis of bacteria by splenic macrophages is not only a major part of nonimmune host defenses, it is also a mechanism for initiating a prompt antibody response in intravascular infections. Several lines of evidence suggest that antibacterial antibodies and,in particular, antibodies directed against the capsular polysaccharide components of the bacteria, play a critical role in prevention of, and recovery from infection. First, in the pre-antibiotic era, type-specific antibodies were used as therapy in pneumococcal bacteremia, with a decrease in the mortality of this disease.[9] The antibodies used were directed against the capsular polysaccharides of the pneumococci; other antibodies against common pneumococcal antigens on the cells wall had no therapeutic effect. This was probably the consequence of the anticapsular antibodies' ability to change the location of C3b deposition from subcapsular, where it is deposited by the alternative pathway, to capsular, the true outer surface of the pneumococcus. Second, vaccination of normal persons with the purified capsular polysaccharides can prevent infection with pneumococcus, *H. influenzae,* and *N. meningitidis;* protection is associated with the development of significant titers of serum antibodies against these antigens. Third, the susceptibility of an individual to infection with *H. influenzae* or *N. meningitidis* has been clearly correlated to the presence or absence of serum antibodies. Studies undertaken in humans and in animal models have shown that the spleen plays a major role in the antibody response to intravenously injected antigens. Moreover, because polysaccharides rapidly enter the bloodstream after intramuscular or subcutaneous injection, the spleen plays a key role in the antibody response to all polysaccharides. There may be additional reasons for the importance of the spleen in the antibody response to polysaccharides, because there is evidence that it is the residence of certain T lymphocytes that are important in the immune response to polysaccharide antigens. For example, there is evidence that the spleen is the site of maturation of a population of T cells that are important in amplifying the immune response to pneumococcal SSSIII.[6] Moreover, there are abnormalities in the subsets of circulating lymphocytes responsible for antibody synthesis in splenectomized humans. Experimental data clearly show that splenectomy results in decreased serum antibody formation in mice immunized with pneumococcal polysaccharide or rats immunized with sheep red blood cells.[120]

The exact role of the spleen in antibody formation in humans is less clear. Several studies have shown that serum IgM levels are lower in splenectomized patients than in normal controls.[7,26,30,125] Studies undertaken in humans to assess the effect of splenectomy on antibody response to pneumococcal polysaccharide vaccine have varied in their conclusions. While some studies have shown normal antibody responses in otherwise healthy splenectomized patients or children with sickle cell disease, others have shown a significantly decreased antibody response as the result of splenectomy.[58,74,111] No study to date has shown that vaccination against pneumococcus results in a decreased incidence of postsplenectomy sepsis in asplenic persons, although the efficacy of the pneumococcal vaccine has been shown for children with sickle cell disease. Thus, no firm conclusion can be drawn about the exact role of the spleen in directing antibacterial antibody synthesis in humans. However, taken together, the weight of the evidence suggests that a defective antibody response in splenectomized persons may be synergistic with the phagocytic defect in leading to the increased propensity of these persons to serious bacteremic infections.

CLINICAL IMPLICATIONS

This brief review of receptor-mediated phagocytosis and of the role of the spleen in host defense suggests that removal of the spleen may have significant clinical implications for the susceptibility of the splenectomized patient to bacteremic infection. In fact, this is the case, and the remainder of the chapter will be devoted to a discussion of the clinical presentation of infections in the splenectomized patient, to their management, and to the management of patients for whom splenectomy is a necessary part of their medical management.

Overwhelming Postsplenectomy Infection (OPSI)

In 1919, Morris and Bullock[99] reported an increased mortality in splenectomized rats that were infected with *Bacterium enteritidis* compared to normal controls. Similar results were reported by Marmorston[92] in 1935 using splenectomized mice. It was not until 1952 that the first cases of postsplenectomy sepsis in humans were reported by King and Shumacker.[82] Since then, numerous case reports and larger retrospective studies have confirmed the increased incidence of OPSI in the congenitally, surgically, or functionally asplenic host.[10, 11, 39, 43, 129]

Incidence

Data on the risk of OPSI are relatively scanty. The incidence of mortality from sepsis in the general population with normal splenic function is very low, about 0.01% (0.3% in <1 year olds; 0.07% in 1 to 5 year olds and 0.02% in 5 to 14 year olds).[129] In asplenic persons, both the incidence of bacteremia and its mortality are increased. In Singer's series,[129] splenectomized patients as a group had an incidence of bacteremia of 4.25%, with a mortality of 2.52%. This is a several hundredfold increase in risk of a septic death in splenectomized patients. The incidence of mortality from OPSI varies with the indication for which the splenectomy is performed. In patients with splenectomy because of traumatic rupture, the incidence of septic death is 58 to 68 times that of the general population. In patients splenectomized for ITP there is a 70- to 140-fold increase in mortality over the general population. The incidence in patients splenectomized for congenital spherocytosis is 200 times that for the general population. An underlying immunologic defect markedly increases the infectious risks of asplenia. Patients splenectomized during workup or therapy of Hodgkin's disease have a very high relative risk of OPSI, although true incidence data have not been accumulated. One of the most dramatic examples of the risk of OPSI is in Wiskott-Aldrich syndrome, a congenital disease characterized by eczema, thrombocytopenia, and immune abnormalities. In these patients, splenectomy is frequently indicated for refractory thrombocytopenia. In the absence of prophylactic antibiotics, the incidence of OPSI in Wiskott-Aldrich patients approaches 100%.[89]

In addition to the nature of the patient's immune system, age is an important determinant of the incidence of OPSI. Children less than 12 months have not only an increased risk of infection, but also a greater mortality from infection.[44, 71, 75] However, OPSI has been reported in patients of all ages. Time since splenectomy is also a factor influencing the incidence of OPSI. About four fifths of cases of OPSI occurs within 2 years of splenectomy,[71, 118, 130] but there are reports of cases up to 31 years after surgery.[153]

Clinical Syndrome

The syndrome of OPSI is typically fulminant, with death occurring within 6 to 24 hours after initial symptoms in 50% to 80% of patients. The hallmark of the septicemic phase of the disease is high-grade bacteremia, often without an obvious infectious source. Prostration, hypotension, and disseminated intravascular coagulation (DIC) rapidly supervene, presumably because of the huge bacterial load in the blood. The bacteremia is often more than 10^6 organisms per ml of blood. A Gram's stain of the buffy coat frequently will reveal the etiologic agent. The initial symptoms are often frighteningly nonspecific: fever, headache, sore throat, vomiting, muscle and joint aches, and upper respiratory tract infection symptoms.[38] In fatal cases, these rapidly progress to shock, meningitis, DIC, adrenal hemorrhage, and death. Of particular interest is the high incidence of a similar syndrome in children with sickle cell disease.

Susceptible children generally have enlarged spleens, because they are in a stage of their disease before total splenic infarction from repeated sickle crises has occurred. These children are considered functionally asplenic, because their spleens are anatomically present but the existence of deformed red blood cells and Howell-Jolly bodies in the peripheral smear suggests that splenic function is not normal. Moreover technetium scanning suggests that blood flow to the enlarged spleen is markedly impaired. These children are at increased risk of OPSI compared with children of the same age splenectomized for trauma, presumably because sickling in other RES organs has made this immune function deficient as well. Moreover, children with sickle cell disease have a poorly characterized opsonic defect related to alternative complement pathway opsonization.[13] Levels of complement components are normal in these children, and the opsonic defect can be corrected with specific antibodies. This suggests that the opsonic complement defect occurs because of abnormal antibody-mediated augmentation of complement function.

Etiology. The vast majority of cases of OPSI are caused by encapsulated bacteria. *Streptococcus pneumoniae* has been implicated in 50% of the cases of OPSI.[39,44,129–131] Many of the remaining cases are caused by *H. influenzae*, type b, and *N. meningitidis. Escherichia coli, Staphylococcus aureus*, other *Streptococcus* species, *Salmonella* species, *Listeria* species, *Pseudomonas aeruginosa*[53] and the gram-negative bacterium DF-2 have also been reported as at least occasional cases of this syndrome.[24,95] Splenectomy also can increase the severity of infection with intraerythrocytic parasites: malaria,[151] babesiosis,[50,51,55,119] and bartonellosis. More severe viral infections,[52] including an increased incidence of disseminated herpes zoster, have been reported in splenectomized patients.

Treatment

Once a splenectomized person becomes infected, treatment consists of supportive measures and rapid institution of antibiotic therapy with a broad enough spectrum of activity to cover the possible etiologic bacteria until isolation of the offending organism. Usually the variety of possible offending agents and the severity of the illness necessitate institution of therapy with more than one antibiotic. If the buffy coat Gram's stain is positive, it may be helpful in guiding the choice of antibiotics. In no circumstance should institution of antibiotics be delayed pending the performance of a diagnostic test such as a radiographic study. Appropriate narrower spectrum antibiotic therapy can then be continued after the sensitivities of the bacteremic organism are known.

As OPSI carries a 50% to 80% mortality even with optimal treatment, emphasis has been placed on prevention of infection in the splenectomized person. These preventive measures fall into three main categories: antibiotic prophylaxis, vaccination, and therapeutic alternatives to total splenectomy.

Antibiotic Prophylaxis. Because *Streptococcus pneumoniae* accounts for 50% of the infections in patients with OPSI, prevention of this syndrome might be possible with prophylactic penicillin. Animal data suggest that prophylactic penicillin reduces the mortality of aerosolized pneumococcal challenge.[40] However, the major issue in prophylaxis of human disease is whether the emergence of organisms resist-ant to penicillin as agents of OPSI in prophylaxed patients would counteract the beneficial effects of prevention of disease with penicillin-sensitive organisms. This is a very difficult question to test in animal models or even in human studies, because incidence figures on the occurrence of OPSI are very inexact and clearly vary with the underlying disease.

Human studies that have been performed on the efficacy of penicillin pro-phylaxis in the asplenic person are generally poorly controlled, with short follow-up periods. Lanzkowsky and co-workers[86] reported on 25 patients undergoing splenec-tomy for staging of Hodgkin's disease. Nineteen of these patients had been on penicillin prophylaxis postoperatively at a dose of 250 mg bid. Of the six patients not on penicillin prophylaxis, two had serious streptococcal infection. One patient died of pneumococcal septicemia, purpura fulminans, and DIC 14 months postsplenectomy. The patient's mother had discontinued the prophylactic penicillin 2 months earlier. The other patient recovered from streptococcal septicemia and polyarthritis. This patient received continuous penicillin for 2 years and developed the infection 3 weeks after stopping the antibiotic. Of note, these authors reported a compliance rate of 94% of patients actually taking their penicillin based on tests of random urine studies. Based on their findings, these authors recommend continuous penicillin prophylaxis in this group of patients. A recent well-controlled study of penicillin prophylaxis in sickle cell disease demonstrated efficacy.[56] However, the physiologic defect in children with sickle cell anemia is not equivalent to splenectomy. These children have a more extensive RES defect, deficient antibody production and poor alternative complement pathway-mediated opsonization as well. Thus, this study is not directly applicable to splenectomized patients.

Despite these caveats, the use of prophylactic penicillin in a dose of 250 mg bid for asplenic patients is common practice. It is most reasonable that this begin at the time of splenectomy, because the incidence of OPSI is highest in the first 2 or 3 years after surgery. Because the incidence of OPSI decreases after this time, prophylaxis is often stopped after 2 years. However, asplenic persons are clearly at somewhat higher risk for sepsis than normals for many years, and there is no clear end point for prophylaxis. Because young children are unable to report symptoms of infection, penicillin should be given up to the age of 5 years.

Potential problems with this form of prophylaxis include emergence of resistant organisms; failure to cover adequately all the organisms implicated in this syndrome (*i.e.*, beta-lactamase producing *Staphylococcus aureus* and *H. influenzae;* patient compliance; cost; and side-effects. The emergence of resistant organisms does not seem to be a problem because no resistant pneumococci have been reported in patients receiving penicillin prophylaxis,[56,78] although no formal study has addressed this question. There are, however, reports of penicillin-resistant pneumococci.[77,96] Use of an antibiotic with a broader spectrum such as amoxicillin or trimethoprim-sulfamethoxazole for prophylaxis might be considered, but the added benefits of these drugs must be weighed against the additional cost.

Patients and their families should be educated about the risk of infection following splenectomy and instructed to seek early medical care with the slightest symptom of a cold or other infection. Institution of antibiotic therapy is indicated even for what appears to be upper respiratory infection, after obtaining blood cultures. The clinical progression of OPSI is so rapid that this may be the only stage of the illness in which antibiotic intervention can affect mortality. If blood cultures are negative, antibiotics can be discontinued. Very responsible patients far from medical care can be instructed to begin antibiotics at the first sign of illness and then seek medical attention. The prompt initiation of antibiotic therapy should not be delayed for any reason in OPSI.

Vaccines

Initial work in animals showed that immunization of splenectomized animals followed by challenge with *Streptococcus pneumoniae* increased the rate of clearance of bacteria and decreased mortality.[33] Vaccines against 23 types of pneumococci,[21] *H. influenzae* type b,[2] and *N. meningitidis* types A,C,X,W-135[1] are presently available. The polyvalent pneumococcal capsular polysaccharide vaccine includes the capsular types responsible for 90% of the pneumococcal types that cause meningitis, pneumonia, and bacteremia in children and adults.[21,83] There have been reports of both normal[137] and impaired antibody responses to the pneumococcal vaccine in patients with sickle cell disease and splenectomy for various reasons.[3,25,27] Patients with Hodgkin's disease who have been splenectomized have an impaired antibody response to vaccine, which is further reduced in those who receive radiation and chemotherapy.[127] Children under 2 years of age show poor response to vaccination with many polysaccharides.[34] Clinical trials with modified polysaccharide vaccines that appear to be more immunogenic in infants are currently underway.

The efficacy of pneumococcal vaccine in splenectomized patients is not established. While vaccination seems to decrease pneumococcal disease in children with sickle cell anemia who respond,[5] these patients are not necessarily analogous to splenectomized patients. Because it is possible that the spleen contributes significantly to the production of an antibody response to pneumococcal polysaccharides, it is generally recommended that patients undergoing elective splenectomy be vaccinated 2 to 4 weeks before surgery. However, because many patients who undergo elective splenectomy are immunosuppressed iatrogenically or by underlying disease, the efficacy of this recommendation is not clear. Moreover, most patients splenectomized for trauma or autoimmune cytopenias cannot wait 2 to 4 weeks before the operative procedure.

Alternatives to Splenectomy

Until recently, splenectomy was considered the only acceptable way to treat splenic injury.[138] In the last few years, interest has been generated in alternatives to splenectomy because of the risk of OPSI. Alternatives include (1) delay in elective splenectomy; (2) conservative management of trauma; (3) hemostasis with topical agents; (4) splenorrhaphy and partial splenectomy; (5) autotransplantation.

Delay in Elective Splenectomy. The immune system may not be fully developed until a child is 7 years old[68] and is certainly very immature in children less than 2 years of age. Pneumococcal vaccines given to children less than 2 years old are usually ineffective.[34] Development of natural immunity to many organisms, particularly the encapsulated bacteria, is also often delayed beyond 2 years of age. For this reason, delay in elective splenectomy as long as possible, and certainly beyond the age of 2, theoretically represents optimal management. No clinical studies have been done to assess whether this management decision actually decreases the incidence of OPSI.

Conservative Management of Trauma. There is an increasing tendency to manage clinically stable patients with splenic trauma without surgery. In several series of children with abdominal injury, 60% or more with splenic trauma avoided surgery.[8,42,79] Interestingly, radioisotope scans are frequently persistently abnormal in medically managed patients, some for as long as 1 year postsurgery.[49] This is not an indication for changes of management. These series show that nonoperative supportive management is successful in the majority of patients with an isolated splenic injury.

Hemostasis with Topical Agents. In unstable patients with multiple abdominal injuries, total splenectomy may be avoidable in some cases. Both Gelfoam and Avitene[14,59,98] have been used to achieve hemostasis in ruptured spleens. However, the use of these agents has been suggested only for superficial splenic lacerations. The clinical utility of this approach has not been systematically evaluated.

Splenorrhaphy and Partial Splenectomy. There are reports of successful splenic repair in some patients with splenic injury.[46,97,108,115,116] Repair in some cases required vessel ligation or partial splenectomy for control of bleeding. Reported series are too small to determine the overall success of these attempts at splenic salvage.

Autotransplantation. In 1978, Pearson and co-workers[110] reported that 13 of 22 children who had undergone splenectomy because of traumatic injury had evidence of splenic function as manifested by a low percentage of pitted red cells and splenic tissue noted on ^{99m}Tc sulfur colloid scans. These findings suggested that the occurence of splenosis was common and might be responsible for the lower frequency of postsplenectomy infection in this group of patients compared to those who underwent elective splenectomy. As a result, several studies have been performed to determine whether deliberate autotransplantation can protect experimental animals for sepsis.

Several studies[33,65,67,73,88,90,123,142] have compared the effect of partial splenectomy, autotransplantation of splenic tissue, and total splenectomy, on survival after IV challenge with pneumococci in experimental animals. These studies showed that, while autotransplantation might confer some increased protection against pneumococcal bacteremia, residual spleen in the anatomically normal location was necessary for efficient protection. This was true both for acute protection against bacteremia and for production of antipneumococcal antibodies. In fact, if 30% to 50% of the spleen was left intact, its host defense factors were essentialy normal. Thus, while the spleen may secrete nonspecific host defense factors such as tuftsin, its primary role in protection against bacteremia seems to be its filter function, which requires that it be

60

located in its anatomically normal site with its usual vascular supply. Clinical case reports also have suggested that splenosis does not protect against OPSI.[103, 117] Thus, deliberate creation of splenosis (autotransplantation) seems an inferior therapeutic modality to partial splenectomy if 30% to 50% of the spleen can be saved.

Conclusions

The data presented in this chapter suggest that the spleen has multiple roles in host immunity. It plays a major role in removal of bacteria from the bloodstream and in their phagocytosis. It also is essential in formation of the antibody response to bloodborne bacteria and viruses, and it is the site of synthesis of phagocytosis modulators such as tuftsin. Based on the observation that the primary problem of splenectomized patients is the occurrence of overwhelming bacteremia, the removal and destruction of bacteria seem to be the major unique, clinically significant function of the spleen. This function is particularly important in nonimmune hosts, which are characterized by the absence of circulating antibody against the bacterial pathogen causing their disease. When antibody is present, the role of the spleen can be assumed, to at least some extent, by the MPS of the liver. The liver can also adequately control bacteremia caused by relatively avirulent organisms. Thus, our knowledge of splenic function to date suggests that the spleen is particularly important in host defense against pathogens of high intrinsic virulence and in the absence of specific immunity.

Because of the occurrence of overwhelming sepsis in some patients after splenectomy, attempts have been made to save splenic tissue whenever possible. Delay of splenectomy in hereditary anemias probably has decreased the incidence of OPSI in these patients. Multiple new approaches to the management of the splenic trauma have been developed, but the efficacy of these new approaches for the prevention of OPSI has not yet been critically evaluated. New approaches to controlling bacteremia will require greater understanding of the regulation of macrophage phagocytosis, with the future promise of therapeutic intervention to eliminate the host defense defect engendered by splenectomy.

REFERENCES

1. ACIP. Meningococcal vaccines. MMWR 1985;34:255.
2. ACIP. Polysaccharide vaccine for prevention of *Haemophilus influenzae* type b disease. MMWR 1985;34:201.
3. Ahonkhai VI, Landesman SH, Fikrig SM, et al. Failure of pneumococcal vaccine in children with sickle-cell disease. N Engl J Med 1979;301:26.
4. Altura BM. Microcirculatory regulation and dysfunction. Relationship to RES function and resistance to shock and trauma. In: Reichard SM, Filkins JP, eds. The reticuloendothelial system. Vol. 7B. New York: Plenum Press, 1985:112.
5. Ammann AJ, Addiego J, Wara DW, et al. Polyvalent pneumococcal-polysaccharide immunization of patients with sickle-cell anemia and patients with splenectomy. N Engl J Med 1977;297:897.
6. Amsbaugh DF, Prescott B, Baker PJ. Effect of splenectomy on the expression of regulatory T cell activity. J Immunol 1978;121:1483.
7. Andersen V, Cohn J, Sorensen SF. Immunological studies in children before and after splenectomy. Acta Paediatr Scand 1976;65:409.

8. Aronson DZ, Scherz AW, Einhorn AH, et al. Nonoperative management of splenic trauma in children: a report of six consecutive cases. Pediatr 1977;60:482.

9. Austrian R, Gold J. Pneumococcal bacteremia with especial reference to bacteremic pneumococcal pneumonia. Ann Intern Med 1964;60:759.

10. Balfanz JR, Nesbit ME Jr, Jarvis C, et al. Overwhelming sepsis following splenectomy for trauma. J Pediatr 1976;88:458.

11. Barrett-Connor E. Bacterial infection and sickle cell anemia. An analysis of 250 infections in 166 patients and a review of the literature. Medicine 1971;50:97.

12. Bar-Shavit Z, Stabinsky Y, Fridkin M, et al. Tuftsin–macrophage interaction: specific binding and augmentation of phagocytosis. J Cell Physiol 1979;100:55.

13. Bjornson AB, Gaston MH, Zellner CL. Decreased opsonization for *Streptococcus pneumoniae* in sickle cell disease: studies on selected complement components and immunoglobulins. J Pediatr 1977;91:371.

14. Bodon GR, Verzosa ES. Incidental splenic injury. Is splenectomy always necessary? Am J Surg 1967;113:303.

15. Bogart D, Biggar WD, Good RA. Impaired intravascular clearance of pneumococcus type-3 following splenectomy. J Reticuloendothelial Soc 1972;11:77.

16. Bohnsack JF, Kleinman HK, Takahashi T, et al. Connective tissue proteins and phagocytic cell function. Laminin enhances complement and Fc-mediated phagocytosis by cultured human macrophages. J Exp Med 1985;161:912.

17. Bradfield JWB. Reticulo-endothelial blockade: a reassessment. In: Wisse E, Knook DL, eds. Kupffer cells and other liver sinusoidal cells. New York: Elsevier/North-Holland, 1977:365.

18. Brown EJ, Hosea SW, Frank MM. The role of the spleen in experimental pneumococcal bacteremia. J Clin Invest 1981;67:975.

19. Brown EJ, Hosea SW, Frank MM. The role of complement in the localization of pneumococci in the splanchnic reticuloendothelial system during experimental bacteremia. J Immunol 1981;126:2230.

20. Brown EJ, Joiner KA, Frank MM. Complement. In: Paul WE, ed. Fundamental immunology. New York: Raven Press, 1984:645.

21. Brunell PA, Bass JW. Recommendations for using pneumococcal vaccine in children. Pediatrics 1985;75:1153.

22. Bussel JB, Hilgartner MW. The use and mechanism of action of intravenous immunoglobulin in the treatment of immune haematologic disease. Br J Haematol 1984;56:1.

23. Bussel JB, Schulman I, Hilgartner MW, et al. Intravenous use of gammaglobulin in the treatment of chronic immune thrombocytopenic purpura as a means to defer splenectomy. J Pediatr 1983;103:651.

24. Butler T, Johnston KH, Gutierrez Y, et al. Enhancement of experimental bacteremia and endocarditis caused by dysgonic fermenter (DF-2) bacterium after treatment with methylprednisolone and after splenectomy. Infect Immun 1985;47:294.

25. Cadman E, Cohen MS, Root RK, et al. Impaired response to pneumococcal vaccine in Hodgkin's disease. N Engl J Med 1978;299:1317.

26. Chaimoff C, Douer D, Pick IA, et al. Serum immunoglobulin changes after accidental splenectomy in adults. Am J Surg 1978;136:332.

27. Chen LT, Moxon ER. Effect of splenic congestion associated with hemolytic anemia on mortality of rats challenged with *Haemophilus influenzae* b. Am J Hematol 1983;15:117.

28. Christensen BE, Jonsson V, Matre R, et al. Traffic of T and B lymphocytes in the normal spleen. Scand J Haematol 1978;20:246.

29. Chu DZJ, Nishioka K, El-Hagin T, et al. Effects of tuftsin on postsplenectomy sepsis. Surgery 1985;97:701.

30. Claret I, Morales L, Mantaner A. Immunological studies in the postsplenectomy syndrome. J Pediatr Surg 1975;10:59.

31. Constantopoulos A, Najjar VA. Tuftsin deficiency syndrome. A report of two new cases. Acta Paediatr Scand 1973;62:645.

32. Constantopoulas A, Najjar VA, Wish JB, et al. Defective phagocytosis due to tuftsin deficiency in splenectomized subjects. Am J Dis Child 1973;125:663.

33. Cooney DR, Dearth JC, Swanson SE, et al. Relative merits of partial splenectomy, splenic reimplantation, and immunization in preventing postsplenectomy infection. Surgery 1979;86:561.

34. Cowan MJ, Ammann AJ, Wara DW, et al. Pneumococcal polysaccharide immunization in infants and children. Pediatrics 1978;62:721.

35. Czop JK, Austen KF. A β-glucan inhibitable receptor on human monocytes: its identity with the

phagocytic receptor for particulate activators of the alternative complement pathway. J Immunol 1985;134:2588.

36. Czop JK, Austen KF. Augmentation of phagocytosis by a specific fibronectin fragment that links particulate activators to the fibronectin adherence receptor of human monocytes. J Immunol 1982;129:2678.

37. Czop JK, Kadish JL, Austen KF. Augmentation of human monocyte opsonin-independent phagocytosis by fragments of human plasma fibronectin. Proc Natl Acad Sci USA 1981;78:3649.

38. Diamond LK. Splenectomy in childhood and the hazard of overwhelming infection. Pediatrics 1969;43:886.

39. Dickerman JD. Bacterial infection and the asplenic host: a review. J Trauma 1976;16:662.

40. Dickerman JD, Bolton E, Coil JA, et al. Protective effect of prophylactic penicillin on splenectomized mice exposed to an aerosolized suspension of type III *Streptococcus pneumoniae*. Blood 1979;53:498.

41. Ehlenberger AG, Nussenzweig V. The role of membrane receptors for C3b and C3d in phagocytosis. J Exp Med 1977;145:357.

42. Ein SH, Shandling B, Simpson JS, et al. Nonoperative management of traumatized spleen in children: how and why. J Pediatr Surg 1978;13:117.

43. Eraklis AJ, Filler RM. Splenectomy in childhood: a review of 1413 cases. J Pediatr Surg 1972;7:382.

44. Eraklis AJ, Kevy SV, Diamond LK, et al. Hazard of overwhelming infection after splenectomy in childhood. N Engl J Med 1967;276:1225.

45. Fehr J, Hofmann V, Kappeler U. Transient reversal of thrombocytopenia in idiopathic thrombocytopenic purpura by high-dose intravenous gamma globulin. N Engl J Med 1982;306:1254.

46. Feliciano DV, Bitondo CG, Mattox KL, et al. A four-year experience with splenectomy versus splenorrhaphy. Ann Surg 1985;201:568.

47. Fidalgo BV, Najjar VA. The physiological role of the lymphoid system. III. Leucophilic ğ-globulin and the phagocytic activity of the polymorphonuclear leucocyte. Proc Natl Acad Sci USA 1967;57:957.

48. Fidalgo BV, Najjar VA. The physiological role of the lymphoid system. VI. The stimulatory effect of leucophilic ğ-globulin (leucokinin) on the phagocytic activity of human polymorphonuclear leucocyte. Biochemistry 1967;6:3386.

49. Fischer KC, Eraklis A, Rossello P, et al. Scintigraphy in the followup of pediatric splenic trauma treated without surgery. J Nucl Med 1978;19:3.

50. Fitzpatrick JEP, Kennedy CC, McGeown MG, et al. Further details of third recorded case of redwater (babesiosis) in man. Br Med J 1969;7:770.

51. Fitzpatrick JEP, Kennedy CC, McGeown MG, et al. Human case of piroplasmosis (babesiosis). Nature 1968;217:861.

52. Forward AD, Ashmore PG. Infection following splenectomy in infants and children. Can J Surg 1960;3:229.

53. Francke EL, Neu HC. Postsplenectomy infection. Surg Clin North Am 1981;61:135.

54. Fries LF, Hall RP, Lawley TJ, et al. Monocyte receptors for the Fc portion of IgG studied with monomeric human IgG1: normal in vitro expression of Fc ğreceptors in HLA-B8/Drw3 subjects with defective Fc-mediated in vivo clearance. J Immunol 1982;129:1041.

55. Garnham PCC, Donnelly J, Hoogstraal H, et al. Human babesiosis in Ireland: further observations and the medical significance of this infection. Br Med J 1969;4:768.

56. Gaston MH, Verter JI, Woods G, et al. Prophylaxis with oral penicillin in children with sickle cell anemia. A randomized trial. N Engl J Med 1986;314:1593.

57. Giebink GS, Foker JE, Kim Y, et al. Serum antibody and opsonic responses to vaccination with pneumococcal capsular polysaccharide in normal and splenectomized children. J Infect Dis 1980;141:404.

58. Giebink GS, Le CT, Schiffman G. Decline of serum antibody in splenectomized children after vaccination with pneumococcal capsular polysaccharides. J Pediatr 1984;105:576.

59. Giuliano AE, Lim RC Jr. Is splenic salvage safe in the traumatized patient? Arch Surg 1981;116:651.

60. Gresham HD, Griffin FM Jr. Induction of phagocytic C3b receptors on human monocytes by lymphokine. Clin Res 1984;32:504A.

61. Griffin FM Jr, Griffin JA. Augmentation of macrophage complement receptor function in vitro. II. Characterization of the effects of a unique lymphokine upon the phagocytic capabilities of macrophages. J Immunol 1980;125:844.

62. Griffin FM Jr, Mullinax PJ. In vivo activation of macrophage C3 receptors for phagocytosis. J Exp Med 1985;162:352.

63. Griffin JA, Griffin FM Jr. Augmentation of macrophage complement receptor function in vitro. I. Characterization of the cellular interactions required for the generation of a T-lymphocyte product that enhances macrophage complement receptor function. J Exp Med 1979;150:653.

64. Griffiss JM. Bactericidal activity of meningococcal antisera. Blocking by IgA of lytic antibody in human convalescent sera. J Immunol 1975;114:1779.

65. Grosfeld JL, Ranochak JE. Are hemisplenectomy and/or primary splenic repair feasible? J Pediatr Surg 1976;11:419.

66. Gudewicz PW, Molnar J, Lai MZ, et al. Fibronectin-mediated uptake of gelatin-coated latex particles by peritoneal macrophages. J Cell Biol 1980;87:427.

67. Haque AU, Hudson P, Wood G, et al. Splenic autotransplant and residual partial spleen: prevention of septicemia. Jpn J Surg 1984;14:407.

68. Heier HE. Splenectomy and serious infections. Scand J Haematol 1980;24:5.

69. Hill HR, Shigeoka AO, Augustine NH, et al. Fibronectin enhances the opsonic and protective activity of monoclonal and polyclonal antibody against group B streptococci. J Exp Med 1984;159:1618.

70. Holzer TJ, Edwards KM, Grewurz H, et al. Binding of C-reactive protein to the pneumococcal capsule or cell wall results in differential localization of C3 and stimulation of phagocytosis. J Immunol 1984;133:1424.

71. Horan M, Colebatch JH. Relation between splenectomy and subsequent infection. A clinical study. Arch Dis Child 1962;37:398.

72. Horsmanheimo A, Horsmanheimo M, Fudenberg HH. Effect of tuftsin on migration of poly-morphonuclear and mononuclear human leukocytes in leukocytes migration agarose test. Clin Immunol Immunopathol 1978;11:251.

73. Horton J, Ogden ME, Williams S, et al. The importance of splenic blood flow in clearing pneumococcal organisms. Ann Surg 1982;195:172.

74. Hosea SW, Burch CG, Brown EJ, et al. Impaired immune response of splenectomized patients to polyvalent pneumococcal vaccine. Lancet 1981;1:804.

75. Huntley CC. Infection following splenectomy in infants and children. Am J Dis Child 1958;95:477.

76. Inada S, Brown EJ, Gaither TA, et al. C3d receptors are expressed on human monocytes after in vitro cultivation. Proc Natl Acad Sci USA 1983;80:2351.

77. Jacobs MR, Koornhof HJ, Robins-Browne RM, et al. Emergence of multiply resistant pneumococci. N Engl J Med 1978;299:735.

78. John AB, Ramlal A, Jackson H, et al. Prevention of pneumococcal infection in children with homo-zygous sickle cell disease. Br Med J 1984;288:1567.

79. Joseph TP, Wyllie GG, Savage JP. The non-operative management of splenic trauma. Aust NZ J Surg 1977;47:179.

80. Kaplan MH, Volanakis JE. Interaction of C-reactive protein complexes with the complement system. I. Consumption of human complement associated with the reaction of C-reactive protein with pneumococcal C-polysaccharide and with the choline phosphatides, lecithin and sphingomyelin. J Immunol 1974;112:2135.

81. Kilpatrick JM, Volanakis JE. Opsonic properties of C-reactive protein. Stimulation by phorbol myris-tate acetate enables human neutrophils to phagocytize C-reactive protein-coated cells. J Immunol 1985;134:3364.

82. King H, Shumacker HB Jr. Splenic studies. I. Susceptibility to infection after splenectomy performed in infancy. Ann Surg 1952;136:239.

83. Klein JO. The epidemiology of pneumococcal disease in infants and children. Rev Infect Dis 1981;3:246.

84. Krumbhaar EB, Lippincott SW. The postmortem weight of the "normal" human spleen at different ages. Am J Med Sci 1939;197:344.

85. Lanser ME, Saba TM, Scovill WA. Opsonic glycoprotein (plasma fibronectin) levels after burn injury. Ann Surg 1980;192:776.

86. Lanzkowsky P, Shende A, Karayalcin G, et al. Staging laparatomy and splenectomy: treatment and complications of Hodgkin's disease in children. Am J Hematol 1976;1:393.

87. Leeson CR, Leeson TS, Paparo AA. Atlas of histology. Philadelphia: WB Saunders, 1985:135.

88. Livingston CD, Levine BA, Sirinek KR. Site of splenic autotransplantation affects protection from sepsis. Am J Surg 1983;146:734.

89. Lum LG, Tubergen DG, Corash L, et al. Splenectomy in the management of the thrombocytopenia of the Wiscott-Aldrich syndrome. N Engl J Med 1980;302:892.

90. Malangoni MA, Dawes LG, Droege EA, et al. Splenic phagocytic function after partial splenectomy and splenic autotransplantation. Arch Surg 1985;120:275.

91. Mantovani B, Rabinovitch M, Nussenzweig V. Phagocytosis of immune complexes by macrophages. Different roles of the macrophage receptor sites for complement (C3) and for immunoglobulin (IgG). J Exp Med 1972;135:780.

92. Marmorston J. Effect of splenectomy on *Bacterium enteritidis* infection in white mice. Proc Soc Exp Biol Med 1935;32:981.

93. Martin SP, Kerby GP. The splanchnic removal in rabbits during fatal bacteremias of the circulating organisms and of superimposed non-pathogenic bacteria. J Exp Med 1950;92:45.

94. Martin SP, Kerby GP, Holland BC. The effect of thorotrast on the removal of bacteria in the splanchnic area of the intact animal. J Immunol 1952;68:293.

95. Martone WJ, Zuehl RW, Minson GE, et al. Postsplenectomy sepsis with DF-2: report of a case with isolation of the organism from the patient's dog. Ann Intern Med 1980;93:457.

96. Meers PD, Matthews RB. Multiply resistant pneumococcus. Lancet 1978;2:219.

97. Mishalany H. Repair of the ruptured spleen. J Pediatr Surg 1974;9:175.

98. Morgenstern L. The avoidable complications of splenectomy. Surg Gynecol Obstet 1977;145:525.

99. Morris DH, Bullock FD. The importance of the spleen in resistance to infection. Ann Surg 1919;70:513.

100. Mosher DF, Williams EM. Fibronectin concentration is decreased in plasma of severely ill patients with disseminated intravascular coagulation. J Lab Clin Med 1978;91:729.

101. Najjar VA. Defective phagocytosis due to deficiencies involving the tetrapeptide tuftsin. J Pediatr 1975;87:1121.

102. Najjar VA, Nishioka K. "Tuftsin": a natural phagocytosis stimulating peptide. Nature 1970;228:672.

103. Navarro C, Kondlapoodi P. Failure of accessory spleens to prevent infection following splenectomy. Arch Intern Med 1985;145:369.

104. Nealon TJ, Beachey EH, Courtney HS, et al. Release of fibronectin-lipoteichoic acid complexes from group A streptococci with penicillin. Infect Immun 1986;51:529.

105. Newland AC, Treleaven JG, Minchinton RM, et al. High-dose intravenous IgG in adults with autoimmune thrombocytopenia. Lancet 1983;1:84.

106. Nishioka K, Constantopoulos A, Satoh PS, et al. Characteristics and isolation of the phagocytosis-stimulating peptide, tuftsin. Biochim Biophys Acta 1973;310:217.

107. Nishioka K, Constantopoulos A, Satoh PS, et al. The characteristics, isolation and synthesis of the phagocytosis stimulating peptide tuftsin. Biochem Biophys Res Commun 1972;47:172.

108. Oakes DD, Charters AC. Changing concepts in the management of splenic trauma. Surg Gynecol Obstet 1981;153:181.

109. Pappas MG, Nussenzweig RS, Nussenzweig V, et al. Complement-mediated defect in clearance and sequestration of sensitized, autologous erythrocytes in rodent malaria. J Clin Invest 1981;67:183.

110. Pearson HA, Johnston D, Smith KA, et al. The born-again spleen. Return of splenic function after splenectomy for trauma. N Engl J Med 1978;298:1389.

111. Pedersen, FK, Henrichsen J, Schiffman G. Antibody response to vaccination with pneumococcal capsular polysaccharides in splenectomized children. Acta Paediatr Scand 1982;71:451.

112. Proctor RA, Mosher DF, Olbrantz PJ. Fibronectin binding to *Staphylococcus aureus*. J Biol Chem 1982;257:14788.

113. Proctor RA, Prendergast E, Mosher DF. Fibronectin mediates attachment of *Staphylococcus aureus* to human neutrophils. Blood 1982;59:681.

114. Quinn TC, Wyler DJ. Intravascular clearance of parasitized erythrocytes in rodent malaria. J Clin Invest 1979;63:1187.

115. Ragsdale, TH, Hamit HF. Splenectomy versus splenic salvage for spleens ruptured by blunt trauma. Am Surg 1984;50:645.

116. Ratner MH, Garrow E, Valda V, et al. Surgical repair of the injured spleen. J Pediatr Surg 1977;12:1019.

117. Rice HM, James PD. Ectopic splenic tissue failed to prevent fatal pneumococcal septicaemia after splenectomy for trauma. Lancet 1980;1:565.

118. Robinson TW, Sturgeon P. Post-splenectomy infection in infants and children. Pediatrics 1960;25:941.

119. Rosner F, Zarrabi MH, Benach JL, et al. Babesiosis in splenectomized adults. Review of 22 reported cases. Am J Med 1984;76:696.

120. Rowley DA. The effect of splenectomy on the formation of circulating antibody in the adult male albino rat. J Immunol 1950;64:289.

121. Saba TM, Blumenstock FA, Scovill WA, et al. Cryoprecipitate reversal of opsonic $_2$-surface binding glycoprotein deficiency in septic surgical and trauma patients. Science 1978;201:622.

122. Saba TM, Jaffe E. Plasma fibronectin (opsonic glycoprotein): its synthesis by vascular endothelial cells and role in cardiopulmonary integrity after trauma as related to reticuloendothelial function. Am J Med 1980;68:577.

123. Scher KS, Wroczynski AF, Scott-Conner C. Intraperitoneal splenic implants do not alter clearance of pneumococcal bacteremia. Am Surg 1985;51:269.

124. Schreiber AD, Frank MM. Role of antibody and complement in the immune clearance and destruction of erythrocytes. I. In vivo effects of IgG and IgM complement-fixing sites. J Clin Invest 1972;51:575.

125. Schumacher MJ. Serum immunoglobulin and transferrin levels after childhood splenectomy. Arch Dis Child 1970;45:114.
126. Shinefield HR, Steinberg CR, Kaye D. Effect of splenectomy on the susceptibility of mice inoculated with *Diplococcus pneumoniae*. J Exp Med 1966;123:777.
127. Siber GR, Weitzman SA, Aisenberg AC, et al. Impaired antibody response to pneumococcal vaccine after treatment for Hodgkin's disease. N Engl J Med 1978;299:442.
128. Simmons BM, Stahl PD, Russell JH. Mannose receptor-mediated uptake of ricin toxin and ricin A chain by macrophages. Multiple intracellular pathways for a chain translocation. J Biol Chem 1986;261:7912.
129. Singer DB. Postsplenectomy sepsis. In: Rosenberg HS, Bolande RP, eds. Perspectives in pediatric pathology. Chicago: Year Book Medical Publishers, 1973:285.
130. Smith CH, Erlandson M, Schulman I, et al. Hazard of severe infections in splenectomized infants and children. Am J Med 1957;22:390.
131. Smith CH, Erlandson ME, Stern G, et al. Postsplenectomy infection in Cooley's anemia. An appraisal of the problem in this and other blood disorders, with a consideration of prophylaxis. N Engl J Med 1962;266:737.
132. Spirer Z, Zakuth V, Bogair N, et al. Radioimmunoassay of the phagocytosis-stimulating peptide tuftsin in normal and splenectomized subjects. Eur J Immunol 1977;7:69.
133. Spirer Z, Zakuth V, Diamant S, et al. Decreased tuftsin concentrations in patients who have undergone splenectomy. Br Med J 1977;2:1574.
134. Spirer Z, Zakuth V, Golander A, et al. The effect of tuftsin on the nitrous blue tetrazolium reduction of normal human polymorphonuclear leukocytes. J Clin Invest 1975;55:198.
135. Springer TA. The LFA-1, Mac-1 glycoprotein family and its deficiency in an inherited disease. Fed Proc 1985;44:2660.
136. Stahl PD, Rodman JS, Miller MJ, et al. Evidence for receptor-mediated binding of glycoproteins, glycoconjugates, and lysosomal glycosidases by alveolar macrophages. Proc Natl Acad Sci USA 1978;75:1399.
137. Sullivan JL, Ochs HD, Schiffman G, et al. Immune response after splenectomy. Lancet 1978;1:178.
138. Thal ER, McClelland RN, Shires GT. Abdominal trauma. In: Shires GT, ed. Care of the Trauma Patient. 2nd ed. New York: McGraw-Hill, 1979:290.
139. Tzehoval E, Segal S, Stabinsky Y, et al. Tuftsin (an Ig-associated tetrapeptide) triggers the immunogenic function of macrophages: implications for activation of programmed cells. Proc Natl Acad Sci USA 1978;75:3400.
140. VanDeWater L, Destree AT, Hynes RO. Fibronectin binds to some bacteria but does not promote their uptake by phagocytic cells. Science 1983;220:201.
141. VanWyck DB, Witte MH, Witte CL. Synergism between the spleen and serum complement in experimental pneumococcemia. J Infect Dis 1982;145:514.
142. VanWyck DB, Witte MH, Witte CL, et al. Critical splenic mass for survival from experimental pneumococcemia. J Surg Res 1980;28:14.
143. Vik DP, Fearon DT. Neutrophils express a receptor for iC3b, C3dg, and C3d that is distinct from CR1, CR2, and CR3. J Immunol 1985;134:2571.
144. Villiger B, Kelley DG, Engleman W, et al. Human alveolar macrophage fibronectin: synthesis, secretion, and ultrastructural localization during gelatin-coated latex particle binding. J Cell Biol 1981;90:711.
145. Volanakis JE, Kaplan MH. Specificity of C-reactive protein for choline phosphate residues of pneumococcal C-polysaccharide. Proc Soc Exp Biol Med 1971;136:612.
146. Warren MK, Vogel SN. Bone marrow-derived macrophages: development and regulation of differentiation markers by colony-stimulating factor and interferons. J Immunol 1985;134:982.
147. Warren MK, Vogel SN. Opposing effects of glucocorticoids on interferon-γ-induced murine macrophage Fc receptor and Ia antigen expression. J Immunol 1985;134:2462.
148. Whitaker AN. The effect of previous splenectomy on the course of pneumococcal bacteremia in mice. J Pathol Bacteriol 1968;95:357.
149. Wright SD, Craigmyle LS, Silverstein SC. Fibronectin and serum amyloid P component stimulate C3b- and C3bi-mediated phagocytosis in cultured human monocytes. J Exp Med 1983;158:1338.
150. Wright SD, Licht MR, Silverstein SC. The receptor for C3d (CR2) is a homologue of CR3 and LFA-1. Fed Proc 1984;43:1487.
151. Wyler DJ. Splenic functions in malaria. Lymphology 1983;16:121.
152. Wyler DJ, Quinn TC, Chen L. Relationship of alterations in splenic clearance function and microcirculation to host defense in acute rodent malaria. J Clin Invest 1981;67:1400, 1981.

153. Zarrabi MH, Rosner F. Serious infections in adults following splenectomy for trauma. Arch Intern Med 1984;144:1421.

BIBLIOGRAPHY

Bohnsack JF, Brown EJ. The role of the spleen in resistance to infection. Annu Rev Med 1986;37:49.

Lockwood CM. Immunological functions of the spleen. Clin Haematol 1983;12:449.

Oakes DD. Splenic trauma. Curr Probl Surg 1981;18:341.

Wright SD, Griffin FM Jr. Activation of phagocytic cells' C3 receptors for phagocytosis. J Leukocyte Biol 1985;38:327.

4

○　　○　　○　　●　　●　　●

TRANSFUSION-RELATED VIRAL INFECTIONS

Paul P. Cook
Mark S. Klempner

Transfusion-related transmission of the retrovirus that causes the acquired immunodeficiency syndrome (AIDS) has poignantly reminded us of the risk of infection by the transfusion of blood products. Indeed, the epidemic occurrence of infections in the posttransfusion setting has provided us with unique insights into AIDS as well as several other viral infections. With the transfusion of over 12 million units of red cells and several million units of blood cell products annually in the United States, it is not surprising that posttransfusion infections are an important concern to the general public as well as to the medical community. With their constant exposure to blood and blood products, surgeons are additionally concerned that transfusion-related infections can be an occupational hazard.

It has become apparent that many infectious agents including viruses, parasites, and bacteria can be transmitted to patients from transfused blood and blood products. However, transfusion of blood products contaminated by bacteria has been dramati-

68

cally reduced by the use of closed systems for collection, and transmission of parasitic infections such as malaria and babesiosis is a rarity. Although rare, transmission of *Trypanosoma cruzi,* the causative agent of Chagas's disease, has recently been reported both in the United States and in Canada.[34,62] Because viruses cause the vast majority of transfusion-related infections, this chapter will review the common viral infections that complicate transfusion therapy.

ROUTINE BLOOD BANK SCREENING

Before discussing the potential pathogens related to blood transfusions, it seems prudent to mention the current methods used by American blood banks to prevent the transfusion of infected blood products. Potential blood donors are given a questionnaire regarding recent health, travel history, medications, and sexual practices. Persons who have traveled recently to an area where malaria is endemic but who did not take antimalarials may donate blood after 6 months from the time of reentry into the United States; those persons who did take antimalarials, who had malaria or who had previously resided in an endemic area, must wait at least 3 years before donating blood.[9] Persons who give a history of homosexual contact or intravenous drug abuse since 1977 are not accepted as blood donors. Persons with fever or anemia are likewise rejected. Once blood is drawn, it is screened for a variety of diseases, including human immunodeficiency virus type 1, human T-cell leukemia virus type 1, hepatitis B, syphilis, and hepatitis C (non-A, non-B hepatitis) (Table 4-1).

RETROVIRAL INFECTIONS

Although human immunodeficiency virus type 1 (HIV-1) is the most renowned of the retroviral infections, two other viruses from the same family (Retroviridae) are potential threats to the blood supply. Human immunodeficiency virus type 2 (HIV-2) and human T-cell leukemia virus type I (HTLV-1) are related retroviruses that may be transmitted via blood transfusions. The hallmark of this family of viruses is the enzyme reverse transcriptase that synthesizes DNA from viral RNA. All retroviruses are enveloped RNA viruses, and all have a tropism for infecting helper (T4 or CD4 +)

Table 4–1
Screening tests on donated blood

Human immunodeficiency virus-1(HIV-1)
Human T-cell leukemia virus-1 (HTLV-1)
Hepatitis B surface antigen (HBsAg)
Alanine aminotransferase (ALT)
Rapid plasma reagin card test for syphilis (RPR)

lymphocytes. The retroviruses have much in common, but there are important differences, which are discussed below.

HUMAN IMMUNODEFICIENCY VIRUS TYPE 1 (HIV-1)

Agent

The major gene products of HIV-1 are listed in Table 4-2. Infection of the T4 cell begins with attachment of the viral surface glycoprotein, gp 120, to the lymphocyte CD4 molecule. Once it is bound, the virus is internalized and uncoated. Viral reverse transcriptase synthesizes DNA from RNA. Activation of the host cell initiates a series of steps that ultimately leads to viral assembly. Unlike other retroviruses such as HTLV-1, HIV-1 is cytopathic for CD4 + cells. The clinical manifestations of the disease are related to the destruction of T4 cells, such that the T4 count is dramatically reduced. Most patients who are infected with HIV-1 and meet the clinical criteria for a diagnosis of acquired immune deficiency syndrome (AIDS) have T4 counts of less than 200 cells/mm^3.

Epidemiology

The Centers for Disease Control (CDC) criteria for the diagnosis of AIDS are given in Table 4-3. The first case of AIDS associated with blood transfusions was diagnosed in 1982.[67] At the time of this writing, there have been over 2600 cases of transfusion-associated AIDS reported to the CDC.[19] It is estimated that 10,000 additional persons were transfused with HIV–1-infected blood prior to institution of the HIV screening test (see below) in 1985.[66] A recent report estimated that 1 in 153,000 units of blood products in this country contains HIV-1.[26] Another study demonstrated that the risk of transmitting HIV-1 via screened blood products was 0.003% per unit.[24] Because over 3 million people in the United States receive transfusions each year, there will continue to be cases of transfusion-related AIDS.

Why should the AIDS virus continue to threaten the blood supply when there appears to be a very sensitive screening test for HIV-1 antibodies? First, the enzyme

Table 4–2
Major genes and gene products of HIV-1

GENE	GENE PRODUCT	PROTEIN FUNCTION
gag (group-specific antigen)	p18, p24, p55	Core antigen
env (envelope)	gp160, gp120, gp41	Surface glycoprotein (gp120) and transmembrane
pol (polymerase)	p66, p51, p31	Reverse transcriptase and endonuclease

Table 4–3
CDC Surveillance Case Definition for AIDS*

I. No laboratory evidence of HIV infection required in absence of other causes of immunodeficiency
    Pneumocystis carinii pneumonia
    Disseminated cytomegalovirus in patients > 1 month old
    Candidiasis of the lungs, esophagus, trachea, or bronchi
    Extrapulmonary crytococcosis
    Mucocutaneous herpes simplex infection > 1 month duration
    Cryptosporidiosis > 1 month duration
    Kaposi's sarcoma in patients < 60 years old
    Disseminated *Mycobacterium avium*
    Primary CNS lymphoma in patient < 60 years old
    Lymphoid interstitial pneumonitis in patient > 13 years old
    Progressive multifocal leukoencephalopathy
    Toxoplasmosis of the brain in patient > 1 month old
II. Laboratory evidence of HIV infection required
    Disseminated histoplasmosis
    Disseminated coccidioidomycosis
    Isosporiasis > 1 month duration
    Extrapulmonary tuberculosis
    Recurrent *Salmonella* septicemia
    Non-Hodgkin's lymphoma
    Primary CNS lymphoma, any age
    Reucrrent pyogenic bacterial infections in patient < 13 years old
    HIV wasting syndrome
    HIV encephalopathy

* *Modified from Centers for Disease Control. MMWR 1987;36 (Suppl): 1.*

immunoassay (EIA or ELISA) test that is used (see below) is not a perfect test. False-negative results, although rare, do occur. Second, there is a latent period from infection to the development of antibodies, the so-called "window" period. Most infected persons will seroconvert within 3 to 12 weeks.[27,42] A recent study demonstrated that many homosexual men with HIV-1 viremia did not seroconvert even after three years following infection.[46] If an infected individual donates blood during this period, the current screening method would be negative even though the blood is highly infectious.

It has been estimated that approximately 1.5 million people in the United States are infected with HIV-1. Over 95% of patients exposed to HIV–1-infected blood will themselves become infected.[92] AIDS will develop in half of these patients within 7 years.[92] This incubation period is highly variable and appears to depend on such factors as viral inoculum size and the recipient's immune status.

Blood products that have been implicated in the transmission of HIV-1 include packed red cells, platelets, plasma, and whole blood.[65] Heat-treated albumin, plasma protein fractions, plasma-derived hepatitis B vaccine, and immune gamma globulin have not been shown to be infectious.

Symptoms

Acute HIV-1 infection may be asymptomatic or may present as a mononucleosis-like syndrome.[27,42,61] The incubation period is 2 to 6 weeks. Fever, malaise, headache, myalgias, sweats, arthralgias, rash, sore throat, and lymphadenopathy are common signs and symptoms of the acute illness. Laboratory features include mild leukopenia and thrombocytopenia, mild elevation of liver transaminase levels, and an elevated sedimentation rate.[27,42] During the acute infection, which is usually self-limited, the virus may be cultured from the blood and, in cases of aseptic meningitis, the cerebrospinal fluid.[42]

The clinical manifestations of AIDS are protean and beyond the scope of this review. Fever, fatigue, weight loss, night sweats, and diarrhea frequently precede the initial opportunistic infection. Generalized lymphadenopathy, oral candidiasis, and dermatomal herpes zoster are frequent prodromal manifestations.

Shortness of breath and dyspnea on exertion may be the presenting symptoms of *Pneumocystis carinii* pneumonia. Headache or mental status changes may be a manifestation of cryptococcal meningitis. Focal neurologic deficits should suggest a diagnosis of toxoplasmosis or of primary central nervous system lymphoma. Loss of vision suggests cytomegalovirus chorioretinitis.

Screening Test

In January 1985, the U.S. Public Health Service recommended screening of all donated blood and plasma for HIV-1 antibody. By March 1985, screening was begun by all American Red Cross regional units. The test uses whole disrupted HIV-1 virus, produced from the H9 cell line, as the ELISA antigen. The sensitivity and specificity of the ELISA test are 97.3% and 98.6%, respectively.[93]

It has been estimated that if the prevalence of HIV-1 antibody in the donor population is 0.1%, then up to 89% of reactive ELISA tests will have false-positive results.[64] It is thought that false-positive reactions are due to the presence of cross-reacting antibodies to HLA-type antigens. Given that, in a low prevalence population, there is a relatively high percentage of false-positive results by ELISA testing, there is a definite need for confirmatory testing.

The test that has been most widely used is the Western blot analysis. For this test, purified, disrupted virus is fractionated and the viral proteins are transferred to a nitrocellulose sheet. Serum is then tested for antibodies to the separated HIV-1 proteins. A reactive Western blot contains at least two of the three major bands (anti-gp 160/120, anti-gp 41, and anti-p 24) (see Table 4-2). An indeterminate Western blot contains one or more viral bands, but insufficient bands to meet the criteria for a positive result.

More sensitive assays for HIV-1 infection include viral culture and the polymerase chain reaction.[30,46] These methods are not commercially available and require technical expertise in research laboratories. The ELISA and Western blot assays are sufficient for most cases. As mentioned previously, blood donation during the so-called "window" period remains a potential threat to the nation's blood supply. The current screening methods will not detect these individuals. Only viral culture or polymerase chain reaction will detect infection, but neither test is practical for screening purposes.

In summary, the risk of HIV-1 infection secondary to blood product transfusion is extremely low and is related to several factors. First, potential donors are given information concerning "high risk" behavior. Those who have had homosexual contacts or who have used intravenous drugs since 1977 are advised not to donate blood. Second, the development of the ELISA screening test with Western blot confirmation of all ELISA-positive specimens has been a major factor in reducing the incidence of transfusion-associated HIV-1 infection. Finally, judicious use of blood products should help to reduce the small risk of transfusion-associated HIV-1 infection.

HIV-2

Human immunodeficiency virus type 2 (HIV-2) is a retrovirus that has many similarities with HIV-1, including mode of transmission and tropism for CD4 + cells. Infection with HIV-2 can lead to depletion of CD4 + cells much like HIV-1 infection. Opportunistic infections result from the depressed T4 cells, resulting in a clinical presentation that is indistinguishable from HIV−1-associated AIDS.

The virus appears to be endemic to West Africa. A recent report of HIV−2-associated AIDS in this country described a patient from the Cape Verde Islands, Africa.[49] American blood banks currently do not screen for the presence of HIV-2 antibodies. This policy may require changes if surveillance testing identifies an increasing incidence of HIV-2.

HTLV-1

Human T cell leukemia virus type 1 (HTLV-1) is another retrovirus that is a threat to the blood supply. Unlike HIV, HTLV-1 does not cause T-helper cell destruction. Rather, infection with HTLV-1 can lead to neoplastic proliferation of T-helper cells resulting in T-cell leukemia-lymphoma. The risk factors for acquisition of the infection are identical to those of HIV, *i.e.*, intravenous drug abuse, transfusion of blood products, and homosexuality.

HTLV-1 is endemic to islands of southwestern Japan, the Caribbean, and the southeastern United States. It may be transmitted by sexual contact, blood transfusion, or by contaminated needles. Seroprevalence rates approach 50% in intravenous drug users in endemic areas.[73] A recent study demonstrated that 2.5 of 10,000 American blood donors were positive for HTLV-1 antibody.[94]

Although HTLV-1 appears to be a relatively common infection, only about 0.1% of carriers will develop T-cell leukemia-lymphoma.[87] There is some suggestion that this figure is much higher in persons who become infected at an early age. Common clinical findings in this disease include lymphadenopathy, hepatosplenomegaly, and characteristic skin lesions. Laboratory findings include an elevated white blood cell count of 10,000 to 100,000 cells/mm^3, and hypercalcemia. Diagnosis is confirmed by a positive serology for HTLV-1, and by demonstrating integration of proviral DNA in the malignant cells.

Blood donors are routinely screened for the presence of HTLV-1 antibody.

HEPATITIS A

Hepatitis A is a 27-nm RNA virus that belongs to the picornavirus class.

Epidemiology

Posttransfusion hepatitis (PTH) secondary to hepatitis A is extremely rare, probably owing to the transient viremic phase of the clinical illness. As shown in Figure 4-1, viremia is first detected approximately 2 to 3 weeks prior to the onset of jaundice. Serum from infected patients has been shown to transmit the virus during this viremic phase.[53] There are several reports of transfusion-acquired hepatitis A,[33,63,77,81] but the actual incidence is probably very small.

Diagnosis

Serologic diagnosis of acute hepatitis A infection requires demonstration of IgM antibodies to hepatitis A.

Prevention

Because adult patients with hepatitis A tend to be more symptomatic during the preicteric phase of their illness,[52] elimination of febrile and symptomatic donors is an effective screening measure.

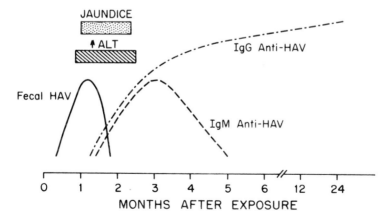

Figure 4–1.
Course of Hepatitis A.

HEPATITIS B

Hepatitis B (HBV) is perhaps the most renowned transfusion-related infection. Advances in serodiagnosis and mandatory screening of all units of blood and plasma have dramatically reduced the incidence of HBV as the cause of PTH. Nevertheless, screening tests do not detect 100% of infectious blood products, and HBV still accounts for 5% to 10% of PTH. This agent also holds a special interest to surgeons because of their occupational risk for infection and the availability of a safe, effective vaccine.

Agent

The hepatitis-B virus is a 42-nM DNA virus that belongs to the Hepadnaviradae virus family. The outer envelope of the virion contains the hepatitis-B surface antigen (HBsAg) which can exist as part of the intact virion (Dane particle) or as part of incomplete particulate viral forms that circulate in the blood of infected individuals. The inner core of the virion contains the hepatitis-B core antigen (HBcAg). Within the core is the viral genome, a partially double-stranded, circular DNA molecule of approximately 3200 base pairs. The core also contains DNA-directed DNA polymerase, protein kinase activity, and possibly the hepatitis-B e antigen (HBeAg).[88] Serodiagnosis is based on detecting these viral antigens or antibodies directed against them.

Epidemiology

There are approximately 300,000 new cases annually of hepatitis-B virus (HBV) infection.[36] Approximately 25% of cases are icteric and nearly 0.1% die of fulminant hepatitis. Almost 90% of cases occur in persons over 20 years of age. Transmission of the virus occurs by way of percutaneous or permucosal routes. Although HBV infection is relatively uncommon in the general American adult population, certain high-risk groups exist (Table 4-4). Whole blood and blood products have been shown to transmit the virus. Heated albumin and plasma apparently do not transmit the virus. Pooled immunoglobulin has not been shown to transmit the virus.[76]

Symptoms

HBV causes a wide spectrum of clinical illness ranging from asymptomatic infection to a fulminant, fatal course. The incubation period of hepatitis B is approximately 7 to 12 weeks (Figure 4-2). While most cases are subclinical, symptomatic patients often present with malaise, loss of appetite, easy fatigability, myalgias and headache. Other more severe signs and symptoms include nausea, vomiting, jaundice, fever, and coma. Between 10% and 20% of patients with acute icteric hepatitis develop a serum sickness-like illness characterized by erythematous maculopapular rash, arthralgias, and occasionally arthritis, urticaria, and fever. These signs and symptoms precede the icteric phase of illness by days to weeks. Dark urine occurs in 94% of icteric cases. Hepatomegaly occurs in 70% and splenomegaly in 20% of symptomatic

Table 4–4
Prevalence of hepatitis B serologic markers in various population groups

POPULATION GROUP	PREVALENCE OF SEROLOGIC MARKERS OF HBV INFECTION	
	HBs Ag (%)	All markers (%)
High Risk		
Immigrants/refugees from areas of high HBV endemicity	13	70–85
Clients in institutions for the mentally retarded	10–20	35–80
Users of illicit parenteral drugs	7	60–80
Homosexually active men	6	35–80
Household contacts of HBV carriers	3–6	30–60
Patients on hemodialysis units	3–10	20–80
Intermediate risk		
Health-care workers—frequent blood contact	1–2	15–30
Prisoners (male)	1–8	10–80
Staff of institutions for the mentally retarded	1	10–25
Low risk		
Health-care workers—no or infrequent blood contact	0.3	3–10
Healthy adults (first-time volunteer blood donors)	0.3	3–5

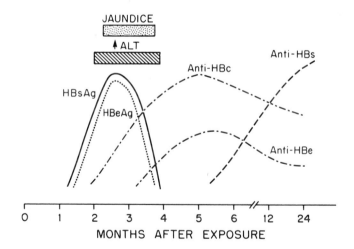

Figure 4–2.
Course of Hepatitis B.

patients, respectively. Right upper quadrant tenderness is common. Cervical lymph-adenopathy and spider angiomata may be seen but are uncommon. Fever, if it occurs, is usually low grade.

Laboratory findings include a normal to slightly decreased hematocrit. Mild hemolysis is occasionally observed. The white cell count is usually normal, but granulocytopenia and relative lymphocytosis may be present. Atypical lymphocytes are common.[56] Liver function tests include an early rise in direct bilirubin when the total bilirubin is normal. Total bilirubin usually peaks at 10 mg% in most icteric cases, but higher bilirubin values can be seen.

Marked elevations of the serum transaminases, alanine aminotransferase (ALT, SGPT), and aspartate aminotransferase (AST, SGOT) are characteristic of viral hepatitis. Peak values above 1000 TU are common. ALT levels usually exceed AST levels. The peak levels are not of any prognostic significance. The serum alkaline phosphatase is usually only mildly elevated and may be normal. The prothrombin time is usually normal or only mildly prolonged (less than 12 seconds).

The clinical course of uncomplicated acute HBV infection is marked by complete recovery 4 to 6 weeks after symptoms appear. Appetite usually returns and malaise resolves as icterus worsens. Serum bilirubin, which rises for approximately 2 weeks, declines to normal over 2 to 4 weeks. Transaminase levels usually begin to decline before the peak in bilirubin. Acute HBV infection may infrequently be complicated by Guillain-Barré syndrome, encephalitis, agranulocytosis, aplastic anemia, thrombocytopenia, and cardiac arrhythmias. Fulminant hepatitis occurs rarely, but is usually associated with a rapid downhill course characterized by hyperexcitability, confusion, asterixis, obtundation, coma, and finally death.

Although most episodes of HBV infection are self-limited, chronic infection occurs and may have morbid consequences. The likelihood of developing chronic HBV infection is inversely related to the age at which infection occurs. Thus, 90% of infected infants versus 10% of infected adults become chronic carriers. In these patients, HBsAg and HBeAg persist in the serum, usually for life. There appears to be a spontaneous clearance of HBsAg in about 2% of chronic carriers per year.[84]

Diagnosis of chronic HBV infection should be considered in patients in whom HBsAg persists in the serum for longer than 6 months. The diagnosis of chronic persistent or chronic active hepatitis depends on liver biopsy. The complications of chronic hepatitis-B virus infection include cirrhosis, hepatocellular carcinoma, and fulminant hepatitis. The risk of developing hepatocellular carcinoma is approximately 200-fold higher in HBsAg carriers than in noncarriers.[11]

Diagnosis

Sensitive serologic testing for HBV antigens and antibodies to HBV proteins has greatly facilitated the diagnosis of this disease. Blood donors are routinely screened for HBsAg. HBsAg-positive blood is discarded. The various antigens and antibodies are listed in Table 4-5, and interpretation of possible results is given in Table 4-6.

The effectiveness of these tests is demonstrated by the reduction in the incidence of PTH secondary to HBV. Prior to serologic testing, 60% of PTH was due to hepatitis B.[7] Since serologic screening has been instituted, only about 11% of cases are due to HBV.[6,7] Presumable, blood from donors who have concentrations of the virus (and HBsAg) too low to be detected by the assay method account for these PTH cases. HBsAg appears in the serum of almost all symptomatic patients and is usually present at the time of clinical illness. Anti-HBc may be the only positive serologic marker of

Table 4–5
Hepatitis Nomenclature

HBV	Hepatitis B virus	Etiologic agent of "serum" or "long-incubation" hepatitis; also known as Dane particle.
HbsAg	Hepatitis B surface antigen	Surface antigen(s) of HBV detectable in large quantity in serum; several subtypes identified.
HBeAg	Hepatitis B e antigen	Soluble antigen; correlates with HBV replication, high titer HBV in serum, and infectivity of serum.
HBcAg	Hepatitis B core antigen	No commercial test available.
Anti-HBs	Antibody to HBsAg	Indicates past infection with and immunity to HBV, passive antibody from HBIG, or immune response from HBV vaccine.
Anti-HBe	Antibody to HBeAG	Presence in serum of HBsAg carrier suggest lower titer of HBV.
Anti-HBc	Antibody to HBcAg	Indicates past infection with HBV at some undefined time.
IgM anti-HBc	IgM class antibody to HBcAg	Indicates recent infection with HBV; positive for 4–6 months after infection.

Table 4–6
HBV Serologic Markers in Different Stages of Infection and Convalescence

STAGE OF INFECTION	HBsAg	ANTI-HBS	ANTI-HBc		HBeAg	ANTI-HBe
			IgG	IgM		
Late incubation period of hepatitis B	+	−	−	−	+ or −	−
Acute hepatitis B	+	−	+	+	+	−
HBsAg negative acute hepatitis B	−	−	+	+	−	−
Healthy HBsAg carrier	+	−	+ + +	+ or −	−	+
Chronic hepatitis B	+	−	+ + +	+ or −	+	−
HBV infection in recent past	−	+ +	+ +	+ or −	−	+
HBV infection in distant past	−	+ or −	+ or −	−	−	−
Recent HBV vaccination	−	+ +	−	−	−	−

HBV infection in a small percentage of patients who have already cleared the HBsAg at the time of presentation. Anti-HBsAg remains detectable for life. In approximately half of the cases, there is a period of 1 to 2 weeks between the disappearance of HBsAg and the appearance of anti-HBs. HBeAg is detectable by radioimmunoassay in almost all cases of hepatitis B infection.

Management

Treatment of acute HBV infection is supportive. Corticosteroids have not been shown to be efficacious and indeed may be harmful.[35,47,71] Steroid therapy for HBsAg positive chronic active hepatitis appears to enhance HBV replication and may have a deleterious effect.[89]

Postexposure Prophylaxis

Use of immune serum globulin (ISG) or hepatitis B immune globulin (HBIG) prophylactically after exposure to blood or secretions of HBsAg-positive persons has been shown to reduce significantly the incidence of infection.[70,78] The decision to give ISG or HBIG must take into account the hepatitis B vaccination status of the exposed person and the HBsAg status (if known) of the source. Recommendations for prophylaxis are summarized in Table 4-7. Note that it is recommended that persons not previously vaccinated with the hepatitis B vaccine be given the initial vaccine dose at the time of exposure. The doses of ISG and HBIG are 0.06 ml/kg and 0.07 ml/kg, respectively.

Table 4–7
Recommendations for Hepatitis B Prophylaxis Following Percutaneous Exposure

SOURCE	EXPOSED PERSON	
	Unvaccinated	Vaccinated
HBsAg-positive	1. HBIG × 1 immediately*	1. Test exposed person for anti-HBs†
	2. Initiate HB vaccine‡ series	2. If inadequate antibody§ HBIG (× 1) immediately plus HB vaccine booster dose
Known source High-risk HBsAg-positive	1. Institute HB vaccine series 2. Test source for HBsAg. If positive, HBIG × 1	1. Test source for HBsAg only if exposed is vaccine nonresponder; if source is HBsAg-positive, give HBIG × 1 immediately plus HB vaccine booster dose
Low-risk HBsAg-positive	Initiate HB vaccine series	Nothing required
Unknown source	Initiate HB vaccine series	Nothing required

* HBIG dose 0.06 ml/kg IM.
† See text for details.
‡ HB vaccine dose 20 μg IM for adults; 10 μg IM for infants or children under 10 years of age. First dose within 1 week; second and third doses, 1 and 6 months later.
§ Less than 10 SRU by RIA, negative by EIA.

Hepatitis B Vaccine

There are currently two vaccine preparations that are commercially available. Plasma-derived, inactivated HBV vaccine (Heptavax-B, Merck Sharp & Dohme, West Point, PA) has been licensed since 1981 and has been found to be safe and effective. The three-step preparation process (urea, pepsin, and formalin) inactivates all classes of virus found in blood, including hepatitis C (non-A, non-B hepatitis) and HIV-1. A recombinant DNA HBV vaccine (Recombivax-HB, Merck Sharp & Dohme) has recently been licensed by the Food and Drug Administration. Both vaccines should be administered in the deltoid region at 0, 1, and 6 months. The dose of the plasma-derived vaccine is 20µg, whereas the dose is 10µg for the recombinant vaccine. The dose is adjusted for children less than 11 years of age (half the adult dose) and for immunosuppressed or hemodialysis patients (twice the adult dose).

Because of the high cost of the hepatitis B vaccine (approximately $120 for the three injections), there has been some interest in using an intradermal inoculation with a lower dose of the vaccine. One recent study demonstrated that an intradermal inoculation of one-tenth the usual dose of plasma-derived hepatitis B vaccine (*i.e.,* 2µg at 0, 1, and 6 months) resulted in the development of protective antibody levels in 95% of healthy medical students.[23]

It is recommended that persons at intermediate or high risk of infection receive either of the vaccines. Table 4-8 lists the persons who should be considered for vaccination. Using either vaccine, anti-HBsAg develops in greater than 90% of healthy individuals. The response is somewhat lower in immunocompromised or hemodialysis

Table 4–8
Persons for Whom Hepatitis B Vaccine Is Recommended

Health care workers:
  Medical technologists
  Operating room staff
  Surgeons
  Pathologists
  Phlebotomists
  Dialysis unit staff
  Dentists
  Dental hygienists
Hemodialysis patients
Homosexual men
Intravenous drug users
Household and sexual contacts of HBV carriers
Clients and staff in institutions for the mentally retarded

patients. Immunity appears to last at least 5 years, but may be less in immunocompromised individuals. The use of a booster vaccine is controversial at the present time, although a recent report advised booster inoculation 5 to 7 years after the last dose of vaccine.[44]

DELTA HEPATITIS

Agent

Hepatitis delta virus (HDV) is a defective RNA virus that requires the presence of hepatitis B virus for its expression. The delta agent is 35 to 37 nm in size. It consists of a low molecular weight RNA and an internal protein (delta antigen) coated with HBsAg as the surface protein.[72] The delta antigen itself is a protein with a molecular weight of 68,000.

Epidemiology

HDV was first discovered in Italy and appears to be endemic to the southern part of that country. The delta agent has a worldwide, but nonuniform, distribution. Besides Italy, endemic foci exist in the Middle East and in parts of Africa and South America. In nonendemic areas, delta infection is confined to polytransfused patients with hemophilia and intravenous drug abusers.

HDV infection can occur simultaneously with hepatitis B or as a superinfection in a hepatitis B carrier. Both types of infection can lead to an acute hepatitis. Recent data have shown that 3% to 12% of American blood donors with HBsAg have antibodies to the delta virus.[75]

Clinical Presentation

The clinical presentation of delta hepatitis is similar to that of the other viral causes of hepatitis. There is substantial evidence that coinfection of chronic HBsAg carriers with the delta agent leads to a more severe hepatitis and to a higher incidence of chronic active hepatitis and cirrhosis as compared with hepatitis B infection alone.[72] The diagnosis should be suspected in chronic carriers of HBsAg who are intravenous drug abusers or who are hemophiliacs receiving pooled blood products.

Diagnosis

Delta infection can be diagnosed by demonstrating delta antigen in the serum or by detecting IgM antibodies to the delta agent. A recent study demonstrated that an ELISA assay for hepatitis delta antigen was more sensitive than anti-HD–IgM for the diagnosis of acute delta infection.[17] The delta antigen has only been detected in serum samples reactive for HBsAg.[75] Therefore, screening for HBsAg should be effective in removing the delta antigen from the nation's blood supply; a recent multicenter study confirmed this hypothesis.[75] It should be kept in mind that prevention of delta infection will only be as effective as the prevention of HBV infection. Because the screening test for HBsAg in blood donors has less than 100% sensitivity, delta infection will continue to be a complication of blood transfusions, albeit a small one. It has been recommended that HBsAg carriers receive blood products from single donors or mini-pool donors in order to reduce their incidence of posttransfusion delta infection.[75]

NON-A, NON-B HEPATITIS (HEPATITIS C)

Despite highly effective detection and control measures for hepatitis B virus, a surprisingly high incidence of PTH has continued. Sensitive serologic tests indicate that cytomegalovirus (CMV), Epstein–Barr virus (EBV), and hepatitis A virus are not the cause of many of these cases. These episodes of hepatitis, which occur both related and unrelated to transfusion and where other etiologies for hepatitis can be excluded, are referred to as non-A, non-B (NANB) hepatitis.

Agents

Non-A, non-B hepatitis is a diagnosis based on exclusion of hepatitis A, hepatitis B, CMV, EBV, and HDV. There are substantial data to suggest that NANB hepatitis is caused by more than one agent. Tabor has suggested that there are three distinct viruses that cause NANB hepatitis.[85] Recently, Choo and colleagues have cloned an agent, an RNA virus, responsible for the majority of cases of NANB PTH. These workers have named this agent hepatitis C virus (HCV) and have developed a radioimmunoassay to detect antibody to the virus (anti-HCV).[54] A recent report by Alter and associates has demonstrated that the radioimmunoassay is highly sensitive in detecting patients with biopsy-proven posttransfusion NANB hepatitis.[8] Unfortunately, there appears to be a long latent period (4 months) from the development of hepatitis to the detection of antibody.

Epidemiology

Non-A, non-B hepatitis is the most common form of PTH, yet it is apparently also transmitted by nonparenteral routes. It is estimated that approximately 150,000 new cases of NANB hepatitis occur in this country each year, but that only 5% to 10% of these cases result from blood transfusions. One report demonstrated that greater than 90% of donors whose blood transmitted NANB hepatitis had themselves never been transfused.[86]

NANB hepatitis is three to five times more common among recipients of commercial blood compared to volunteer blood. In fact, elimination of paid donors is felt to be the most important factor in reducing the incidence of PTH. The average incidence of posttransfusion NANB hepatitis is approximately 7% in recipients of volunteer blood.[43] When at least one of the transfused units is commercial blood, the incidence rises to 28.1%. Because these studies preceded current screening methods for NANB (see below), the actual incidence may be lower.

Symptoms

The incubation period of hepatitis C virus is approximately 5 to 10 weeks. Most patients with NANB hepatitis are asymptomatic. Only about 25% of cases develop jaundice.[1,79] Symptomatic cases are clinically similar to cases of type B hepatitis. Between 20% and 60% of patients with NANB hepatitis develop chronic liver disease. The risk of developing chronic hepatitis is inversely correlated with the severity of acute NANB hepatitis. Anicteric cases and cases with serum ALT values less than 300 IU tend to progress to chronic active hepatitis.[13]

Diagnosis

An assay for detection of antibodies to hepatitis C virus (anti-HCV) has recently been developed.[54] At present, blood banks routinely screen blood for ALT, because the risk of acquiring PTH secondary to NANB is directly related to the ALT level of the donor blood.[2] For example, donor blood with an ALT value greater than 60 IU/L is associated with a greater than fourfold increased risk of PTH, as compared with donor units with ALT values less than 45 IU/L (21.7% versus 4.8%, respectively).[83] It is unclear what effect anti-HCV testing will have on the incidence of PTH. Because of the prolonged "window period" (*i.e.,* the time between infection and the development of anti-HCV antibodies), the test will certainly not identify all units of blood that are infected.

Prevention

Prevention of PTH requires judicious use of blood products. Properly heat-treated albumin and plasma do not transmit NANB hepatitis. Immune globulin prophylaxis was shown to be somewhat effective in decreasing the incidence of NANB PTH,[53] but a subsequent randomized study failed to confirm this finding.[80] At present, although no specific recommendation can be made, it may be reasonable to administer ISG (0.06 ml/kg) to persons who have had percutaneous exposure to blood from a patient with NANB patients.[69] Perhaps the most important means of reducing NANB PTH is to use only volunteer blood.

Treatment

Two recently published studies demonstrated the effectiveness of recombinant interferon α in the treatment of chronic hepatitis C infection.[28,29] Improvement was usually transient, however, and relapse was common after treatment was terminated.

CYTOMEGALOVIRUS

Agent

Cytomegalovirus (CMV) is the largest member of the herpesvirus family. It is a DNA virus consisting of a 64-nm core that contains the viral genome. The core is enclosed by a 110-nm icosahedral capsid, which itself is enclosed by an envelope containing 25 to 30 virally coded proteins.[5]

Infection by the virus involves adherence, perhaps to specific cell–surface receptors, followed by viral uncoating in the cytoplasm and transport of the nucleocapsids to the nucleus. Once in the nucleus, transcription of viral DNA, translation of viral proteins, and replication of viral DNA take place.

CMV can infect virtually any organ system, but it most commonly infects the parotid gland, kidney, gastrointestinal tract, lung, liver, and brain. Like other herpes viruses, CMV can produce latent infections. It is believed that the latent virus is harbored within leukocytes, probably both mononuclear cells and neutrophils. Attempts to culture the virus from seropositive-banked blood have been largely unsuccessful, suggesting that the virus is transmitted in a latent state. It has been suggested that allogeneic stimulation of latently infected lymphocytes (as occurs when antigenically dissimilar leukocytes are transfused) may induce transformation to an active state.[20]

Epidemiology

CMV infection occurs in 7% to 30% of patients receiving blood transfusions.[3] The incidence of infection is related both to the number of donors and to the volume of blood transfused.[3] Transmission of the agent has occurred with transfusion of whole blood, packed red cells, and leukocytes. Leukocyte transfusions have been especially associated with CMV infections in immunocompromised hosts.[39,95] Patients at high risk for developing CMV disease are pregnant women and premature neonates who are CMV-seronegative prior to transfusion. Seronegative recipients of organ transplants from seropositive donors are also at high risk, as are seronegative immunosuppressed oncology patients (Table 4-9).

Table 4–9
**Individuals At Risk for Serious
CMV Infection**

Premature infants
Organ transplant recipients
Seronegative pregnant women
Oncology patients receiving chemotherapy

These are three possible types of CMV infection. Primary infection occurs in patients who are CMV seronegative. Secondary infection may be either reactivation of a latent virus or reinfection that occurs in CMV-seropositive patients but involves a different exogenous strain. The distinction between reactivation and reinfection can be made using restriction endonuclease methodology, which gives characteristic DNA "fingerprints" unique to each strain.[45]

There is considerable geographic variation in the distribution of CMV-seropositive blood donors. In Third World countries, virtually 100% of donors are CMV-seropositive.[51] In the United States, the prevalence of seropositive donors is inversely related to the socioeconomic status of the donor population.

Symptoms

While most transfusion-associated CMV infections are asymptomatic, the incubation period for those who do develop clinical illness is approximately 2 to 6 weeks. The manifestations in symptomatic patients depend largely on the host. Immunocompetent patients may develop a mononucleosis-like syndrome consisting of fever, splenomegaly, hepatomegaly, malaise, and myalgias.[3,25] Lymphadenopathy is said to be less common in CMV mononucleosis compared to EBV mononucleosis[5] (Table 4-10). CMV mononucleosis rarely causes more serious illness in immunocompetent persons, but pneumonia, myocarditis, pericarditis, aseptic meningitis, retinitis, encephalitis, hemolytic anemia, and the Guillain–Barré syndrome have all been reported.[10,12,16,18,76]

The duration of symptoms is variable, lasting from a few days up to 6 weeks, with a mean duration of 3 weeks. Laboratory findings include a relative and absolute lymphocytosis with numerous atypical lymphocytes. Abnormal liver function tests occur in more than 90% of patients and are usually mild (AST < 100 IU; bilirubin < 2 mg/dl).

Immunosuppressed patients usually exhibit more malignant manifestations of CMV infection. Primary and recurrent infections as well as reinfections occur, although the relative frequency of each type is unknown. Primary infections tend to be more virulent. Mortality rates as high as 40% occur in premature infants with primary infections.[40] Approximately 85% of transplant recipients with primary infections, compared to only 20% to 40% of these patients with recurrent infections, are symp-

Table 4–10
Clinical Findings in CMV Versus EBV Infection

	SORE THROAT	LYMPH-ADENOPATHY	LYMPHO-CYTOSIS	ATYPICAL LYMPHOCYTES	HETEROPHILE ANTIBODY
EBV	Common	Common	Common	Common	Positive
CMV	Uncommon	Rare	Common	Common	Negative

tomatic.[41] Pneumonia is the most common complication in immunosuppressed patients and has a mortality rate approaching 85% in bone-marrow transplant recipients.[59] Other complications include esophagitis, enteritis, pancreatitis, retinitis, and hepatitis. Fever is an almost universal finding. Other physical findings include hepatomegaly and splenomegaly. Patients with retinitis frequently have decreased visual acuity. Laboratory findings include lymphocytosis and elevated transaminases. Atypical lymphocytosis is less common than in immunocompetent persons.[59] The virus is more likely to be cultured from the blood in immunosuppressed patients. The chest radiograph in patients with CMV pneumonia usually shows unilateral or bilateral interstitial infiltrates that start peripherally and extend centrally.[5]

Diagnosis

Tissue sections demonstrating characteristic intranuclear inclusions are diagnostic of CMV infection. Serologic methods, including complement fixation, indirect hemagglutination, indirect immunofluorescence, and enzyme-linked immunosorbent assay, are the most common means of making a diagnosis; a fourfold or greater increase in antibody titer between acute and convalescent sera is necessary for diagnosis. Seroconversion proves primary infection. Distinguishing reactivation from reinfection requires restriction endonuclease analysis of viral DNA.[45] CMV can be cultured from the urine, saliva, and from the buffy coat of blood; the virus produces characteristic cytopathic changes of infected human diploid fibroblasts but the slow rate of growth (up to 4 to 6 weeks) makes tissue culture impractical in many situations. Rapid diagnostic tests include electron microscopy of urine[53] and DNA hybridization using a radiolabeled, cloned fragment of CMV DNA to detect CMV in urine.[22]

Documentation of infection by virus isolation or a fourfold rise in serology does not necessarily imply a causal relationship to illness. Asymptomatic persons frequently shed virus in the urine for months after primary or recurrent infection. Therefore, isolation of CMV from the urine of a patient with a pulmonary infiltrate does not necessarily mean that the pneumonia is caused by CMV. Clearly, better diagnostic techniques are needed.

Prevention

There is substantial evidence that transfusion-associated CMV infection can be prevented. Exclusive use of CMV-seronegative blood has been shown to essentially eliminate posttransfusion CMV infections in seronegative neonates.[4,96] A recent study of seronegative bone-marrow recipients who were given bone marrow from seronegative donors demonstrated a significant decrease in the incidence of CMV infection in those patients receiving only CMV-seronegative blood products (1 of 32 compared to 8 of 25 in recipients from unscreened blood products).[14] This protective effect was not seen in patients who had received CMV-seropositive donor marrow. Because 45% to 79% of donors are CMV-seropositive, use of only CMV-seronegative blood would severely limit the number of acceptable units. An alternative is to use frozen, deglycerolized blood products.[15,90] This technique removes 98% to 100% of viable leukocytes.[48,58] Brady and coworkers[15] demonstrated that none of 106 CMV-seronegative neonates developed virologic or serologic evidence of CMV infection 3 months after receiving frozen deglycerolized red blood cells. The major drawback of this procedure is the expense.

Because most CMV infections are mild in immunocompetent persons,[3] there is no justification for transfusing only CMV-seronegative blood or frozen, deglycerolized blood to the general population. Persons in whom transfusion of CMV-seronegative or deglycerolized blood products should be used include seronegative premature infants and pregnant women, and seronegative transplant recipients receiving organs (*i.e.,* kidney, heart, bone marrow) from seronegative donors.[3] This form of transfusion should also be considered in seronegative immunocompromised oncology patients.[3]

Treatment

Cytomegalovirus infection in the immunocompetent host is usually self-limited. In immunocompromised patients the disease can be life threatening. Ganciclovir, an acyclovir analog, has good *in vitro* activity against CMV, but is associated with significant bone marrow suppression and leukopenia. Clinical trails have shown ganciclovir to be efficacious in immunocompromised solid organ transplant recipients with serious CMV infection.[31] However, clinical improvement frequently necessitates removal of immunosuppressive agents, which may risk the organ transplant.

EPSTEIN–BARR VIRUS

Epstein–Barr virus (EBV) is a member of the herpesvirus group. Transfusion-associated EBV infection is rare; only a few cases have been reported.[32,82,91] It is estimated that 75% of posttransfusion EBV infections produce no symptoms.[32,37] The incubation period of the virus is approximately 3 to 7 weeks, but an incubation period of 2 days has been reported in one patient.[82] The clinical presentation is similar to that of CMV infection. The mono spot test detecting heterophile antibodies is usually positive. More sensitive serologic tests include antibodies to viral capsid antigen (VCA) and early antigen (EA), which appear at the time of clinical presentation. Antibodies to nuclear antigen (EBNA) appear 3 to 4 weeks after clinical presentation.

Because most of the adult population has protective antibodies, there is no need for screening of donor blood.

REFERENCES

1. Aach RD, Kahn RA. Post transfusion hepatitis: current perspectives. Ann Intern Med 1980;92:539.
2. Aach RD, Szmuness W, Mosely JW, et al. Serum alanine aminotransferase of donors in relation to the risk of non-A, non-B hepatitis and recipients. The Transfusion-Transmitted Viruses Study. N Engl J Med 1981;304:989.

3. Adler SP. Transfusion-associated cytomegalovirus infections. Rev Infect Dis 1983;5:977.
4. Adler SP, Chandrika T, Lawrence L, et al. Cytomegalovirus infections in neonates acquired by blood transfusions. Pediatr Infect Dis 1983;2:114.
5. Alfred CA, Britt WJ. Cytomegalovirus. In Fields BN (ed). Virology. New York: Raven Press, 1985;629.
6. Alter HJ, Holland PV, Purcell RH. The emerging pattern of post-transfusion hepatitis. Am J Med Sci 1976;270:329.
7. Alter HJ, Purcell RH, Holland PD, et al. Clinical and serological analysis of transfusion-associated hepatitis. Lancet 1975;2:838.
8. Alter HJ, Purcell RH, Shih JW, et al. Detection of antibody to hepatitis C virus in prospectively followed transfusion recipients with acute and chronic non-A, non-B hepatitis. N Engl J Med 1989;321:1494.
9. American Association of Blood Banks. Standards for Blood Banks and Transfusion Services. 12th ed. Arlington, VA, 1987.
10. Back E, Hoglund C, Malmlund HO. Cytomegalovirus infection associated with severe hepatitis. Scand J Infect Dis 1977;9:141.
11. Beesley RP, Lin CC, Hwang LY, et al. Hepatocellular carcinoma and hepatitis B virus: a prospective study of 23,707 men in Taiwan. Lancet 1981;2:1129.
12. Berlin BS, Chandler R, Greene D. Anti-"i" antibody and hemolytic anemia associated with spontaneous cytomegalovirus mononucleosis. Am J Clin Pathol 1977;67:459.
13. Berman M, Alter HJ, Ishak KG, et al. Clinical sequelae of non-A, non-B hepatitis. Ann Intern Med 1979;91:1.
14. Bowden RA, Sayers M, Flournoy M, et al. Cytomegalovirus immune globulin in seronegative blood products to prevent primary cytomegalovirus infection after marrow transplantation. N Engl J Med 1986;314:1006.
15. Brady ET, Milam JD, Anderson DC, et al. Use of deglycerolized red blood cells to prevent posttransfusion infection with cytomegalovirus in neonates. J Infect Dis 1984;150:334.
16. Browning JD, More I, Boyd JF. Adult pulmonary cytomegalic inclusion disease: report of a case. J Clin Pathol 1980;33:11.
17. Buti M, Esteban R, Jardi R, et al. Serological diagnosis of acute delta hepatitis. J Med Virol 1986;18:81.
18. Causey JQ. Spontaneous cytomegalovirus in mononucleosis-like syndrome and aseptic meningitis. South Med J 1976;69:1384.
19. Centers for Disease Control Statistics. Aids 1989;3:733.
20. Cheung KS, Lang DJ. Transmission and activation of cytomegalovirus with blood transfusion: a mouse model. J Infect Dis 1977;135:841.
21. Choo Q-L, Kuo G, Weinger AJ, et al. Isolation of a cDNA clone derived from a blood-borne non-A, non-B viral hepatitis genome. Science 1989;244:359.
22. Chow S, Merrigan TC. Rapid detection and quantitation of human cytomegalovirus in urine through DNA hybridization. N Engl J Med 1983;308:921.
23. Clark JA, Hollinger FB, Lewis E, et al. Intradermal inoculation with Heptavax-B: immune response and histologic evaluation of injection sites. JAMA 1989;262:2567.
24. Cohen ND, Muñoz A, Reitz BA, et al. Transmission of retroviruses by transfusion of screened blood in patients undergoing cardiac surgery. N Engl J Med 1989;320:1172.
25. Conrad ME. Diseases transmissible by blood transfusion: viral hepatitis and other infectious disorders. Semin Hematol 1981;18:122.
26. Cumming PD, Wallace EL, Schorr JB, Dodd RY. Exposure of transfused patients to human immunodeficiency virus through the transfusion of blood components that test antibody-negative. N Engl J Med 1989;321:941.
27. Cooper DA, Gold J, MacLean P, et al. Acute AIDS retrovirus infection: definition of a clinical illness associated with seroconversion. Lancet 1985;1:537.
28. Davis GL, Balart LA, Schiff EF, et al. Treatment of chronic hepatitis C with recombinant interferon alfa: a multicenter randomized, controlled trial. N Engl J Med 1989;321:1501.
29. DiBisceglie AM, Martin P, Kassianides C, et al. Recombinant interferon alfa therapy for chronic hepatitis C: a randomized, double-blind, placebo-controlled trial. N Engl J Med 1989;321:1506.
30. Eisenstein BI. The polymerse chain reaction: a new method of using molecular genetics for medical diagnosis. N Engl J Med 1990;322:178.
31. Erice A, Jordan C, Chace BA, et al. Ganciclovir treatment of cytomegalovirus disease in transplant recipients and other immunocompromised hosts. JAMA 1987;257:3082.
32. Gerber P, Walsh JH, Rosenblum EN, et al. Association of EB-virus infection with the post-perfusion syndrome. Lancet 1969;1:593.
33. Goodman RA. Nosocomial hepatitis A (editorial). Ann Intern Med 1985;103:452.

34. Grant IH, Gold JWM, Wittner M, et al. Transfusion-associated acute Chagas disease acquired in the United States. Ann Intern Med 1989;111:849.
35. Gregory PB, Knauer CM, Kempson RL, et al. Steroid therapy in severe viral hepatitis: a double-blind, randomized trial of methyl-prednisilone vs. placebo. N Engl J Med 1976;294:681.
36. Guidelines for prevention of transmission of human immunodeficiency virus and hepatitis B virus to health-care and public safety workers. MMWR 1989;38:5.
37. Henle W, Lenle G, Scriba M, et al. Antibody responses to the Epstein-Barr virus and cytomegalovirus after open-heart and other surgery. N Engl J Med 1970;282:1068.
38. Hepatitis-B vaccine: evidence confirming lack of AIDS transmission. MMWR 1984;33:685.
39. Hersman J, Meyers JD, Thomas ED, et al. The effect of granulocyte transfusions on the incidence of cytomegalovirus infection after allogeneic marrow transplantation. Ann Intern Med 1982;96:149.
40. Ho M. Epidemiology of cytomegalovirus infection in man. In Greenough WP, Merigan TC (eds). Cytomegalovirus, virology and infection: current topics in infectious disease. New York: Plenum, 1982:47.
41. Ho M. Human cytomegalovirus infections in immunosuppressed patients. In Greenough WP, Merigan TC (eds). Cytomegalovirus, virology and infection: current topics in infectious diseases. New York: Plenum, 1982:171.
42. Ho DD, Sarngadharan MG, Resnick L, et al. Primary human T-lymphocytic virus infection. Ann Intern Med 1985;103:880.
43. Hollinger FB, Melnick JL. Viral hepatitis: epidemiology. In Fields BN (ed). Virology. New York: Raven Press, 1985:1145.
44. Hollinger FB. Factors influencing the immune response to hepatitis B vaccine, booster dose guidelines, and vaccine protocol recommendations. Am J Med 1989;87(suppl 3A):36S.
45. Huang ES, Alford CA, Reynolds TW, et al. Molecular epidemiology of cytomegalovirus infection in women and their infants. N Engl J Med 1980;303:958.
46. Imagawa DT, Lee MH, Wolinsky SM, et al. Human immunodeficiency virus type 1 infection in homosexual men who remain seronegative for prolonged periods. N Engl J Med 1989;320:1458.
47. Johnson BE, Reed JS. Prolongation of the prodrome to acute hepatitis B infection by corticosteroids. Arch Intern Med 1983;143:1810.
48. Kivitz SR, Valeri DA, Melaragno AJ, et al. Leukocyte-poor red blood cells prepared by the addition and removal of glycerol from red blood cell concentrates stored at 4°C. Transfusion 1981;21:435.
49. Klosner PC, Mangia AJ, Leonard J, et al. HIV-2-associated AIDS in the United States: the first case. Arch Intern Med 1989;149:1875.
50. Knodell RG, Conrad ME, Ginsberg Al, et al. Efficacy of prophylactic gamma globulin in preventing non-A, non-B posttransfusion hepatitis. Lancet 1976;1:557.
51. Krech U. Complement-fixing antibodies against cytomegalovirus in different parts of the world. Bull WHO 1973;49:103.
52. Krugman S, Giles JP, Hammond J. Infectious hepatitis: evidence for two distinctive clinical, epidemiological and immunological types of infection. JAMA 1967;200:365.
53. Krugman S, Ward R, Giles JP. The natural history of infectious hepatitis. Am J Med 1962;32:717.
54. Kuo G, Choo Q-L, Alter HJ, et al. An assay for circulating antibodies to a major etiologic virus of human non-A, non-B hepatitis. Science 1989;244:362.
55. Lee FK, Nahmias HA, Stagno S. Rapid diagnosis of cytomegalovirus infection in infants by electron microscopy. N Engl J Med 1987;299:1266.
56. Litwins J, Leibowitz S. Abnormal lymphocytes and virus diseases other than infectious mononucleosis. Acta Haematol 1951;5:223.
57. Marker SC, Howard RJ, Simmons RL, et al. Cytomegalovirus infection: a quantitative perspective study of 320 consequent renal transplants. Surgery 1981;89:660.
58. Meryman HT, Hornblower M. The preparation of red cells depleted of leukocytes: review and evaluation. Transfusion 1986;26:101.
59. Meyers JD, Flowinoy N, Wade JC, et al. Biology of interstitial pneumonia after marrow transplantation. In Gale RP (ed). Recent advances in bone marrow transplantation. New York: Alan R. Liss, 1983;405.
60. Murray HW. CMV retinitis. Br Med J 1976;2:1071.
61. Needlestick transmission of HTLV-III from a patient infected in Africa [editorial]. Lancet 1984;2:1376.
62. Nickerson P, Orr P, Schroeder M-L, et al. Transfusion-associated *Trypanosoma cruzi* infection in a non-endemic area. Ann Intern Med 1989;111:851.
63. Noble RC, Kane MA, Reeves SA, et al. Post infusion hepatitis A in a neonatal intensive care unit. JAMA 1984;252:2711.

64. Osterholm MT, Bowman RJ, Chopek MW, et al. Screening donated blood and plasma for HTLV-III antibodies: facing more than one crisis? [editorial] N Engl J Med 1985;312:1185.

65. Peterman TA, Jaffe HW, Feorino PM, et al. Transfusion-associated acquired immunodeficiency syndrome in the United States. JAMA 1985;254:2913.

66. Peterman TA, Lui KJ, Lawrence DN, Allen JR. Estimating the risks of transfusion-associated acquired immune deficiency syndrome and human immunodeficiency virus infection. Transfusion 1987;27:371.

67. Possible transfusions-associated acquired immune deficiency syndrome—California. MMWR 1982;31:652.

68. Provisional public health service agency recommendations for screening donated blood and plasma for antibody to the virus causing acquired immunodeficiency syndrome. MMWR 1985;34:1.

69. Recommendations for protection against viral hepatitis. MMWR 1985;34:313.

70. Redecker AJ, Mosely JW, Gocke DJ, et al. Hepatitis B immune globulin as a prophylactic measure for spouses exposed to acute type B hepatitis. N Engl J Med 1975;293:1055.

71. Redecker AB, Schweitzer IL, Yamahiro HA, et al. Randomization of corticosteroid therapy in fulminant hepatitis. N Engl J Med 1976;294:728.

72. Rizzetto M. The delta agent. Hepatology 1983;3:729.

73. Robert-Guroff M, Weiss SH, Giron JA, et al. Prevalence of antibodies to HTLV-I–II and -III in intravenous drug abusers from an AIDS endemic region. JAMA 1986;255:3133.

74. Rosina F, Saracco G, Rizzetto M. Risk of post-transfusion infection with the hepatitis delta virus: a multicenter study. N Engl J Med 1985;312:1488.

75. Safety of therapeutic immune globulin preparations with respect to transmission of human T lymphotrophic virus type III/lymphadenopathy-associated virus infection. MMWR 1987;35:231.

76. Schmitz H, Enders G. Cytomegalovirus as a frequent cause of Guillain–Barré syndrome. Gen Med Virol 1977;1:21.

77. Seeberg S, Brandberg A, Svante H, et al. Hospital outbreak of hepatitis A secondary to blood exchange in a baby. Lancet 1981;1:1115.

78. Seeff LB, Wright EC, Zimmerman HJ, et al. Type B hepatitis after needlestick exposure: prevention with hepatitis B immune globulin. A final report of the Veterans Administration Cooperative Study. Ann Intern Med 1978;88:285.

79. Seeff LB, Wright EC, Zimmerman HJ, et al. VA cooperative study of post transfusion hepatitis; 1969–1974: incidence and characteristics of hepatitis and responsible risk factors. Am J Med Sci 1975;270:355.

80. Seeff LB, Zimmerman HJ, Wright EC, et al. Randomized double-blind controlled trial of the efficacy of immune globulin for the prevention of post transfusion hepatitis. Gastroenterology 1977;72:111.

81. Sheretz RJ, Russell BA, Reuman PD. Transmission of hepatitis A by transfusion of blood products. Arch Intern Med 1984;144:1599.

82. Solem JH, Jorganson W. Accidentally transmitted infectious mononucleosis. Acta Med Scand 1969;186:433.

83. Stevens CE, Aach RD, Hollinger FB, et al. Hepatitis B virus antibody and blood donors and the occurrence of non-A, non-B hepatitis and transfusion recipients: an analysis of the Transfusion-Transmitted Viruses Study. Ann Intern Med 1984;101:733.

84. Sumpliner RE, Hamilton FA, Iseri OA, et al. The liver histology and frequency of clearance of the hepatitis B surface antigen (HBsAg) in chronic carriers. Am J Med 1979;277:17.

85. Tabor E. The three viruses of non-A, non-B hepatitis. Lancet 1985;1:743.

86. Tabor E, Hoofnagle JH, Smallwood LA, et al. Studies of donors who transmit post transfusion hepatitis. Transfusion 1979;19:725.

87. Tajima K, Kamura S, Ito S, et al. Epidemologic features of HTLV-I carriers and incidence of ATL in and ATL-endemic island: a report of the community-based cooperative study in Tsushima, Japan. Int J Cancer 1987;40:741.

88. Takahashi K, Alkahane Y, Gotanda T, et al. Demonstration of hepatitis e antigen in the core of Dane particles. J Immunol 1979;122:275.

89. Tam KC, Tai CL, Trepo C, et al. Deleterious effect of prednisolone and HBeAg-positive chronic active hepatitis. N Engl J Med 1981;304:380.

90. Tolkoff-Rubin NE, Rubin RH, Kelleher EE, et al. Cytomegalovirus infections in dialysis patients and personnel. Ann Intern Med 1978;89:625.

91. Turner AR, McDonald RN, Cooper BA. Transmission of infectious mononucleosis via transfusion pre-illness plasma. Ann Intern Med 1972;77:751.

92. Ward JW, Bush TJ, Perkins HA, et al. The natural history of transfusion-associated infection with human immunodeficiency virus: factors influencing the rate of progression to disease. N Engl J Med 1989;321:947.
93. Weiss SH, Goedert JJ, Sarngadharnan MD, et al. Screening test for HTLV-III (AIDS agent) antibodies: specificity, sensitivity and applications. JAMA 1985;253:221.
94. Williams AE, Fang Chyang CT, Slamon DJ, et al. Seroprevalence and epidemological correlates of HTLV-I infection in U.S. blood donors. Science 1988;240:643.
95. Winston DJ, Ho WG, Howell CL, et al. Cytomegalovirus infections associated with leukocyte transfusions. Ann Intern Med 1980;93:671.
96. Yeager AS, Grumet FC, Hafleigh EB, et al. Prevention of transfusion-acquired cytomegalovirus infections in newborn infants. J Pediatr 1981;98:281.

5

○   ○   ○   ●   ●   ●

ABDOMINAL ABSCESSES

Clifford M. Herman
C. James Carrico

It is easy to gain the erroneous impression that the results of treating abdominal abscesses are improving, especially when compared with three or more decades ago. However, there are few convincing data to support this optimistic view. In fact, the reported experience suggests a more sobering reality. From the 1938 review of 3608 instances of abdominal sepsis by Ochsner and DeBakey[57] to more recent reports,[20,63] the overall mortality remains at 25% to 40%. There is, of course, a variation that depends on several features of the patient populations described. For example, there is 8% mortality in patients younger than 20 years of age with an abdominal abscess, compared with a 41% mortality rate for patients older than 40 years of age.[20]

The impact of computed tomography (CT) and ultrasonography (US) on facilitating earlier diagnosis and treatment has not yet become clear. It is also unclear whether the growing array of antibiotics has shortened the course or altered the outcome to a significant degree.

Abscesses in the abdomen continue to be a serious challenge to the surgeon and a major source of prolonged suffering and death to the patient. They remain difficult to control and eliminate, and especially those associated with the pancreas and bowel still tax the resources of everyone who cares for them.

Compounding the difficulties is the effect of abdominal infection on organs not directly involved in the infectious process. The growing attention to this problem, now commonly known as multiple organ failure, attests to its importance. This importance can be seen in the potential for a fatal outcome. One recent prospective study[62] of surgical patients with abdominal sepsis found a 3% mortality with no failed major organ (heart, lungs, kidney, or central nervous system [CNS] coma unrelated to head trauma). Mortality climbed to 10% with one failed major organ, 50% with two, and a 100% in patients with failure of three major organs. These data agree closely with other reports in the literature.[21,26,27]

Part of the lethal implication of remote organ failure associated with abdominal sepsis is the fact that a failing organ system will almost always remain refractory to treatment until the septic source is eliminated. For example, acute renal failure was one of the first described in septic patients.[25] While the nephrotoxic antibiotics commonly given to septic patients are partly responsible, sepsis itself remains the leading cause of acute renal failure. The responsible mechanisms are not well understood, and even the use of dialysis is usually ineffective in altering the patient's overall course. The development of renal failure with intra-abdominal infection is a grave prognostic sign, carrying a mortality of 80%.

A similar relationship has been described for the adult respiratory distress syndrome (ARDS). Abdominal sepsis is the leading cause of this problem, occurring as the underlying etiologic factor in 26 of 44 patients in one study.[28] The death rate for septic patients with ARDS remains as high as 77% to 90% in reported series.[1,61]

The consequences of hepatic failure in patients with intra-abdominal sepsis that does not directly involve the liver or biliary tract are also severe. Mortality from hepatic failure in these patients is about 50%.[32]

The frequent association of multiple organ failure with intra-abdominal sepsis, and the attendant high mortality in these patients, have led to the recommendation to reexplore all patients who develop organ system failure after abdominal operations.[65] Carrying out such exploration in a timely fashion also seems to be important. A recent study of laparotomy performed for potential or presumed intra-abdominal sepsis[74] found the best accuracy (89%) and survival (51%) rates when exploration was done before the onset of septic shock or bacteremia. Once these two grave problems had developed, there was 90% mortality, regardless of the findings at exploration. It was suggested that the early use of sensitive detection techniques that permit directed laparotomy before septic deterioration should improve survival. Another report[60] of experience with patients with peritonitis found a 29% mortality when planned re-laparotomy was performed within 2 or 3 days after the initial operation. This contrasted with a 73% mortality in a group whose reexploration was carried out only after clear clinical signs of further deterioration occurred, usually about 6 days later.

With this background in mind, this chapter will concentrate on the detection and management of abdominal abscesses. The general plan will be to review the clinical settings and early signs that make an abdominal abscess likely. We will then present a reasonable diagnostic approach. We will end with a scheme for guiding the appropriate selection of percutaneous or open surgical drainage for the individual patient.

The selection and use of antibiotics are important aspects of the treatment of intra-abdominal abscesses and will be discussed in detail in other sections of this book. The pathophysiology is thoroughly reviewed elsewhere[3,34] and will not be discussed here.

THE CLINICAL SETTING

One might think that in this age of new and increasingly more sensitive radiographic technologies there is no longer any need for the history and physical exam. It might seem that one should be able simply to order a battery of studies from the radiology and nuclear medicine departments for a suspect patient; the reports then could detect the specific location of an abscess and determine the underlying course.

In fact, while these special diagnostic procedures are certainly useful, they cannot substitute for astute clinical judgment. They are most likely to pinpoint a diagnosis when guided by the total clinical picture, and they tend to show the most unequivocal diagnosis only when the condition is very far advanced. Therefore, the workup of a patient suspected of abdominal sepsis should begin with consideration of the clinical setting. In particular, a careful and detailed review of the preceding events can help significantly in establishing the initial differential diagnostic list to be considered.

The underlying causes and the resulting location of intra-abdominal abscesses have changed over the last 40 years. This is most likely due to the impact of more effective antibiotics, better supportive care, earlier diagnosis, and improved operative approaches.[70] Early studies[4,57] found that most of these abscesses developed from spontaneous disease processes such as perforated appendicitis, colonic diverticulitis, or perforated gastroduodenal ulcers. Today, the most common etiology is a prior abdominal operation.[2] Spontaneous or traumatic perforation of the gastrointestinal tract is now less often responsible.

This changing etiology and location can be seen clearly with respect to subphrenic abscesses. Prior to the 1950s, abscesses in the spaces immediately below the diaphragm (including the subhepatic area) most frequently developed from a spontaneous intra-abdominal infectious process.[70] More recently, septic complications of abdominal operations cause 90% of all subphrenic and subhepatic abscesses.[13,58] A detailed analysis[18] of one series found that the overwhelming majority developed after gastric (44%) or biliary tract (21%) operations.

THE SIGNS OF AN
INTRA-ABDOMINAL ABSCESS

The clinical picture of a patient with an abdominal abscess depends on the stage in its development. It also depends on its location within the abdomen. Both the stage and location will become increasingly apparent as the infection progresses over time. The early, subtle systemic signs, often with no direct evidence pointing to an abdominal problem, gradually evolve into the full-blown derangements of septic shock. This clinical course is described in more detail elsewhere in the book, but it is worth brief emphasis here because of the importance of finding and eliminating the abscess in its early stage, and the dismal consequences of delayed diagnosis.

The proper approach to a patient suspected of developing abdominal sepsis is first to confirm the suspicion of infection, as suggested by the indirect signs mentioned below. The location then must be sought, keeping in mind that the demonstration of infection in such common sites as the respiratory or urinary tracts does not obviate the need to investigate the abdomen as well. Once having established the presence of an abdominal abscess, the challenge becomes deciding the best means for draining it. This decision must take into consideration all of the relevant factors present in each individual patient. It requires firm knowledge of the reported experience, tempered and enhanced by experienced surgical judgment.

Early Indirect Systemic Signs
Fever and leukocytosis
Mental confusion (or decreased alertness), especially in ICU patients
Mild respiratory alkalosis
Decreased platelet count
Positive bacterial cultures from blood or other sites

These signs may progress to hemodynamic instability requiring massive intravenous volume support, inadequate oxygen extraction with metabolic acidosis, and the gradual development of organ system failure.

Indirect Abdominal Signs
New development of abdominal distention
Ileus in patient with previous bowel function
Increasing nasogastric (NG) tube output
Pleural effusion
Rising serum amylase
Rising serum bilirubin

LOCATING AN INTRA-ABDOMINAL ABSCESS

The most effective approach to the patient with a suspected abdominal abscess is the same as that for any problem. One should proceed in a logical fashion from the information that is quickest to obtain to the later use of complex invasive technology.

HISTORY

The proper sequence begins with a complete history. This should include the points emphasized above under "Early Indirect Systemic Signs" and "Indirect Abdominal Signs." It has been said that after a week, all patients in a surgical intensive care unit look alike. There is a tendency to pay less attention to the original incident and clinical course that led up to it because the ravages of sepsis are a greater leveler. It seems to make less and less difference whether the patient started with a gunshot wound of the duodenum or a ruptured abdominal aortic aneurysm.

However, it is important to avoid this pitfall. A history of the preceding abdominal operation or injury, in a patient with the developing systemic signs and indirect abdominal signs of an abscess, provides a significant aid in defining the next steps.

PHYSICAL EXAMINATION

While the classic signs of a tender mass with erythema of the overlying skin are often absent, the evidence of infection must be sought. Purulent drainage from an incision should be investigated for an underlying abscess. The wound must be examined closely for any signs of pus exuding between fascial sutures. Demonstration of this problem requires surgical exploration to open all intra-abdominal sources of the infection, to investigate the possibility of communication with the bowel, and to establish adequate drainage.

Because abdominal abscesses can be so elusive, one must use every means available to detect them. This includes thorough digital exploration through any enterostomies that may be present, using bimanual palpation where possible to examine for an abscess, which may be etiologically related to the stoma. An abscess between loops of bowel or mesentery is less likely to be apparent on physical exam. However, an abscess in this location is quite likely to cause localized effects to adjoining viscera. This should be pursued by use of the radiographic imaging techniques.

Abscesses in the upper or lower extremes of the abdomen commonly present minimal or no physical signs. For example, an abscess deep in the pelvis may be clinically "silent" or may produce only such nonspecific signs as diarrhea, which, in turn, can be overlooked or misinterpreted in a seriously sick patient on antibiotics and parenteral nutrition.

The digital rectal exam offers an important diagnostic potential that is too often overlooked. This should be performed every day on a patient with any reason to suspect abdominal sepsis. It is more than the cursory insertion of a finger. The goal is to reach as high into the rectum as possible. This is facilitated greatly by positioning the patient supine and flexing the hips to the fullest extent possible. This spreads the buttocks and allows insertion of the maximum length of examining finger. An early pelvic abscess may show only a slight induration of the anterior rectal wall, which is usually tender in a cooperative patient. As it progresses, a mass will develop. In its most advanced state, a fluctuant center will be palpable. This picture is not often seen in this era of wide use of potent antibiotics, but it must be kept in mind, because this close adherence to the rectum allows effective transrectal drainage.

THE USE OF CONVENTIONAL RADIOGRAPHY

After considering the clinical setting, the history, and the physical exam findings, it is important to continue logically in the workup of the patient. The next step should be a review of the x-rays such patients usually accumulate. These should include upright or at least lateral decubitus views to demonstrate extraluminal air/fluid levels. Soft tissue densities, segmental ileus, or intestinal displacement and distortion on these roentgenograms are useful indirect signs of localized infection. A chest film, upright if possible, adds considerably to the diagnosis of subphrenic infection by showing pleural effusion, basilar atelectasis, or elevation or obliteration of the diaphragm.

It should be obvious that the maximum value of these studies will come from careful personal review of serial x-rays side-by-side with the radiologist. Addition of the surgeon's chronologic clinical history is a valuable guide to interpretation of the films. One is more likely to find such subtle signs as a developing or persistent air/fluid density that appears to be outside the intestine only when compared with serial films in the context of the history. This can be especially important for the upper abdomen and subphrenic areas, where an abscess is often silent and highly lethal. Like all diagnostic tests, a normal result does not rule out a problem, but an abnormal finding is a valuable guide for further study.

At any point in this progressive workup, the clear demonstration of an abscess should signal the end of the search. Further diagnostic tests are redundant. They should not be allowed to delay treatment. Only if percutaneous drainage is being considered should one proceed to the use of ultrasound (US) or computed tomography (CT), only as needed to guide the procedure. If surgery is indicated, that should be the next step.

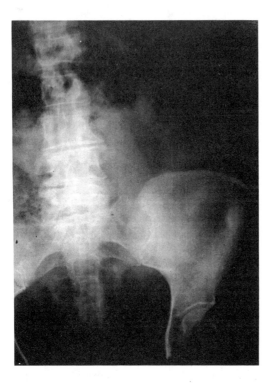

Figure 5–1.
Diffuse extraluminal gas on a plain film of an elderly woman.

This is emphasized by considering one recent case. An 87-year-old woman was admitted from a nursing home after having been found obtunded and hypotensive. She had a fever and an apparently tender abdomen. The plain film seen in Fig. 5-1 showed diffuse extraluminal gas, which could have come only from a GI tract perforation. After a brief period of cardiovascular resuscitation, she should have been taken directly to the operating room, where the problem could have been quickly found and treated. No further diagnostic workup was needed. Instead, the CT scan in Fig. 5-2 was obtained, which only confirmed the diagnosis and unneccessarily delayed her treatment.

This study was totally inappropriate, but it is worth relating the case because it illustrates a principle that should be self-evident but sometimes isn't. Before any test is ordered, it should be clearly understood just how the results will influence the patient's management. If the results will not make any difference, then the test should not be done. To do it under those circumstances is a sign of imprecise thinking and can only confuse the situation.

If the plain films suggest but do not confirm an abscess, the next consideration should be dye-contrast x-rays directed at the area in question. Appropriate contrast material in the GI tract can help distinguish intraluminal gas from an extraluminal abscess. It can also show leaks or distortion from an inflammatory mass. Advantage should also be taken of drainage tubes, fistulas, or stomas for contrast injection for the same purpose.

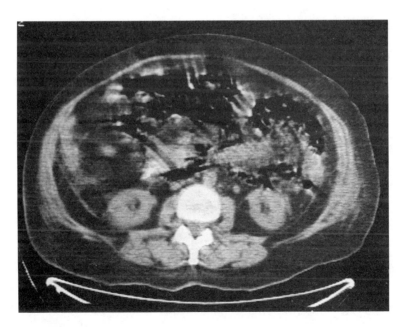

Figure 5–2.
CT scan of the same patient as in Fig. 5-1, showing the extraluminal gas.

THE USE OF SPECIAL
IMAGING TECHNIQUES

Before discussing the increasingly widespread and varying experience with the special imaging methods available for demonstrating abdominal abscesses, it is important to review the objective characteristics of each. This is necessary to avoid unrealistic expectations and excessively subjective interpretations of results.

Clinicians often find themselves looking at complex images on a film viewbox or a small photographic print and having to rely on a specialist to translate the image into a diagnosis relevant to the patient in question. This is not, however, analogous to the physician's confident use of a biochemical laboratory data (*e.g.,* blood gas, or serum saline) produced by methods he doesn't understand. For such laboratory test results, the confidence limits of a single number are well defined within a normal distribution.

Most radiographic and radionuclide scans are pictorial displays of anatomy constructed by a computer. They may contain an entire spectrum of tissue radiodensity, US responses, or emission of radioactivity. These are displayed in a black and white format that contains all shades of grey. They may also incorporate normal intrinsic variations of human anatomy. The interpretation, therefore, requires a high degree of knowledge and extensive experience.

The pictures produced by newer imaging methods resemble the internal anatomy of the abdomen well enough to become believable. Because surgeons tend to be quite oriented toward visual and tactile input, it is easy to be persuaded that one is actually looking at a living situation and not a computer-generated representation acquired by indirect techniques.

The interpretation of these images may also be quite subjective. Therefore, it is important that one must never rely on a report of a scan, whether written, by telephone, or through another intermediary. What may be reported indirectly as a pancreatic duct leak, for example, may be finally labeled as a hematoma when the clinical history is incorporated into the reading. It is imperative that the surgeon who will use the results view the images side-by-side with the specialist and review the rest of the clinical story with him so that the interpretation becomes a composite of the clinical and radiographic experts.

Computed Tomography

The pertinent biophysics of CT are discussed clearly in several excellent reviews.[12,38,81] This technique uses the same radiation source as plain roentograms or fluoroscopy, but the results differ because of several significant factors. The beam is confined for each individual image to a thin transverse "slice" of the body. These images are more readily comprehended than conventional x-ray images, because confusion caused by superimposed structures is eliminated. The tight collimation of the beam markedly decreases the registration of scattered x-rays, thus improving the contrast of the image. The definition is greatly enhanced by computer analysis of the graded differences between tissues in their interference with passage of the rays. It can display tissue attenuation differences as small as 0.5%, sufficient to discriminate between white and gray matter in the brain.

The diagnostic limits of CT are clearly defined. At radiation doses that are practical, spatial distinctions cannot be improved beyond about 0.5 mm. Because all x-ray techniques visualize electron densities of tissues, they delineate organ boundaries (where contrasts are great) more clearly than they detect abnormalities within an organ.

One of the greatest limitations of CT is its inability to differentiate among various types of fluid. One elegant study[12] of fluid from cysts, abscesses, and ascites examined these fluids *in vivo* and then *in vitro* after removal from the patients. Small differences in attenuation were found on the *in vitro* samples, but these could not be duplicated on the *in vivo* scans of the patients from whom the sample fluids were obtained.

In a related study,[22] various concentrations of blood, blood products, and solutions of albumin and chondroitin sulfate were analyzed by CT and by US (in a phantom with characteristics of liver). On the CT scans, fluids with CT numbers close to those of their surroundings were poorly detected. There was variation from one fluid to the others in the change in radiodensity in relation to change in concentration. This emphasizes the clinical reality that a fluid collection seen on CT scan is still an unknown in important ways that affect diagnosis. The fluid can be blood, ascites, bile, urine, pus, or a normal postoperative collection of sterile peritoneal transudate. There are still no good data to describe what constitutes a normal CT for a postoperative abdomen at various times after surgery. A decision to operate on a fluid collection remains a clinical one based on all signs and symptoms.

Advantages of CT

The greatest advantage of CT is its high resolution. Based on the physical characteristics of this methodology pointed out briefly above, it can detect fine detail and small differences between tissues and display these details reproducibly on the screen and in photographic prints. This reproducibility is a feature of the computer storage of each bit, or pixel, of information from which the image is constructed. It can distinguish reliably between solid and cystic structures and can differentiate solid organs or lesions that have only slightly differing radiodensities.

Its elimination of anatomical distractions, due to the thinness of each slice, enhances and refines its precision. Furthermore, the bowel gas that so often limits the ability to see clearly the structural details one seeks with US is not a problem with CT. With CT, gas constitutes just one of the differential radiodensities that enhance its effectiveness.

While the interpretation of a CT image requires considerable skill and experience, the generation of that image is quite well standardized. A well-trained technician will reliably be able to produce excellent images for the interpreter to evaluate.

Limitations of CT

Computed tomography takes place in a separate room with fixed equipment, so the patient must go to the machine. This can be a major problem for an unstable ICU patient, who will have to be moved and who will be difficult to monitor and treat in the radiology facility. For the critically ill septic patient, this may be one of the most important obstacles to its use. One must balance the risk of the trip to the scanner against the potential benefits to be gained.

Good resolution in a CT scan requires the patient to lie as still as possible during the exposures; slight motion will introduce a small loss of resolution that may or may not be important for a particular patient. Just as the decision to make the trip to the scanner is a balancing of risks and benefits, this is a judgment based on the whole clinical picture. If the information is expected to be valuable enough, an intubated patient who can't cooperate sufficiently can be paralyzed and his ventilation controlled for the few minutes necessary to get a CT scan.

The value of CT can also be limited by the presence of metallic surgical clips, which scatter the x-ray beams and obscure some important details. The newer scanners and techniques have lessened this but not eliminated this effort.

Another factor to be considered is the dose of ionizing radiation used to produce the CT images. Modern equipment limits this as much as possible, but the radiation exposure by CT is cumulative in entirely the same manner as is true for any x-ray imaging method. While the danger of repeated exposure is small, CT should be used only when it offers the best chance for making the diagnosis.

Cost is often mentioned as a limitation to the use of CT. However, especially when dealing with very sick patients, cost must be considered in relation to benefits. It is more meaningful to discuss cost within the clinical context of each specific case. For example, the intensive care required by many of the patients suspected of abdominal sepsis costs $2,000 to $3,000 per day. A $700 CT that hastens the diagnosis and treatment of an abdominal abscess by even 1 day, correspondingly shortening the ICU stay by that 1 day, is obviously an excellent investment. This is a common clinical situation. So, on financial grounds alone, an appropriately ordered abdominal CT should offer an unquestionable advantage. It should go without saying that an unnecessary CT, like any procedure not clinically indicated, is an unwarranted expense.

The benefits in human terms are more difficult to quantify, but it seems very likely that earlier detection and surgical treatment of abdominal sepsis will increase a patient's chance of survival. When used judiciously, CT will facilitate earlier diagnosis and drainage, lessening the mortality of this serious problem. On both human and financial grounds, the benefits of CT and any special tests that will help the patient are substantial. These benefits must not be denied solely on the basis of potential saving of money for the tests themselves without considering the larger potential for saving days of treatment and even life itself.

The beneficial and disadvantageous characteristics of CT, along with the clinical condition of the patient, must be considered in deciding on its use in locating an abdominal abscess. The practical choice for this purpose is usually between CT and US. A comparative tabulation of the relative strengths and weaknesses of these two techniques is set forth below.

Ultrasonography

The medical use of US is based on the reflection of high-frequency mechanical sound waves by successive tissue interfaces. The outlining of anatomical structures depends on the ability of the piezoelectric crystal (transducer) to detect and display differences in acoustic impedance by different body tissues and fluids. The detailed physical and clinical characteristics are reviewed in several publications.[5,22,23,37,40,47,68] It will be sufficient for our purposes here to comment on the clinically relevant features that should guide its use for patients suspected of abdominal infection.

Advantages of US

The greatest advantage of US is its ease of application relative to CT, especially in an unstable ICU patient. Several features make this so. First, the excellent capability of current equipment makes it feasible to obtain high quality studies at the patient's bedside. This offers real savings in time and effort for nursing personnel as well as the safety of keeping the patient in the more protected care environment. Secondly, the images are immediately visible on the display screen. The patient's physician can (and should) help guide the ultrasonographer's examination as it takes place; this kind of direct participation is not normally possible for CT.

A third advantage is the US display of motion as it occurs. This is often more important for such studies as echocardiography, but it can still be useful in looking for indirect signs of an abdominal abscess. Altered diaphragm movement seen on US can be a helpful clue to infection or fluid collections not otherwise visible in the region. A fourth advantage, shared with CT, is its ability to distinguish between solid and cystic structures and lesions.

A fifth advantage is the lower cost of US than of CT for examining the same body region. However, just as in the discussion above for CT, the cost of US must be viewed within the context of potential benefit in the complete clinical setting of each individual patient. A misleading US study can be worse than useless when compared to a more expensive CT scan that could have led to an earlier and more accurate diagnosis. These factors should clarify the reasons why cost cannot be the primary consideration when investigating a serious problem such as the possibility of undrained infection in the abdomen. The basis for choosing a strategy to use imaging techniques in the septic abdomen will be detailed later in the chapter.

A final advantage of US is its avoidance of ionizing radiation. The nonionizing radiation of US has no known biologic effects, allowing unlimited studies in a patient without concern about the risks from the cumulative effects of x-radiation.

Limitations of US

An important limitation of US is its heavy reliance on the skill and experience of the ultrasonographer. This is true both for executing the test and for interpreting the images. Intrinsic to this is the highly subjective nature of this technology.

Resolution of the final images obtained is an example of this subjectivity. The resolution along the axis of the acoustic beam is best at high frequencies and is about 0.5 mm for most equipment. Resolution perpendicular to this axis is not so easily defined. In fact, it is quite variable, depending on distance from the transducer and on the characteristics of each tissue and anatomical interface through which the direct and reflected beams pass in both directions. Therefore, the minimum size limits of any object or lesion that can be reliably detected are different for various types of tissue. This fact, plus the need for an intimate knowledge of the many normal and pathologic anatomical variations to be expected in any part of the body, constitute part of the "art" of this modality.

Along with operator dependence and variable resolution, another limitation is the interference of strong anatomical boundaries with the acoustic beam. These boundaries, such as those between tissue and bone or tissue and air, reflect most of the incident acoustic energy. This prevents acquisition of data from structures lying beyond them. The resulting poor penetration of bone, and its rapid attenuation in air, makes US relatively useless for conditions affecting the brain or lungs. It is also responsible for the interference by bowel gas that often limits the ability of US to detect an abdominal abscess. Similarly, interference by the air in the lung limits its utility for detecting fluid under the diaphragms.

Still another factor that can interfere with the use of US for the patient with suspected abdominal sepsis is the condition of the abdominal wall. Optimal use of US requires an expanse large enough to allow wide movement of the transducer over intact skin. The abdominal wall must also be pliable enough for repositioning and invaginating the transducer to obtain the best angle for aiming the acoustic beam at suspected areas. The presence of wounds, drains, fistulas, and stomas, so common in the patients to be studied, will limit severely the ability of the ultrasonographer to carry out an adequate exam.

Ultrasound vs Computed Tomography

As discussed above, the differences and similarities between these two techniques are not necessarily mutually exclusive. Each has its proper place, and the decision to use one or the other, or both, must be based on careful evaluation of each individual patient's clinical situation. Table 5-1 summarizes the main features to be considered.

Table 5–1
Features of Ultrasound Compared with Those of Computed Tomography

US	CT

Non-ionizing acoustic radiation
  No known biologic effects
	Ionizing radiation
	  Cumulative ill effects

Heavily operator-dependent	Less operator-dependent
Portable	Fixed facility
Allows study of motion	Fixed views
Limited by gas, bone, obesity, barium, motion	Limited by ileus, inanition, barium, metal, motion
Requires intact skin for transducer placement	Not limited by skin defects (wounds, drains, stomas)
Distinguishes solid tissue from fluid	Distinguishes solid tissue from fluid, as well as some solid organ abnormalities

A number of gamma-emitting radioisotopes have been attached to larger molecules in attempts to demonstrate abdominal abscesses. They all rely on the affinity of these materials for areas of inflammation, where their concentration would be detectable as a sign of localized infection. In general, however, the poor sensitivity and specificity, the length of time required to obtain results, and the expensive equipment and intensive technician time involved have decreased the enthusiasm for these techniques. The increasing availability and quality of CT and US have further diminished isotope use. Because of some continuing reported usage, and because of the value of special applications, a short review is included.

Liver–Spleen–Lung Scans

For indirect signs of a subphrenic abscess, or to differentiate one from a subpulmonic collection, a combined liver–spleen–lung scan can be useful. Technetium-labeled albumin (for the lung) and technetium-labeled sulphur colloid (for the liver and spleen) are injected intravenously. Scanning 1 to 4 hours later can show an abnormally widened separation of lung from liver or spleen. In the absence of pleural effusion, this finding suggests a subphrenic abscess. This technique has largely been replaced by US and CT for this purpose, but it can be useful for the occasional problem patient. It has similarly been displaced for locating intrahepatic or intrasplenic abscesses.

Gallium Scans

Scanning for uptake of [67]gallium citrate has been widely used to locate intra-abdominal infection. It depends on the isotope concentrating in an area of inflammation containing large numbers of acute inflammatory cells. Several studies illustrate the use of this technique, none in a controlled fashion that assigns a level of precision or accuracy in comparison with the other modalities evaluated. In two reports,[45,72] gallium scans detected abdominal infection with about the same accuracy as did CT or US. However, there was no attempt made to compare the two by any prospective study design. In fact, most of the patients had both studies done. The authors recommend gallium as a screening procedure to guide the subsequent use of CT, but the data do not clearly support the suggestion.

Another retrospective review[54] of the use of US, CT, and gallium scan for diagnosing abdominal abscess produced a little more concrete data. In 75 patients, they found the sensitivity of US to be 82%, gallium 96%, and CT 100%. The specificity was 91% for US, 65% for gallium, and 100% for CT. All diagnoses were confirmed by aspiration or surgical drainage. The perfect sensitivity and specificity of CT speaks for itself. While these features for gallium seem accurate in the report, the real role for this modality is still not clear. When one adds its shortcomings—concentrating in the liver and colon, requirement for serial scans over 48 to 72 hours, failure to distinguish an abscess from normal inflammatory tissue—it is difficult to make a case for its use in the sick patient with suspected abdominal sepsis.

Leukocyte Scans

A more recently developed technique uses another approach. A patient's own polymorphonuclear leukocytes are incubated with [111]indium and reinjected. The test depends on the radiolabeled neutrophil concentrating in an area of inflammation containing large numbers of acute inflammatory cells. Accumulation of the isotope is determined by scanning, with a localized concentration felt to indicate an abscess. In one report[14] of 68 scans done in 53 patients with clinically suspected abdominal abscesses, all of the 14 surgically proven abscesses were associated with abnormal leukocyte images. Thirty-nine studies demonstrated normal leukocyte distribution in the abdomen, and in none of these did clinical evidence of an abdominal abscess develop. Abnormal scans were noted in an additional 15 studies but did not suggest abscesses. In these, the abnormalities resulted from wound infection, colonic accumulation, or accessory spleens. This illustrates some of the pitfalls of this method, as well as its apparent ability to demonstrate an abscess when other causes for isotope accumulation are eliminated.

A special application of this WBC-labeling technique has been reported[8] in a small series. Eight patients were studied in an attempt to differentiate a pancreatic abscess from a pseudocyst. In all four with an abscess, the scan was positive and led to successful surgical drainage. In the four with pseudocysts, three of the scans were negative and one showed diffuse uptake suggestive of pancreatitis but none in the area of the cysts. This small experience suggests a potential use in differentiating fluid collections associated with the pancreas, where one needs to drain an abscess but might choose to wait for a more appropriate time to operate on a pseudocyst. Its exact reliability for this problem needs wider study.

While this leukocyte labeling technique is a little faster (24 versus 48 hours) and avoids the intestinal excretion of gallium, it is extremely expensive in terms of technician time. Even the reports cited seem to show only that it usually correlates with CT findings.

Biliary Tract Radioisotope Scans

Unlike the isotope scans intended to screen the entire abdomen for sepsis, with unproven success, techniques for imaging the biliary tract have earned a more definite place for specific clinical situations. When investigating the possibility of acute cholecystitis in a patient with right upper abdominal pain and signs of sepsis, the studies mentioned above have important limitations. US can demonstrate stones in the gallbladder and ducts very reliably, but it cannot indicate whether there is acute inflammation associated with them. The same is true of CT. Estimates of such factors as thickness of the gallbladder wall are unreliable indicators of acute infection. Both of these radiographic techniques leave unanswered the possibility that the cholelithiasis is an asymptomatic, incidental finding that is not responsible for the clinical picture of acute infection.

The radioisotope studies reviewed above are not practical for rapid diagnosis and have not been thoroughly evaluated for detection of acute cholecystitis. The increasing use of early cholecystectomy for acute cholecystitis increases the importance of early diagnosis. For this purpose, the use of various derivatives of technetium-99m-labeled iminodiacetic acid has proven helpful. A comparison of HIDA scan with US in 144 patients suspected of having acute cholecystitis[82] found 98% sensitivity and 79% specificity for both techniques. Nonvisualization of the gallbladder on HIDA scan and cholelithiasis on US were applied as diagnostic criteria. The remaining 21% had chronic cholecystitis.

Another study[49] compared diagnostic sensitivity and specificity of HIDA scan, US, and CT in 75 patients with right upper quadrant abdominal pain. The findings were subsequently confirmed operatively and histologically. Ninety-three percent of the 58 patients proven to have acute cholecystitis had positive isotope studies (nonvisualization of the gallbladder but prompt visualization of the common bile duct and duodenum). There were 6.9% false-negative and no false-positive isotope scans, giving an overall accuracy of 93% for this technique. This compared to 86.2% true-positive, 14% false-negative, and 0% false-positive rates for US in the same patients. The overall accuracy rate for US was calculated to be 86%.

In addition to the above estimates of accuracy, the isotope scans offer the advantage of safe use in acutely ill patients with elevated bilirubin and amylase levels, without inaccuracies from body habitus, intestinal gas, or pancreatitis.

One extensive review of biliary tract imaging[42] also discusses clearly the methods for using true-positive, true-negative, false-positive, and false-negative ratios for any test to determine specificity, sensitivity, and accuracy. These calculations are set forth here because of their general applicability to any complete set of data and their importance in analyzing the significance of reports of treatment modalities.

$$TP = \text{True positive}$$
$$FP = \text{False positive}$$
$$TN = \text{True negative}$$
$$FN = \text{False negative}$$

$$\text{Sensitivity (true-positive ratio)} = \frac{TP}{TP + FN}$$

$$\text{Specificity (true-negative ratio)} = \frac{TN}{TN + FP}$$

$$\text{Repeatability (accuracy)} = \frac{TP + TN}{TP + FN + TN + FP}$$

The strict criteria for interpretation of the biliary isotope scans, regardless of which of the technetium-99m materials used (PIPIDA, HIDA, DISIDA, or Diethyl-IDA) are shown in Table 5-2.

Table 5–2
Criteria for Interpretation of Biliary Isotope Scans

Normal	Gallbladder fills in 30 min and isotope in the duodenum within 30 min
Hypofunctioning gallbladder	Gallbladder fills in over 30 min
Blocked gallbladder	Gallbladder not visualized in 2 h
Incomplete biliary obstruction	Isotope in duodenum within 60–180 min
Complete biliary obstruction	No isotope in duodenum in 24 h *and* duct size increased
Hepatocellular disease	Poor liver image *and* increased renal excretion

As with any of these imaging techniques, radiologists and nuclear medicine specialists will vary in their interpretation of a particular study as they gain increasing experience. However, the tabulated findings above are a strict set of criteria the clinician can use as a baseline to evaluate the findings for an individual patient.

Magnetic Resonance Imaging

This technique was formerly known as nuclear magnetic resonance, a reflection of its earlier use to obtain information about atomic and biologic organization in tissue samples studied *ex vivo*. Because of its increasing application for generating tomographic images of structures *in vivo* as they reside within the intact body, it has acquired the name magnetic resonance imaging (MRI). This perhaps reflects a more clinical orientation and a tacit acknowledgement of possible lay public concern about the term "nuclear" applied to human subjects. The characteristics of this technique are detailed elsewhere[38] so they will only be summarized briefly here. It depends on the fact that a magnetic force applied to a cell will cause magnetic alignment of the hydrogen nuclei, as well as of other nuclei with odd numbers of protons and neutrons, causing the particles to spin (the process was originally called nuclear spin resonance).

In its clinical application, the patient is inserted into a body-size chamber in a large magnet producing a powerful magnetic field. This causes the magnetic alignment of his cell nuclei. When the proper amount of energy and correct radio frequency are applied, the spins of these nuclei can change direction, absorbing energy in the process. This energy is subsequently re-emitted at a radio frequency that is unique for each type of cell. A computer then plots the distribution of the nuclei responsible for the emission, furnishing precise definition of the tissue and variations within the tissue, as from a tumor or ischemic area.

An understanding of the clinical usefulness of this modality is still evolving. Its limitations are also becoming better defined. Up to this time, it seems clear that ferromagnetic material contained in such devices as surgical clips, prostheses, and pacemakers are probably contraindications to its use. The need for rather prolonged imaging times, during which the patient must not move, also can limit its usefulness for many patients. At this point, it has not been thoroughly evaluated for ability to identify an intra-abdominal focus of infection, so its discussion is largely academic for that purpose.

Summary of the Imaging Techniques

For managing intra-abdominal sepsis, the major contribution of the newer imaging modalities described above has been to locate an abscess precisely enough to guide the choice of drainage approach. Increasingly, this has come to mean the facilitation of percutaneous catheter drainage wherever feasible. US and CT have emerged as the most clearly useful for guiding the placement of these catheters. In fact, this use has been largely responsible for the increasing skill and experience by interventional radiologists in helping with these difficult patient problems. The predominance of US and CT in this role is reflected in the following section.

CHOOSING THE METHOD FOR DRAINAGE

The Need to Drain

Once an abdominal abscess has been located with as much certainty as possible, it must be drained expeditiously and effectively. This may seem self-evident to the experienced and skilled general surgeon, who often assumes that other physicians share this basic understanding of the principles that apply to this problem. However, perhaps nowhere else does the old adage "the patient is too sick to operate on" pose a worse trap for the clinician. If the patient is sick because of his undrained abscess, then obviously the only chance for improvement is to drain the abscess. A short period of intensive resuscitation, emphasizing aggressive intravascular volume support, may be necessary to ensure against circulatory collapse in the operating room. This should never be allowed to extend over more than a few hours, even for the patient whose status is so unstable as to require placement of central lines for guiding cardiac support.

Even for the patient whose sepsis exists along with other seemingly more urgent problem, the undrained abscess will certainly be contributing to his overall difficulties. A typical example is the elderly diabetic being cared for in the intensive care unit for an evolving myocardial infarction. When fever, leukocytosis, abdominal pain, and hemodynamic instability develop, there is real danger in evoking the "too sick to operate on" philosophy. Certainly there is considerable risk in carrying out major abdominal surgery on such a patient, and it is unfortunate if no septic source is found. However, when the strong likelihood of abdominal sepsis is based on sound clinical judgment, using all appropriate diagnostic aids, the risk must be taken. The patient will not survive with untreated gangrenous cholecystitis, cholangitis, or dead bowel. The increasing application of an intensive care unit level of support in the operating room should give the maximum chance of surviving the operation.

Making a Plan

There are three approaches to abscess drainage now available:

○ Complete surgical exploration of the abdomen
○ Local (extraserous or transperitoneal) drainage
○ Percutaneous catheter drainage

The extraserous or local transperitoneal drainage of an intra-abdominal abscess has a long history of success. This method is used much less today. The availability of appropriate antibiotics, and better understanding of the effectiveness of vigorous irrigation of the peritoneal cavity, have lessened the fear of contaminating clean areas of the abdomen by releasing the contents of an abscess. Experience has also contributed the knowledge that up to 30%[33] of intra-abdominal abscesses are multiple. This is a problem not completely managed by limited local drainage.

The effectiveness of US and CT in both detecting and guiding the drainage of abdominal abscesses has largely displaced the use of local surgical drainage. A possible exception is the extraperitoneal approach to draining a localized well-established appendiceal abscess, which is still rather commonly employed. For the most part, the rest of the discussion will be based on choosing drainage either by open surgical exploration or by percutaneously placed catheters. It should be well understood that appropriate antibiotics given in adequate doses are an essential accompaniment to any method of drainage.

The Goals of Percutaneous Drainage

A comparison of percutaneous and surgical drainage of abdominal abscesses should begin by considering the realistic goals for each approach. For surgical drainage, the goal is to obtain debridement and drainage adequate to cure the abscess. Where such underlying problems as a leaking intestinal anastomosis exist, the surgery is also intended to correct that problem as well.

The goals for percutaneous drainage are somewhat different. In order to judge true success, as a guide to its application, the result must be measured against the intended outcome.

Complete elimination of an abdominal abscess is only one potential goal. Increasing experience with this procedure is teaching us that it has considerable additional utility. The potential purposes for this method of drainage include:

Cure of the abscess
Conversion of a GI tract leak into a controlled external fistula to:
    Allow time for a patient's condition to improve
      without a major immediate operation
    Facilitate a single, definitive future operation
    Possibly obviate the need for any operation
Control one abscess, allowing more limited surgery for another

Given this variety of goals for percutaneous abdominal abscess drainage, it seems clear that any study that judges its efficacy only on the basis of "cure" is misleading and not very useful as guidance. When the intended purpose is stated more specifically, evaluation of its success in meeting this purpose is more helpful. This perspective should be kept in mind as we proceed to a consideration of the factors involved in choosing this approach.

Factors Involved in Choice of Drainage Approach

Just as with any surgical procedure, proper selection of patients is the main determinant of success. The effectiveness of either method for draining an abdominal abscess cannot be judged by itself. It must be evaluated in terms of appropriateness for each individual patient with a particular clinical problem. Failure to follow this principle will only lead to unwarranted pessimism or unsupported enthusiasm, a weakness in some of the reports of results. One must be careful to avoid attributing either the success or failure of percutaneous drainage to the method rather than to its injudicious use for the wrong kind of patient.

The choice between percutaneous or surgical drainage is based on the interplay of a number of factors (see Table 5-1). They will be discussed in the appropriate context below.

With rare exceptions, such as liver abscesses and pancreatic fluid collections, no single factor by itself can determine the decision. These two exceptions will be discussed first.

SPECIAL CASES

Intrahepatic Abscesses

Abscesses in the liver represent a rather special case, which doesn't follow the plan to be presented separately below. The main point is that there are two fundamentally different kinds of liver abscesses that require different approaches to management. Pyogenic or parasitic abscesses, whether cryptogenic or associated with infection elsewhere in the abdomen, are usually managed successfully by percutaneous drainage. On the other hand, abscesses with biliary tract disease require an additional attack on the bile duct problem as well.

The main factor determining success with percutaneous drainage of a liver abscess is whether or not it is associated with infection in the biliary tract. The data are somewhat confused, but a brief review of some of the pertinent studies will help illuminate the issues. In one study[52] of 106 patients, a relatively high proportion (31%) of the pyogenic liver abscesses were due to cholangitis secondary to extrahepatic biliary obstruction. There was a much higher death rate in those treated percutaneously (95%) than for those treated surgically (26%). There are at least two reasons these results should not be accepted without much more examination. First, it has been well shown that infected bile in the common duct from distal obstruction (ascending cholangitis) requires more complete drainage than can be achieved indirectly by a percutaneously placed intrahepatic catheter. Even drainage by a large cholecystostomy tube may not be as effective as a large T-tube in the common duct for treating this problem. Second, this report suffers from an apparent dissimilarity between the patient groups treated by the two methods—a problem shared by most of the reports cited in this chapter. They seem to have selected the sickest patients for percutaneous drainage. The poor outcome then led them to recommend percutaneous drainage only for high-risk patients, a scheme likely to produce a self-fulfilling prophecy. We cannot know what the relative success of percutaneous or surgical drainage would have been if the study had been carried out prospectively, with random assignment of similar patients to both kinds of treatment. The lesson from such a study is not that percutaneous drainage is not good—it is only that percutaneous drainage may not be adequate for draining an infected obstructed common bile duct.

Another report of 10 patients illustrates the confusion that results from considering hepatic abscesses as a single disease.[24] The authors described a selected group of patients whose liver abscesses were known to be associated with biliary tract disease. Percutaneous catheter drainage was used only as an adjunct to surgical correction of the biliary tract problem. It would obviously be incorrect to cite this report as an argument against percutaneous drainage of liver abscesses.

The experience with percutaneous drainage of hepatic abscesses that are not associated with biliary tract disease has been significantly different. While again there are no randomized prospective studies, the experience has been extensive. In one report of 192 cases with pyogenic hepatic abscesses due to bacteria or parasites (mainly amoebiasis), success was much greater and mortality much lower with percutaneous aspiration or catheter drainage than with surgical drainage.[19] A small series of six patients described 100% success in curing pyogenic liver abscesses by percutaneous drainage, and encouraged the use of large 18F catheters.[71] Another report of 82 patients advocates percutaneous drainage for both pyogenic and amebic hepatic abscesses.[15] One particularly useful reference presents an 89% success rate with percutaneous drainage of liver abscesses.[30] That report also contains an extensive review of the literature on that subject, and so is an excellent source of all the major references on percutaneous drainage of pyogenic liver abscesses.

The description of a group of 10 patients makes several key points.[11] Their high proportion (50%) of biliary tract problems as the underlying cause emphasizes the need to evaluate the biliary tract in any patient with a liver abscess. The other critical point is that most liver abscesses are a result of an infection somewhere in the portal drainage area. Fifty years ago, appendicitis was the principal cause. More aggressive early surgery and more effective antibiotics have diminished that problem, and biliary tract disease has taken its place.

Other etiologic factors are apt to be less apparent, and the diagnosis is often simply labeled as "idiopathic." However, a thorough search for such inciting infectious foci as colon diverticulitis must be made before a liver abscess is called "cryptogenic." This will allow definitive treatment of the primary problem, even though the liver abscess itself may well be managed successfully by percutaneous drainage. The reported experience with many series seems to be that about 30% of liver abscesses will not be found to have any identifiable primary cause. This seems to be an irreducible number, but it should not dissuade one from a search for the cause.

A final point to be considered, largely in the internal medicine literature, is the great success from treating liver abscesses with antibiotics alone, without any kind of drainage. These experiences are undoubtedly true, but the cases seem highly selected, and there is usually no review of the entire patient population from which they came. Based on the large body of data that emphasize the high mortality for patients with liver abscesses, and the efficacy of percutaneous drainage in properly selected cases, treatment with antibiotics alone cannot be recommended.

Pancreas-Associated Collections

Fluid collections associated with inflammation or injury to the pancreas represent another special case not lending itself to the more general guidelines presented below. Here the central problem is to distinguish between a sterile pseudocyst, which one would like to drain internally in a definitive operation at the appropriate time, and a pancreatic abscess (or infected pseudocyst), which requires adequate external drainage immediately.

Our recent review of 22 patients having percutaneous drainage of abscesses in the postoperative abdomen that is difficult to explore illustrates the reality of pancreatic collections.[78] Whereas 69% of the nonpancreatic collections were cured by percutaneous drainage, only 33% of those associated with the pancreas responded well to this approach. This was because the pancreatic collections contained thick material loaded with cellular debris, which required open surgical debridement and wide drainage not achievable with a percutaneous catheter.

The inadequacy of percutaneous drainage for pancreatic abscesses or infected pseudocysts seems well accepted. However, initial needle aspiration guided by US or CT can be very useful in making the diagnosis. Aspiration of sterile fluid indicates a pseudocyst, which should not be drained by catheter. If pus is aspirated, surgery is required for debridement and adequate external drainage. Even with prompt surgical drainage,[16] the mortality for pancreatic abscess is about 40%, so percutaneous catheter drainage has no place for this deadly problem.

GENERAL CASES

Except for liver and pancreatic abscesses discussed above, principles have been evolving that can be applied to the choice of drainage route for abscesses elsewhere in the abdomen. It is apparent that this choice usually depends on the interplay among several separate considerations. However, in the hope of clarifying this complex topic, the individual factors that determine this choice for each patient will be discussed separately. Following this, an overall scheme for management will be presented.

The factors to be considered are:

- Condition of the abdomen—simple or complex
- Condition of the patient—age, overall health and stability
- Location of the abscess—accessibility to percutaneous catheter
- Number of abscesses present—single or multiple
- Communication of the abscess with GI tract or pancreas
- Nature of abscess contents—thin fluid or thick debris

Condition of the Abdomen

This factor has rarely been studied as a distinct entity in determining the choice of the most feasible and effective for draining an abdominal abscess. Yet it is often the main issue on which the choice is made.

On one end of the scale is the abdomen that has had:

- Only one prior surgical operation
- No generalized peritonitis
- No GI tract ostomies or stomas
- No loss of abdominal wall integrity

Such an abdomen can be anticipated to be easy and safe to explore, with normal anatomy and tissue planes except for the abscess itself. There should be little danger of injuring organs such as bowel, biliary tract, or pancreas during exploration, and consequently little chance of ending with fistulas and other severe new problems after the surgery. In these cases, one has a free choice of either percutaneous or surgical drainage. The decision can be made on the basis of the accessibility of the abscess to a percutaneously placed catheter and the radiologist's experience and skill with the procedure.

On the other end of the scale is the abdomen characterized by:

- Multiple prior operations
- Prior generalized peritonitis with dense adhesions
- Intestinal stomas and drain tracts
- Pancreatic-cutaneous fistula
- Abdominal wall defects from fascial necrosis, perhaps closed with plastic mesh now densely adherent to the underlying viscera.

In this worst possible case, well-known to all surgeons, one is extremely reluctant to operate once again. The risks of creating new enterotomies likely to fistulize, possibly damaging other vital and unforgiving organs, and potentially ending with an even more difficult abdominal wall defect to control, are great indeed. Percutaneous drainage of an abscess buried under and within such problems can offer great advantage.[78] The goal of percutaneous drainage is not necessarily to cure the abscess. In fact, percutaneous drainage can be used to gain control of a bowel leak, making possible a single future operation to correct the underlying problem. Based on the limited goal, the use of percutaneous drainage was successful 69% of the time when the abscess was not associated with the pancreas.

Condition of the Patient

The condition of the patient and the condition of his abdomen often go hand-in-hand and must be considered together. It is not enough to say that a patient who is very sick from an abdominal infection would face great risk from surgical drainage of the abscess. If his abdomen were easy to explore, then that should be the treatment of choice. If his abdomen presents a challenge for surgery, it may be better to attempt percutaneous drainage followed by surgical exploration if there is no improvement in 24 hours

Location of the Abscess

Percutaneous drainage originally had been recommended only for an abscess in direct contact with the abdominal wall.[31,80] That was to avoid the possibility of traversing bowel with the drainage catheter. Increasing experience with percutaneous placement of catheters has indicated that the exact location of an abscess within the abdomen is less important. There are now few places that are inaccessible to the invasive radiologist. The radiology literature contains many reports of success with percutaneously draining fluid collections buried beyond loops of bowel. It is commonly recommended that one can safely traverse bowel with a small needle on the way to draining an abscess. This seems to be a cavalier attitude, mentioned here only to be condemned.

Accessibility alone is not sufficient for choosing this approach. Puncturing bowel, even with the thin needle initially placed to guide percutaneous drainages, must be avoided, lest the procedure produce a bigger problem than it is intended to solve. Especially with the larger sump catheters now being used for this purpose, the percutaneous approach must not add a leak from the GI tract to the existing problem.

There are similar concerns about placing a percutaneous drainage catheter through a previously sterile space. This is probably not a problem in the abdomen, where a catheter tract usually becomes sequestered quickly as occurs with a surgically placed drain. The issues are different regarding the pleural space, where the danger from seeding infection is greater. The risk of creating empyema is too serious to warrant placing a percutaneous drainage catheter into an abdominal abscess by way of the pleural space.

Number of Abscesses Present

From the earliest experience with US- or CT-guided percutaneous drainage came a recommendation that the technique be reserved for only a single abscess. This was based on the fear of missing the additional abscesses to be expected in those patients that could be found by complete surgical exploration.

The main danger is to overlook one of the abscesses. Once this is understood, there is no intrinsic reason that one of a number of abscesses in an abdomen cannot be drained percutaneously, allowing a more limited surgical approach to others present. This could work well for an intrahepatic abscess associated with perforated diverticulitis. The liver abscess could be drained effectively by percutaneous catheter, and the bowel problem could be managed by the surgical approach dictated by the circumstances.

In other multiple abscess situations, percutaneous drainage of one could facilitate a more localized approach to another, possibly avoiding tedious and treacherous dissection in a complex abdomen. This is another illustration of the need to consider all aspects of any patient's problem in choosing the best way to manage the abdominal abscess.

Presence of GI or Pancreatic Fistulas

Longstanding experience has taught that the proper treatment of an abdominal abscess communicating with the GI tract of pancreas is surgical exploration. The visceral leak could be managed by whatever was needed and feasible, including resection and/or repair where possible. Either correction or well-controlled egress to the outside was the goal. Additional drainage of the abscess area was established.

Increasing experience with percutaneous drainage has developed new understanding of the utility and limitations of this method for abscesses associated with internal visceral fistulas. Like all of the factors discussed above, the presence of a visceral communication is not enough by itself to mandate for or against percutaneous drainage. The location of a GI tract hole plays a key role, because the duodenum is much less amenable to direct surgical repair than is the jejunum or ileum. The expected condition of the internal abdominal anatomy is likewise important. A problem that would otherwise be easy to correct in a normal peritoneal cavity could be impossible when exploring an abdomen that resembles "infected concrete." It is helpful to look at some extreme conditions to illustrate the issues.

At the simpler end of the spectrum is a small leak from a repaired stab wound of the mid-ileum in a previously normal abdomen. Because small bowel lends itself to resection and primary anastomosis of a localized problem area, this situation is solved readily by immediate resection and reanastomosis. This same approach applies to an acute foreign body perforation of a normal stomach. In both of these situations, even when the presentation has been delayed for several days and the leak is locally contained, there is no role for percutaneous drainage. Definitive surgical correction of the problem can be accomplished readily and should be undertaken immediately.

At the other extreme are such complex problems as a small breakdown of the repair of a gunshot wound of the duodenum. One knows from experience and understanding surgical principles that a surgical exploration of the area would be carried out for the purpose of establishing controlled drainage. Diversion of the GI contents might also be attempted. Repair of the leak would not be expected to hold up in the face of infection from the outside and pancreatic juice, gastric contents, and bile from the inside, so it would not be attempted. Also, the anatomy of the duodenum does not allow excision of damaged areas except for a small part of the most distal portion.

For this problem, an attempt to obtain the same control over the leakage by placing a draining catheter percutaneously would be worth considering. The effectiveness could be monitored by the patient's clinical condition. Periodic x-rays with radiopague dye injected through the catheter would determine how well the duodenal drainage was being led to the outside. If this succeeded, one could end with a narrow drain tract that should close as the drain was gradually withdrawn. If, on the other hand, the patient did not improve clinically and dye studies showed leakage over an unacceptably wide area, one would proceed directly to the operating room to gain better control.

A situation that presents the same considerations would be a leak from the tail of the pancreas that had sustained unrecognized damage during splenectomy. If this had been present for several days, there would be such intense inflammation in the area that surgical excision of the tail and closure of the stump might not be reliably possible. One could be faced with another leak and the same situation after the surgery. For this problem percutaneous drainage is a reasonable choice. If it produces a controlled fistula to the outside, and if the drainage is managed carefully to protect the skin, the fistula can be expected to close around the catheter. Provided the remainder of the gland, including the duct system, is normal, this should solve the problem definitively. It may require several months, but it is well worth the attempt.

As with any percutaneous drainage application, it should be pursued only as long as it is accomplishing the intended purpose. The patient must be monitored closely, especially during the first week after catheter placement. As long as there are no signs of sepsis or interference with function of the stomach and other adjacent organs, and as long as the serum amylase level does not rise to indicate inadequate external drainage of the leaking pancreatic juice, this course can be continued. Periodic x-rays taken after injection of radiopaque dye into the catheter are helpful in assessing how well the catheter is controlling the leak. At any time that signs of inadequate control develop, surgical drainage should be carried out.

A report of radiologic management of enterocutaneous fistulae[51] illustrates the potential of aggressive application of percutaneous drainage techniques. Twelve patients with high-output duodenal or proximal small bowel enterocutaneous fistulae occurring after radiation of upper GI tract surgery were managed by percutaneous insertion of a large T-tube into the bowel opening. Additional sump drains were placed into the abscess usually associated with the leak. In all cases, the fistulae were well-controlled and the abscesses resolved within 6 weeks. Except in one patient with radiation bowel injury requiring 3 months of drainage, the fistulae closed within 2 weeks after removal of the T-tubes.

Like all such reports, this was a description of experience, not a controlled study. However, the results were impressive enough to warrant considering this kind of approach for the patient with a difficult upper GI fistula that does not close after a reasonable course of parenteral nutrition.

Nature of the Abscess Contents

The nature of an abscess' contents determines how effectively it can be drained by a percutaneous catheter of a limited size. An abscess containing only thin liquid pus should drain well and resolve after management with an adequate size catheter. One that contains considerable necrotic tissue debris will need debridement and more effective drainage than can ordinarily be obtained by the percutaneous route.

One of the principal areas where this arises as an important issue is abscesses involving the pancreas. The considerable tissue necrosis from exposure to the caustic pancreatic juice probably explains why these abscesses must be cleaned out and drained surgically. Even that approach is not always effective, and the unconventional methods devised to secure adequate surgical drainage of a pancreatic abscess are detailed below.

The ineffectiveness of percutaneous drainage of pancreatic collections referred to in our study[78] has been described by others[6,67] as well. Despite the most vigorous surgical management, the mortality for patients with severe pancreatitis and a pancreatic abscess remains high. Percutaneous drainage has no place in the management of this problem.

In considering the best method of drainage, the nature of abscess contents is usually less of a factor in an abscess not associated with the pancreas. As reviewed above, even an abscess related to an upper GI tract fistula can be managed by percutaneous drainage.

The important considerations in treating fistulas of the colon are the location (right versus left colon), the size of the leak, and how well-contained the associated abscess is. A small leak, evidenced only by the periodic emission of the bowel gas through the fistula, with a small abscess effectively contained in the area immediately adjacent to the leak, can sometimes be managed successfully by percutaneous placement of a catheter. If the patient is eating well, maintaining his weight, and having normal bowel function, precutaneous catheter management should be considered. Assuming no distal bowel obstruction or the presence of malignancy in the area, this method is well worth the attempt. The leak and the fistula may resolve without direct surgical attack, which otherwise requires two stages of surgery. Nonsurgical management may require weeks or even months for conclusion. As long as progress is evident, as documented by periodic catheter dye studies showing decreasing size of the abscess cavity and eventual closure of the communication to the bowel—and provided the patient remains clinically free of clinical signs of infection—pursuit of this course can be rewarded with success. Patients who meet these criteria may by managed outside the hospital, with checkups every 1 or 2 weeks.

One recent report describes an experience with 17 patients with a diverticular abscess of the colon.[69] CT-guided needle aspiration demonstrated pus in 11 patients. Three of these patients had abscesses that were either too small to warrant drainage or presented no safe access route for percutaneous catheter placement. Seven of the remaining eight patients underwent a single-stage resection 1 to 3 weeks later, with no complications.

This method has been used successfully for leaks from either the proximal or distal colon. The condition of the abdomen is an important factor influencing choice of drainage route. The more difficult the abdomen would be to operate on, the more seriously percutaneous drainage should be considered.

AN OVERALL SCHEME FOR THE PATIENT

The many factors discussed above and the need to individualize so carefully will now be combined into an overall scheme for guiding the management of each patient suspected of an abdominal abscess. The question in the left upper corner box in Fig. 5-3 ("Is the patient infected?"), and the next three in sequence beneath it have been reviewed early in the chapter. Beginning at the points in the diagram where an abscess has been clearly demonstrated by plain x-ray, dye-contrast x-ray, or by CT or US, the decisions become more complex. That area of the scheme is enlarged in Fig. 5-4. We will first review the pathways that lead to percutaneous drainage.

Percutaneous Catheter Drainage

As discussed above, the expected ease or difficulty in surgically exploring an abdomen is a key point in deciding on surgical or percutaneous drainage. For an uncomplicated abdomen, either method will be feasible and likely to succeed. Other factors, such as the patient's age and ability to withstand surgery, overall medical condition, and occasionally ability to cooperate by leaving a drainage catheter in place, can be used to help decide on the drainage method (Fig. 5-5).

For the abdomen that would be difficult to explore, and especially when it would be even more difficult to secure any kind of satisfactory closure of an abdominal wall riddled with stomas and fascial defects, percutaneous drainage is attractive. Some of the specific experience cited above during consideration of the factors governing the choice of drainage route should help make the decision to attempt percutaneous drainage.

There is a growing body of literature supporting the efficacy of that method for a wide range of abdominal abscess situations. One series showed 80% success by percutaneous drainage in a group of patients selected on the basis of having no more

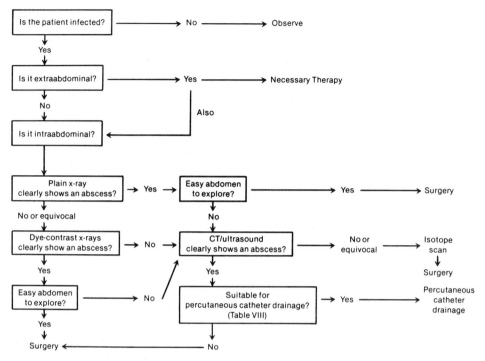

Figure 5–3.
An overall scheme for managing the patient suspected of having an abdominal abscess.

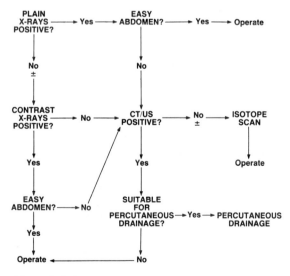

Figure 5–4.
Expanded view of the same scheme as in Fig. 5-3, showing
the further examination of patient with abdominal abscess.

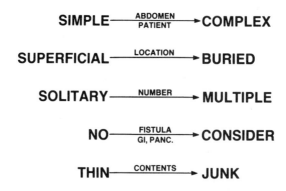

Figure 5-5.
The spectrum of factors to be considered in determining feasibility of percutaneous drainage of abdominal abscess.

than two abscesses, good accessibility, absence of a contaminating GI tract source, and containing no fungi as causative organisms.[2] It seems apparent that if one expands the potential goal to include gaining control over a bowel fistula so as to enhance future surgery, or to include limiting the number of operations on a very difficult abdomen, good results may have been obtained for a less strictly limited group of patients.

Another report described complete resolution of abdominal abscess or postoperative fluid collection in each of 66 patients treated by percutaneous catheter drainage alone.[59] That series contained a number of patients with infected or sterile fluid collections following biliary tract surgery. These patients were part of a larger group, of whom the remainder underwent surgery instead. The report suffers from offering no explanation of how the patients were selected for the percutaneous drainage procedure, but it describes 100% success by careful patient selection.

A study of 55 patients at a leading university teaching center found 96% of pyogenic, nonfungal, nonfistulous abscess were cured by percutaneous drainage.[66] Their complete failure to cure any abscess containing yeast as a major component or with necrotic tumor confirms the experience of others with these two problems.

Additional studies are worth a brief reference, not because they are either well-controlled or different in any major way, but simply to offer more data. In one, 27 patients had their abdominal abscesses treated percutaneously over the preceding 5 years.[39] These were compared with 43 having surgical drainage over the preceding years. With no explanation of how patients were chosen for each approach, and with one method covering only half the time period of the other, this should be considered an "experience" rather than a "study." However, if the details are taken into consideration, the results are interesting. The percutaneously drained group had fewer complications (4% versus 16%), a smaller incidence of inadequate drainage (11% versus 21%), and shorter duration of drainage (17 days versus 29 days) than those drained surgically. One could infer that the surgically drained group were more complicated or sicker patients, which could explain the differences in results. However, by eliminating patients with pancreatic abscesses or infected pseudocysts, and those with diverticular, perirectal, and abdominal wall abscesses, the series offers some illumination on the topic.

Still another report relates an unusually broad experience with percutaneous catheter drainage of a wide variety of abscesses of the abdomen and mediastimum.[41] These included abscesses in the liver, retroperitoneal space, and in subphrenic, subhepatic, and pelvic locations. Four patients with postoperative bowel anastomic leaks were also included, two of whom were managed successfully with percutaneous drainage. This experience was too uncontrolled to allow any estimate of relative efficacy, but it is interesting in its detailed discussion of experience with increasingly large and multiple-lumen catheters. Two more reports are worth mentioning for the same reasons.[48,53]

One report from one group that has led the way with percutaneous drainage of abdominal abscesses has updated their earlier experience.[29] They describe their results with that method applied to 125 abscesses in 113 patients. Their latest expanded criteria for selection included multiple abscesses, complex abscesses (loculated, ill-defined, or extensively dissecting), abscesses with enteric fistulas or whose drainage routes traversed normal organs, as well as complicated abscesses (appendiceal, splenic, interloop, and pelvic). Nonoperative success was achieved in 73.6% of the whole group. Cure was achieved in 82% of simple abscesses but in only 45% of those that were complex. They found no correlation among size, depth, drainage route, or etiology (spontaneous versus postoperative) with either cure or complications. They recommended a trial of percutaneous drainage for all simple and most complex abscesses, with clinical response as the key determinant of the need for operative intervention.

That recommendation is a fitting way to end this section on percutaneous drainage. When that method is used, the patient must be watched closely for signs of failure. If there is no improvement within 24 hours in fever, white blood cell count, hemodynamic stability, or the other signs of sepsis, the patient must proceed to surgical drainage. The principle is no less true for primary surgical management, but a surgeon who has thoroughly explored an abdominal abscess and dealt with any inciting factors can probably be more certain that he has done everything possible. No such certainty is possible when one has relied only on a catheter placed through the skin into an abscess seen only on a CT or US screen.

SURGICAL DRAINAGE

We have concentrated on the factors involved in deciding whether to drain an abscess percutaneously or by open surgical exploration. We have also emphasized how the anticipated ease or difficulty of surgery exploration plays an important role in making the choice of drainage method.

It needs to be emphasized and reemphasized that the decision to carry out limited drainage, whether percutaneously or through a localized surgical approach, is never considered to be the final solution to the patient's problem. The patient must be watched closely after a limited drainage procedure. If the systemic signs of sepsis improve during the ensuing 24 to 48 hours, as evidenced by decreasing fever and WBC count and improving hemodynamic stability and pulmonary function, continued monitoring can be planned. However, any clinical deterioration, even after initial improvement, means that the limited drainage is failing. Thorough surgical exploration, even with its risks and difficulties, remains the definitive management and must be carried out expeditiously at this point.

From here on, the discussion will concentrate on the principles of surgical drainage. First, we will discuss localized surgical drainage, then complete abdominal exploration including various adjunctive measures, and finish with management of the difficult abdominal wall after exploration.

Localized Surgical Drainage

Once having decided that an abscess needs to be managed surgically, the next choice is between total exploration of the abdomen or a limited, local approach to the abscess area. An extensive historic review[55] of indications for drainage, selection of drainage device, and choice of drainage route is well worth considering.

There is a large body of literature describing various special approaches for localized drainage of abscesses in particular locations in and around the abdomen. As is typical for this whole subject, there are few data that are more than simply descriptions of an experience. However, one report[77] of randomized, prospective selection of patients for either extraperitoneal or transperitoneal drainage of intra-abdominal abscesses is interesting. Sixty patients, comparable in all respects, were drained by either route (31 transperitoneally and 29 extraperitoneally). The transperitoneal approach produced more hollow viscus injuries with subsequent enterocutaneous fistulae. Furthermore, the need to reoperate for another or persistent abscess was the same in both groups. Overall, there were more deaths and complications in the group drained transperitoneally, although the differences were not statistically significant. The authors felt that their data refute the professed superiority of a transperitoneal approach, both from the requirement for reoperation and from incidence of intestinal fistula formation. There seem to be no other reliable studies on this point.

Our general preference is for total abdominal exploration where possible rather than the limited, and often indirect, approach. This is because total exploration offers potentially greater safety by allowing direct exposure of more of the anatomy, with less risk of injuring organs unintentionally. It also ensures that an additional, unexpected abscess is not overlooked. In the proper circumstances, it also allows one to correct a bowel leak or other such problem that may be associated with the infection. The tradeoff, of course, is that the whole peritoneal cavity is exposed to the infecting organisms that had been confined to one localized area.

Abscesses in certain locations lend themselves to a limited drainage procedure. Those around the periphery of the abdominal cavity—the upper, lateral, and pelvic extremities—are most amenable to that approach. In that regard, there are similarities to percutaneous drainage, in that both methods are least suitable to an abscess between loops of bowel in the midabdomen.

Localized surgical drainage is the most effective procedure for an abscess deep in the pelvis adjoining the rectum. Transrectal drainage avoids the danger of creating a tract from the rectum into the peritoneal cavity. It also offers a direct drainage path not available by an intra-abdominal approach.

Similarly, an established appendiceal abscess can be well managed by draining through a lateral extraperitoneal approach. Provided there are no systemic signs of sepsis or bowel obstruction, this method will usually allow the abscess to resolve; an elective appendectomy can be carried out several months later. The concern here is the possibility one may be dealing with a different kind of problem, such as a perforated colon malignancy, which requires direct surgical management. If there is any doubt of the diagnosis, as in an elderly person with several months of bowel symptoms, the abdomen should be explored through a standard midline incision rather than by the limited, blind extraperitoneal approach.

Abscesses in the upper abdomen have also been managed by a variety of limited surgical approaches. Those in the right upper abdomen, above or below the liver, can be approached through an anterior or anterolateral transverse incision. Drains should then be placed through separate small incisions situated as far laterally as possible to allow dependent drainage. However, this approach is still rather blind. Especially in an obese patient, exposure can be very difficult to gain, which limits severely the ability to dissect and demonstrate safely the duodenum, biliary tract, pancreas, and other vital structures in the area. One can find, at the end of a struggle through this limited approach, that it would have been better to begin with a true exploratory incision.

Ordinarily, these infra- or suprahepatic abscesses will have been located by US or CT. If an expert invasive radiologist is available, a better approach might be to attempt percutaneous catheter drainage. If this is unsuccessful or proves inadequate (by the patient's early clinical response), our preference would be to bypass the limited local surgical approach and proceed directly to a wide surgical exploration.

Abscesses in the central epigastric region are usually in the lesser sac and are associated with a pancreatic problem. In this circumstance, the most logical surgical approach is through a standard upper midline incision, extended to the length necessary for safe visualization of all the important structures in the area. As discussed earlier, percutaneous drainage has no place in the treatment of pancreas-associated abscesses.

The left upper abdomen presents some other factors to be considered. An abscess under the left diaphragm is accessible either from the front or the back. If it is situated more anteriorly, it can be approached by a left subcostal incision carried through a subperitoneal plane along the diaphgram until the abscess is entered. For one situated posteriorly, a posterior approach through the bed of the 12th or 11th rib allows direct access, wide exposure, and dependent drainage. However, this approach carries one to the blind side of the stomach, colon, pancreas, and the spleen, if present. It is difficult to be certain one has opened all ramifications of the abscess without endangering these organs. If one is too vigorous, one can end with gastric or colon contents, or pancreatic juice, draining from the cavity.

Posterior drainage through the bed of a rib is indeed very effective for a left subphrenic abscess. However, we have employed a variation of this method. The patient's skin is prepped from the right anterior axillary line all the way around the left side to the spine and from nipples to pubis, finishing with the patient lying supine on a sterile drape inserted from the left. The left arm is also wrapped sterilely, and the abdomen is entered through a long midline incision. The stomach, colon, and spleen (if present) are mobilized so as to open the abscess widely and expose the area over the 11th and 12th ribs. We have managed enough cases in which the stomach, and sometimes the colon or spleen as well, is densely adherent to the posterior rib cage due to the infection to appreciate that a dissection made blindly from the outside only could easily have produced injury to these organs. Having thus mobilized everything necessary, a large suture needle is passed outward through the 11th interspace to the outside, marking the desired location.

While one surgeon keeps a hand inside the abdomen touching the rib to be resected, and with moist towels holding the viscera in place, the patient is rolled up onto his right side. An incision about 10 cm long is made over the posterior rib marked by the previously placed suture. An 8-cm section of the 12th rib is then removed subperiosteally from the outside, beginning just lateral to the transverse process of the vertebra. The fingertips of the surgeon's hand inside the abdomen are easily felt through the rib bed, and the incision through the peritoneum can be made precisely while the viscera are held safely out of the way. The opening into the peritoneal cavity should then be extended to admit the width of the hand.

There is a variety of devices available, some commercial and some favorite self-styled contrivances, for draining through such a pathway. Given the wide open course to the outside and the assistance from gravity for this route, the actual nature of the drains may well not be critical. The important principle seems to be that multiple large drains should be used to keep the incision widely open.

However, a word of caution is pertinent. There are many multiple-lumen sump drains on the market, which seem less likely to become obstructed and will allow for irrigation. These are probably worthwhile goals, but all of these sump drains are quite firm. They will all erode tissues, even those made of supposedly "soft" materials like silicon. We have seen gastrocutaneous and colocutaneous fistulas created by sump drains placed through the bed of the rib into a left subphrenic abscess. Such drains have also eroded the tail of the pancreas, resulting in prolonged drainage of pancreatic juice and perpetuation of the abscess. Similar injury occurs to the spleen when it is present in that circumstance.

The safest procedure is probably to place multiple large Penrose drains when there is potential danger to adjacent viscera. They function effectively to carry the drainage passively to the outside, especially when the pathway is dependent. The common practice of cutting sideholes in the drains and placing straight catheters inside has not been conclusively shown to add any advantage, although a catheter does allow performing dye-contrast x-ray studies to monitor the size of the abscess space.

Abdominal Exploration for Drainage

When one chooses to carry out exploratory laparotomy for an abscess, the commitment is to:

- ○ Explore the abdomen thoroughly
- ○ Secure any initiating source such as a bowel perforation or disrupted anastomosis
- ○ Debride infected material where indicated and feasible
- ○ Consider establishing antibiotic or antiseptic solution lavage
- ○ Establish effective external drainage
- ○ Close the abdomen as securely as possible

Surgical Exploration

Thorough exploration of an abdomen that is infected and has been operated on before is a challenge that will tax the skill of any surgeon. We will not detail the approach for defining free peritoneal cavity and proceeding from the more nearly normal areas to the site of the abscess. We will only emphasize that the task is to open all areas and define all of the anatomy possible—while avoiding to the maximum extent possible injury to any organs. Such injury cannot always be avoided, so it is equally important to search for and find any unintended damage. The worst outcome is the catastrophic delayed presentation of an undetected enterotomy created during the prior search for sepsis.

Securing the Inciting Focus

Securing any inciting focus of infection depends on the anatomical situation. A disrupted small bowel anastomosis can be excised back to normal, well-vascularized tissue and rejoined without tension. A colon perforation in the presence of established peritonitis or abscess, on the other hand, must be either resected with proximal diversion or treated by colostomy as close to the problem area as possible in the case of the distal sigmoid colon or rectum. The obvious variations of such problems and their many kinds of solutions are beyond the scope of this discussion.

Debridement

Debridement of the infected abdomen is a subject about which it is difficult to make general statements. Certainly an attempt should be made to remove loose necrotic debris from an abscess cavity, by irrigation and manual means that are gentle enough to avoid damage to the viscera. Vigorous removal of the necrotic material associated with a pancreatic abscess is a special case that will be discussed separately below. One approach that has enjoyed some attention is the radical debridement of peritoneum involved in established peritonitis. A report of a randomized prospective clinical trial described no difference in hospital mortality or frequency of reoperation for abscess between 31 patients undergoing radical peritoneal debridement and 29 having standard surgical management.[64] Previous reports of success from the radical debridement approach have not been otherwise confirmed, and the procedure cannot be recommended for general use.

Adjunctive Irrigation

Irrigation of the peritoneal cavity with various antibiotic and antiseptic solutions likewise has not found wide acceptance. Wide dispersion of the solutions for up to 3 days has been demonstrated experimentally in rabbits,[73] and continuous irrigation with antibiotics has lowered the mortality from peritonitis in rats.[43] An interesting study[46] in dogs found no improvement in survival from experimental peritonitis. Coupled with a significant metabolic acidosis in those lavaged with povidone–iodine solution, the authors felt these findings argued against the safety and efficacy of this procedure in humans. Despite several reports in the clinical literature,[7,50,56] and the fact that earlier concerns about respiratory depression due to absorption of uncontrolled amounts of certain antibiotics have been dismissed, the data remain unconvincing, and this procedure is not recommended.

Peritoneal lavage (or "dialysis" as it is sometimes labeled) for acute pancreatitis is a somewhat special case that has received separate attention. The controversies and uncertainties concerning this procedure can perhaps best be summarized by reference to a published review[79] of a clinical report. The absence of persuasive results of controlled studies seems to be responsible for the lack of general acceptance of this technique for acute pancreatitis. Vigorous circulatory and pulmonary support, optimum nutrition, a careful search for and surgical decompression of unrecognized choledocholithiasis and cholangitis, and surgical drainage and debridement of pancreatic abscesses, continue to be the foundation of management of this difficult problem.

Establishing Effective External Drainage

The principles presented above for local surgical drainage apply equally well for draining an abscess that has been uncovered by open surgical exploration. The pathway should take maximum advantage of the effect of gravity wherever possible. Except for the subphrenic and flank areas, this is often not possible. For areas that do not lend themselves to dependent drainage, a suction drain seems to be effective. Provided the dangers of tube drains reviewed above are heeded, small sump drains served by low levels of suction will serve the purpose. The passive soft rubber Penrose type of drain should still be considered where a wide pathway to the skin is available, especially where a harder tube might endanger nearby viscera.

The ultimate scheme for truly effective external drainage would logically seem to be an abdomen left totally open to the outside. Variations of this scheme have been described, in efforts to achieve maximum open drainage while avoiding evisceration and attempting to minimize the damage to exposed bowel. The inevitable abdominal wall fascial defects resulting from this approach have also been managed subsequently in several ways.

A recent report compared the results of controlled open drainage with closed drainage for severe intra-abdominal sepsis.[10] Thirty-one patients had their abscesses packed with gauze in a plastic intestinal bag or rubber glove, with wound closure only to the degree needed to prevent evisceration. Any bowel left exposed was covered with plastic sheeting sewn to the wound edges, covered with petrolatum gauze, and kept damp with saline-soaked dressings. The gauze packing was left in place a minimum of 4 to 5 days, then slowly removed at the bedside in small daily increments. Plastic sheeting, if used in the wound, was retained until granulation tissue covered the bowel and was then removed at the bedside. No other attempts at wound closure were made. Eighteen other patients underwent drainage with soft rubber or sump drains and complete fascial closure of the wound. While not selected for either treatment in a random fashion, the two groups were similar in most respects reported.

The mortality was lower for the open drainage group (23% versus 45%), and they also had a shorter mean hospital stay (22 days versus 41 days). One patient developed a small-bowel fistula after open drainage, which closed without surgical intervention. While the number of study patients was small, and the results were weakened somewhat by the absence of truly randomized, prospective assignment of patients to the two treatment groups, it does point out an important principle of abscess management. The walls of an intra-abdominal fluid collection or abscess tend to collapse when drained with any type of drainage device. This often allows septic foci in the depths of the abscess to become walled off from the drain and sets the stage for recurrence of the abscess. Open drainage is designed to prevent this collapse and to keep the cavity walls separated until sufficient granulation has formed to stabilize them in this position. This should prevent sequestration of purulent material in the depths of the abscess and promote healing from below upward. It seems to require at least 4 or 5 days for this stabilization of the abscess walls to occur, beyond which time the packing can be removed in small increments.

This open controlled method of abdominal abscess drainage has found aggressive application to abscesses involving the pancreas. Experience with 17 patients undergoing surgery for pancreatic abscess[17] found no deaths in the 6 patients managed by open packing of the abscess and a 55% death rate in the 11 undergoing sump drainage with closure of the incision. Both groups had vigorous debridement of necrotic debris. The wounds in the open drainage group were packed with gauze to prevent evisceration. That experience was updated more recently[9] with similar results in a somewhat larger group of patients.

While it is clear that open drainage is effective, the disadvantages are considerable and must be weighed in the decision process. For the short term, evisceration can be prevented by some method of packing. The danger to exposed bowel is less easily managed. In many of these patients, the greater omentum is not readily available as a protective barrier, and even coverage with Silastic or other plastic films is not totally reliable. Despite all measures, all of which should include keeping the bowel moist, one can probably expect an irreducible incidence of enterocutaneous fistula formation. There is also an unmeasured but real loss of heat and protein-containing peritoneal fluid from the abdomen left open. These are not insurmountable but should be kept in mind in managing the patient's nutritional and fluid support. Purulent exudate is rich in albumin and other proteins, and while the loss is a necessary part of the intended effective drainage of the abscess, it must be taken into account in planning the patient's alimentation needs.

A related situation is presented by the patient whose abdominal wall fascia cannot be closed primarily after surgery for intra-abdominal sepsis, which often requires debridement of necrotic fascia. The use of synthetic mesh sutured to the skin about the defect is described in a review[36] of this technique. Some have advocated removal of the mesh after about 1 week, before it becomes incorporated into the granulation tissue forming on the underlying viscera, before it erodes into the bowel, but after the organs have become well enough stabilized that evisceration is unlikely. The mesh is then replaced with autologous skin graft as a covering until much later, when repair of the defect can be considered. Others have left the mesh in place, covering it with grafted skin when a suitable granulating bed has developed.

A variation of this approach has been described in which a zipper is incorporated into the mesh used in the manner described above to prevent evisceration and to allow wide drainage for abdominal sepsis.[35] The authors describe opening the zipper and carrying out debridement and irrigation as a bedside procedure not requiring anesthesia or a trip to the operating room.

All of these techniques should be in the repertoire of the general surgeon. The selection of the appropriate patients for their application remains a matter of judgment based on experience. A few generalities seem reasonable. First, some abscesses contain a large amount of necrotic debris, most notably those involving the pancreas, in which the ongoing leakage of pancreatic juice feeds the process. This is the single condition in which open drainage, allowing easy access for frequent debridement and irrigation, should be considered most strongly, because closed drainage with sump tubes and even continuous lavage irrigation are so often ineffective.

The second applicable generality is that most other abscesses will respond satisfactorily to closed drainage after abdominal exploration, allowing closure of the incision and avoiding the complications of open drainage detailed above. This brings us to the third principle, which is that the best chance for success in managing abdominal sepsis lies in close evaluation of results from whatever method of drainage was used. In fact, in patients such as those with multiple areas of infection found at exploratory laparotomy, it is very reasonable to plan a second-look operation at the time of the initial procedure. This is attractive even in the absence of uncertainty about the viability of bowel left in place, and poses a reasonable alternative to the more aggressive use of totally open drainage with all its disadvantages.

We have pointed out earlier that a limited approach, whether by percutaneous catheter placement or local surgical drainage, should be abandoned and surgical exploration should be done if a patient fails to show clear signs of clinical improvement within the first 24 to 48 hours.

There are similar principles for evaluating success beyond the first few days of improvement following any method of drainage. Assuming one has seen clear and progressive improvement in the patient's clinical condition over the subsequent week or more, including periodic dye-contrast studies showing decreasing size of the abscess cavity, one must decide when to stop the antibiotics that are part of all such patients' management. Several studies can help guide this decision. In one report of 65 patients with postoperative intra-abdominal sepsis, 51 were afebrile when antibiotics were stopped.[44] Intra-abdominal infection developed or recurred in one third of those who had a persistent leukocytosis and in none whose WBC remained normal. The development of nosocomial infection showed a similar relationship to the white cell count. The authors concluded that those at risk of developing a postoperative infection after responding to treatment for intra-abdominal sepsis are those who are afebrile with a persistent leukocytosis, or who remain febrile, after antibiotics are stopped.

These findings were reinforced and expanded somewhat in a retrospective review of 2,567 patients studied to identify reliable predictors of sepsis eradication.[76] After stopping antibiotic therapy, sepsis recurred in 19% of those who were afebrile, in 3% of those with normal temperature and WBC count, and in none who, in addition, had fewer than 73% granulocytes and fewer than 3% immature forms on a differential blood smear. At the time of hospital discharge, the comparable rates for recurrence of sepsis were 8%, 2%, and 0%.

From beginning to end, the price of successful management of abdominal sepsis is eternal vigilance at each step. Failure early after limited drainage requires a trip to the operating room for complete abdominal exploration. Failure to achieve normal temperature and white cell count at the time antibiotics are stopped means a significant chance that the abdominal infection will recur or that a nosocomial infection will ensue.

Determining Severity of Sepsis

One factor that has been missing as an aid to managing abdominal sepsis is a method of quantitating the severity of a patient's illness in terms of some standard index. In managing an individual patient, it is, of course, crucial to evaluate his responses to treatment in relation to his preceding clinical course. However, for epidemiologic studies of severe intra-abdominal sepsis, and particularly for trials of therapy, classification of patients according to mortality risk is essential. Furthermore, the ability to prognosticate about expected outcome with some degree of certainty is a great help in making final decisions about continuing or withdrawing life support and preparing families for this process.

Several scales, such as the APACHE score, are probably too broadly based on a wide spectrum of medical conditions to be optimum for septic surgical patients. Some success has been reported recently with applying two illness severity indices to a selected group of 58 patients with secondary bacterial peritonitis.[75] The authors compared Sepsis Severity Score (SSS), which measures organ dysfunction, with the well-documented Acute Physiology Score (APS). They evaluated the prognostic ability of the two indices and studied the relationships of the methods to each other and to other prognostic determinants. The two were equally effective in predicting survival rates for the patients. While it is important to emphasize that no index of illness is directly applicable for making decisions about an individual patient, such measurements are necessary for evaluating trials of selected treatment regimens. They may have their greatest usefulness in ensuring that therapeutic trials involving several separate institutions would have an appropriate type of stratification of the patients' illness, to allow comparability among different groups and, therefore, comparability among institutions. An appreciation of these issues is important for anyone who is managing seriously sick patients and who must understand the validity and potential pitfalls in new experiences reported in the published literature.

REFERENCES

1. Adult respiratory distress syndrome. Lancet February 1986:301.
2. Aeder MI, Wellman JL, Haaga JR, et al: The role of surgical and percutaneous drainage in the treatment of abdominal abscesses. Arch Surg 1983;118:273.
3. Ahrenholz DH, Simmons RL: Peritonitis and other intra-abdominal infections. In: Simmons RL, Howard RJ (eds). Surgical infectious diseases. Norwalk: Appleton-Century-Croft. 1982;34:795.
4. Altemeier WA, Culbertson WR, Fullen WD, et al. Intra-abdominal abscesses. Am J Surg 1973;125:70.
5. Amstey MS, Schaffer DL: Ultrasound in the identification of true pelvic abscesses. Infect Surg 1984:190.
6. Aranha GV, Prinz RA, Greenlee HB. Pancreatic abscess: an unresolved surgical problem. Am J Surg 1982;144:534.
7. Aune S, Norman E. Diffuse peritonitis treated with continuous peritoneal lavage. Acta Chir Scand 1970;136:401.
8. Bicknell TA, Kohatsu S, Goodwin DA: Use of indium-111 labeled leukocytes in differentiating pancreatic abscess from pseudocyst. Am J Surg 1981;142:312.
9. Bradley EL, Fulenwider JT. Open treatment of pancreatic abscess. Surg Gynecol Obstet 1984;159:509.
10. Bradley SJ, Jurkovich GJ, Pearlman NW, et al. Controlled open drainage of severe intra-abdominal sepsis. Arch Surg 1985;120:629.
11. Buchman TG, Zuidema GD. The role of computerized tomographic scanning in the surgical management of pyogenic hepatic abscess. Surg Gynecol Obstet 1981;153:1.
12. Bydder GM, Kreel L: Attenuation values of gluid collections within the abdomen. J Comput Assist Tomogr 1980;4:145.
13. Cater R, Brewer LA III: Subphrenic abscess: a thoracoabdominal clinical complex. Am J Surg 1964;108:165.
14. Coleman RE, Black RE, Welch DM, et al: Indium-111 labelled leukocytes in the evaluation of suspected abdominal abscesses. Am J Surg 1980;139:99.
15. Conter RL, Pitt HA, Tompkins RK, et al. Differentiation of pyogenic from amebic hepatic abscesses. Surg Gynecol Obstet 1986;162:114.
16. Crass RA, Meyer AA, Jeffrey RB, et al. Pancreatic abscess: impact of computerized tomography on early diagnosis and surgery. Am J Surg 1985;150:127.
17. Davidson ED, Bradley EL. "Marsupialization" in the treatment of pancreatic abscess. Surgery 1981;89:252.
18. DeCosse JJ, Poulin TL, Fox PS, et al: Subphrenic abscess. Surg Gynecol Obstet 1974;138:841.
19. Dietrick RB. Experience with liver abscess. Am J Surg 1984;147:288.
20. Doberneck RC, Mittelman J: Reappraisal of the problems of intra-abdominal abscess. Surg Gynecol Obstet 1982;154:875.
21. Eiseman B, Beart R, Norton L. Multiple organ failure. Surg Gynecol Obstet 1958;66:426.
22. Ferrucci JT Jr: Body ultrasonography. N Engl J Med 1979;11:538.
23. Filly RA, Sommer FG, Minton MJ: Characterization of biological fluids by ultrasound and computed tomography. Radiology 1980;134:167.
24. Fischer MG, Beaton HL: Unsuspected hepatic abscess associated with biliary tract disease. Am J Surg 1983;146:658.
25. Fischer RP, Polk HC Jr. Changing etiologic patterns of renal insufficiency in surgical patients. Surg Gynecol Obstet 1975;140:85.
26. Fry DE, Garrison RN, et al. Determinants of death in patients with intra-abdominal abscess. Surgery 1980;88:517.
27. Fry DE, Pearlstein L, Fulton RL: Multiple system organ failure: the role of uncontrolled infection. Arch Surg 1980;115:136.
28. Fulton RL, Jones CE: The cause of post-traumatic pulmonary insufficiency in man. Surg Gynecol Obstet 1975;140:179.
29. Gerzof SG, Johnson WC, Robbins AH, et al. Expanded criteria for percutaneous abscess drainage. Arch Surg 1985;120:227.
30. Gerzof SG, Johnson WC, Robbins AH, et al. Intrahepatic pyogenic abscesses: treatment by percutaneous drainage. Am J Surg 1985;149:487.
31. Gerzof SG, Robbins AH, Johnson WC, et al. Percutaneous catheter drainage of abdominal abscesses: a five-year experience. N Engl J Med 1981;305:653.
32. Goris, RJ, Boekhorst, TPA, Nuytinck, KE, et al. Multiple-organ failure. Arch Surg 1985;120:1109.
33. Halsz N: Synchronous intraabdominal abscesses. JAMA 1970;214:724.

34. Hau T, Haaga JR, Aeder MI: Pathophysiology, diagnosis, and treatment of abdominal abscesses: anatomy of the peritoneal cavity. Curr Probl Surg 1984;21:8.

35. Hedderich GS, Wexler MJ, McLean APH, et al. The septic abdomen: open management with Marlex Mesh with a zipper. Surgery 1986;99:399.

36. Hiatt JR, Calabria RP, Wilson SE. Septic dehiscence of the abdominal wound. Infect Surg 1986:429.

37. Hildell J, Aspelin P, Wehlin L: Gray scale ultrasound and endoscopic ductography in the diagnosis of pancreatic disease. Acta Chir Scand 1979;145:239.

38. Jaffe CC: Medical imaging: many different techniques compete for attention, but each has unique strengths and applications. Am Scientist 1982;70:576.

39. Johnson WC, Gerzof SG, Robbins AH, et al. Treatment of abdominal abscesses: comparative evaluation of operative drainage versus percutaneous catheter drainage guided by computed tomography or ultrasound. Ann Surg 1981;194:510.

40. Kane RA.: Ultrasonographic diagnosis of gangrenous cholecystitis and empyema of the gallbladder. Radiology 1980;124:191.

41. Karlson KB, Fankuchen EI, Casarella WJ. Percutaneous abscess drainage. Surg Gynecol Obstet 1982;154:44.

42. Krishnamurthy GT: Acute cholecystitis: the diagnostic role for current imaging tests. West J Med 1982;127:87.

43. Lally KP, Trettin JC, Torma MJ. Adjunctive antibiotic lavage in experimental peritonitis. Surg Gynecol Obstet 1983;156:605.

44. Lennard ES, Dellinger EP, Wertz MJ, et al. Implications of leukocytosis and fever at conclusion of antibiotic therapy for intra-abdominal sepsis. Ann Surg 1982;195:19.

45. Levitt RG, Biello DR, Sagel SS, et al. Computed tomography and ^{67}Ga citrate radionuclide imaging for evaluating suspected abdominal abscess. AJR 1979;132:529.

46. Lores ME, Ortiz JR, Rosello PJ. Peritoneal lavage with povidone–iodine solution in experimentally induced peritonitis. Surg Gynecol Obstet 1981;153:33.

47. Mahony BS, Callen PW: Sonography in the detection of intra-abdominal abscesses. Infect Surg 1984:691.

48. Mandel SR, Boyd D, Jacques PF, et al. Drainage of hepatic, intra-abdominal, and mediastinal abscesses guided by computerized axial tomography. Am J Surg 1983;145:120.

49. Matolo NM, Stadalnik RC, McGahan JP: Comparison of ultrasonography, computerized tomography and radionuclide imaging in the diagnosis of acute and chronic cholecystitis. Am J Surg 1982;144:676.

50. McKenna JP, Currie PJ, McDonald JA. The use of continuous post-operative peritoneal lavage in the management of diffuse peritonitis. Surg Gynecol Obstet 1970;130:254.

51. McLean GK, Mackie JA, Freiman DB, et al. Enterocutaneous fistulae: interventional radiologic management. AJR 1982;138:615.

52. Miedema BW, Dineen P: The diagnosis and treatment of pyogenic liver abscesses. Ann Surg 1984;200:328.

53. Miller MH, Frederick PR, Tocino I, et al. Percutaneous catheter drainage of intraabdominal fluid collections including infected biliary ducts and gallbladders. Am J Surg 1982;144:660.

54. Moir C, Robins RE: Role of ultrasonography, gallium scanning, and computed tomography in the diagnosis of intraabdominal abscess. Am J Surg 1982;142:582.

55. Moss JP. Historical and current perspectives on surgical drainage. Surg Gynecol Obstet 1981;152:517.

56. Moukhtar M, Romney S. Continuous intraperitoneal antibiotic lavage in the management of purulent sepsis of the pelvis. Surg Gynecol Obstet 1980;150:548.

57. Ochsner A, DeBakey M: Suphrenic abscess: collective review and an analysis of 3608 collected and personal cases. Surg Gynecol Obstet 1938;66:429.

58. Ozeran RS: Subdiaphragmatic abscess: diagnosis and treatment. Am Surg 1967;33:65.

59. Palestrant AM, Vine HS, Sacks BA, et al. Nonoperative drainage of fluid collections following operations on the biliary tract. Surg Gynecol Obstet 1983;156:305.

60. Penninckx FM, Kerremans RP, Lauwers PM: Planned relaparotomies in the surgical treatment of severe generalized peritonitis from intestinal origin. World J Surg 1982;7:762.

61. Pepe PE, Hudson LD, Carrico CJ: Early application of positive end-expiratory pressure in patients at risk for the adult respiratory-distress syndrome. N Engl J Med 1984;311:281.

62. Pine RW, Wertz MJ, Lenneard ES, et al. Determinants of organ malfunction or death in patients with intra-abdominal sepsis. Arch Surg 1983;118:2442.

63. Pitcher WD, Musher DM: Critical importance of early diagnosis and treatment of intra-abdominal infection. Arch Surg 1983;117:328.

64. Polk HC, Fry DE. Radical peritoneal debridement for established peritonitis. Ann Surg 1980;192:350.

130

65. Polk HC, Shields CL: Remote organ failure: a valid sign of occult intra-abdominal infection. Surgery 1977;81:310.
66. Pruett TL, Rothstein OD, Crass J, et al. Percutaneous aspiration and drainage for suspected abdominal infection. Surgery 1984;96:731.
67. Ranson JHC, Balthazar E, Caccavale R, et al. Computed tomography and the prediction of pancreatic abscess in acute pancreatitis. Ann Surg 1985;201:656.
68. Rose JG, Hiatt JR: Noninvasive methods for detection of intra-abdominal abscess. Infect Surg 1983:347.
69. Saini S, Mueller PR, Wittenberg J, et al. Percutaneous drainage of diverticular abscess. Arch Surg 1986;121:475.
70. Sanders RC: The changing epidemiology of subphrenic abscess and its clinical and radiological consequences. Br J Surg 1970;57:449.
71. Sheinfeld AM, Steiner AE, Rivkin LB, et al. Transcutaneous drainage of abscesses of the liver guided by computed tomography scan. Surg Gynecol Obstet 1982;155:662.
72. Shimshak RR, Korobkin M, Hoffer PB, et al: The complementary role of gallium citrate imaging and computed tomography in the evaluation of suspected infection. J Nucl Med 1978;19:262.
73. Silenas R, O'Keefe P, Gelbart S, et al. Mechanical effectiveness of closed peritoneal irrigation in peritonitis. Am J Surg 1983;145:371.
74. Sinanan M, Maier RV, Carrico CJ: Laparotomy for intra-abdominal sepsis in patients in an intensive care unit. Arch Surg 1984;119:652.
75. Skau T, Nystrom PO, Carlsson C. Severity of illness in intra-abdominal infection. Arch Surg 1985;120:152.
76. Stone HH, Bourneuf AA, Stinson LD. Reliability of criteria for predicting persistent or recurrent sepsis. Arch Surg 1985;120:17.
77. Stone HH, Mullins RJ, Dunlop WE, et al. Extraperitoneal versus transperitoneal drainage of the intra-abdominal abscess. Surg Gynecol Obstet 1984;159:549.
78. Walters R, Herman CM, Neff R, et al. Percutaneous drainage of abscesses in the postoperative abdomen that is difficult to explore. Am J Surg 1985;149:623.
79. Warshaw AL. Surgical pros and cons. Surg Gynecol Obstet 1980;151:547.
80. Welch CE. Catheter drainage of abdominal abscesses. N Engl J Med 1981;305:694.
81. Whalen JP: Radiology of the abdomen: impact of new imaging methods. AJR 1979;133:585.
82. Zeman RK, Burrell MI, Cahow CE, et al: Diagnostic utility of cholescintigraphy and ultrasonography in acute cholecystis. Am J Surg 1981;1414:446.

6

○   ○   ○   ●   ●   ●

ANTIBIOTIC PROPHYLAXIS IN GASTROINTESTINAL SURGERY

Robert E. Condon

Antibiotic prophylaxis in surgery refers to the administration of antibiotic or antimicrobial drugs to patients who do not have evidence of an established infection. The objective is to reduce the risks of postoperative infectious complications. Nearly half of all antibiotics administered are given for prophylaxis, and nearly all of these antibiotic prescriptions are written by surgeons.

At one time, administration of antibiotics for prophylaxis was a very controversial issue and was a practice condemned by many surgeons. During the past two decades, however, surgeons have had the benefit of the results from a relatively large number of properly organized and controlled clinical trials that have addressed the issue of antibiotic prophylaxis. Although all of the debate in this arena is by no means resolved, we are presently in a position to answer the major question positively. Antimicrobials definitely have a place in the management of patients undergoing selected operations on the gastrointestinal tract. Appropriately administered antibiotic prophylaxis will, in the typical case, reduce the risk of infection by about half.

Antibiotics cannot completely eliminate all risk of infection, however, and sterility or total absence of sepsis is not an appropriate objective of prophylactic antibiotic administration. Further, antibiotics are not a substitute for good surgical practices. Low infection rates are best obtained by strict adherence to exquisite surgical technique. Other factors that will help to keep the infection risk at a minimum include a short preoperative stay in the hospital, preoperative bathing with an antiseptic soap, minimizing the duration of the operation and anesthetic, and avoiding shaving or clipping hair until just prior to the operative skin preparation.

Residual controversy under active discussion today is focused on the duration of antibiotic prophylaxis, the selection of competing drugs and, in the context of colorectal operations, the choice of oral versus parenteral administration of antibiotic prophylaxis.

PRINCIPLES OF PARENTERAL PROPHYLAXIS

In order for parenterally administered antimicrobial agents to be fully effective in achieving the objectives of prophylaxis, adherence to the following principles is important:

1. *Choose a fully effective drug.* The antibacterial spectrum of the antibiotic or combination of antibiotics chosen for prophylaxis should be effective against all of the major potential pathogens likely to be encountered during the operation. While administration of antibiotics effective against only a portion of the spectrum of pathogens often will improve the end results and lower the incidence of infections, such incomplete treatment is not as effective as covering the entire bacterial spectrum.

2. *Administer a fully effective dose.* In certain quarters there is a notion that minimal, or even suboptimal, doses of antibiotics are sufficient for prophylactic purposes. This is not correct. When administered for prophylaxis, fully effective doses of an antibiotic should be administered. Usually, maximal doses are chosen, particularly if antibiotic prophylaxis is to be only a single dose or be administered only on the operative day.

3. *Short duration of antibiotic administration.* Prophylactic antibiotics need not be administered for more than 3 days in any case. In most surgical contexts, a single preoperative dose of antimicrobial is sufficient; in nearly all clinical situations, antibiotic prophylaxis limited to the operative day has been demonstrated to be as effective as administration of antibiotics for longer periods.

4. *Choose the least toxic drug.* Obviously, the least toxic drug or drug combination is to be preferred among those alternatives that will cover the required antibacterial spectrum.

5. *Avoid drugs that are useful for treatment of serious sepsis.* Whenever possible, the drugs chosen for prophylaxis should be those that are less essential for treatment of complicated infections in hospitalized patients. For example, prophylactic administration of ampicillin is preferable to administration of an aminoglycoside. Similarly, prophylactic administration of a first-generation cephalosporin is much preferred over administration of a third-generation cephalosporin.

In addition to following the principles enumerated above, constant updating of information concerning the current antibiotic sensitivities of bacteria recovered in each hospital in which the surgeon works is essential to provide the basis for an optimal choice of drugs for prophylaxis.

INDICATIONS FOR ANTIBIOTIC PROPHYLAXIS

As is true in other clinical situations, a judgment to employ antibiotic prophylaxis results from consideration of the relative risks and benefits. The obvious benefit is a reduction in the incidence of infections and their consequences. The concomitant risks involve the possible appearance of toxic or allergic reactions, superinfection in the patient by bacteria or fungi, and alteration of the hospital flora toward predominance of resistant strains as a result of more widespread institutional antibiotic use.

The incidence of both toxic and allergic reactions to most antibiotics that would be considered for prophylactic administration is sufficiently small that, when appropriate, antibiotic prophylaxis should not be withheld. Similarly, bacterial and fungal overgrowth in a patient requires relatively long-term administration of antibiotics. Bacterial superinfection has not been a problem in patients receiving antibiotics as a single dose or only on the operative day. Alteration of the bacterial flora in the hospital environment is a probable consequence of antibiotic use and is seen most clearly in those hospital locations, such as an intensive care unit, in which prolonged antibiotic administration is a regular practice.

Whether the administration of high doses of antibiotics is the essential factor leading to emergence of resistant bacterial strains, or whether the chronic presence of even tiny amounts of antibiotic in the hospital environment is sufficient to induce bacterial mutation, is an unsettled matter. But, it has been a regular observation that bacterial resistance evolves and increases as antibiotics are introduced into hospital practice; this appears to be a consequence that is not easily avoided. Therefore, avoidance of use for prophylactic purposes of antibiotics that are essential for treating more serious forms of established sepsis is important and reinforces adherence to this principle of antibiotic prophylaxis.

The accepted indications for antibiotic prophylaxis are conduct of a clean–contaminated operation and operations involving the insertion of a prosthesis. Less well accepted indications include clean operations in patients with impaired host defenses or in patients in whom the consequences of infection may be very morbid.

Clean–Contaminated Operations. For shorthand purposes, these can be thought of as those operations that may open into one of the hollow visceral systems of the body that harbor an endogenous bacterial flora. In addition, operations for trauma in which spillage from a hollow viscus is absent also are viewed as clean–contaminated cases.

In this class of operations, the bacterial density in the wound may exceed the threshold of 10^6 organisms per gram of tissue at which increased risk of infection begins to occur. The bacterial concentrations actually found in clean–contaminated wounds, however, are rarely much higher than 10^8 or 10^9 organisms per gram of tissue. Thus, tissue contamination in clean–contaminated operations can be sufficiently heavy to produce an increased risk of septic complications, but the contamination is not so dense as to make suppuration inevitable.

Clean Operations Involving Insertion of a Prosthesis or Other Foreign Body. The presence of a prosthesis (foreign body) disables wound healing and local wound defense mechanisms and results in an increase in the underlying wound infection risk. For most operations, the presence of the prosthesis doubles the infection risk compared to a similar operation not involving the insertion of a foreign body. In effect, the insertion of a prosthesis moves the infection risk from that associated with a clean operation to that of the clean–contaminated class. Administration of effective antibiotic prophylaxis will reduce the infection risk associated with insertion of a prosthesis to that obtained with an otherwise clean operation not involving the insertion of a prosthesis.

Clean Operations in Patients with Impaired Host Defenses. The evidence supporting this indication is indirect and derives from the treatment of patients undergoing chemotherapy and who have associated severe leukopenia. Treatment of these compromised patients with continuous administration of antibiotics and provision of in-hospital care under conditions of protective isolation both are associated with a reduction in the incidence of septic episodes. Because antibiotic administration reduces the risks of sepsis in a compromised host, it is assumed by extrapolation that antibiotics administered to patients with less severely impaired host defense mechanisms will also be efficacious.

Clean Operations in which Infection Constitutes a Disaster. This indication remains the most controversial for antibiotic prophylaxis. It has not been possible to establish the efficacy of antibiotic prophylaxis in this setting. The difficulty arises from the fact that the incidence of infection in these clean cases is already sufficiently low that inordinately large numbers of patients would have to be studied under strictly controlled conditions in order to demonstrate possible efficacy. The studies would require such large numbers of patients that they are unmanageable in any practical clinical sense. Therefore, the known efficacy of antibiotic prophylaxis in clean–contaminated operations has been extrapolated to clean operations in neurosurgery, cardiac surgery, and ophthalmology.

TIMING, DURATION, AND ROUTE OF ADMINISTRATION OF ANTIBIOTIC PROPHYLAXIS

Timing

The classic work of Miles, Miles, and Burke[10] established that prophylactic antibiotics needed to be present in tissue at the time bacterial contamination occurs. In his experiments, Burke[2] showed that administration of antibiotics before or at the time of tissue contamination was associated with a negligibly increased infection risk. But, as antibiotic administration was delayed, infection risk increased; antibiotics administered more than 4 hours after tissue contamination had no effect. Burke's observations were of *Staphylococcus aureus* and have long been believed to be applicable to all aerobic organisms. More recently, the fact that this principle applies also to prophylaxis against anaerobic organisms was established by the work of Shapiro and colleagues,[14] studying a similar experimental model in which the pathogen inoculated was *Bacteroides fragilis*. Numerous clinical studies have confirmed the experimental observations. For example, Stone's study[15] recorded a decrease in wound infection rate from 14% in controls to 3.5% in patients receiving timely antibiotic prophylaxis in association with a variety of abdominal operations.

Parenteral antibiotics in fully effective doses generally should be administered as an intravenous infusion beginning 30 minutes before the operation begins, or 1 to 2 hours before potential intraoperative tissue contamination is likely to occur. This timing interval results in the presence of therapeutic drug levels in the wound and related tissues during operation and at the time of tissue contamination, but does not readily allow the development of bacterial resistance to the antibiotic.

Duration

The duration of antibiotic prophylaxis is a much less settled matter because data concerning many classes of operations are lacking. But, whenever this issue has been examined critically, short-term prophylaxis has been shown to be as effective as longer term prophylaxis. Several studies have established the efficacy of short-term prophylaxis in orthopedic surgery, as well as in gynecologic operations and in cardiac surgery. Recently, the report of Strachan and colleagues[16] has demonstrated that short-term prophylaxis is as effective as longer term therapy in patients undergoing cholecystectomy. Dellinger and associates[7] have shown that 12 hours of doxycycline and penicillin prophylaxis was as effective in patients with penetrating abdominal trauma as was 5 days of this antibiotic therapy.

When prophylaxis is accomplished with orally administered antibiotics, as is the usual practice in elective colon and rectal resection operations, the oral antibiotic agent should be administered during the 24-hour period immediately prior to operation. Longer periods of preoperative oral antibiotic administration are not necessary and have been associated with the isolation of resistant organisms within the colonic lumen at the time of resection.[4,9,11]

Route

Among the various routes by which parenteral prophylactic antibiotics can be administered, intravenous administration is preferred in most surgical patients. Alexander and Alexander[1] have studied the kinetics of distribution in tissue fluid following administration of antibiotics by various routes. Administration of antibiotics intravenously in a relatively small volume of diluent over a short (20- to 30-minute) period of time results in high serum levels, which are reflected in more rapid entry and higher early concentration of antibiotics in wound fluid and, presumably, wound tissues. Administration of parenteral antibiotics by other routes produces lower peak blood levels and retarded entry of antibiotics into tissue.

Topical application of antibiotics to wound surfaces and body cavities is an arena in which theory and practice are not in consonance. Because antibiotics inhibit bacterial growth by interfering with metabolism and replication, rather than by acting as a topical microbicide (as does iodine), it is difficult to explain on theoretical grounds the effectiveness of topically applied antibiotics in controlling wound infections. The studies of Edlich[8] and of Robson[12] demonstrated that systemic absorption of antibiotics and, indeed, penetration of antibiotics into wound tissues is limited following topical application to the wound. Perhaps, topically applied antibiotics are effective because they establish a high local concentration of drug within the wound. By whatever mechanism topically applied antibiotics do act, they have been demonstrated in some clinical contexts, particularly in patients undergoing appendectomy for acute appendicitis, to reduce significantly the incidence of wound infection and other septic complications of operation.

TYPICAL PATHOGENS

Three major groups of bacteria may be encountered in the course of a gastrointestinal operation: the organisms derived from the environment (exogenous flora), and the two major groups of endogenous gastrointestinal organisms (the oral and the fecal flora). The solid organs, such as the liver and spleen, do not harbor a resident microflora. It is the hollow visceral systems that house bacteria.

Knowledge of the specific bacteria that constitute the exogenous or environmental flora, together with knowledge of those bacteria constituting the endogenous flora at various body sites, is the basis on which the bacteria likely to be associated with a septic surgical complication can be anticipated. Additionally, up-to-date knowledge concerning the antimicrobial sensitivity of the major pathogens within each of these flora is essential to guide a rational choice of antibiotics for prophylaxis.

The bacterial flora of the environment and of various body sites are relatively predictable and are summarized in Table 6-1. In Table 6-1, the most common pathogens of concern are indicated by boldface type. No single antibiotic can be relied on for effective prophylaxis in all clinical settings. The antibiotic or antibiotics employed must be chosen on the basis of their efficacy against the microorganisms that usually cause infectious complications in association with a specific operation.

Table 6–1
Typical Pathogens

AEROBES	ANAEROBES
ENVIRONMENTAL (Exogenous)	
Staphylococcus aureus	Clostridium sp.
Staphylococcus epidermidis group	
E. coli	
Pseudomonas sp.	
Citrobacter sp.	
Enterobacter sp.	
MOUTH-PHARYNX (Oral)	
Streptococcus viridans	**Peptostreptococcus sp.**
Streptococcus salivarius	**Bacteroides (oral) sp.**
Neisseria sp.	Veillonella sp.
Candida sp.	Fusobacterium sp.
Staphylococcus aureus	
Actinomyces sp.	
BILIARY TRACT	
E. coli	Clostridium sp.
Klebsiella sp.	Peptostreptococcus sp.
Enterococcus group	Bacteroides sp.
Proteus sp.	
COLON (including appendix and distal small bowel)	
E. coli	**B. fragilis** group
Klebsiella sp.	**Peptostreptococcus sp.**
Proteus sp.	**Clostridium sp.**
Pseudomonas sp.	B. melaninogenicus
Enterococcus group	other Bacteroides sp.
Streptococcus sp.	Eubacterium sp.
Enterobacter sp.	Fusobacterium sp.
Staphylococcus aureus	
Candida sp.	

Environmental Flora. The environmental flora is composed predominantly of aerobic organisms, because most anaerobes are unable to survive in the oxygen concentration of room air. Regular representation is present of the various members of the *Staphylococcus epidermidis* group, as well as of *Staphylococcus aureus* and the coliforms, predominantly *Escherichia coli.* In hospitals, particularly in intensive care units and in other settings where antibiotic treatment pressure enhances the emergence of resistant organisms, additional aerobic organisms will be found regularly in the environmental flora. These latter bacteria include *Pseudomonas* *aeruginosa* and other *Pseudomonas* species, *Citrobacter* species and *Enterobacter* species.

In wounds that have been contaminated by soil, *Clostridium* species are the only anaerobes that regularly affect humans. The reason that clostridia are able to survive in the oxygen concentration of our environment is that they readily form spores. There are, of course, literally hundreds of other different bacterial species present in the environment, mostly soil saprophytes. But, these organisms usually do not act as pathogens (*i.e.*, become tissue invasive) in humans.

Oral Microflora. The mouth and pharynx normally harbor a luxuriant microflora composed of both aerobic and anaerobic microorganisms. The concentration of bacteria in saliva is approximately 10^6 organisms per milliliter. This mixed flora includes aerobic species such as streptococci, staphylococci, and *Branhamella*, as well as *Candida* and *Actinomyces*. The anaerobic component is composed predominantly of peptostreptococci and the oral *Bacteroides* group, with lesser numbers of fusobacteria and *Veillonella.*

Extremely anaerobic conditions (Eh below -300 mv) exist in dental plaque and in the gingival sulcus, providing an ideal environment for the growth of oral anaerobes. Good dental hygiene and adequate nutrition contribute to prevention of overgrowth of these organisms. Conversely, if oral hygiene is poor, periodontal disease develops due to tissue invasion by these anaerobic bacteria. Additionally, decaying teeth and similar attributes of poor dental hygiene provide an opportunity for aerobic coliforms from the environment to lodge and become a part of the oral flora.

The oral flora transiently contaminates the esophagus during swallowing, and organisms derived from the oral and the environmental flora regularly become resident in the esophagus if obstruction or stasis are present. The swallowed organisms of the oral and the environmental flora ordinarily are killed rapidly by the acid normally present in gastric juice. Thus, the normal stomach does not harbor a resident flora, and the effluent from the fasting stomach does not ordinarily bring about bacterial contamination of the upper small bowel. In patients with an impaired ability to secrete hydrochloric acid, and in patients who have been treated with H_2 blocker drugs, swallowed oral and environmental organisms may become resident in the stomach.

Fecal Microflora. In most patients, the distal ileum harbors a resident microflora that is thought to result from backwash of bacteria from the cecum and colon through the ileocecal valve. Concentrations of bacteria average 10^4 to 10^5 per milliliter of distal ileal content. *Bacteroides fragilis* and other fecal anaerobes first appear as residents at this level of the bowel. Beyond the ileocecal valve, a striking increase occurs in the numbers of both aerobic and anaerobic organisms. *Escherichia coli*, the most prevalent of the aerobes, is found in concentrations of 10^6 to 10^9 bacteria per gram of colon content. *Bacteroides fragilis*, the most frequently encountered anaerobe, is isolated in concentrations of 10^8 to 10^{11} organisms per gram of colon content.

The predominance of anaerobes in the large bowel is because of the ideal environment, which includes both stasis and low oxidation-reduction potential (Eh of -150 mv or below). Fungi, especially *Candida*, and staphylococci are also regularly present in feces, although in low concentrations. The normally luxuriant flora in the colon, in terms of both its aerobic and anaerobic organisms, increases in concentration even further whenever mechanical obstruction is present. Concentrations of bacteria approaching 10^{12} organisms per gram of intestinal content, the theoretical upper concentration limit if fecal bacteria are optimally packed, are recovered regularly from obstructed bowel. In addition, the character of the stool above an obstruction tends to become somewhat more fluid.

The principal aerobic bacteria of the fecal flora include coliforms, streptococci, lactobacilli, and fungi. The anaerobic organisms include *B. fragilis* and other members of the *Bacteroides* group, as well as oral *Bacteroides*, peptostreptococci, bifidobacteria, fusobacteria, clostridia, and eubacteria.

Biliary Microflora. The biliary tract, including the liver, rarely harbors bacteria in normal persons. In the presence of chronic calculous cholecystitis, bacteria can be isolated in up to two thirds of patients. The older the patient with chronic calculous cholecystitis, the greater the chance of a positive bile culture. Almost all patients 80 years of age or older will have a positive bile culture. Cultures of the gallbladder wall will yield a higher percentage of positive cultures than will culture only of gallbladder bile. Quantitative bile cultures have shown concentrations of bacteria in most biliary disease states to be less than 10^5 viable organisms per milliliter of bile; patients with cholangitis may harbor higher concentrations, however, ranging up to 10^9 to 10^{11} bacteria per milliliter of bile.

Of patients found to have acute cholecystitis at operation, about half will have positive cultures of gallbladder bile or gallbladder wall, while in advanced acute disease, such as empyema of the gallbladder, nearly all will have positive cultures. Common duct obstruction due to stone or stricture will result in a positive culture of common duct bile in more than 85% of patients. When the common duct obstruction is due to neoplasm or pancreatitis, on the other hand, only about 10% of patients have a positive common duct bile culture.

The bacteria isolated from bile in all disease states of the biliary tract are primarily gram-negative enteric aerobic coliforms. *E. coli,* alone or mixed with other organisms, is present in more than half of positive cultures. Other coliforms, principally *Klebsiella,* also are regularly present; *Proteus* and *Enterobacter* are less commonly isolated. Organisms of the group-D enterococcal group (*Enterococcus faecalis, Enterococcus faecium*) are aerobic gram-positive cocci that also are frequently isolated from bile. Their pathogenic role remains somewhat controversial.

Anaerobic microorganisms are isolated only rarely in patients with cholecystitis. In the presence of common duct stone or stricture, anaerobic organisms still are isolated infrequently, being present in about 20% of cases. *Clostridium perfringens* is the most commonly isolated anaerobic organism. A polymicrobial infection, caused by both aerobic and anaerobic organisms, and in which *B. fragilis* and other fecal anaerobes will sometimes be found to participate, is present in liver abscess, long-standing common duct obstruction due to choledocholithiasis, and in patients with suppurative acute cholangitis.

SPECIFIC CONSIDERATIONS IN GASTROINTESTINAL OPERATIONS

Many of the published controlled trials of antibiotic efficacy involve relatively small numbers of patients. These studies typically fail to demonstrate any difference between two drug regimens under study, primarily because of the small size of the denominator. Sometimes, erroneously, the failure to demonstrate a difference is interpreted as indicating that the two regimens are equally efficacious. This is a type II error, because failure to demonstrate a difference never indicates identity.

The data from these multiple studies of small numbers of patients can be useful, however, to help establish the relative efficacy of various antibiotic regimens through techniques of pooling[13] in which identical treatment regimens from multiple studies are taken together, increasing the size of the denominator and, sometimes, making relative judgments about efficacy possible. Although certain precautions need to be taken when data are pooled, the technique is useful and has been used in evaluation of data presented in Tables 6-2, 6-3, and 6-5 through 6-8.

Esophagus

The esophagus lacks a serosa and has a poor blood supply so that leaks of esophageal anastomoses are relatively frequent. Cyclic negative intrathoracic pressure exerted on the postoperative esophagus also promotes anastomotic leakage. Careful studies demonstrate that about 40% of all esophageal anastomoses and closures of esophageal wounds develop at least a minor leak; up to 10% have a major leak causing some degree of clinical mediastinitis. Therefore, the potential for mediastinal contamination following operations on the esophagus is great.

The esophagus does not have a resident flora but is regularly contaminated by swallowed oral and environmental microorganisms. If the patient has been receiving antibiotics for more than 4 or 5 days, the numbers of *Candida* swallowed also markedly increase. Effective peristalsis sweeps most of these organisms into the stomach. Postoperatively, however, the degree of oral contamination is increased and the effectiveness of esophageal swallowing–sweeping is reduced, thereby enhancing the infection risk. In the presence of esophageal obstruction—either mechanical or functional—the esophagus rapidly acquires a resident flora composed of a mixture of fecal aerobes plus oral aerobes and anaerobes.

We employ a single preoperative IV dose of 2 g of cefazolin in elective operations on the unobstructed esophagus. In the presence of obstruction—mechanical or functional—we decompress the esophagus above the obstruction with a nasogastric tube, and irrigate the lumen of the esophagus preoperatively with 1% kanamycin solution. In emergency operations for esophageal perforation, IV cefazolin is administered preoperatively and is continued postoperatively as clinically indicated.

Stomach

The normal stomach is an effective sterilizer of swallowed bacteria. Indeed, 30 minutes of contact with normal gastric acid juice serves to kill even relatively protected encapsulated organisms, such as *Mycobacterium tuberculosis*. The transit time across the normal fasting stomach is 30 minutes. Thus, no resident flora occupies the lumen of the normal stomach and essentially no microorganisms are passed into the duodenum or upper small bowel in the fasting state in a patient whose gastric acid barrier is intact.

Diseases involving the gastric mucous membrane—chronic gastritis, gastric ulcer, gastric carcinoma, pernicious anemia—are all associated with diminished to absent secretion of hydrochloric acid and consequent impairment of the gastric barrier. Administration of drugs that block acid secretion (cimetidine, ranitidine) also disables the normal gastric bacterial barrier mechanism. In patients with an impaired gastric barrier, viable bacteria are transmitted across the stomach and contaminate the duodenum and upper small bowel in the fasting state, and a resident flora comes to occupy the lumen of the stomach. Other patients may have acute disorders that also interfere with the acid gastric barrier. Patients with a bleeding duodenal ulcer and those with gastric outlet obstruction (abnormal motility) may be capable of acid secretion, but nonetheless have an ineffective gastric barrier due to dilution or buffering.

Experience with antibiotic prophylaxis is summarized in Table 6-2. Clinically, all patients with gastric mucosal disease, those with gastric outlet obstruction or hemorrhage as an indication for operation, and all those treated with H_2 blocker drugs, are at increased risk of postoperative infection. The organisms involved in these "failed barrier" patients are the aerobic and anaerobic oral bacteria together with moderate numbers of fecal aerobes, especially *E. coli.* In such patients, we administer 2 g IV

Table 6–2
Antibiotic Prophylaxis in Esophago-Gastro-Duodenal Operations*

TREATMENT	NO. STUDIES	NO. PATIENTS	NO. INFECTED	% INFECTED
None (placebo)	12	307	103	33
Cephaloridine	5	145	3	2†
Cefuroxime	2	47	3	6†
Cefamandole	2	44	1	2†
Aminoglycoside-clindamycin	2	39	4	10
Penicillins	2	55	7	13
Cephalothin	1	33	0	†
Cefazolin	1	49	2	4†
Moxalactam	1	9	1	11
Cefotaxime	1	30	3	10
Cefuroxime-metronidazole	1	21	2	10

* *Pooled data of 16 reports, 1969–1984; 779 patients, all indications.*
† *Indicates significant reduction in infections compared with no antibiotic prophylaxis.*

cefazolin with induction of anesthesia, and repeat this dose every 8 hours during the day of operation.

Small Bowel

Because of the effective gastric acid barrier in normal persons, the upper small bowel in the fasting state possesses no resident flora. The upper small bowel is transiently contaminated with swallowed microorganisms during and for 1 to 2 hours after ingestion of a meal, but then the normal state of near sterility is restored. Beginning in the mid-ileum, the distal small bowel acquires a flora due to backwash from the cecum through the ileocecal valve. In the distal 2 feet of ileum, a fecal aerobic–anaerobic microflora is always resident.

Obstructed small bowel rapidly accumulates a large volume of luminal secretion, which, essentially, can be viewed as fluid feces. The source of the microorganisms in small bowel obstruction is not precisely known, but most of the bacteria probably are derived from distal small bowel and contaminate proximal small bowel retrogradely just prior to complete bowel obstruction. Every effort should be made intraoperatively in the management of small bowel obstruction *not to open* the bowel. Bowel decompression by open suction, or by any enterotomy, is associated with a sixfold increase in the risk of septic complications. As an alternative, a long tube can be passed through the nose preoperatively. Or, a tube such as the Nelson-Baker tube can be passed through a gastrostomy. On occasion, entry into obstructed small bowel or resection of obstructed segments is necessary; in such cases, the operation should be viewed as contaminated, and the skin and subcutaneous tissues should be left open.

In operations on normal small bowel, no antibiotic prophylaxis is needed. In patients with a failed gastric barrier having an elective operation, and in all emergency operations on obstructed small bowel, we administer cefoxitin, 2 g IV preoperatively and then 1 g IV every 4 hours to the end of the operative day. If intraoperative contamination occurs, antibiotics are continued as clinically indicated.

Appendix

The appendix contains a rich fecal flora, identical to that of the rest of the colon and rectum. Aerobic coliforms, especially *E. coli,* seem to predominate in appendix-related wound infections while fecal anaerobes, particularly *Peptostreptococcus* and *B. fragilis* group organisms, have a more important role in appendiceal abscess, peritonitis, and postoperative intra-abdominal infections. A variety of antibiotics have been prescribed for prophylaxis in association with appendectomy; nearly all of them seem to have some positive effect (Table 6-3).

Our practice is to administer 2 g of cefoxitin IV with induction of anesthesia. If the appendix is normal, no further antibiotics are given. If the appendix is inflamed but not gangrenous or perforated, a second 2-g IV dose of cefoxitin is given 4 hours after the first dose; no further antibiotics are administered. If the appendix is perforated or gangrenous, the subcutaneous wound is not closed and antibiotics are administered as clinically indicated.

Table 6–3
Antibiotic Prophylaxis of Appendicitis*

TREATMENT	NO. STUDIES	NO. PATIENTS	NO. INFECTED	% INFECTED
None (placebo)	53	4,094	722	17.6
Ampicillin	2	114	34	20
Cefazolin	4	312	88	28
Cephaloridine	4	191	22	12
Cefamandole	4	184	33	18
Cefoxitin	3	152	27	18
Cefoperazone	2	89	13	15
Metronidazole	28	2,701	319	11†
Clindamycin	3	262	34	13
Aminoglycoside-clindamycin-penicillin	8	387	23	6†
Aminoglycoside-metronidazole	2	61	15	25
Aminoglycoside-penicillin	2	108	12	11
Cefotaxime-metronidazole	2	265	29	11
Ceforanide-clindamycin	1	34	3	9
Cefamandole-carbenicillin	1	45	0	
Ampicillin-metronidazole	1	142	19	13
Amoxicillin clavulanate	1	115	13	11
Ticarcillin	1	92	8	9
Tetracycline	1	83	1	2†
Imipenem	1	33	1	3†
Moxalactam	1	27	1	4†
Cefotaxime	1	103	13	13

* *Pooled data of 77 reports, 1956–1986; 11,756 patients, all stages.*
† *Indicates significant reduction in infections compared with no antibiotic prophylaxis.*

Colon

The colon contains a dense aerobic–anaerobic microflora. Operations on the colon without prophylactic antibiotic cover are associated with a 40% risk of wound infection or other major septic complication. Achieving a reduction in the risk of infectious complications associated with elective colorectal operations involves two linked actions: thorough mechanical cleansing of gross feces from the colon lumen followed by administration of antibiotics. Both mechanical cleansing and antibiotic administration are essential; either alone is less effective. Indeed, mechanical preparation alone without antibiotics is almost as risky as no preparation at all.

Our preference, supported by our own clinical trials[3,6] as well as the experience of others, is for oral antibiotic preparation in elective cases (Table 6-4). Combination chemotherapy with an aminoglycoside (neomycin or kanamycin) together with a

Table 6–4
Regimen for Oral Antibiotic Prophylaxis for Colorectal Operations

Mechanical Colon Cleansing (lavage method)

Pre-op day 1 Pass NG tube, weigh patient, determine serum potassium.
Start polyethylene glycol by NG tube at 9 A.M. Initial rate 1000 ml/20 min; adjust rate to minimize cramps and distention.
Place patient on commode. Continue lavage to (a) minimum volume of 10 liters, and (b) until anal effluent clear.
At end of lavage: weight patient, determine serum potassium; order IV fluids or diuretics, if needed.

Catharsis Method (an alternative to lavage)

Pre-op day 3 Minimum residue or clear liquid diet.
Bisacodyl, 1 capsule orally at 6 P.M.

Pre-op day 2 Minimum residue or clear liquid diet.
Magnesium sulphate, 30 ml of 50% solution (15 g) orally at 10 A.M., 2 P.M., 6 P.M.
Saline enemas in evening (modified three-position technique) until final returns are clear.

Pre-op day 1 Clear liquid diet.
Magnesium sulphate (in dose above) at 10 A.M. and 2 P.M.
Supplemental IV fluids as needed.
No enemas.

Antibiotic Preparation

Pre-op day 1 Neomycin, 1 g, and erythromycin base, 1 g, together orally at 1 P.M., 2 P.M., and 10 P.M.

Operative day Evacuate rectum at 6:30 A.M.
Operation scheduled for 8 A.M.

drug effective against anaerobes (erythromycin base, metronidazole, tetracycline) is effective (Table 6-5). Our personal experience with oral neomycin–erythromycin base preparation indicates this regimen is associated with a 5% to 6% risk of postoperative wound infection.[5] Parenteral administration of antibiotics has a more mixed record (Table 6-6). The data in Tables 6-5 through 6-7 have been pooled from 112 studies, published between 1960 and 1986, involving elective colorectal operations in 13,912 patients.

We do not use parenteral antibiotics in patients who can be successfully prepared with oral antibiotics for elective abdominal operations, reserving parenteral administration of antibiotics for patients who have high-grade colon obstruction, who are undergoing an emergency operation that obviates oral bowel preparation, or who are having an extraperitoneal low anterior resection of the rectum. However, we recognize that most surgeons employ both oral and parenteral antibiotic prophylaxis for all colorectal operations (Table 6-7). Administration of parenteral antibiotics has little impact on the incidence of those infectious complications directly related to intraoperative fecal contamination from the colon, but does reduce the overall inci-

Table 6–5
Oral Antibiotic Prophylaxis in Elective Colorectal Operations

TREATMENT	NO. STUDIES	NO. PATIENTS	NO. INFECTED	% INFECTED
None (placebo)	52	2149	833	39
Aminoglycoside-erythromycin	23	1658	165	10.0*
Aminoglycoside-metronidazole	12	314	52	17*
Aminoglycoside-tetracycline	6	787	171	22*

* Indicates a significant reduction in infections compared with no antibiotic prophylaxis.

Table 6–6
Parenteral Antibiotic Prophylaxis in Elective Colorectal Operations

TREATMENT	NO. STUDIES	NO. PATIENTS	NO. INFECTED	% INFECTED
"1st generation" cephalosporins	13	461	110	24
Cephaloridine	9	399	71	18
Cefamandole	2	72	13	18
Cefoxitin	8	339	35	10*
Moxalactam	4	171	13	8*
Cefuroxime-metronidazole	6	129	15	12*
"1st generation" cephalosporins-clindamycin	2	63	7	11*

Table 6–7
Combined Oral Neomycin-Erythromycin and Parenteral (as listed) Antibiotic Prophylaxis for Elective Colorectal Operations

TREATMENT	NO. STUDIES	NO. PATIENTS	NO. INFECTED	% INFECTED
Neomycin-erythromycin plus:				
Cefazolin	4	238	15	6*
Cephalothin	4	712	51	7*
Cefamandole	2	121	5	4*
Cefoxitin	2	153	9	6*
Ceftizoxime	1	30	2	7*
Ticarcillin	2	73	2	3*
Gent-clinda-pen	2	70	3	4*

* Indicates a significant reduction in infections compared with no antibiotic prophylaxis.

dence of postoperative infections, mainly by decreasing the incidence of pneumonia and urinary tract infection.

Biliary Tract

The flora of importance in the biliary tract varies with the state of disease. Although a variety of fecal organisms can be recovered from gallbladder mucosa or from fluid gallbladder bile, *E. coli* is the organism that causes nearly all infectious complications associated with cholecystectomy. The risk of infection in cholecystectomy also depends on whether or not acute cholecystitis is present or has recently subsided; the risk is higher in such cases. Further, in chronic cholecystitis, the risk of infection is dependent on the patient's age, and also on whether or not the gallbladder is removed intact. Several studies have shown that the risk of infection correlates with the presence of bactibilia, which progressively increases from 10% to 20% below age 60 to 100% at and above 80 years of age.

In patients with common duct obstruction, particularly those in whom the obstruction is due to stone or stricture, the flora is more varied. In addition to *E. coli*, *Klebsiella*, and enterococci, the usual organisms recovered from the gallbladder, *Proteus* and *Clostridium* species are regularly associated with septic complications of common duct disease.

In cholangitis (temperature + 101°F, bilirubin + 3.0 mg%, chills), bile should be viewed as dilute fluid feces. Although aerobes still are the numerically predominant organisms, anaerobes also are more numerous in this clinical situation than in other forms of biliary tract disease. The anaerobic microflora includes not only *C. per-fringens,* but relatively high numbers of peptostreptococci and, occasionally, *B. fragilis.*

Experience with antibiotic prophylaxis in biliary tract operations is displayed in Table 6-8. We give a preoperative IV dose of 2 g of cefazolin to all patients having biliary tract operations unless clinical cholangitis is present. In cholangitis, we administer an aminoglycoside, usually gentamicin, 2 mg/kg every 8 hours initially, plus high-dose penicillin, 4 million units every 4 hours; both drugs are given intravenously. The objective in the patient with suspected cholangitis is to provide antibiotic coverage of clostridia and enterococci.

Pancreas

The normal pancreas is sterile. Edematous (acute or relapsing) pancreatitis, the usual form of alcohol-related pancreatitis, is not a septic disease. Hemorrhagic–necrotic pancreatitis, on the other hand, is associated with a high incidence of pancreatic abscess; indeed, one fourth of deaths associated with this serious form of pancreatitis are due to septic complications.

Controlled clinical trials that have looked at the issue of antibiotic prophylaxis in pancreatitis have all been conducted in patients with chronic relapsing edematous alcohol-related pancreatitis, in which infection is rarely a clinical consideration. Not suprisingly, these trials have indicated that antibiotics are unwarranted in the man-

Table 6–8
Prophylactic Antibiotics in Biliary Surgery*

TREATMENT	NO. STUDIES	NO. PATIENTS	NO. INFECTED	% INFECTED
None (placebo)	22	963	194	10.2
Cefazolin	9	557	8	1†
Cephaloridine	4	144	7	5†
Cefamandole	5	184	4	2†
Cefoxitin	3	100	4	4†
Cefurox-metron	4	97	2	2†
Cefuroxime	3	72	2	3†
Ceftriaxone	3	75	0	†
Moxalactam	2	66	2	3†
Mezlocillin	2	234	6	3†
Cephalothin	1	50	2	4†
Cefotaxime	1	54	0	†
Cephradine	1	50	0	†
SMX-TMP	1	48	2	4†

* *Pooled data of 33 reports, 1967–1986; 3,208 patients, all stages.*
† *Indicates a significant reduction in infections compared with no antibiotic prophylaxis.*

agement of this form of pancreatitis. Unfortunately, principally because the number of cases is relatively small, the issue of whether or not to prescribe antibiotics in patients with the more serious necrotic forms of pancreatitis remains unsettled.

My personal practice is to administer antibiotics if patients are hemodynamically unstable, require blood transfusion or albumin infusion as part of resuscitation, or require peritoneal lavage as part of their therapy. The organisms usually involved in infectious sequelae of hemorrhagic–necrotic pancreatitis are aerobic coliforms. Anaerobes are not commonly a part of the infecting flora unless the colon becomes involved in the ongoing pancreatic necrosis. Administration of cefazolin, 1 to 2 g IV every 8 hours, provides appropriate antibacterial coverage of hemorrhagic–necrotic pancreatitis.

REFERENCES

1. Alexander JW, Alexander NS. The influence of route of administration on wound fluid concentration of prophylactic antibiotics. J Trauma 1976;16:488.
2. Burke JF. The effective period of preventive antibiotic action in experimental incisions and dermal lesions. Surgery 1961;50:161.
3. Clarke JS, Condon RE, Bartlett JG, et al. Preoperative oral antibiotics reduce septic complications of colon operations: results of prospective, randomized, double-blind clinical study. Ann Surg 1977;186:251.

4. Cohn I Jr. Intestinal antisepsis. Springfield, IL: Charles C Thomas, 1968.
5. Condon RE. Antibiotic coverage for bowel surgery. Int Adv Surg Oncol 1984;7:1.
6. Condon RE, Bartlett JG, Greenlee H, et al. Efficacy of oral and systemic antibiotic prophylaxis in colorectal operations. Arch Surg 1983;118:496.
7. Dellinger EP, Oreskovich ME, Wertz MJ, et al. Risk of infection following laparotomy for penetrating abdominal injury. Arch Surg 1984;119:20.
8. Edlich RF, Smith QT, Edgerton MT. Resistance of the surgical wound to antimicrobial prophylaxis and its mechanisms of development. Am J Surg 1973;126:583.
9. Keighley MRB, Arabi Y, Alexander-Williams J, et al. Comparison between systemic and oral prophylactic antimicrobial prophylaxis in colorectal surgery. Lancet 1979;1:894.
10. Miles AA, Miles EM, Burke J. The value and duration of defence reactions of the skin to the primary lodgement of bacteria. Br J Exp Pathol 1957;38:79.
11. Nichols RL, Condon RE, Gorbach SL, et al. Efficacy of preoperative antimicrobial preparation of the bowel. Ann Surg 1972;176:227.
12. Robson MC, Edstrom LE, Krizek TJ, et al. The efficacy of systemic antibiotics in the treatment of granulating wounds. J Surg Res 1974;16:299.
13. Sacks HS, Berrier J, Reitman D, et al. Meta-analyses of randomized controlled trials. N Engl J Med 1987;316:450.
14. Shapiro M, Shimon D, Freund U, et al. A decisive period in the antibiotic prophylaxis of cutaneous lesions caused by *Bacteroides fragilis* in guinea pigs. J Infect Dis 1980;141:532.
15. Stone HH, Haney BB, Kolb LD, et al. Prophylactic and preventive antibiotic therapy. Timing, duration and economics. Ann Surg 1979;189:691.
16. Strachan CJL, Black J, Powis SJA, et al. Prophylactic use of cephazolin against wound sepsis after cholecystectomy. Br Med J 1977;1:1254.

7

○   ○   ○   ●   ●   ●   ●

THE EPIDEMIOLOGY
OF SURGICAL WOUND
INFECTIONS

Richard L. Gamelli
Susan E. Pories

I was getting sick, and you came at once,
Together with a hundred students, O Symmachus;
A hundred frosty fingers probed me;
I had no fever, O Symmachus; now I have.[59]

HISTORIC PERSPECTIVES

The ancient Egyptians believed the same god could both cause and cure a disease.[2] Perhaps this could be said of infection, as both *Staphylococcus* and a penicillin producing dermatophyte have been found on the skin of the New Zealand hedgehog.[105] Presumably the gods had a sense of irony—the *Staphylococcus* was already equipped with penicillinase. Despite the gods' sure knowledge of the proximity of cure to disease, humans' understanding of the problem has been less sure. Wound infections and the surgeon's efforts to treat them effectively are an integral part of the history of surgery.

Hippocrates (460 to 377 BC) described gas gangrene and staphylococcal lesions.[4] He advised the use of wine for dressing wounds.[3] Similar use of antiseptics is mentioned in the biblical parable of the Good Samaritan who is depicted as dressing

150

wounds with oil and wine.[58] Until Lister's principles of antisepsis were introduced and adopted, however, progress in infection control was painfully slow.

In 1536, Paré experimented with the treatment of military wounds without the use of boiling oil, the conventional therapy at the time.[2] Largely by accident, since he was out of hot oil, he rediscovered Hippocrates' gentle treatment of wounds and began using a mixture of eggs, oil of roses, and turpentine to dress wounds. To his amazement, this resulted in less inflammation and pain with improved healing.

The role of "invisible organisms" in infection was proposed by Fracastoro in 1546.[23,112] He described and analyzed smallpox, measles, bubonic plague, syphilis, typhus, and leprosy. Van Leeuwenhoek, following the invention of the microscope in 1676, was the first to actually visualize microorganisms.[23]

Oliver Wendell Holmes published his treatise "On the Contagiousness of Childbed Fever" in 1843. Holmes postulated that puerperal infections were spread to women from infected autopsy material or other infected women by the hands of caregivers.

In 1862, Pasteur introduced the germ theory of infection, disproving the theory of spontaneous generation with his studies on the process of fermentation.[4] He showed conclusively that the microbes causing fermentation and putrification were effectively killed by heat.

Semmelweis in Vienna noted in 1861 that women who bore children delivered by physicians became infected four times as often as those who delivered their babies at home by midwives.[3] He showed the infection could be prevented by treating rabbits' vaginas with chlorinated lime. Semmelweis then introduced handwashing and disinfectants into use, virtually eliminating puerperal sepsis in the Vienna hospital.

Despite Semmelweis' work, infection remained a major killer. Eighty percent of all operations were followed by "hospital gangrene" and almost half of all patients died after undergoing major operation.[2] Surgical practices of the time were almost unimaginable. Instruments were reused without cleaning, and patients' skin and surgeons' hands were unwashed. Hospitals had poor sanitation practices and were noted for their stench. Sick patients were bedded together in giant beds, and bandages were routinely reused.

Lister, in 1867, was the first to realize the logical connection between the suppurative process in wounds and the fermentation process described by Pasteur.[3] He introduced the use of carbolic acid as an antiseptic and decreased the mortality of amputation from 45% to 15%.

Koch expanded on Pasteur and Lister's work by separating and identifying bacteria and showing that individual microbes caused specific disease. Koch's famous postulates sketch the means of establishing the pathogenicity of bacteria as causative agents of disease. He also introduced steam sterilization.[4]

In the early 1900s, Halsted and Reid stressed the importance of technical factors as determinants of infection and cleanliness. Halsted introduced gloves 20 years after Neuber and von Bergmann advocated gowns and caps for surgical attire.[4]

In 1929, Sir Alexander Fleming discovered penicillin. The practical development of the drug was accomplished by Florey and Chain in 1939.[2] Sulfonamides were introduced in 1935 by Gerhard Domagk who was commissioned by Hitler to find a chemotherapeutic agent effective against streptococcal infections.[2]

The medical community in the 1940s entered what has been referred to as the "antibiotic" period when general and indiscriminate antibiotic use prevailed. Antibiotic-resistant microbes developed, and the complications of antibiotic usage began to be recognized. The prevalence of gram-negative infections, fungemias, and secondary or superimposed infections in today's hospitals is due, in part, to the indiscriminate antibiotic use established during this period.

THE CHANGING RELATIONSHIP BETWEEN NOSOCOMIAL AND COMMUNITY INFECTIONS

Nosocomial infections develop within a hospital or are produced by microorganisms acquired during hospitalization. Community-acquired infections are present before admission to the hospital.

The distinctions have somewhat blurred between hospital and community strains of pathogens. For instance, the staphylococcal mastitis seen commonly in nursing mothers has been attributed to colonization of the infant in the newborn nursery with subsequent transmission of the organism to the mother at home.[95] In Detroit, intravenous drug users have been reported to take black market oral cephalosporins along with illicit drugs to prevent infections.[93] Unfortunately, staphylococcal endocarditis still occurs in this population, but the pathogens are now often cephalosporin and methicillin resistant. Patients on home total parenteral nutrition and home dialysis also extend the hospital environment into the community.

The hospital community today is an increasingly susceptible population. As the trend toward early discharge or outpatient care for routine procedures in relatively healthy patients continues, those people in the hospital for significant periods of time, such as premature or low-birth-weight infants, the elderly, patients with cancer or chronic illness, transplant patients, cardiac surgical patients, patients who have undergone prosthetic implantation, or major trauma victims, are more susceptible to infectious complications.

Accordingly, there is a large population of patients receiving steroids, immunosuppressive agents, or hyperalimentation, all of which are associated with an increased incidence of infection. There has also been a marked increase in the use of invasive devices for hemodynamic monitoring, which provide a portal of entry for microbes. Many of these patients receive antibiotics some time during their hospitalization, setting the stage for the hospital to become a reservoir of antibiotic-resistant bacteria. Areas of consideration are not only the wards, intensive care unit, and dialysis unit, but also the kitchen, water supply, and pharmacy.

THE THREE DETERMINANTS OF INFECTION

A multitude of factors have been implicated in the development of infection (Fig. 7-1). They can be broken down into three major areas to consider: the environment, the host, and the bacteria.

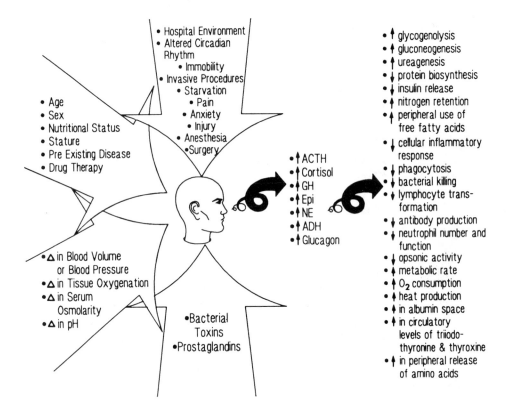

Figure 7–1.
The determinants and effects of infection.

The Environment

The effects of the hospital environment have been examined extensively. Microbes can survive in almost any environment, and, while it is easy to assess their prevalence, it is difficult to establish the role of these organisms as a direct cause of disease. Clearly, decisions about culturing practices and cleaning methods may have considerable financial impact on a hospital. Most experts now agree that routine culturing of the environment is not cost-effective and is not recommended except when a cluster of infections appears.[65] Most outbreaks of nosocomial infection are associated with person-to-person spread or due to contamination of a sterile item.

In a series of classic experiments to examine the infectivity of contaminated articles, Rammelkamp and Perry studied streptococcal transmission in army barracks.[81] Army blankets were issued to each service man on the military base upon his arrival and then reissued to the next individual without washing, unless the blankets were grossly soiled. When recruits had streptococcal illness or pharyngeal colonization, their personal effects as well as air and dust in the barracks were often contaminated with group A streptococci. No significant difference could be demonstrated in the incidence of streptococcal infection between recruits issued *Streptococcus*-contaminated blankets and recruits issued freshly laundered blankets.

In some instances, however, fomites do play an important role in transmission of disease. Outbreaks of *Staphylococcus aureus* and *Staphylococcus pyrogenes* have been conclusively linked to airborne spread from dispersers in the operating room and the newborn nursery.[87] Increases in bacteremia and respiratory tract infection have been demonstrated with increases in air contamination by *Klebsiella* or *Pseudomonas aeruginosa*.[36,48] Airborne transmission of *Legionella pneumophila* and *Aspergillus* has also been implicated in outbreaks, although nosocomial *Legionella* infections are more strongly associated with contamination of potable water supply.[87,88] At least one outbreak of *Pseudomonas* wound infections has been linked to contaminated hydrotherapy tanks, and outbreaks of *Legionella pneumophila* have been associated with contaminated water systems.[63,66,70,88]

Operating room design, traffic patterns, scheduling, and air supply all have the potential for influencing patterns of infection. It is difficult to prove the effect of operating room design and traffic flow on infection, but an effort is made in most hospitals to separate "clean" from "dirty" traffic. Predictably, the human element involved has ensured that most operating suites are not really used as planned by the architect.[54,55] As in many areas of infection control, large amounts of money and resources are spent on operating room design without much supporting data to guide decisions.

Laminar air flow has been suggested as a method to decrease wound infection rates. Laminar flow units, which are very expensive, deliver air in an undirectional manner and can be horizontally or vertically directed. This has been shown to decrease ambient bacterial counts, but there is no evidence this has a significant effect on the incidence of surgical wound infections.[54] It has been used in "ultra clean" protective environments for patients undergoing bone marrow transplantation or intensive chemotherapy.[82] Some proponents have suggested this type of air-handling system for joint replacements. However, the only large multicenter study to address the use of laminar flow in joint replacements was not controlled for perioperative antibiotic use.[57] In addition, the organisms cultured from wound infections following joint replacements correlated poorly with those found in the operating room suite, suggesting that more likely sources of infection in these patients are their own skin flora or person-to-person transmission.

In general, floors, walls, and other surfaces are not a significant source of clinical disease.[62] However, respiratory synctial virus, *Clostridium difficile* and hepatitis B virus have all been transmitted to hospital workers and patients by way of fomites.[27,42,53]

At present, routine culturing is recommended for renal dialysis fluids, infant formula prepared in the hospital, and spore strips used to monitor autoclave function.[87] Biologic monitoring of autoclaves with spore strips is the most effective way to determine successful sterilization. Microorganisms chosen for spore strips are more resistant to sterilization than most naturally occurring pathogens. They are provided in relatively high concentrations to ensure a margin of safety. After sterilization, the test strips are cultured in broth.

Water used for preparation of dialysis fluid should be tested by colony counts once a month and should contain no more than 200 viable organisms per milliliter, and the dialysate should contain less than 2000 per milliliter. The rationale behind this comes from studies indicating pyrogenic reactions did not occur when the dialysate had less than 2000 organisms per milliliter.[26] Bacteria cannot cross an intact dialysis membrane, but endotoxin can. The viable bacterial concentration is a rough measure of the endotoxin concentration.

Overall, nosocomial infection rates have been found to differ substantially from one hospital to another. In the mid-19th century, Sir James Simpson found that death from infected amputations varied directly with the size of one hospital, with higher infection rates in larger hospitals.[102] He called this phenomenon "hospitalism."

The Study on the Efficacy of Nosocomial Infection Control (SENIC) data initially seemed to support this premise. They reported an infection rate of 3.7% in small nonteaching hospitals (less than 200 beds); 5.1% in larger nonteaching hospitals (greater than 200 beds); 7.6% in nonprofit teaching hospitals; and 8.5% in municipal teaching hospitals.[37] However, when these data were analyzed further, the differences were found to be due largely to differences in the mix of patients treated. When controlled for patient risk factors, length of stay, and completeness of diagnostic workup, the difference in average infection rates disappeared.

Seasonal variations have been noted in the occurrence of nosocomial infections with certain gram-negative rods. Peaks are seen in the summer and early fall in *Klebsiella, Enterobacter, Serratia, Acinetobacter,* and *Pseudomonas aeruginosa.*[46] In contrast, *Staphylococcus* and *Streptococcus* show no significant seasonal variation in the nosocomial setting. *Escherichia coli, Enterococcus, Enterobacter,* and anaerobes also do not demonstrate seasonal variation. Nosocomial viral respiratory infections seem to follow the same seasonal patterns noted in the community.[41]

For some time, researchers have had great interest in ultraviolet (UV) radiation because it is highly bactericidal and markedly reduces any airborne contamination in the operating room. The comprehensive National Research Council report done from 1958 to 1964 showed a one third reduction in clean-wound infection rate with the use of UV light, but it had no statistically significant benefit in contaminated cases.[43,73] Five hospitals participated in this study to investigate the efficacy of UV irradiation for control of postoperative infections. By random selection, one half of the cases were done under UV radiation. The clean-wound infection rate fell by one third when performed under UV radiation. At the same time, Duke University carried out a parallel study comparing the Duke Medical Center, which was equipped with UV irradiation, with their Veterans Administration (VA) Hospital, which did not have UV lighting installed.[43] These investigators found the clean-wound infection rate in the VA hospital to be 5 times higher than at Duke Medical Center. Wright and Burke reported a decline in postoperative sepsis following craniotomy (5.3%) and laminectomy (4.1%) to 0.7% and 0.3%, respectively, after a 36-month trial of UV light at Massachusetts General Hospital.[122] One of the drawbacks to the use of UV light is the need for goggles and hoods for the operating room (OR) team, but, with suitable protection, direct UV irradiation is safe for OR personnel and patients.

The next obvious area of concern is hospital staff as part of the hospital environment. Fifteen percent of normal non-hospital-associated persons carry *Staphylococcus aureus* in their nasopharynx.[5,98] Roughly 40% to 60% of hospital workers are staphylococcal carriers, and the incidence of penicillin-resistant strains may reach 90% in such a population. Gram-negative bacilli can also be harbored in the nares or the gastrointestinal tract of hospital personnel.

Yu recently carried out a 5-year prospective controlled study to link nasal and skin *Staphylococcus aureus* infection in dialysis patients.[123] Seventy percent of the patients studied were staphylococcal carriers. Half of the carriers were treated every 3 months with 5 days of oral rifampin and topical bacitracin. The other half were treated with placebo. The 3-month period was chosen, because preliminary studies showed it took approximately 3 months for the carrier state to return. Yu found a significant difference between the two groups. During the study period, 11.5% of noncarriers became infected. Forty-six percent of carriers who did not receive prophylaxis became infected, and only 11% of carriers who received prophylaxis became infected. The phage type of the infection isolate matched the carrier isolate in 93% of infections.

Cross contamination between patients in a hospital setting poses a significant and serious risk. Handwashing is widely considered the most important means of minimizing the spread of infection.[107] The purpose of handwashing in patient care is to remove transient microbial contamination acquired by recent contact with infected or colonized patients. There are essentially two types of organisms on the hands: resident and transient flora. Resident flora survive and multiply on the skin and can be cultured repeatedly. Transient flora do not survive and multiply and can only be cultured for a short time. Resident flora are of low virulence and are not easily removed by scrubbing but can be inactivated with antiseptics. Most resident organisms are found on the superficial skin surface, but 10% to 20% are in skin crevices where lipid and superficial cornified epithelium make their removal difficult and complete sterilization of the skin impossible. Transient flora are not attached firmly to the skin and can be removed quickly and effectively by washing with soap and water for 30 seconds.

A variety of soaps and antiseptics have been used for handwashing. Iodine is an outstanding antiseptic with a wide range of action, but it can burn, chap, and discolor skin.[107] The most commonly used solutions today are iodophors or hexachlorophene. An iodophor is formed by water-soluble complexes of iodine and organic compounds. Because the iodine is bound and released slowly, there are less adverse skin reactions and staining but also decreased antibacterial potency. Hexachlorophene antiseptics are as effective as iodophors in reducing resident skin flora. However, hexachlorophene has minimal activity against gram-negative bacilli and fungi. *Pseudomonas aeruginosa*, *Serratia marcescens*, and *Alcaligenes faecalis* have been found to grow in hexachlorophene.[107] There have also been reports that blood levels of hexachlorophene of 2.3 μg per milliliter or greater have been associated with vacuolization of gray and white matter of the brain in newborn monkeys bathed in hexachlorophene.[49] Newborn babies bathed with hexachlorophene 3 weeks or longer developed blood hexachlorophene concentrations of 0.21 to 1.1 μg per milliliter. Hexachlorophene, for this reason, is no longer recommended for neonates.

Liquid soap dispensers have been associated with nosocomial outbreaks and should be emptied, cleaned, and refilled on a regular basis.[107] In contrast, no outbreaks secondary to contaminated bar soap have been reported. Organisms inoculated on bar soap die quickly; although, if the soap is left in pools of water, bacterial growth can occur.

An adequate handwashing policy consists of washing with antiseptics before surgery or an invasive procedure, and washing with soap and water between routine patient contacts. Antiseptics are not recommended for routine handwashing because they lead to dryness, cracking, and dermatitis. Colonization with *Staphylococcus aureus* and gram-negative organisms is more common on dermatitic skin, and bacterial counts are more difficult to reduce.

Because surgical wound infections constitute a large and costly problem, surgeons have looked repeatedly at how to manipulate the environment to decrease the infection rate. All such research necessarily separates surgical wounds into clean, clean–contaminated, contaminated or dirty, and infected, using the definitions given by the American College of Surgeons (Table 7-1).[5] The clean-wound infection rate is most useful for examining differences in methodology and is a valuable reflection of the quality of surgical care (Table 7-2).

Probably the most useful and complete data on determinants of clean-wound infection rates come from the 10-year prospective study of 62,939 surgical wounds done by Cruse and Foord at the Foothills Hospital in Calgary, Canada.[15] Cruse's data showed a wide variation in clean-wound infection rates of various surgical services but could not demonstrate statistical significance. Urology and general surgery had the highest infection rates at Foothills Hospital while neurosurgery and plastic surgery had the lowest rates. In contradistinction, analysis of the clean-wound infection rates at the Medical Center Hospital of Vermont shows a significant difference (p 0.001) between departments: cardiac surgery, 5.3%; general surgery, 3.0%; neurosurgery, 1.4%; gynecologic surgery, 1.2%; thoracic surgery, 1.0%; orthopedics and ear, nose and throat surgery, 0.6%; urologic surgery, 0.5%; and plastic surgery 0.0%.[67]

The choice of surgical scrub and duration of the scrub time have been evaluated for effect on wound infection rates by several investigators. Dineen was unable to show any significant difference between a 5- and 10-minute scrub.[19] Cruse's data were similar. Cruse also looked at the choice of an iodophor preparation versus hexachlorophene and found no effect on the rate of clean-wound infections.[15] In a study of wound infection rates done at the Medical Center Hospital of Vermont, we were also unable to show that the method of skin disinfection influenced clean or clean–contaminated wound infection rates.[67]

Cruse's data showed an increase in clean-wound infection rate with the use of plastic drapes.[15] He found a wound infection rate of 1.5% when cotton drapes were used and a rate of 2.3% when plastic drapes were used.

Gloves have been a standard part of the operating room garb since Halsted introduced them, not to protect his patients but rather his nurse's hands from the harsh antiseptics used at the time.[2] Protection of the surgeon and nurses may still be one of the most important reasons to wear gloves. Wise and colleagues showed that up to 1.8×10^5 organisms can be cultured from inside the gloves after a surgical procedure.[121] However, using an electronic device to detect glove punctures,[80] Cruse found that although 11.6% of gloves were punctured at the end of surgery, this had no discernable effect on the wound infection rate.[15]

Table 7–1
Wound Classification—Guidelines of Surgical Wounds Provided by the
American College of Surgeons

Clean
Nontraumatic
No inflammation encountered
No break in technique
Respiratory, alimentary, genitourinary tract not entered
Clean-contaminated
Gastrointestinal or respiratory tracts entered without significant spillage
Appendectomy
Oropharynx entered
Vagina entered
Genitourinary tract entered in absence of infected urine
Biliary tract entered in absence of infected bile
Minor break in technique
Contaminated
Major break in technique
Gross spillage from gastrointestinal tract
Traumatic wound, fresh
Entrance of genitourinary or biliary tracts in presence of infected urine or bile
Dirty and Infected
Acute bacterial inflammation encountered, without pus
Transection of "clean" tissue for the purpose of surgical access
to a collection of pus
Perforated viscus encountered
Traumatic wound with retained devitalized tissue, foreign bodies, fecal
contamination and/or delayed treatment, or from dirty source

Table 7–2
Infection Rate by Degree of Wound Contamination

| WOUND CLASSIFICATION | MCHV* | | CRUSE AND FOORD (%) |
	No. of Wounds	No (%) Infected	
Clean	5,927	87(1.5)	1.5
Clean-contaminated	1,494	46(3.1)	7.7
Contaminated	607	50(8.2)	15.2
Dirty	446	52(11.7)	40.0
Total	8,474	235(2.8)	4.7

* *MCHV indiates Medical Center Hospital of Vermont, Burlington.*
(Mead PB et al. Arch Surg 1986; 121:458)

Interestingly, the gloves themselves may cause problems because pyrogens have been noted on sterile latex surgical gloves. In one study, the incidence of febrile reactions following cardiac catheterization was decreased from 11.6% to 0.6% when rinsing of gloves before catheterization was made routine.[52]

The Host

The second area of consideration is the host. In a state of good health, we coexist fairly happily with the large amount of normal flora in and on our bodies. This is primarily due to excellent local and systemic defenses, which are compromised in the hospitalized patient who has been subjected to burns, trauma, drugs, anesthetics, surgery, blood transfusions, invasive procedures, and/or malnutrition.[1,6,9,23,45,60,83,85,113]

The skin serves as a thick mechanical barrier to microbes. The number of bacteria residing in the skin surface is kept down by the dry conditions that make a hostile environment for growth. In areas protected from drying, such as skinfolds and axillary and genital regions, the number of bacteria increases markedly. The acid mantle is a thin film coating the outer skin surface, and its *p*H is too low for the growth of many pathogens.[8] The keratinized layer of the epidermis has restricted attachment sites for primarily nonpathogenic organisms.[103] Normal flora compete with pathogens and inhibit their attachment. Other microorganisms are capable of colonizing the skin but only transiently because of their lack of attachment.

The cleansing and flushing mechanisms of the respiratory, gastrointestinal, and genitourinary tracts serve to remove the majority of microorganisms. Decreased motility and stasis increase bacterial overgrowth. Antimotility drugs for infectious diarrhea, therefore, are counterproductive. Between meals, when salivary flow is decreased, the number of bacteria in the saliva increases fourfold.[45] Dehydration, radiation to the salivary glands, and certain diseases reduce salivary flow resulting in a marked increase in the number of oral bacteria. In addition to the flushing action of urine, the acidic *p*H of urine inhibits bacterial growth.

The mucosal immune system is a first-line defense against invasion by potentially pathogenic microorganisms and viruses.[109] The essential element in this defense system is the large number of lymphoid and plasma cells that lie in intimate anatomical proximity to the basement membrane of mucous membranes. Plasma cells produce primarily IgA antibodies. The IgA system of the gut is especially extensive, with 20 IgA-producing cells for each IgG or IgM cell. IgA neutralizes viruses in the absence of complement, coats bacteria, and prevents their adherence to mucous surfaces. The gut is equivalent to the spleen in terms of numbers of immunoglobulin containing lymphoid cells. There is also a predominance of IgE cells in secretory sites such as respiratory and gastrointestinal tracts. Immunoglobulins IgG and IgA and IgM are also found in urine and impair microbial attachments to bladder epithelial cells. In addition, saliva and mucus contain antimicrobial substances, such as lysozyme, which splits the muramic acid -B(1−4)-N-acetyl-glucosamine linkage in bacterial cell walls.

Drying also impairs the efficiency of mucociliary defense systems. Thickened mucus is more difficult for the ciliated epithelium to move toward the mouth. Furthermore, drying damages the epithelial cells of the trachea and bronchi and leads to decreased ciliary action, predisposing to infection.

Any break in the integument will predispose patients to infection. Certainly the increasing incidence of invasive procedures and frequent placement of monitoring devices and implants, such as ventricular shunts, have increased the nosocomial infection rate. It has been shown that 10% to 20% of patients undergoing ventricular shunt insertion or revision develop shunt infections.[96] Infections in patients with ventricular shunts are primarily caused by *Staphylococcus,* probably due to incomplete eradication of normal skin flora. Thirty-five percent of patients with ventriculoureteral shunts develop infections from gram-negative enterics.[96] Arterial lines yielded positive cultures in 4% of patients and were responsible for 12% of all sepsis in one intensive care unit.[7,32] With elimination of a static inline fluid column and scrupulous asepsis, the positive arterial catheter tip culture rate has been reduced to 0.85% at the Medical Center Hospital of Vermont.[100] Transducers have also been a source of bacteremia and candidemia.

Deep wound infections following total hip replacements are a debilitating problem.[28] *Staphylococcus epidermidis* is the leading cause. The implant materials may inhibit host ability to deal effectively with contaminating organisms.[29] Polymethylmethacrylate is most strongly incriminated. Bone necrosis secondary to the surgical insult, the heat of polymerization, and the toxicity of methylmethacrylate work together to create favorable growth conditions for microorganisms.

Host defense mechanisms are also altered by therapeutic interventions, stress, illness, malnutrition, and age.[11,91,104,106,108,118] In the majority of critically ill patients who die, sepsis remains the most common cause of death. Cruse showed that patients 66 years or older were six times more likely to develop infections than patients 1 to 14 years of age.[15] Our data also showed a significant increase in the clean-wound infection rate in the older population (greater than 50 years old) and the very young (less than 1 year of age).[67] B-lymphocyte function decreases in the elderly with a corresponding decrease in IgG, IgM, and IgD and a decreased antibody response to antigens.[91] Additionally, decreased T-lymphocyte function has been described in the elderly.[115]

Diabetes is associated with defects in leukocyte mobilization, which can be corrected by control of blood glucose. Increased glucose levels predispose to hyperosmolarity and mycotic overgrowth with inhibited phagocytosis. Ketoacidosis can lead to invasive pulmonary infections with rhizopus.

Steroid use depresses all functions of leukocytes. Rinehart looked at the effects of a short course of high-dose corticosteroid therapy.[90] A transient decrease in the number of circulating monocytes was seen, which returned to normal in 24 hours. After 3 days of treatment, a marked impairment was seen in bactericidal and fungicidal activity. A recent study by DeMaria showed that steroid use in seriously injured head trauma patients significantly increases infectious complications.[18] In patients with an injury severity score greater than 20, 47% of patients treated with steroids developed infectious complications as opposed to 14.5% of those not receiving steroids.

The presence of cancer is often associated with alterations in cell-mediated immunity. Brugarolas correlated anergy with extent of disease, response to chemotherapy, and survival time in patients with cancer.[10] Those patients with widespread disease were anergic, while those with limited disease showed a moderate to good reaction to skin testing.

Chronic renal failure is associated with decreased immune responsiveness and defective cell-mediated immunity, decreased circulating lymphocytes, thymic atrophy, and IgA deficiency.[119] Obesity has also been associated with an increased infection rate in patients undergoing operative intervention.[84]

Nutritional imbalances have profound effects on immunity.[6,94] Protein and calorie deprivation decreases cellular immunity and leads to thymic involution, lymphoid hypoplasia, lymphopenia, decreased antibody response, and decreased complement levels. These patients may also demonstrate decreased E rosette forming T lymphocytes and decreased response of T lymphocytes to phytohemaglutinin. Chronic nutritional deprivation leads to microbiocidal and chemotactic defects of granulocytes.

Using an experimental model, Dionigi studied the effects of intravenous nutritional repletion on immunodepression secondary to malnutrition.[20] He found that nutritional repletion would return IgG, IgM, C3 levels, hemagglutinin titers, and neutrophil chemotaxis to normal or supernormal levels. Parenteral nutrition did not improve absolute lymphocyte counts, the response to phytohemagglutinin (PHA) (an indicator of T-cell function), leukocyte migration, or phagocyte function.

The relationship between anergy and mortality from infectious complications has been shown to be statistically significant. MacLean prospectively studied patients and found a significant difference in the incidence of septicemia between anergic patients and normals as well as an increased mortality in anergic patients.[60]

In hospitalized trauma patients, approximately one fifth of all deaths have been attributed to infection or multiorgan failure that often starts with infection.[110] Nichols has shown that, at least in penetrating injuries, the probability of infection developing correlated well with gastrointestinal soilage of the peritoneum.[75] In patients with such leakage, the risk of infection increased with the severity of injuries, increasing age and left colon injury.

Infection after trauma can contribute significantly to morbidity. Roth has looked at the problem of post-traumatic extremity infection and osteomyelitis.[92] He noted that organisms recovered in cultures from open fractures were more likely to be hospital-acquired rather than stemming from initial contamination of the fracture. This suggests that the pathogens primarily responsible for infection may have been introduced during open management of the fracture.

Burn patients are a subset of trauma patients with an increased risk of infection.[95] Nearly two thirds of all patients with burns that are over 30% who die do so as a result of infection.[61] There is a direct association between the size of the burn injury and death from infection (Fig. 7-2). Infection affects nearly all patients with greater than 40% of the total body surface area burned.

The necessarily immunocompromised transplant patient constitutes a relatively new and rapidly growing group of patients at risk for serious injection. Usually, the site of infection problems is related to the specific type of allograft.[9] For instance, pneumonia is the most common site of infection in heart and lung transplant recip-

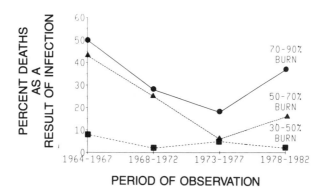

Figure 7–2.
Infection related deaths in burn patients. There is a direct association between the size of the burn injury and death from infection. This figure represents data from the University of Cincinnati Hospital Burn and Trauma Unit and Cincinnati Shriner's Hospital in 1964–1982. Overall mortality caused by infection dropped from 26% in 1964–67 period to 12% in 1978–82 period. (MacMillan BG. In: Hospital Infections. 2nd ed. Boston: Little Brown + Co, 1986:466)

ients. Septicemia occurs more frequently in liver transplant and bone marrow transplant patients.[71,72] The urinary tract is the most common site of infection in renal transplant patients.

Anesthetic agents cause a broad range of changes in the immune system.[16,17,22,23,47,78,89,120] General anesthesia inhibits cell replication and leukocyte mobility.[16,69] Local anesthetics affect granulocyte migration. Chemotaxis is affected by narcotics, induction agents, muscle relaxants and volatile anesthetics. Narcotics have also been shown to decrease interferon elaboration.[47] Park measured the reactivity of peripheral blood lymphocytes using PHA in patients receiving general anesthesia.[79] The response to PHA fell within 2 hours of surgery, then rose steadily reaching preoperative levels within a week. Donovan noted decreased reticuloendothelial function in postoperative patients.[21] There are also nonimmunologic influences of anesthesia on host defense mechanisms, such as impaired mucociliary function and bacterial clearance, altered respiratory mechanics, and decreased coughing.

There is a direct relationship between the length of time of an operation and the infection rate. Cruse showed that the rate of clean-wound infections roughly doubles with every extra hour in the operating room.[15] Our data also show increased length of surgery to increase significantly the risk of infection in both clean and clean–contaminated categories (Table 7-3).[67]

Cruse did show that a preoperative shower with hexachlorophene decreased the infection rate of clean wounds.[15] Those who did not shower had a wound infection rate of 2.3%, those who showered with soap had a wound infection rate of 2.1%, and those who showered with hexachlorophene had an infection rate of 1.3%.

Table 7–3
Duration of Surgery and Infection Rates*

| | CLEAN WOUNDS | | CLEAN-CONTAMINATED WOUNDS | |
DURATION, HR	No. of Cases	Percent Infected	No. of Cases	Percent Infected
<1	368	0.0	29	0.0
1–2	2,466	0.8	654	1.8
2–3	1,557	1.7	393	2.3
3–4	736	3.0	200	3.0
>4	800	2.4	218	8.7

* For both groups, p<0.001. Medical Center Hospital of VT, Burlington
(Mead PB et al. Arch Surg 1986; 121:458)

In addition, Cruse showed that increasing the length of preoperative hospitalization clearly increases the clean-wound infection rate.[15] Those patients in the hospital only 1 day preoperatively had a clean-wound infection rate of 1.2%. Those patients who were in the hospital a week preoperatively had a rise in their infection rate to 2.1%, and those in the hospital longer than 2 weeks preoperatively had an infection rate of 3.4%. Mead corroborated this in both clean and clean–contaminated categories (p 0.001 for both categories).[67]

Shaving has been shown to increase the infection rate. In Cruse's study, patients who were shaved with a razor had a clean-wound infection rate of 2.5%.[15] When clippers were used, the infection rate was 1.7%. Patients who were shaved with an electric razor had a clean-wound infection rate of 1.4%. Patients who were neither shaved or clipped had a clean-wound infection rate of 0.9%

We recently looked at the timing of operative site shaving and found no significant difference in clean-wound infection rates.[67] Patients shaved in the operating room had a trend toward higher clean-wound infection rates (1.9%) than those shaved the night before surgery (1.4%). The lowest infection rate was found in patients who were not shaved at all. Olson looked at the effect of preoperative hair removal with clippers and was unable to show any change in the clean-wound infection rate as compared with shaving or depilatory agents.[76]

The Pathogen

The final area of consideration is the microbe. While gram-positive organisms have traditionally been the cause of hospital epidemics and were the impetus behind the hospital infection control programs conceived in the 1950s, gram-negative organisms have been implicated more frequently in recent times. This is not to say that gram-positive organisms are no longer a threat because there is now a resurgence of methicillin resistant *Staphylococcus.*[34,98,99]

As part of the National Research Council study on UV light done in 1964, frequencies of recovery of organisms from wound infections were recorded.[73] Coagulase-positive and negative *Staphylococcus* led the list with a 61% frequency of recovery. They were followed by *Escherichia coli* (22%), *Proteus* (12%), *Pseudomonas* (13%), nonhemolytic *Streptococcus* (9.7%), and *Klebsiella* (8.7%). The same information was recorded as part of the National Nosocomial Infection Study (NNIS) from 1970 to 1973. Overall, *Escherichia coli* led the list with 18.7%, followed by *Staphylococcus aureus* (18.6%), *Pseudomonas* (8.8%), and *Proteus* (5.6%). On the surgical services, *Staphylococcus aureus* was still predominant (19%) with *Escherichia coli* running a close second (18%).

Similar information was again collected as part of the NNIS from 1980 to 1982.[46] *Escherichia coli* predominated overall as the most commonly isolated pathogen in nosocomial infections at all sites. *Staphylococcus aureus* still predominated on adult and pediatric surgical services. However, *Escherichia coli*, *Enterococcus*, and *Bacteroides* were predominant in wound infections on obstetric and gynecologic services.

Increases in fungal infections, especially *Candida* and *Aspergillus*, have occurred as well as anaerobic infections and mixed infections. There has been an increase in infections caused by bacteria of low virulence and atypical bacterial forms such as L forms. In addition, outbreaks by multiply resistant gram-negative organisms have increased. Several newly recognized nosocomial pathogens have also emerged as virulent threats during the past decade, such as *Legionella pneumophila*, *cinetobacter*, *Pseudomonas*, *Flavobacterium*, and *Citrobacter.*[31] Bacteria newly recognized as nosocomial pathogens share several characteristics: they have relatively slow growth on agar, demonstrate fastidiousness of nutritional and atmospheric requirements, and resemble bacteria considered to be commensals.

The mere presence of virulent microorganisms in a wound does not make infection inevitable. Equally as important are the local conditions, the patient's general condition, and underlying disease processes and immune status. In a study done by Elek and Conen, the forearms of British medical students were injected with measured numbers of *Staphylococcus aureus.*[24] They found that 6.5 million staphyloccoci were needed to produce an abscess. However, if the organisms were injected into an area with a subcutaneous silk suture, only 100 organisms were necessary. Miles and Niven showed that shocked experimental animals with a decrease in wound perfusion required 10,000-fold fewer organisms to initiate a wound infection.[68] Inadequate hemostasis, retained blood clots, necrotic or traumatized tissue allow small numbers of bacteria to create a suppurative wound infection.

From animal research done by Burke and others, there seems to be a "decisive period," probably the first 3 hours after bacterial contamination, which ultimately decides the fate of the wound.[13] If host resistance is decreased during this time, lesions are increased in size and severity, suggesting value for augmenting host resistance with antibiotics during this time when there is a high probability that a patient's natural resistance to invasion will not overcome the combined bacterial and physiologic challenge of a surgical procedure.

THE PROBLEM OF ANTIBIOTIC RESISTANCE

As a result of the changing patient populations and increasing antibiotic resistance, nosocomial infections are increasingly serious and increasingly difficult to control.[12,39,74] Resistance to penicillin G appeared rapidly after its introduction. In 1945, Fleming, Chain, and Florey shared the Nobel Prize for the discovery of penicillin.[2] By 1949, 40% of strains isolated at Boston City Hospital were resistant to penicillin G. Today there are very few hospital isolates of staphylococcus susceptible to penicillin G. Since the 1960s, reports of antibiotic-resistant bacteria in hospitals have appeared with increasing frequency.[64] Burn wounds demonstrate clearly the changing character of pathogens over the years since antibiotic therapy was introduced and resistances have developed (Fig. 7-3).[61]

Patients with chronic respiratory or urinary tract infections who have frequent admissions and transfers from other hospitals or nursing homes are likely to bring resistant organisms into the hospital. It has been estimated that 15% to 25% of patients colonized or infected with aminoglycoside-resistant gram-negative bacilli have brought these strains with them into the hospital.[33] The NNIS data from 1975 to

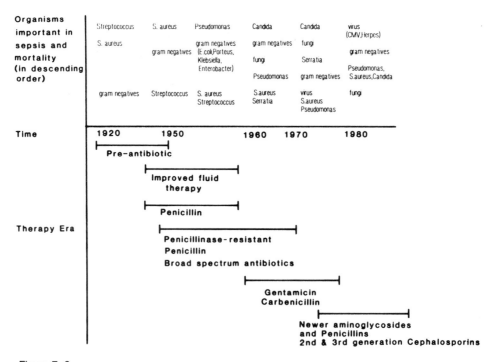

Figure 7–3.
The changing patterns of burn infections. Burn wounds demonstrate the changing character of pathogens over the years since antibiotic therapy was introduced. (MacMillan BG. In: Hospital Infections. 2nd ed. Boston: Little Brown + Co, 1986:467)

1982 showed that 52% of the 340,000 nosocomial infections were caused by gram-negative organisms. Five percent of *Enterobacteriaceae* were resistant to gentamicin and/or tobramycin, as well as 14% of *Pseudomonas.*[114]

There are often many colonized patients for each patient with recognized infections. This is referred to as the "iceberg" effect.[114] Colonization with hospital flora happens within a few days of admission (Fig. 7-4).[97] The resistant bacteria are spread by way of transient carriage on the hands of personnel, contributing to the "iceberg" of colonized patients.

Data indicate that 25% to 35% of hospitalized patients receive systemic antibiotics at any given time and there is a trend toward increasing antibiotic use within hospitals.[50] Several studies have shown that only 38% of patients receiving antibiotics had recorded evidence of infection. At the University of Virginia in a 3-month survey of antibiotics used on the medical-surgical service, 58% of antibiotics given were for prophylaxis.[51] At the Medical Center Hospital of Vermont, a survey of antibiotic usage on the surgical service during a typical month (April 1985) indicated that in patients given antibiotics, 47% were given antibiotics for prophylaxis, 23% of the patients had documented infection, and in 30% antibiotics usage was as empiric therapy for presumed infection (Harry D. Antibiotic usage at the Medical Center Hospital of Vermont. 1985. Personal communication). Of the prophylactic antibiotics given, 49% were administered for a 24- to 48-hour period.

Bacterial resistance can develop by way of several different mechanisms. Chromosomal resistance occurs by spontaneous mutation and Darwinian selection of organisms resistant to single or closely related agents. Bacteria may also acquire resistance rapidly through accrual of R factors or resistance plasmids, which encode multiple resistances to unrelated drugs.[30] Plasmids are extra chromosomal DNA

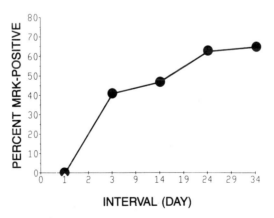

Figure 7–4.
Colonization of patients with resistant organisms often occurs within a few days of admission to the hospital. This figure represents patients positive for multiply resistant *Klebsiella* on rectal culture, by interval from admission. (Selden R, et al. Ann Intern Med 1971; 74:647.)

molecules that replicate independent of the chromosome. Transposons, the molecular level portion of plasmids, may hitchhike from one plasmid to another or between the plasmid and the bacterial chromosome. Transposons carrying genes for resistance may align with elements encoding virulence or colonization factors, creating R factors with an impressive potential for mischief. Resistance determinants are linked to plasmids that specify other traits essential for bacterial survival. They require only small amounts of DNA. Even with the absence of antibiotic selection, resistance genes remain with the plasmids and are lost only at a very slow rate. Resistant bacteria have the growth advantage and may ultimately become the predominant organism.

Evidence suggests that the proportion of bacteria resistant to a given antibiotic increases as use of the drug increases and may decrease with decreased use or cessation of the drug. Antibiotic auditing is now required by the Joint Council on Accreditation of Hospitals.

Another insidious problem is the large amount of antibiotics used in animal feed.[56] For over 30 years, subtherapeutic amounts of broad-spectrum antibiotics have been added to feed in an attempt to promote growth. It has been shown that bacteria from the animal gut can find its way into the gastrointestinal tract of humans and cause disease. In England and other European countries, realization of the problem led to removal of antibiotics from animal feed after serious disease in humans was caused by multiply resistant *Salmonella typhimurium* type 20 originally found in cattle.[44]

THE COST OF NOSOCOMIAL INFECTIONS

Nosocomial infections are a major public health problem and represent a severe financial drain on hospitals. In addition, nosocomial infections are one of the ten leading causes of death in the United States. Most authorities would agree that surgical wound infections represent the most serious and costly nosocomial infections. Surgical wound infections account for only 29% of nosocomial infections, but they account for 57% of the extra hospital days secondary to nosocomial infections and 42% of the extra costs.[38] In comparison, pneumonia accounts for 24% of extra hospital days and 39% of the extra costs. Urinary tract infections represent 11% of extra hospital days and 13% of the extra costs. Bloodstream infections account for 4% of extra hospital days and 3% of the extra costs.

There are three traditional ways to estimate the cost of infections: length of stay, hospital costs, and patient mortality attributable to infections. Litigation is another measure of costs, and recent figures indicated that surgical wound infections are one of the ten leading causes of medical malpractice claims in the state of Florida.[111] The lowest estimate in the literature for average extra length of stay necessitated by a surgical wound infection is 7 days.[14,35,40,86] It is estimated that over 8 million extra hospital days a year are necessitated nationwide for nosocomial infections.[38] It is difficult to measure the number of deaths truly attributable to nosocomial infections, because many of these patients are seriously ill with underlying conditions or have weakened immunity. However, the Centers for Disease Control (CDC) has shown that

10% of patients with nosocomial infections die in the hospital, and, of these, 10% die as a direct result of nosocomial infection. In another 30%, the nosocomial infection substantially contributes to death. When these figures are projected on a nationwide basis of the 2 million or more nosocomial infections a year, 20,000 deaths are directly attributable to the infection while 60,000 are attributable in part.

The allotted length of stay and charges allowed by the Diagnosis Related Groupings (DRG) are only a small fraction of what nosocomial infections actually cost.[38] In addition, nosocomial infections occur most often in patients who have other complications. After the first comorbidity or complication, the DRG payment cannot be further increased for additional complications such as nosocomial infections.[116]

INFECTION PREVENTION THROUGH SURVEILLANCE

Surveillance is the collection, tabulation, and dissemination of data on the occurrence of nosocomial infections for the purpose of preventing and controlling them. Several systems of surveillance have been described, such as Wenzel's Kardex system and surveillance by objective as described by Haley.[25,38,117] Reduction in the wound infection rate with a surveillance program has been well shown.[15,38,67,77]

The SENIC project was started in 1974 by the Centers for Disease Control to study the effectiveness of surveillance and control[38,39]. Infection control program activities were assessed in 6,000 U.S. hospitals; 80% of the nation's hospitals participated. Three hundred and thirty-eight hospitals were then chosen randomly for further study. The hospitals were divided into 16 groups according to surveillance and control activities. Twenty-one hospitals were chosen from each group, and the study group was, therefore, representative of all approaches to infection control being practiced. Each of the 16 groups were also subgrouped by categories of hospital size and medical school affiliation.

Four components were found essential for an infection control program to decrease nosocomial infection rates significantly and are described below:[38]

1. A high level of surveillance activity was found to decrease significantly the rate of infection. However, in surgical wound infections, surveillance was effective only if surgical wound infection rates were routinely reported to the surgeons.
2. A well-executed system of infection prevention and control
3. Ensuring that there is one infection control nurse for each 250 beds
4. A physician with appropriate interest and training in epidemiology and infection control

Hospitals that had all four of the essential components decreased their surgical wound infection rate 35%.[38] Hospitals without the four components actually increased their nosocomial infection rates by 18% over the 5-year period, which was statistically significant and true in all regions of the country and all types and sizes of hospitals.

168

The increase in nosocomial infections in hospitals that did not practice effective surveillance and control was felt to be secondary to the introduction of invasive and immunocompromising technology into hospital medicine.

In 1983, the CDC repeated their survey of U.S. hospitals to update their findings. If all U.S. hospitals had adopted the four components, 32% of infections could have been prevented as opposed to the actual figure of only 9%, which reflects the large gap between real and ideal investment of resources.[38]

At the Minneapolis VA Hospital, Olson was able to show a decrease in the overall infection rate from 4.2% to 1.9% and a decrease in the clean-wound infection rate by 64% with a surveillance and control program.[77] Cruse demonstrated a steady fall in the clean-wound infection rate at Foothills Hospital in Calgary with the institution of a surveillance and notification program.[15] At the Medical Center Hospital of Vermont, we demonstrated a reduction of 42% in the clean-wound infection rate with a surveillance notification program.[67] Reporting surgeon-specific surgical wound infection rates to surgeons is the only procedure shown to reduce substantially infection rates.[38,39]

The economic savings with a successful infection surveillance and control program are substantial. The CDC cost–benefit ratio analysis adapted for 1985 dollars for every 250 occupied hospitals beds is $60,000/year.[38] Breakdown of the $60,000/year is as follows:

$28,000 for infection control nurse salary
$8,000 for a physician consultant
$9,000 for clerical assistance
$5,000 for supplies and miscellaneous costs
$10,000 for indirect costs

A 6% decrease in the infection rate pays for the surveillance and control program. A 32% decrease in the infection rate saves the hospital $260,000. A 50% decrease in the infection rate will save a 250-bed hospital $440,000 annually.

SUMMARY

The interactions necessary for wound infection can be viewed as three intersecting spheres, representing the host, the pathogen, and the environment. Although each area was considered separately here, they are in reality closely linked and in dynamic balance.

The conscientious surgeon can manipulate aspects of all three spheres, but a critical determinant of whether a wound becomes infected remains surgical technique. Traumatized, irritated, and dead tissues support and enhance bacterial growth. Increased pressure and tension on tissues decrease circulation and lymphatic flow, which facilitates bacterial growth. Inadequate hemostasis with retained blood and clot inhibit bacterial eradication by the host and may enhance bacterial growth. It is necessary to ensure adequate debridement in wounds of trauma and violence, to excise necrotic and devitalized tissue, and to remove foreign bodies while preserving blood supply.

It remains, however, impossible to perform truly aseptic surgery, and our armamentarium of antibiotics may not be able to keep pace with the pathogens' Darwinian potential for resistance. Our susceptibility to infection from previously peaceful microbes increases with today's escalating technical and chemical manipulation of immune status along with our efforts to perform surgery on higher risk patients with major underlying alterations in their immune status.

It is in the face of these ever larger challenges that our vigilance as surgeons must improve to at least maintain if not lessen infectious complications and deaths. Vigilance today entails not only technical skills but institution of a support for infection surveillance, notification and control activities, intelligent antibiotic use, and nutritional support in compromised patients.

GLOSSARY

Airborne Spread—Dissemination of organisms by way of a true airborne route within droplet nuclei or dust particles.

Antiseptic—Chemical agent applied to the body that kills or inhibits growth of pathogenic microorganisms so long as there is contact between agent and the microorganism.

Carrier—Individual colonized with a microorganism from whom the organism can be recovered, but without overt expression of the presence of the microorganism, although the individual may have a previous history of disease secondary to the organism:

    (a) *Transient*—short-term.
    (b) *Intermittent*—occasional.
    (c) *Chronic*—persistent.

Case Control Study—Comparison of a study group, affected with a given disease, and a comparison control group and determining the differences between them to ascertain the cause of the disease.

Cohort Study—Comparing a group of people who have certain characteristics or who have received a certain intervention with a control group to determine the effect of the intervention or characteristics that might be related to outcome.

    (a) *Concurrent Cohort Study*—the cohort is assembled in the present and followed into the future.
    (b) *Historic Cohort Study*—identifying the cohort from past records and following forward from that time up to the present.

Colonization—Growth and multiplication of a microorganism in or on a host without overt clinical expression or detected immune reaction.

Common Vehicle Spread—A contaminated inanimate vehicle serves as the vector for transmission to multiple persons.

Contact Spread—The victim has contact with the source—either direct, indirect, or by droplets.

Contamination—Microorganisms transiently present on the body surface without tissue invasion or physiologic reaction.

Disease—Illness caused by presence and activity of a microbial agent.

Disinfectant—Germicidal chemical substance used on inanimate objects to kill pathogenic microorganisms.

Dissemination—Shedding of microorganisms from the carrier into the environment. Usually only a fraction of colonized persons are disseminating.

Dose—The number of organisms available to cause infection.

Endemic—Disease that occurs with ongoing frequency in specific geographic areas in a finite population and over a defined time period.

Endogenous—Infection caused by an infectious agent already present in the body (*i.e.*, the patient's own flora).

Entrance—Sites of deposition or entry into the host.

Epidemic—Increase in incidence of a disease above its expected endemic occurrence.

Epidemiology—Discipline concerned with the distribution and determinants of disease in populations.

Exit—Portal of exit for organisms from the host.

Exogenous—Infections induced by organisms from a source other than the patient.

Fomite—An inanimate object that may be contaminated with microorganisms and serve in their transmission.

Hyperendemic—Gradual increase in occurrence of a disease in a defined area beyond the expected number of cases.

Incidence—Fraction of a group that develops an outcome over a given period of time.

Index Case—The first case in an outbreak.

Infection—Multiplication of microorganisms in the host tissues.

Infectivity—The ability of an organism to spread from a source to a host.

Invasiveness—The ability of microorganisms to invade tissues.

Nosocomial—Infections that develop within a hospital or are produced by microorganisms acquired during hospitalization.

Outbreak—Increased rate of occurrence but not at levels as serious as an epidemic.

Pathogenicity—Measure of the ability of microorganisms to induce disease.

Prevalence—Fraction of a group possessing a clinical outcome at any given point in time.

Reservoir—Place where the organism maintains its presence, metabolizes, and replicates.

Source—Place from which the infectious agent passes to the host.

Specificity—Referring to the range of hosts susceptible to a particular microorganism.

Sporadic—Cases that occur occasionally and irregularly without any specific pattern.

Sterilization—The process of killing all microorganisms by physical or chemical agents.

Subclinical Infection—Interaction between host and microorganism resulting in a detectable immune response but no overt symptoms.

Transmission—Interaction between an infectious agent and a susceptible host.

Vectorborne Spread—

I. *External*—mechanical transfer of microorganisms on the body or appendages of the vector.

II. *Internal*

   (a) *Harborage*—no biologic action between the vector and the agent.

   (b) *Biologic Transmission*—the agent goes through biologic changes within the vector.

Virulence—Measure of severity of the disease caused by a microorganism.

REFERENCES

1. Abraham E. Immunologic mechanisms underlying sepsis in the critically ill surgical patient. Surg Clin North Am 1985;65:991.
2. Ackerknecht EH. A short history of medicine. Baltimore: Johns Hopkins University Press, 1982.
3. Alexander JW. The contributions of infection control to a century of surgical progress. Ann Surg 1984;201:423.
4. Altemeier WA. Sepsis in surgery. Arch Surg 1982;117:107.
5. Altemeier WA, Burke JF, Pruitt BA, et al. Manual on control of infection in surgical patients. Philadelphia: JB Lippincott, 1984.
6. Anderson CF, Mosness K, Meister J, et al. The sensitivity and specificity of nutrition related variables in relationship to the duration of hospital stay and the rate of complications. Mayo Clin Proc 1984;59:477.
7. Band JD, Maki DG: Infections caused by arterial catheters used for hemodynamic monitoring. Am J Med 1979;67:735.
8. Bickers DR, Kappas A. Metabolic and pharmacologic properties of the skin. Hosp Pract 1974;9:97.
9. Brooks RG, Remington JS. Transplant related infections. In: Bennett JV, Brachman PS, eds. Hospital infections. 2nd ed. Boston: Little, Brown & Co, 1986;581.
10. Brugarolas A, Takita H. Immunologic status in lung cancer. Chest 1973;64:427.
11. Buckley CE, Dorsey FC. The effect of aging on human serum immunoglobulin concentrations. J Immunol 1970;105:964.
12. Buckwold FJ, Ronald AR. Antimicrobial misuse—effects and suggestions for control. J Antimicrob Chemother 1979;5:129.
13. Burke JF. Risk factors predisposing to wound infection and means of their prevention. In: Dineen P, Hildick-Smith G, eds. The surgical wound. Philadelphia: Lea & Febiger, 1981;132.
14. Clarke SKR. Sepsis in surgical wounds with particular reference to *Staphylococcus aureus*. Br J Surg 1967;44:592.
15. Cruse PJE, Foord R. The epidemiology of wound infection. Surg Clin North Am 1980;60:27.
16. Cullen BF. The effect of halothane and nitrous oxide on phagocytosis and human leukocyte metabolism. Anesth Analg 1974;53:531.
17. Cullen BF, Van Belle G. Lymphocyte transformation and changes in leukocyte count: effects of anesthesia and operation. Anesthesiology 1975;43:563.
18. DeMaria EJ, Reichman W, Kenney PR, et al. Septic complications of corticosteroid administration after central nervous system trauma. Ann Surg 1985;202:248.
19. Dineen P. An evaluation of the duration of the surgical scrub. Surg Gynecol Obstet 1969;129:1181.
20. Dionigi R, Zonta A, Dominioni L, et al. The effects of total parenteral nutrition on immunodepression due to malnutrition. Ann Surg 1977;185:467.
21. Donovan A. The effect of surgery on reticuloendothelial function. Arch Surg 1967;94:247.
22. Duncan PG, Cullen BF. Anesthesia and immunology. Anesthesiology 1976;45:522.
23. Duncan PG, Mathieu A, Mathieu D. Effects of anesthesia and surgery on mechanisms of immune defense. In: Mathieu A, Burke JF, eds. Infection and the perioperative period. New York: Grune & Stratton, 1982;37.
24. Elek SD, Conen PE. The virulence of *Staphylococcus pyrogenes* for man: a study of the problems of wound infection. Br J Exp Pathol 1957;38:573.

172

25. Evans RS, Larsen RA, Burke JP, et al. Computer surveillance of hospital acquired infections and antibiotic use. JAMA 1986;256:1007.
26. Favero MS, Peterson NJ, Carson LA, et al. Gram negative bacteria in hemodialysis systems. Health Lab Sci 1975;12:321.
27. Fekety R, Kim YH, Brown D, et al. Epidemiology of antibiotic associated colitis: isolation of *Clostridium difficile* from the hospital environment. Am J Med 1981;70:906.
28. Fitzgerald RH, Jones DR. Hip implant infection. Am J Med 1985;78(suppl 6B):225.
29. Fitzgerald RH, Peterson IFA, Washington JA, et al. Bacterial colonization of wounds of sepsis in total hip arthroplasties. J Bone Joint Surg (Am) 1973;55:1242.
30. Foster TJ. Plasmid-determined resistance to antimicrobial drugs and toxic metal ions in bacteria. Microbiol Rev 1983;47:361.
31. Fraser DW. Bacteria newly recognized as nosocomial pathogens. Am J Med 1981;70:432.
32. Gardner RM, Schwartz R, Wong HC, et al. Percutaneous indwelling radial artery catheters for monitoring cardiovascular function. N Engl J Med 1974;290:1227.
33. Gaynes RP, Weinstein RA, Smith J, et al. Control of aminoglycoside resistance by barrier precautions. Infect Control 1983;4:221.
34. Goldmann, DA. Epidemiology of *Staphylococcus aureus* and group-A streptococci. In: Bennett JV, Brachman PS, eds. Hospital infections. 2nd ed. Boston: Little, Brown & Co, 1986;483.
35. Green JW, Wenzel RP. Postoperative wound infection: a controlled study of the increased duration of hospital stay and direct cost of hospitalization. Ann Surg 1977;185:264.
36. Grieble HG, Bird TJ, Nidea HM, et al. Chute hydropulping waste disposal system: a reservoir of enteric bacilli and pseudomonas in a modern hospital. J Infect Dis 1974;130:602.
37. Haley RW. Incidence of nature of endemic and epidemic nosocomial infections. In: Bennett JV, Brachman PS, eds. Hospital infections. 2nd ed. Boston: Little, Brown & Co, 1986;359.
38. Haley RW. Managing hospital infection control for cost effectiveness. Chicago: American Hospital Publishing, 1986.
39. Haley RW, Culver DH, White JW, et al. The efficacy of infection surveillance and control programs in preventing nosocomial infections in US hospitals. Am J Epidemiol 1985;121:182.
40. Haley RW, Schaberg DR, Von Allmen SD, et al. Estimation of the extra charges and prolongation of hospitalization due to nosocomial infections: a comparison of methods. J Infect Dis 1980;141:248.
41. Hall CB. Nosocomial viral respiratory infections: Perennial weeds on pediatric wards. Am J Med 1981;70:670.
42. Hall CB, Douglas RG. Modes of transmission of respiratory syncytial virus. J Pediatr 1981;99:100.
43. Hart D, Postlethwait RW, Brown IW, et al. Postoperative wound infections: a further report on ultraviolet irradiation with comments on the recent (1964) National Research Council cooperative study report. Ann Surg 1968;167:728.
44. Holmberg SD, Osterholm MT, Senger KA, et al. Drug-resistant salmonella from animals fed anti-microbials. N Engl J Med 1984;311:617.
45. Howard RJ. Host defense against infection—Parts 1 and 2. Curr Probl Surg 1980;17:267.
46. Hughes JM, Culver DH, White JW. Nosocomial infections surveillance 1980–1982. MMWR 1983;32:155.
47. Hung CY, Lefkowitz SS, Geber WF. Interferon inhibition by narcotic analgesics. Proc Soc Exp Biol Med 1973;142:106.
48. Kelsen SG, McGuckin M. The role of airborne bacteria in the contamination of fine particle neutralizers and the development of nosocomial pneumonia. Ann NY Acad Sci 1980;353:218.
49. Kopelman AE. Cutaneous absorption of hexachlorophene in low birth weight infants. J Pediatr 1973;82:972.
50. Kunin CM. Evaluation of antibiotic usage: A comprehensive look at alternative approaches. Rev Infect Dis 1981;3:745.
51. Kunin CM, Tupasi T, Craig WA. Use of antibiotics. A brief exposition of the problem and some tentative solutions. Ann Intern Med 1973;79:555.
52. Kure R, Grendahl H, Paulssen J. Pyrogens from surgeon's sterile latex gloves. Acta Pathol Microbial Immunol Scand 1982;90:85.
53. Lauer JL, Van Drunen NA, Washburn JW, et al. Transmission of hepatitis B virus in clinical laboratory areas. J Infect Dis 1979;140:512.
54. Laufman H. The operating room. In: Bennett JV, Brachman PS, eds. Hospital infections. 2nd ed. Boston: Little Brown & Co, 1986:315.
55. Laufman H. What's wrong with our operating rooms? Am J Surg 1971;122:322.
56. Levy SB. Playing antibiotic pool: time to tally the score (editorial). N Engl J Med 1984;311:663.

57. Lidwell OM, Owburg EJL, Whyte W, et al. Effect of ultraclean air in operating rooms on deep sepsis in the joint after total hip or knee replacement. A randomised study. Br Med J 1982;285:10.
58. Luke 10:34, The Bible.
59. Lyons AS, Petrucelli RJ. Medicine: an illustrated history. New York: Harry N Abrams, 1978.
60. MacLean LD, Meakins JL, Taguchi K, et al. Host resistance in sepsis and trauma. Ann Surg 1975;182:207.
61. MacMillan BG, Holden IA, Alexander JW. Infections of burn wounds. In: Bennett JV, Brachman PS, eds. Hospital infections. 2nd ed. Boston: Little, Brown & Co, 1986:465.
62. Maki DG, Alvarado CJ, Hassemer CA, et al. Relation of the inanimate hospital environment to endemic nosocomial infection. N Engl J Med 1982;307:1562.
63. Marshall W, Foster RS, Winn W. Legionnaire's disease in renal transplant patients. Am J Surg 1981;141:423.
64. McGowan JE. Antimicrobial resistance in hospital organisms and its relation to antibiotic use. Rev Infect Dis 1983;5:1033.
65. McGowan JE, Weinstein RA, Mallison GF. The role of the laboratory in control of nosocomial infection. In: Bennett JV, Brachman PS, eds. Hospital infections. 2nd ed. Boston: Little, Brown & Co, 1986:113.
66. McGuckin MB, Thorpe RJ, Abrutyn E. An outbreak of pseudomonas wound infections related to Hubbard tank treatments. Arch Phys Med Rehabil 1981;62:283.
67. Mead PB, Pories SE, Hall P, et al. Decreasing the incidence of surgical wound infections. Arch Surg 1986;121:458.
68. Miles AA, Niven JSF. The enhancement of infection during shock produced by bacterial toxins and other agents. Br J Exp Pathol 1950;31:73.
69. Moudgil GC, Allan RB, Russell RJ, et al. Inhibition, by anaesthetic agents, of human leucocyte locomotion towards chemical attractants. Br J Anaesth 1977;49:97.
70. Muder RR, Yu VL, McClure JK, et al. Nosocomial Legionnaire's disease uncovered in a prospective study: implications for underdiagnosis. JAMA 1983;249:3184.
71. Murphy JF, McDonald, Dawson M, et al. Factors affecting the frequency of infection in renal transplant recipients. Arch Intern Med 1976;136:670.
72. Myerowitz RL, Medeiros AA, O'Brien TF. Bacterial infection in renal homotransplant recipients. Am J Med 1972;53:308.
73. National Academy of Sciences. National Research Council Division of Medical Sciences, Ad Hoc Committee of the Committee on Trauma. Postoperative wound infections: the influence of ultraviolet irradiation of the operating room and of various other factors. Ann Surg 1964;160(suppl):1.
74. Neu HC. Antimicrobial activity, bacterial resistance, and antimicrobial pharmacology. Am J Med 1985;78(suppl 6B):17.
75. Nichols RL, Smith JW, Klein DB, et al. Risk of infection after penetrating abdominal trauma. N Engl J Med 1984;311:1065.
76. Olson MM, MacCallum J, McQuarrie DG. Preoperative hair removal with clippers does not increase infection rate in clean surgical wounds. Surg Gynecol Obstet 1986;162:181.
77. Olson M, O'Connor M, Schwartz ML. Surgical wound infections. A 5-year prospective study of 20,193 wounds at the Minneapolis VA Medical Center. Ann Surg 1984;199:253.
78. Oyama T. Endocrine responses to anaesthetic agents. Br J Anaesth 1973;45:276.
79. Park SK, Brody JI, Wallace HA, et al. Immunosuppressive effect of surgery. Lancet 1971;1:53.
80. Penikett EJK, Gorrill RH. The integrity of surgical gloves tested during use. Lancet 1958;2:1042.
81. Perry WD, Siegel AC, Rammelkamp CH, et al. Transmission of group A streptococci. I. The role of contaminated bedding. Am J Hyg 1957;66:85.
82. Pizzo PA. The value of protective isolation in preventing nosocomial infections in high risk patients. Am J Med 1981;70:631.
83. Polk HC, George CD, Wellhausen SR, et al. A systematic study of host defense processes in badly injured patients. Ann Surg 1986;204:282.
84. Postlethwait RW, Johnson WD. Complications following surgery for duodenal ulcer in obese patients. Arch Surg 1972;105:438.
85. Pruitt BA. Host opportunist interactions in surgical infection. Arch Surg 1986;121:13.
86. Public Health Laboratory Service. Incidence of surgical wound infection in England and Wales. Lancet 1960;2:659.
87. Rhame FS, The inanimate environment. In: Bennett JV, Brachman PS, eds. Hospital infections. 2nd ed. Boston: Little, Brown & Co, 1986:223.
88. Rhame FS, Streifel AJ, Kersey JH, et al. Extrinsic risk factors for pneumonia in the patient at risk. Am J Med 1984;76(5A):42.

174

89. Riddle PR. Disturbed immune reactions following surgery. Br J Surg 1967;54:882.
90. Rinehart JJ, Sagone AL, Balcerzak SP, et al. Effects of corticosteroid therapy on human monocyte function. N Engl J Med 1975;292:236.
91. Roberts-Thompson IC, Whittingham S, Youngchaiyud U, et al. Aging, immune response and mortality. Lancet 1974;2:368.
92. Roth AI, Fry DE, Polk HC. Infectious morbidity in extremity fractures. J Trauma 1986;26:757.
93. Saravolatz LD, Pohlod DJ, Arking LM. Community acquired methicillin resistant *Staphylococcus aureus* infections: a new source for nosocomial outbreaks. Ann Intern Med 1982;97:325.
94. Schackert HK, Betzler M, Zimmermann GF, et al. The predictive role of delayed cutaneous hypersensitivity testing in postoperative complications. Surg Gynecol Obstet 1986;162:563.
95. Schaffner W. The relationship between the hospital and the community. In: Bennett JV, Brachman PS, eds. Hospital infections. 2nd ed. Boston: Little, Brown & Co, 1986;135.
96. Schoenbaum SC, Gardner P, Shillito J. Infections of cerebro-spinal fluid shunts: epidemiology, clinical manifestations and therapy. J Infect Dis 1975;131:543.
97. Selden R, Lee S, Wang WLL, et al. Nosocomial *Klebsiella* infections: intestinal colonization as a reservoir. Ann Intern Med 1971;74:657.
98. Sheagren JN. *Staphylococcus aureus*, the persistent pathogen. Part I. N Engl J Med 1984;310:1367.
99. Sheagren JN. *Staphylococcus aureus*, the persistent pathogen. Part II. N Engl J Med 1984;310:1437.
100. Shinozaki T, Deane RS, Mazuzan JE, et al. Bacterial contamination of arterial lines. A prospective study. JAMA 1983;259:223.
101. Silverman SH, Ambrose NS, Youngs DJ, et al. The effect of peritoneal lavage with tetracycline solution on postoperative infection. Dis Colon Rectum 1986;29:165.
102. Simpson JY. Our existing system of hospitalism and its effects. Part I. Edinburgh Med J 1869;14:816.
103. Smith JK. Mechanisms of host defense against infection: aging and immunity. In: Mathiew A, Burke JF, eds. Infection and the perioperative period. New York: Grune & Stratton, 1982:3.
104. Smith JK, Wiener SL. Aging, immunity and antibiotics. Drug Ther 1978;3:19.
105. Smith JMB, Marples MJ. A natural reservoir of penicillin resistant stains of *S. aureus*. Nature 1964;201:844.
106. Solomon GF, Amkraut AA, Kasper P. Immunity, emotions and stress. Ann Clin Res 1974;6:313.
107. Steere AC, Mallison GF. Handwashing practices for the prevention of nosocomial infections. Ann Intern Med 1975;83:683.
108. Thoren L. General metabolic response to trauma including pain influence. Acta Anaesth Scand [Suppl] 1974;55:9.
109. Tomasi, TB. Mucosal immune system. Ann Otol Rhino Laryngol 1976;85:87.
110. Trunkey DD. Trauma. Sci Am 1983;249:28.
111. Walker JW. Medical malpractice claims causes and prevention. J Fla Med Assoc 1982;69:167.
112. Wangensteen OH, Wangensteen SD, Klinger CF. Surgical infection and history. In: Simmons RL, Howard RJ, eds. Surgical infectious diseases. New York: Appleton Century Crofts, 1982;1.
113. Ward CG. Influence of iron on infection. Am J Surg 1986;151:291.
114. Weinstein RA. Multiple resistant strains: epidemiology and control. In: Bennett JV, Brachman PS, eds. Hospital infections. 2nd ed. Boston: Little Brown & Co, 1986;483.
115. Weksler ME, Hutteroth TH. Impaired lymphocyte function in aged humans. J Clin Invest 1974;53:99.
116. Wenzel RP. Nosocomial infections, diagnosis related groups, and study on the efficacy of nosocomial infection control. Economic implications for hospitals under the prospective payment system. Am J Med 1985;78(suppl 6B):3.
117. Wenzel RP, Osterman CA, Hunting KJ, et al. Hospital acquired infections. I. Surveillance in a university hospital. Am J Epidemiol 1976;103:251.
118. Wilmore DW, Long JM, Mason AD, et al. Stress in surgical patients as a neurophysiologic reflex response. Surg Gynecol Obstet 1976;142:257.
119. Wilson WEC, Kirkpatrick CH, Talmage DW. Suppression of immunologic responsiveness in uremia. Ann Intern Med 1965;62:1.
120. Wingard DW, Lang R, Humphrey LJ. Effect of anesthesia on immunity. J Surg Res 1967;7:430.
121. Wise RI, Sweeney FJ, Haupt GJ, et al. The environmental distribution of Staphylococcus aureus in an operation suite. Ann Surg 1958;149:30.
122. Wright RL, Burke JF. Effect of ultraviolet radiation on postoperative neurosurgical sepsis. J Neurosurg 1969;31:533.
123. Yu VL, Goetz A, Wagener M, et al. *Staphylococcus aureus* nasal carriage and infection in patients on hemodialysis. Efficacy of antibiotic prophylaxis. N Engl J Med 1986;315:91.

8

○　　○　　○　　•　　•　　•

ANTIMICROBIAL AGENTS

Barry Jay Hartman
R. Gordon Douglas, Jr.

Surgical infections may occur spontaneously as in intestinal perforation, or secondarily as seen with wound infections following surgical procedures. Antibiotics play a major role in treating such infections, although often they are an adjunct to surgical drainage, debridement, or amputation. Not infrequently, the infections are polymicrobial requiring broad-spectrum agents or a combination of agents. An understanding of the spectrum of action, side-effects, toxicities, and costs of the major antibiotics has become a necessity for all surgeons. The rapid expansion of available agents has made this task difficult, and the number of agents that will be available in the future will surely increase this difficulty.

In this chapter, major antibiotic groups will be reviewed, including their mechanisms of action, means by which resistance develops, spectrum, pharmacokinetics, side-effects and toxicities, and surgical indications.

THE CHOICE OF AN APPROPRIATE ANTIBIOTIC

The spectrum of activity of an antibiotic is ultimately the most crucial factor in the choice of an antimicrobial agent. There are often multiple antibiotics that are effective, making other factors very important as well.[26,80] Generally, it is best to choose an agent with a narrower spectrum if possible, because it will preserve more of the body's normal bacterial flora and will have less adverse impact on bacterial resistance in hospitals.

One must also consider the overall condition of the patient and the toxicities of the antibiotic. For example, if a patient has severe renal disease, one should choose an agent that has minimal nephrotoxicity. If several agents are necessary to treat a polymicrobial infection, one should choose antibiotics with varying toxicities so that additive or synergistic effects on toxicity will not occur.

Infections such as meningitis or prostatitis require agents that adequately achieve levels in the spinal fluid and prostatic tissue, respectively. Infections in some sites such as the abdomen or pelvis are usually polymicrobial and, therefore, may require multiple antibiotics or a single agent with a broad spectrum of activity.

The allergic history of the patient must also be considered. The most common antibiotic allergies are to penicillin and sulfonamides. In patients with such a history, one should avoid agents that are related to the prior offending agent. If the history of penicillin allergy is only minimal or questionable, one might choose a cephalosporin or related beta-lactam, but observe the patient carefully for any serious allergic reactions.

Lastly, but of increasing importance, is the factor of cost in the choice of an antibiotic treatment. In a situation where multiple agents with similar efficacies or toxicities are available, one should choose the agent that is least expensive. In general, the newer agents such as the third-generation cephalosporins and carbapenems are expensive. Although they are very active, they may not be more efficacious in many situations than older, narrower spectrum cephalosporins or penicillins. Implicit in the cost of an antibiotic are the costs of administration. Agents used in the hospital that require multiple daily doses result in greater utilization of supplies, as well as pharmacy and nursing staff time. Table 8-1 lists factors in the choice of an antibiotic.

GENERAL CONSIDERATIONS

Mechanism of Action

There are four major mechanisms of action for all currently available agents and for those being studied as investigational agents. The beta-lactam antibiotics (penicillins, cephalosporins, carbapenems, monobactams), vancomycin, bacitracin, cycloserine, and others affect cell wall synthesis, thereby disrupting the normal cell wall formation required for the osmotic stability of the organism. The aminoglycosides, clindamycin, erythromycin, tetracyclines, and chloramphenicol inhibit protein synthesis by binding to one of the two ribosomal subunits. The sulfonamides, tri-

Table 8–1
Factors in Choosing an Antibiotic

Spectrum of activity
Underlying condition of the patient
Specific infectious agent
Site of infection
Specific toxicity of the antibiotic
Allergic history
Pharmacokinetic properties of the antibiotic
Cost of the antibiotic

---

methoprim and pyrimethamine, inhibit enzymes in the folic acid pathway leading to purine synthesis. Rifampin and the newer quinolones inhibit nucleic acid synthesis and packaging in the replicating bacteria.

Mechanisms of Resistance

The most effective means for bacteria to resist the action of an antibiotic is for the bacteria to destroy the antibiotic prior to its effect on its site of action.[74] Beta-lactamases,[103] aminoglycoside-inactivating enzymes,[45] and chloramphenicol amino-transferase[65] either destroy or modify their substrate antibiotic so that it is no longer active against the bacterium.

The site or target of action of an antibiotic can also be altered so that the agent does not bind to it and thereby is prevented from exerting its normal action.[65] For beta-lactams, the enzymatic targets on the cell membrane are altered. Ribosomal subunits can be changed to prevent binding of protein inhibitors. Enzymes in the folic acid pathway can be modified or changed to prevent the action of sulfonamides and other folate antagonists.[21,110]

Permeability of the membrane structure of the bacterium can be decreased so that antibiotics can no longer reach their specific target from the environment external to the bacteria. This is particularly true for gram-negative bacteria in which there is a complex outer membrane structure.

Lastly, in some bacteria such as *Staphylococcus aureus*, the beta-lactams inhibit the growth of the organism but do not effectively kill and lyse the bacteria.[38] This inability to kill the bacteria effectively is termed *tolerance*.

Antibiotic Susceptibility Testing

Most clinical laboratories determine susceptibility or resistance of a bacterium to a group of antibiotics using the Kirby-Bauer disc technique. In this procedure, the organism is grown to a standard inoculum and then spread over an agar plate. Discs containing given concentrations of antibiotics are placed on top of the agar plate containing the bacteria. The plate is then incubated for 18 to 24 hours to allow the bacteria to grow and the antibiotics in the discs to diffuse circumferentially. A specific zone diameter of bacteria-free agar around the disc is measured, and its size is correlated with susceptibility or resistance. This zone varies for each antibiotic tested. The Kirby-Bauer disc method is inexpensive, efficient, and best-suited for commercial laboratories.

Other methods of determining antibiotic susceptibility are also available. The tube (Broth) method or agar dilution method uses a series of test tubes or agar plates with serial twofold dilutions of an antibiotic in culture medium to which a given inoculum of an organism is added. The tubes or plates are incubated overnight for 18 to 24 hours, and the minimum antibiotic concentration that inhibits growth by visual inspection is referred to as the minimal inhibitory concentration (MIC). By applying a specific volume of medium from the visually negative dilutions used to determine MIC to fresh agar plates without any antibiotic present, one can determine the minimal bactericidal concentration (MBC).[76,91] The MBC is that concentration of antibiotic that kills 99.9% of the starting inoculum after 18 to 24 hours.

Significance of Serum Bactericidal Levels

To determine that amount of antibiotic in the serum of a patient, twofold dilutions of the serum are incubated with a given inoculum of the offending organism being treated. In a manner similar to the tube dilution method, the serum inhibitory level is that dilution of serum that inhibits growth of the bacteria. By plating a given volume of the twofold dilutions on fresh agar plates, the serum bactericidal titer can be ascertained.

In 1977, bacterial endocarditis was shown to be more effectively treated in the rabbit model when the serum level of antibiotic was at least eightfold above that necessary to inhibit the organism.[15] This has also been shown to improve outcome for human endocarditis. Using the rabbit model of meningitis, cerebrospinal fluid (CSF) levels of antibiotic of at least tenfold the inhibitory level improved survival. Recently, Klastersky[51] has shown that neutropenic patients do better when serum levels are 16-fold above the inhibitory level for gram-negative bacteria. Some infectious disease experts feel that eightfold or greater serum levels should be achieved for optimal outcome in osteomyelitis and other conditions. However, these are unproven, and there is no evidence that serum levels eightfold or higher must be achieved for infections such as intra-abdominal sepsis, urosepsis, or pneumonia.

BETA-LACTAM ANTIBIOTICS

Mechanism of Action

All beta-lactam antibiotics prevent the terminal steps in cross-linking of the bacterial cell wall.[114] To do this, these antibiotics must reach enzymes on the cyto-plasmic membrane that are responsible for this terminal cross-linking. Beta-lactam agents covalently bind to these enzymes, which are referred to as penicillin-binding proteins (PBPs).[113,115] All bacteria have multiple PBPs, which are in part responsible for the ultimate shape of the bacteria and which have varying affinities for different beta-lactams.

The exact consequences of the binding of the beta-lactam to the PBPs are unknown. However, some bacteria, such as pneumococci, are quickly killed and lysed. Other bacteria, such as GpA beta-hemolytic streptococci, are killed rapidly but fail to lyse. A third group of bacteria are easily inhibited from growth but are not effectively killed or lysed (*Streptococcus sanguis, Staphylococcus aureus*).[44] This latter group of bacteria are referred to as "tolerant." It is speculated that autolytic enzymes present in bacteria and used routinely to assist the bacteria in division and multiplication are released in an uncontrolled manner following the binding to the PBPs. Tolerant bacteria appear to have a reduced quantity of the autolytic enzymes or an increased amount of autolytic enzyme inhibitor.[38]

PENICILLINS

Spectrum

The natural penicillins, such as penicillin G and penicillin V, have a spectrum of activity primarily against gram-positive cocci such as the aerobic and anaerobic streptococci. A few gram-negative aerobic organisms, such as *Neisseria gonorrhea, N. meningitidis, Eikenella corrodans,* and *Pasteurella multocida,* are also exquisitely sensitive.

Because 90% of *Staphylococcus aureus* now produce penicillinase that can destroy the natural penicillins, the penicillinase-resistant penicillins are used primarily to treat these organisms. These agents are also very narrow spectrum with somewhat reduced activity against most organisms sensitive to the natural penicillins.

The aminopenicillins, such as ampicillin and amoxicillin, are destroyed by penicillinase and, therefore, are not usually effective against *Staphylococcus aureus.* However, these agents have an extended spectrum against gram-negative organisms such as *Hemophilus influenzae, Escherichia coli, Proteus mirabilis, Salmonella* sp. and *Shigella* sp.

To expand the spectrum of the aminopenicillins to include *Pseudomonas,* carboxypenicillins, such as carbenicillin and ticarcillin, and the newer ureidopenicillins, such as piperacillin, azlocillin and mezlocillin,[25] were developed. These agents maintain the spectrum of the natural and aminopenicillins but are destroyed by some beta-lactamases, such as the penicillinase produced by *Staphylococcus aureus.*[126] Table 8-2 lists surgical indications for administering penicillins.

Pharmacokinetics

Most penicillins are excreted and secreted by the kidney,[6] thereby requiring dosage adjustment for renal failure. (See Appendix C.) Only the penicillinase-resistant penicillins, such as nafcillin, oxacillin, and dicloxacillin, are primarily metabolized by the liver and require little or no adjustment for renal failure.[68]

Table 8–2
Surgical Indications for Penicillins

Cellulitis/furuncles/carbuncles (penicillin or penicillinase-resistant penicillins)
Septic arthritis (penicillin ± penicillinase-resistant penicillin)
Osteomyelitis (penicillinase-resistant penicillins)
Brain abscess (penicillin)
Acute epididymo-orchitis from *Neisseria gonorrheae*
Gas gangrene (penicillin)
Pseudomonas infections (anti-pseudomonal penicillin ± aminoglycoside)
Antibiotic prophylaxis for infective endocarditis (penicillin or ampicillin ± aminoglycoside)

All penicillins also achieve excellent tissue levels in most tissues including CSF. However, they must be given in high dosage to achieve adequate levels in both the CSF and prostatic tissues. The agents vary in their protein binding, but this does not seem to affect clinical efficacy significantly.

Toxicity

The most common toxicity with all beta-lactams are hypersensitivity reactions.[89,94] These reactions can vary from a severe and potentially fatal anaphylactic reaction to a mild, maculopapular rash. Anaphylactic reactions are mediated by IgE and occur in up to 5 of every 10,000 penicillin courses. Less severe reactions are generally mediated by IgG or IgM. Rarely, a serum sickness reaction manifested by fever, arthritis, and rash can occur secondary to IgG, as well.

All penicillins occasionally cause bone marrow toxicity with isolated suppression of white cell precursors leading to neutropenia.[75] Occasionally, isolated thrombocytopenia may occur. More commonly, anemia secondary to a peripheral destruction of red cells from a Coombs-positive hemolytic anemia can develop. This hemolysis is mediated by IgG that binds to a penicillin–protein complex on the red cell membrane usually in the setting of both high dose and prolonged therapy.[50] Bleeding complications may occur with carboxypenicillins[12] or ureidopenicillins due to inhibition of platelet aggregation by inhibiting the action of adenosine diphosphate (ADP).

All penicillins, particularly aqueous penicillin G in doses above 20 million units daily in patients with renal failure,[8] can produce seizures and other neurologic complications in animals, but very few have caused them clinically. Most penicillins have also been reported to cause interstitial nephritis, but this complication has been seen most often with methicillin. Drug fever, hepatitis, and gastrointestinal symptoms including pseudomembranous colitis from *Clostridium difficile* have all been reported infrequently. The carboxypenicillins are disodium salts and, therefore, can lead to fluid overload and hypokalemia. The ureidopenicillins are monosodium salts and have less problems with fluid and electrolyte abnormalities.

CEPHALOSPORINS

Spectrum

Cephalosporins (Table 8-3) have been divided into first, second, and third generations based primarily on their spectrum of activity against aerobic gram-negative bacilli (Table 8-4).

Table 8–3
Surgical Indications for Cephalosporins

Surgical prophylaxis (cefazolin, cefoxitin, others)

Staphylococcal and streptococcal infections in mildly penicillin-allergic patients (cefazolin)

Community-acquired polymicrobial infections of the abdomen and pelvis (cefoxitin, cefotetan)

Nosocomial infections (third-generation cephalosporins)

Pseudomonas infections (ceftazidime or cefoperazone ± aminoglycoside)

Table 8–4
Newer Parenteral Beta-Lactam Antibiotics Specific Advantages and Disadvantages

	ADVANTAGES	DISADVANTAGES
Penicillins		
Carboxypenicillins		
Carbenicillin	Very good for *pseudomonas* Synergy with aminoglycosides	High sodium content Anti-platelet activity No *Klebsiella* activity
Ticarcillin	Slightly better *Pseudomonas* activity than carbenicillin	High sodium content Anti-platelet activity No *Klebsiella* activity
Ticarcillin/clavulanic acid	Penicillinase-producing *Staphylococcus aureus* activity Good *Klebsiella* activity Good *Bacteroides fragilis* activity	Same as ticarcillin
Ureidopenicillins		
Azlocillin	Excellent *Pseudomonas* activity Low sodium content	Potential anti-platelet effect
Mezlocillin	Very good *Pseudomonas* activity Very good *Bacteroides fragilis* activity Best *Klebsiella* activity of all penicillins Low sodium content	Potential anti-platelet effect

(continued)

Table 8–4 (continued)

	ADVANTAGES	DISADVANTAGES
Piperacillin	Best *Pseudomonas* activity of all penicillins Very good *Bacteroides fragilis* activity Low sodium content	Potential anti-platelet effect High cost
Cephalosporins		
Second Generation		
Group 1—Excellent Hemophilus Influenzae Activity		
Cefuroxime	Only first or second generation cephalosporin approved for meningitis	
Cefamandole		MTT side chain and potential bleeding problems Antabuse effect with alcohol
Cefonicid	Long half-life for once or twice daily dosing	
Ceforanide	Long half-life for twice daily dosing	
Group 2—Excellent Anaerobic Activity		
Cefotetan	Longer half-life for twice daily dosing Lower cost	Limited clinical experience MTT side chain and potential bleeding problems Reduced activity against Bacteroides species other than *Bacteroides fragilis*
Cefoxitin	Extensive clinical experience Excellent *Bacteroides fragilis* and *Bacteroides* spp. activity	
Third Generation		
Group 1—Excellent Enteric Bacillary Activity		
Cefotaxime	Most clinical experience for meningitis	Frequent daily dosing Beta-lactamase induction High cost
Ceftizoxime	Fair to good *Bacteroides fragilis* activity	Beta-lactamase induction High cost
Ceftriaxone	Longest half-life for once daily dosing Much clinical experience for meningitis at twice daily dosing No adjustments for renal failure	Beta-lactamase induction High cost
Group 2—Anti-Pseudomonal Agents		
Cefoperazone	Twice daily dosing Good enteric bacillary activity No adjustments for renal failure Synergistic with aminoglycosides	MTT side chain and potential bleeding problems Antabuse effect with alcohol Not approved for pediatrics Not approved for meningitis High cost

(continued)

Table 8–4 (continued)

	ADVANTAGES	DISADVANTAGES
Ceftazidime	Excellent enteric bacillary activity Most synergistic agent with amino- glycosides for *Pseudomonas*	Poor gram-positive activity Poor *Bacteroides fragilis* activity High cost
Cefsulodin*	Excellent *Pseudomonas* activity Good *Staphylococcus* activity	Investigational agent Minimal activity against other gram-negative, gram-positive or anaerobic organisms
Oxabetalactams		
Moxalactam	Excellent enteric bacillary activity Fair *Pseudomonas* activity Very good *Bacteroides fragilis* activity Much clinical experience with meningitis	Poor *Streptococcus* *pneumoniae* activity Poor *Staphylococcus* *aureus* activity MTT side chain and po- tential bleeding problems from hypoprothrom- binemia Antabuse effect with alcohol Anti-platelet effect Enterococcal super- infections
Carbapenems		
Impipenem/cil- astatin	Broadest spectrum of any available agent Excellent *Pseudomonas* activity	High cost Relatively high incidence of CNS side effects *Pseudomonas* resistance may develop when used alone
Monobactams		
Aztreonam	Excellent gram-negative bacillary action Excellent *Pseudomonas* activity Minimal cross-reactivity to other beta- lactams	No gram-positive activity No anaerobic activity

* *Indicates investigational agent*

First-generation cephalosporins such as cephalothin and cefazolin[83] are very active against all aerobic gram-positive cocci including streptococci, penicillin-sensitive and penicillinase-producing staphylococci. These agents also have activity to a lesser extent than penicillin G against anaerobic mouth bacteria such as peptostreptococci and *Bacteroides* species in the mouth. *Bacteroides fragilis* is usually resistant. Aerobic gram-negative, enteric rods such as *Escherichia coli, Klebsiella, Proteus* sp. and *Enterobacter* sp. are frequently susceptible to these agents. However, similar organisms isolated in the hospital have an increased rate of resistance to first-generation agents.

Second-generation agents are divided into two groups. The first group includes those agents (cefamandole, cefuroxime, cefonicid, and ceforanide) with excellent activity against *H. influenzae,* both non-penicillinase and penicillinase-producing strains.[84] These agents also retain good activity against streptococci and staphylococci, but to a lesser degree than first-generation agents. This group also has a greater spectrum against some additional enteric bacilli such as some *Enterobacter* and *Klebsiella* strains that may be resistant to first-generation agents.[59]

The second group of second-generation cephalosporins includes cefoxitin[85] and cefotetan.[78] Both these agents are very effective against *Bacteroides fragilis.* Cefoxitin also is very active against other *Bacteroides* species; whereas cefotetan is often ineffective against these other species. Both agents have increased activity against enteric gram-negative organisms resistant to first-generation cephalosporins including *Serratia marcescens.* Gram-positive aerobic cocci are less susceptible to these agents than either the first generation or first group of second-generation cephalosporins.

Third-generation cephalosporins can also be divided into two major groups. In the first group are those agents (cefotaxime, ceftizoxime, cetriaxone, and moxalactam) that are most effective against the majority of enteric gram-negative bacilli including those strains that are resistant to first- and second-generation cephalosporins and aminoglyosides, as well.[29] These agents are also very effective against nosocomial gram-negative bacilli including *Serratia marcescens* and multiply resistant enteric bacilli. Only moxalactam has fair anti-*Pseudomonas* activity, but it is rarely used because of the bleeding complications associated with it. Less than 20% to 30% of *Pseudomonas* strains are susceptible to maximum doses of the other three agents in this group, and they are, therefore, not recommended for *Pseudomonas* infections. Anaerobes such as *Bacteroides fragilis* and gram-positive cocci such as streptococci and staphylococci are often susceptible but require high levels of antibiotics making them less effective than the first-generation cephalosporins or penicillins. Cefoxitin and cefotetan are also considerably more active against *Bacteroides fragilis* than these third-generation cephalosporins.[104] All these agents are extremely effective against all *H. influenzae, N. gonorrhea,* and *N. meningitidis* strains.

The second group of third-generation cephalosporins is composed of cefoperazone[11] and ceftazidime.[123] These agents have a very similar spectrum to the first group but also possess excellent activity against *Pseudomonas aeruginosa.*

Pharmacokinetics

All cephalosporins achieve excellent serum and tissue levels. However, only cefuroxime and most of the third-generation cephalosporins achieve adequate CSF levels with inflamed meninges to be approved for meningitis therapy.[73] Levels within the prostate are also marginal but are adequate for prostatitis when given as high dose parenteral therapy.

Most cephalosporins are excreted primarily by the kidneys, and serum levels can be increased using probenecid. Cefoperazone and ceftriaxone are metabolized primarily by the liver and achieve very high biliary tract and gastrointestinal levels. These agents do not require significant adjustments in dosage for renal disease.

Presently, most cephalosporins are available in the parenteral form. Only first-generation cephalosporins such as cephalexin, cefadroxil, and the second-generation agent, cefaclor, are available in oral forms. Cefixime, a recently approved third-generation agent with broad-spectrum gram-negative activity excluding *Pseudomonas*, is also available as an oral preparation.

Adverse Reactions

The cephalosporins have similar adverse reactions to penicillins. There is a 5% to 20% cross-reactivity to the penicillins regarding hypersensitivity reactions.[77] However, they can be used with caution in penicillin-allergic patients provided that the reaction was not mediated by IgE (anaphylaxis or hives).

Several cephalosporins (cefamandole, cefoperazone, cefotetan, and moxalactam) with the methylthiotetrazole (MTT) side chain cause two specific adverse reactions: elevation in the prothrombin time[88] and a disulfuram reaction. The mechanism by which these occur is unknown; however, it is postulated that the MTT side chain may competitively inhibit a carboxylase enzyme system in the liver necessary to produce vitamin K-dependent factors. Others believe that the effect is secondary to high concentrations of the antibiotic in the bowel reducing the bowel flora that are necessary to produce vitamin K. The mechanism by which it produces the disulfuram reaction in the presence of alcohol is also unknown but may be due to the effect of the MTT side chain on the aldehyde dehydrogenase enzyme system. These agents should be used with caution in those patients with postoperative bleeding problems and those receiving anticoagulation. Moxalactam, unlike the other agents with the MTT side chain, also has antiplatelet effects preventing platelet aggregation and thereby having a greater propensity for producing severe bleeding complications.

OTHER BETA-LACTAM ANTIBIOTICS

Carbepenems

Imipenem

Spectrum—Thienamycins belong to a class of new beta-lactam agents called the penems (carbapenems) and are represented by a specific agent called imipenem. Imipenem is metabolized by an enzyme produced by the human kidney tubule, thereby preventing active urinary level of the drug. To counteract this, cilastatin has been combined with imipenem to inhibit the action of this tubular enzyme. The product is marketed as a combination of these two agents, which are mixed together at the time of administration.

Imipenem is the broadest spectrum parenteral agent now available.[5] Staphylococci, streptococci, *Neisseria* species, anaerobes including *Bacteroides*, and gram-negative bacilli including *Pseudomonas aeruginosa* are usually exquisitely susceptible to imipenem. However, *Pseudomonas cepacia, Pseudomonas maltophilia,* methicillin-resistant *Staphylococcus aureus* and *Staphylococcus epidermidis, Streptococcus faecium* and some corynebacterium are usually resistant.[46]

Pharmacokinetics

Imipenem is excreted by the kidney and must be significantly reduced in dosage for severe renal disease.[35] It is available as a parenteral preparation only. It achieves excellent tissue levels including the CSF but is not yet approved for the treatment of meningitis.

Although data are lacking, it is assumed that imipenem cross-reacts with penicillins to a similar degree as the cephalosporins and has other side-effects similar to the penicillins and cephalosporins. However, imipenem also has a higher incidence of central nervous system (CNS) toxicity than many other beta-lactams.[14] It is estimated that up to 0.4% of patients will show muscle twitching, myoclonus, or even generalized seizures. Those CNS complications usually occur in patients with severe underlying renal disease, who also have a prior history of seizures and who are markedly debilitated and malnourished. Strict dosage recommendations must be followed in the above setting. If CNS events occur, the antibiotic should either be reduced in dosage or stopped.

MONOBACTAMS

The newest group of beta-lactams possess only the beta-lactam ring and are called monobactams.[102] Aztreonam, the best-studied agent in this group, has a very broad gram-negative bacillary spectrum including most *Pseudomonas aeruginosa.* However, it has no significant activity against gram-positive cocci or anaerobes. *Acinetobacter* and some *Pseudomonas* species are also resistant. Thus, Aztreonam has a spectrum similar to the aminoglycosides, but without the toxicity.

This agent is excreted by the kidney and must also be adjusted for reduced renal function.[101] It is available in only the parenteral form and also achieves excellent tissue levels.

Aztreonam has similar adverse reactions as other beta-lactams.[41] However, several studies have shown that it does not cross-react with penicillins and cephalosporins, and may be safe to use in patients who are severely allergic to other beta-lactams.[90]

BETA-LACTAMASE INHIBITORS

Clavulanic acid[69, 124] and sulbactam are beta-lactam agents with little intrinsic antibacterial activity of their own, but with very high affinity for many classes of beta-lactamases. When combined with other beta-lactamase sensitive antibiotics these inhibitors allow the active antibiotic to reach its target and kill the organism without being hydrolyzed by the beta-lactamase. Presently, there are three commercially available preparations. Amoxicillin-clavulanic acid is an oral preparation that expands the spectrum of amoxicillin to cover *Staphylococcus aureus, Klebsiella, Bacteroides fragilis,* and some other amoxicillin-resistant organisms.

Ticarcillin-clavulanic acid[81] is a parenteral combination preparation that broadens the activity of ticarcillin to include *Staphylococcus aureus, Klebsiella* and most *Bacteroides fragilis.* Ampicillin-sulbactam is the newest parenteral agent which offers a considerably expanded spectrum of activity for ampicillin.

VANCOMYCIN

Mechanism of Action

Vancomycin (Table 8-5) inhibits the synthesis of bacterial cell walls at steps that precede those inhibited by beta-lactam agents.

Spectrum

Vancomycin has activity primarily against gram-positive organisms.[34] No strain of *Staphylococcus aureus* has been found to be resistant to vancomycin. Recently, vancomycin-resistant *Staphylococcus epidermidis* has been reported.[92] Virtually all streptococci including viridans streptococci, enterococci, and *Streptococcus pneumoniae* are sensitive, including those that are resistant to penicillin.[125] Vancomycin also has activity against most gram-positive anaerobic bacteria including *Clostridium perfringens* but is not the therapy of choice for any of these organisms.

Vancomycin is the treatment of choice for methicillin-resistant *Staphylococcus aureus*[97] and *Staphylococcus epidermidis.*[48] It is also the therapy of choice in combination with an aminoglycoside in penicillin-allergic patients who have enterococcal endocarditis. In penicillin-allergic patients, vancomycin is frequently used for antibiotic prophylaxis prior to cardiothoracic, orthopedic, and neurosurgical pro-

Table 8–5
Surgical Indications for Vancomycin

Methicillin-resistant *Staphylococcus aureus* and *Staphylococcus epidermidis* (± aminoglycoside; ± rifampin)

Enterococcal endocarditis in penicillin-allergic patients (with an aminoglycoside)

Surgical prophylaxis in penicillin and cephalosporin-allergic patients

Antibiotic prophylaxis for infective endocarditis in penicillin-allergic patients (± aminoglycoside)

Pseudomembranous colitis (oral form)

---

cedures and as prophylaxis for endocarditis in penicillin-allergic patients. Oral vancomycin is the therapy of choice for pseudomembranous colitis secondary to *Clostridium difficile.*[95]

Vancomycin is also the treatment of choice for some species of dipheroids and corynebacterium such as CDC-JK.

Pharmacokinetics

Vancomycin is available primarily as an intravenous preparation. It achieves excellent levels in most tissues but only reaches therapeutic levels in the CSF when the meninges are inflamed. An oral form is also available for therapy of *Clostridium difficile* colitis because it is poorly absorbed but achieves very high levels in the bowel.

Vancomycin is almost completely excreted in the urine. Dosage must be markedly reduced for increasing renal failure.[62] In those who require dialysis, it can be given as a 1-g dose every 5 to 7 days, which maintains adequate serum levels. It is not hemodialyzed or peritoneally dialyzed to any extent.

Adverse Reactions

Vancomycin has only minimal nephrotoxicity when used alone.[1,27] However, in combination with aminoglycosides, it acts synergistically to produce increased nephrotoxicity.

Vancomycin also has produced ototoxicity similar to the aminoglycosides.[57] It is usually associated with very high serum levels. Infrequent side-effects include leukopenia and neutropenia, eosinophilia, and rash.

A red flush of the face, neck, and upper chest due to vasodilation can occur when vancomycin is infused too rapidly. This is called the "red-man" or "red-neck" syndrome.[70] In severe cases, hypotension may occur. To prevent this, infusion must be over a minimum of 1 hour. Slow infusion rates also decrease phlebitis from local irritation at the infusion site.

AMINOGLYCOSIDES

Mechanism of Action

Aminoglycosides (Table 8-6) are bactericidal antibiotics that act as protein synthesis inhibitors at the 30s ribosomal subunit. Resistance to aminoglycosides is generally mediated by the production of aminoglycoside-modifying enzymes (AME).[45] There are three groups of AMEs, which acetylate, adenylate, or phosphorylate the aminoglycoside and thereby prevent its action at the 30s subunit. Each aminoglycoside has varying abilities to be modified by these enzymes. Amikacin is the most difficult to modify, and this accounts for its broad activity even against organisms that are resistant to other aminoglycosides. In addition, gram-negative bacilli can also alter their target on the 30s ribosomal subunit. This resistance mechanism can

Table 8–6
Surgical Indications for Aminoglycosides

Nosocomial gram-negative bacillary infections
Mixed gram-negative and anaerobic infections (with clindamycin or metronidazole)
Elective colorectal surgery (oral neomycin)
Pseudomonas infections (often with an anti-pseudomonal penicillin or anti-pseudomonal cephalosporin)

---

act in association with AMEs and potentially make an organism resistant to all aminoglycosides.

Spectrum

The spectrum of activity for all the aminoglycosides is primarily directed against gram-negative aerobic bacilli.[61] Streptomycin, kanamycin, and neomycin are excellent for enteric organisms but have virtually no intrinsic activity against *Pseudomonas aeruginosa*. Agents such as gentamicin, tobramycin, netilmicin, and amikacin also possess excellent activity against *Pseudomonas aeruginosa*. Many *Staphylococcus aureus* are susceptible to aminoglycosides; yet, these agents are ineffective in eradicating *Staphylococcus aureus* infections when used alone because of the rapid emergence of resistance. In combination with penicillinase-resistant penicillins or vancomycin, aminoglycosides act synergistically against most *Staphylococcus aureus* and *Staphylococcus epidermidis*. Aminoglycosides are not very active against streptococci, but do act synergistically with penicillins against most streptococci, particularly, viridans streptococci and enterococci (*Streptococcus faecalis, Streptococcus faecium*). In fact, the combination of penicillin (or ampicillin) with gentamicin (or streptomycin) is the treatment of choice for endocarditis caused by enterococci.

Streptomycin is specifically used in the treatment of tuberculosis (*Mycobacterium tuberculosis*) and is bactericidal. Other aminoglycosides including gentamicin and amikacin also posses some antimycobacterial properties, but are rarely used for this purpose. Streptomycin is also a very active and useful agent in brucellosis, tularemia, and the plague. Kanamycin is not used much now because of its inherent lack of *Pseudomonas* activity. Neomycin is used primarily as an oral agent for bowel "clean-out" often in combination with other oral agents prior to elective gastrointestinal surgery. It is also used in irrigation solutions and topical ointments and creams.

Pharmacokinetics

Streptomycin is available only as an intramuscular preparation. Neomycin is available both as an oral preparation and in topical ointments and creams. When given orally in routine doses, up to 10% of neomycin is absorbed into the bloodstream. This is not enough, however, to allow oral neomycin to be used in the therapy of systemic infection, but may cause toxicity in some situations.

Gentamicin, tobramycin, netilmicin, and amikacin are available as parenteral preparations for intramuscular and intravenous administration. Excellent serum levels are achieved by either route, and the intramuscular route is well tolerated.

All systemic aminoglycosides are excreted and concentrated by the kidneys achieving high urinary levels that can be tenfold greater than serum levels. The doses of these agents must, therefore, be significantly reduced in patients who have renal insufficiency. These agents are removed by both hemodialysis and peritoneal dialysis. Administration of gentamicin, tobramycin, netilmicin, or amikacin into peritoneal dialysis solution in appropriate concentrations can maintain serum levels for many days without continued parenteral administration once a loading dose of the aminoglycoside has been given parenterally (Table 8-7).

Side-effects

Nephrotoxicity is the major side-effect that limits the use of amino-glycosides.[55,64] All aminoglycosides can produce an increase in blood urea nitrogen and serum creatinine. Streptomycin and neomycin are least and most nephrotoxic, respectively. However, there is no universal agreement whether there is a significant difference in nephrotoxicity among other aminoglycosides. Various nomograms and computer programs have been developed to predict serum levels of aminoglycosides based on renal function, age, weight, and anticipated serum levels. However, various methods of measuring serum levels are available and remain the most accurate way to ensure adequate and safe dosing. Nephrotoxicity is usually reversible and rarely is severe enough to cause end-stage renal disease, if levels are monitored.

Toxicity to the eighth cranial nerve may occur with all aminoglycosides and may involve auditory or vestibular dysfunction.[47,63] The specific incidence of toxicity varies and is dependent on how carefully patients are followed. The most common effect is loss of high-frequency hearing noted only by formal audiographic evaluation. Neo-

Table 8–7
Dosing of Aminoglycosides in Patients on Peritoneal Dialysis (PD)

AMINOGLYCOSIDE	INTRAVENOUS LOADING DOSE (mg/kg)	PD CONCENTRATION/LITER (mg)
Gentamicin	2	5–10
Tobramycin	2	5–10
Netilmicin	2	5–10
Amikacin	7.5	20–40

mycin is the most toxic to the auditory component, while streptomycin is most toxic to the vestibular system. Once toxicity occurs, it may not be reversible in all cases.

Other side-effects are very uncommon but include neuromuscular blockade producing a curarelike effect. This toxicity may occur with administration into large serosal cavities in the presence of underlying diseases such as myasthenia gravis.

CHLORAMPHENICOL

Chloramphenicol (Table 8-8) is a protein inhibitor acting at the 50s ribosomal subunit. It is usually bacteriostatic against enteric gram-negative and anaerobic organisms.

Spectrum

Chloramphenicol has a very broad spectrum of activity.[4] It is active against most enteric gram-negative bacilli such as *Escherichia coli, Klebsiella, Proteus,* and *Enterobacter. Shigella* and *Salmonella* are also frequently susceptible. It has almost uniform efficacy against all anaerobes including *Bacteroides fragilis* and other *Bacteroides* species.

Chloramphenicol provides excellent coverage for the organisms causing most cases of meningitis. It is bactericidal against *H. influenzae, Streptococcus pneumoniae* and *N. meningitidis.*[79] Rickettsiae, mycoplasma, chlamydia, and most spirochetes are also susceptible.

Chloramphenicol is never effective against *Pseudomonas aeruginosa* but is

Table 8–8
Surgical Indications for Chloramphenicol, Clindamycin, Erythromycin, and Tetracyclines

---

Chloramphenicol
Brain abscess (often with penicillin)
Clindamycin
Intra-abdominal infections (with aminoglycosides)
Nonvenereal pelvic inflammatory disease (with aminoglycosides)
Other mixed aerobic–anaerobic infections such as decubitus ulcers (with aminoglycosides)
Erythromycin
Chlamydial infections in pregnant women
Elective colorectal surgery (orally with neomycin for bowel clean-out)
Tetracycline
Chlamydial infections (PID)

---

often active against other *Pseudomonas* species such as *Pseudomonas cepacia* and *Pseudomonas maltophilia.* It is also rarely efficacious against the enterococci. Although it may have *in vitro* activity against most staphylococci, it is often ineffective *in vivo* and, therefore, rarely used for severe staphylococcal infections.

Pharmacokinetics

Very high serum levels are achieved after oral or intravenous administration.[52,96] The intramuscular route is not recommended because of unpredictable absorption and poor serum levels. The antibiotic is almost entirely metabolyzed by the liver and, therefore, requires no adjustment for severe renal disease. However, those patients with severe hepatic failure with jaundice must have the dosage adjusted. Very little drug is protein bound, and, therefore, chloramphenicol achieves excellent levels in serum, tissues, and CSF.

Adverse Reactions

Chloramphenicol generally has few adverse reactions. However, in one patient out of 25,000 to 40,000 patients, an idiosyncratic, irreversible aplastic anemia may occur leading to death of the patient.[128] These cases have occurred almost entirely after oral administration, but a few cases of parenteral-induced aplastic anemia have also been reported. More commonly, a reversible bone marrow suppression occurs following high-dose prolonged therapy, which resolves when chloramphenicol is reduced or discontinued. By following serum iron and iron-binding capacity at weekly intervals while on chloramphenicol one can often predict this reversible toxicity by detecting increasing values due to the inhibition of iron utilization by red cell precursors.

Optic neuritis, peripheral neuropathy, delirium, and coma are infrequently reported neurologic side-effects of chloramphenicol. In newborns given high doses of chloramphenicol, cardiovascular collapse can occur[17] secondary to the inability of the immature liver to metabolize the antibiotic (gray-baby syndrome). Levels of warfarin, oral hypoglycemics, and phenytoin are increased in the presence of chloramphenicol due to an inhibition in the normal hepatic metabolism of these agents.

CLINDAMYCIN

Clindamycin (see Table 8-8) inhibits protein synthesis by binding to the 50s ribosomal subunit in a similar location to erythromycin.

Spectrum

Clindamycin has its principal activity against gram-positive and anaerobic organisms.[56] It has virtually no activity against gram-negative organisms. Its spectrum includes streptococci including *Streptococcus pneumoniae, Staphylococcus au-*

reus, and *Staphylococcus epidermidis.* Those *Staphylococcus aureus* strains that are resistant to erythromycin may develop resistance to clindamycin due to a mechanism called cross-dissociative resistance. Therefore, these *Staphylococcus aureus* strains should not be treated with clindamycin. Clindamycin has no activity against enterococci and rarely is effective for methicillin-resistant *Staphylococcus aureus.*

Clindamycin is one of the most active agents against a broad array of anaerobic cocci and bacilli.[100] About 95% of *Bacteroides fragilis* and *Bacteroides* species are sensitive to clindamycin.[74] Virtually all other anaerobes, such as peptostreptococci and clostridia, are susceptible although clostridial species other than *Clostridium perfringens* may be resistant.

Pharmacokinetics

Clindamycin is available orally and parenterally. It achieves excellent serum levels by either route.[22, 56] It does not reach adequate levels in the CNS or CSF at routine doses and is, therefore, not used in CNS infections. However, high doses have recently been used to treat CNS toxoplasmosis in AIDS patients who are allergic to sulfonamides and in others who have ocular toxoplasmosis. Bone levels of clindamycin are high,[72] making clindamycin an excellent alternative in the therapy of grampositive osteomyelitis.

Doses do not have to be altered in renal failure because most of the drug is metabolized in the liver. Moderate adjustments are required in severe hepatic failure.

Adverse Reactions

The major side-effect of both oral and parenteral clindamycin is diarrhea. Up to 20% of patients may have mild diarrhea,[93, 107] but 1% to 2% develop severe diarrhea, cramps, bloody discharge, and fever secondary to the production of a heat-labile toxin produced by *Clostridium difficile.*[108] This severe diarrhea has a pseudomembrane over the intestinal mucosa, referred to as pseudomembranous colitis (PMC), and may rarely be fatal. Although PMC may occur with other broad-spectrum agents such as ampicillin, cephalosporins, and tetracycline, the greatest incidence occurs with clindamycin. Treatment of PMC consists of discontinuing the offending antibiotic, fluid replacement, and the administration of either oral vancomycin or oral metronidazole.[106]

Infrequent adverse reactions such as mildly elevated liver function tests, allergic reactions such as rash, neuromuscular blockade and bone marrow toxicity may also occur.

ERYTHROMYCIN

Erythromycin (see Table 8-8) is a macrolide antibiotic that binds to the 50s ribosomal subunit and inhibits protein synthesis.

Spectrum

Erythromycin's activity is primarily against gram-positive aerobic organisms.[118] It is very active against most *Staphylococcus aureus* and some *Staphylococcus epidermidis.* However, it is rarely active against methicillin-resistant *Staphylococcus aureus.* In addition, those *Staphylococcus aureus* strains that are sensitive to erythromycin but resistant to clindamycin will rapidly develop resistance to erythromycin because of *cross dissociative resistance.*[33] The same phenomenon occurs in the reverse when clindamycin is used to treat an erythromycin-resistant, clindamycin-sensitive *Staphylococcus aureus.*

Erythromycin is also very effective against most streptococci including viridens streptococci, *Streptococcus pyogenes* (GpA Beta-strep) and *Streptococcus pneumoniae.* Enterococci, however, are usually resistant.

Gram-positive aerobic bacilli such as *Corynebacterium diphtheriae,* and *Listeria monocytogenes* are also susceptible to erythromycin as are both *N. gonorrhea* and *N. meningitidis.* Most other gram-negative aerobes and most anaerobes are usually resistant. *Campylobacter jejeuni* remains a susceptible organism and erythromycin remains its treatment of choice.

Recently, the use of erythromycin has increased significantly[67] because of its excellent clinical activity against atypical pneumonia agents, primarily *Legionella pneumophila,*[24] *Legionella* species, and *Mycoplasm pneumoniae.*

Pharmacokinetics

Both oral and parenteral preparations of erythromycin are available. Oral erythromycin is absorbed well and achieves adequate serum and tissue levels.[71] However, for severe *Legionella* pneumonia, parenteral therapy is recommended. Because the agent is metabolized by the liver, its dosage does not have to be altered significantly in the setting of renal inefficiency. Erythromycin is one of only a few antibiotics that achieves high concentrations in the prostate, but its spectrum is not appropriate for most prostate infections.

Adverse Reactions

Erythromycin frequently causes upset stomach, nausea, vomiting, abdominal pain or diarrhea following oral administration. Giving the medication with food may alleviate some of the upper gastrointestinal symptoms. Parenteral erythromycin often causes phlebitis secondary to local inflammation. When given in high doses to patients with renal insufficiency, transient hearing loss may rarely occur.[39]

Lastly, erythromycin estolate may cause a cholestatic hepatitis secondary to a hypersensitivity reaction. Patients develop jaundice, abdominal pain, enlarged liver, and peripheral eosinophilia.[9] This reaction is extremely uncommon with other salts of erythromycin. Because of this problem, the estolate salt is rarely used in adults.

TETRACYCLINES

These are a group of agents that act as protein synthesis inhibitors at the 30s ribosomal subunit (see Table 8-8). These agents are bacteriostatic and not bactericidal.

Spectrum

All tetracyclines have a similar spectrum of activity so that one antibiotic disc will represent the activity of all the agents in the group. Most streptococci and many staphylococci are sensitive to tetracycline[32] although up to 10% of *Streptococcus pneumoniae* and *Streptococcus pyogenes* and 30% to 50% of *Staphylococcus aureus* are resistant.

Tetracyclines also have excellent activity against *N. meningitidis* and *N. gonorrhea.*[43] However, penicillinase-producing *N. gonorrhea* (PPNG), intrinsically resistant *N. gonorrhea* and the recently described tetracycline-resistant gonorrhea are resistant.[109] Their activity is good against mouth anaerobes but up to two thirds of *Bacteroides fragilis* are now resistant.[104]

Many enteric gram-negative bacilli such as *Escherichia coli* and *Klebsiella*, as well as *Salmonella* and *Shigella* are also susceptible. However, increasing resistance has developed, and, therefore, sensitivity patterns must be examined before depending on tetracyclines to treat serious infections with these organisms.

Tetracycline has become the therapy of choice in several situations. All rickettsial, mycoplasma, and chlamydial infections may be treated effectively with tetracycline. *Borrelia burgdorferi*, the spirochete responsible for Lyme disease,[98] *Treponema pallidum*, the spirochete causing syphilis, and *Borrelia recurrentis*, the responsible spirochete of Borreliosis, are all effectively treated with tetracycline. Because of its excellent activity against *Chlamydia*, it is recommended as adjunctive therapy in those being treated for gonorrhea because of the 20% to 50% association with *Chlamydia*. It is also commonly used by gynecologists to treat pelvic inflammatory disease (PID) caused by chlamydia.

Pharmacokinetics

Tetracyclines are available in oral and parenteral forms but are usually used orally.[20] The agents are adequately absorbed on an empty stomach achieving good tissue, serum, and urinary levels. Food and calcium-containing products such as milk and antacids prevent absorption from the GI tract. Only doxycycline absorption is unaffected by food and antacids. Intravenous tetracycline is most commonly used to treat seriously ill females with PID caused by *Chlamydia* and severely ill patients with rickettsial infections.

Most tetracyclines are excreted by the kidneys and should either be reduced in dosage or not used in the setting of severe renal disease. However, doxycycline is metabolized by the liver and may be used, if necessary, in patients with severe renal disease.[122]

Adverse Reactions

Tetracyclines are contraindicated in children under 8 years old and in pregnant women because of the potential deleterious effects on teeth[10] and developing bones.[16] An unusual and potentially lethal side-effect, fulminant fatty degeneration of the liver, can also occur in pregnant women who take tetracycline, particularly, in the parenteral form.[112]

Tetracyclines produce frequent gastrointestinal side-effects when given orally including nausea, vomiting, cramps, and diarrhea. PMC secondary to *Clostridium difficile* toxin has also been reported. Hypersensitivity reactions such as rashes, hives, drug fevers, and fixed drug eruptions have occurred. In some patients, exposure to the sun causes a photosensitivity reaction. Outdated tetracycline can lead to a reversible Fanconi syndrome, but only demeclocycline can cause nephrogenic diabetes insipidus.[122]

SULFONAMIDES

All sulfonamides (Table 8-9) inhibit the enzyme, tetrahydropteroic acid synthetase, early in the folic acid pathway to purine metabolism. They act as competitive antagonists to para-aminobenzoic acid (PABA).

Spectrum

Sulfonamides have a broad range of activity against both gram-positive and gram-negative aerobic organisms.[3] They are effective against many strains of streptococci, *N. gonorrhea* and *N. meningitidis*. Many strains of enteric gram-negative

Table 8–9
Surgical Indications for Sulfonamides and Trimethoprim

Sulfonamides
Urinary tract infections (cystitis)
Trimethoprim
Urinary tract infections
Prostatitis
Urinary suppression
Trimethoprim/Sulfamethoxazole
Upper and lower urinary tract infections
Prostatitis

---

bacilli such as *Escherichia coli, Klebsiella, Enterobacter,* and *Proteus* are also susceptible. Sulfonamides generally have no significant activity against staphylococci, enterococci, *Serratia* and *Pseudomonas.*

Sulfonamides have intrinsic activity against *Actinomyces, Nocardia,* and *Chlamydia.* They also are used in combination with pyrimethamine or trimethoprim in the therapy of protozoal infections such as toxoplasmosis, malaria, and *Pneumocystis carinii* pneumonia.

Pharmacokinetics

Most sulfonamides are available in the oral form and are well absorbed. Usage is primarily for the treatment of simple, uncomplicated urinary tract infections. Azulfidine is poorly absorbed but achieves very high levels in the gut and is used in the therapy of ulcerative colitis.

Parenteral forms of sulfonamides are used for severe cases of nocardiosis or toxoplasmosis in those patients who are unable to take oral medication. Sulfonamides are excreted by the kidneys after metabolism in the liver, and, therefore, dosage must be adjusted in severe renal disease.[18]

Adverse Reactions

The most common side-effects are hypersensitivity reactions leading to rash, eosinophilia, fever, and serum sickness. Rarely, rashes may progress to a fatal Stevens-Johnson syndrome.[2]

Bone marrow toxicity can also be seen primarily with suppression of the granulocyte series. In those with G6PD deficiency, sulfonamides may cause a severe hemolysis and should, therefore, not be used in these patients. In large doses, crystalluria and renal damage may occur, but can be prevented by combining several different sulfonamides into a combination product and by alkalinizing the urine. Multiple other toxicities occur rarely and include elevated liver function tests and cholestatic hepatitis, headache, and tinnitus.

Sulfonamides are approved for use in children but can cause kernicterus in the newborn child of a mother taking the medication. This occurs by displacing bilirubin from protein binding sites. This same process of displacement from protein binding sites leads to a potentiation of the effects of coumadin, thiazides, and other agents.

In relationship to surgery, some local anesthetics such as procaine can decrease the effectiveness of sulfonamides due to the derivation of these anesthetics from PABA, which antagonizes sulfa drugs.

TRIMETHOPRIM

Trimethoprim (see Table 8-9) is a folic acid antagonist that inhibits the dehydrofolate reductase enzyme in a similar manner to pyrimethamine. This agent is used alone or may be combined with sulfamethoxazole to achieve synergy against many bacteria. As a single agent, trimethoprim is used primarily to treat urinary tract infections and prostatitis.

Spectrum

Trimethoprim is very active against most aerobic gram-negative bacilli except *Pseudomonas aeruginosa*.[3] It is also effective against most aerobic gram-positive organisms such as staphylococci and streptococci (including some enterococci). It is not usually used clinically, however, either alone or in combination with sulfamethoxazole to treat enterococcal urinary tract infections. Anaerobes are usually resistant to trimethoprim.

Pharmacokinetics

Trimethoprim alone is available only in an oral form. It is well absorbed from the GI tract and achieves good levels in all tissues including the prostate and prostatic secretions. Up to 80% of the drug is excreted in the urine with a serum half-life of 9 to 11 hours. The dosages should be reduced in severe renal disease.[18, 120]

Side-effects

Trimethoprim may cause bone marrow toxicity including anemia, thrombocytopenia, and leukopenia. Rashes may also occur but are more common when it is used in combination with sulfamethoxazole, and may, therefore, be due to the sulfamethoxazole.

TRIMETHOPRIM/SULFAMETHOXAZOLE (TMP/SMX)

TMP/SMX (see Table 8-9) is a fixed combination of two antibacterial agents in a ratio of one part trimethoprim to five parts sulfamethoxazole. These agents work synergistically by inhibiting two sequential steps in the folic acid pathway to purine synthesis.

Spectrum

This combination agent is a very broad-spectrum antibiotic against most gram-positive and gram-negative aerobic organisms.[82] Many organisms that are resistant to either sulfonamides or trimethoprim alone are sensitive to the combination. Most staphylococci and streptococci are susceptible including methicillin-resistant *Staphylococcus aureus* and *Staphylococcus epidermidis*. There is, however, limited clinical information on treatment of methicillin-resistant staphylococcal infections with this agent.

Neisseria meningitidis and *N. gonorrheae* are usually susceptible. It is an excellent agent against *H. influenzae* including penicillinase-producing strains. Most enterobacteriaceae such as *Escherichia coli*, *Klebsiella*, *Proteus*, and *Enterobacter* are sensitive. *Shigella* and *Salmonella* are also well-treated with TMP/SMX. *Pseudomonas aeruginosa* is invariably resistant, although *Pseudomonas* species such as *Pseudomonas maltophilia* and *Pseudomoans cepacia* are frequently susceptible.

Pharmacokinetics

TMP/SMX is available as an oral tablet and a parenteral combination preparation. Tablets and ampules have 80 mg of TMP and 400 mg of SMX. A double-strength tablet is also available. The oral preparation is very well-absorbed and achieves excellent serum and tissue levels including CSF and prostatic tissues. It is one of the most effective treatments for prostatitis because of its high prostatic levels.[58]

Renal excretion of the both agents requires adjustment in dosage for renal insufficiency.

Adverse Reactions

All adverse reactions seen with sulfonamides are also seen with this combination. In addition, the increased blockade of the folic acid pathway may lead to added bone marrow toxicity when given in large doses.[37] Some have used folinic acid (leucovorin factor) to bypass the blockade and prevent bone marrow toxicity. This has neither a deleterious effect on the desired action of the combination nor a proven protective effect on the marrow.[82] Intravenous usage in high doses may also have greater adverse effects on liver function tests than sulfonamides alone.[66,54]

METRONIDAZOLE

The mechanism of action for metronidazole, a nitroimidazole compound, is not entirely known, but it must be in the reduced form in anaerobic bacteria before it can be effective.[60] It is believed that the ultimate effect is to disrupt DNA transcription and replication.

Spectrum

The antibacterial effect of metronidazole is entirely limited to anaerobic organisms.[105] It is the only uniformly bactericidal agent against all *Bacteroides fragilis* and *Bacteroides* species. It is also very active against most mouth anaerobes and clostridial species but has only limited activity against other gram-positive anaerobic bacilli such as *Proprionobacterium acnes*. Although not active against most aerobic bacteria, it is the treatment of choice for bacterial vaginosis secondary to *Gardnerella vaginale*. Many protozoan infections such as trichomoniasis, amebiasis, and giardiasis are also very effectively eradicated with this antibiotic.

Pharmacokinetics

Metronidazole is available in oral and parenteral forms. It is very well absorbed orally and achieves excellent serum and tissue levels including the CNS. It is metabolized by the liver and need not be reduced in patients with renal inefficiency.

Adverse Reactions

Nausea and a metallic taste in the mouth may occur with oral therapy.[31] Various neurologic side-effects such as headaches, dizziness, peripheral neuropathies, and even seizures have been reported with high dose therapy. An antabuse (Disulfiram) reaction may occur if metronidazole is given simultaneously with alcohol-containing beverages or medications. Patients should be warned not to ingest alcohol until metronidazole has been discontinued for at least 48 hours.

THE NEW QUINOLONES

Recently, a new generation of quinolones (Table 8-10) has been studied and marketed.[30] These new agents are fluorinated piperazinyl quinolones, which have a very broad spectrum of activity. The antibiotics inhibit the DNA gyrase enzyme necessary to package DNA properly in dividing bacteria.

Many quinolones are now being developed. Norfloxacin and Ciprofloxacin are presently FDA approved. Ofloxacin, enoxacin, pefloxacin, and others are currently being studied.

Spectrum

These agents possess a broad spectrum of activity against gram-positive and gram-negative aerobes and have some activity against anaerobes as well.[42] *Pseudomonas aeruginosa*, enterococci, some methicillin-resistant *Staphylococcus aureus* and *Staphylococcus epidermidis*, *Listeria monocytogenes*, *Chlamydia*, *Mycoplasma*, and *mycobacteria* are often susceptible. Ciprofloxacin has greater activity against *Pseudomonas* than the other related compounds. Because these agents are

Table 8–10
Surgical Indications for the Newer
Quinolones

Urinary tract infections
Prostatitis
Osteomyelitis
Oral therapy for *Pseudomonas aeruginosa* infections

unrelated to the other major groups of antibiotics, organisms resistant to other agents are often susceptible.[60a]

The new quinolones are available primarily in the oral form. However, some of the investigational agents also have a parenteral form available. All are well absorbed orally. Levels in most tissues including the prostate are excellent, and they may be used for prostatitis.[53] These agents are primarily metabolized by the liver but must be slightly adjusted for severe renal insufficiency.

Adverse Reactions

Gastrointestinal side-effects such as nausea, vomiting, abdominal pain, or diarrhea may occur in 1% to 2% of patients taking oral therapy.[42] Mild abnormalities in liver function tests and hematologic parameters have also been reported with both oral and parenteral preparations. Unanticipated adverse reactions may still occur due to the relatively short time that these agents have been investigated.[15a]

OLDER QUINOLONES

Naladixic acid and oxalonic acid are older quinolones used for many years. They achieve adequate levels in the urine and are used only for urinary tract infections, primarily cystitis. They are rarely used in serious urinary tract infections because levels are poor in the kidney and prostate. They are used in suppression of recurrent infections.

These agents have their primary activity against most gram-negative bacilli but have no *Pseudomonas* activity. Resistance may develop over prolonged periods of use.

Side-effects may occur in the elderly and include headaches, vertigo, inability to concentrate, and rarely seizures. Photosensitivity, photophobia, and mild hemolytic anemia have also been reported.

RIFAMPIN

Rifampin (see Table 8-11) blocks RNA synthesis by inhibiting DNA-dependent RNA-polymerase.

Spectrum

Rifampin has a broad range of activity and is usually an extremely potent antibiotic.[28] However, bacteria may rapidly become resistant if used as a single agent.

Although rifampin is a primary bactericidal agent against *M. tuberculosis*, it may also be employed in combination with penicillinase-resistant penicillin or vancomycin to treat *Staphylococcus aureus* and *Staphylococcus epidermidis*.[111] Whether the combination is synergistic or additive remains conjectural. Several studies, however, have shown antagonism of rifampin in combination with these

Table 8–11
Surgical Indications for Metronidazole and Rifampin

Metronidazole
Brain abscess
Intra-abdominal infections (with aminoglycosides)
Nonvenereal pelvic inflammatory disease (with aminoglycosides)
Prophylaxis in elective colorectal surgery
Pseudomembranous colitis
Rifampin
Prosthetic device infections of the heart, joints, and central nervous system
(always in combination with other agents such as penicillinase-resistant
penicillins, vancomycin ± aminoglycosides)

---

agents against *Staphylococcus aureus*, but not *Staphylococcus epidermidis*. Rifampin is also very active against *N. meningitidis* and *H. influenzae* and is used to eradicate the meningococcal and *Hemophilus* carrier states. Occasionally, when combined with an oral anti-staphylococcal agent, rifampin has also eliminated the staphylococcal carrier state.[121]

Pharmacokinetics

Rifampin is used primarily in the oral form.[86] It has a long half-life and can be given once or twice daily. It achieves excellent levels in all tissues including CSF and may be used in therapeutic regimens for CSF shunt infections.[127] Most of the drug is metabolized by the liver and excreted in the feces, although some is also excreted in the urine. The urine, spinal fluid, and tears may be changed to an orange-yellow color confirming the absorption of the agent.

An intravenous preparation is available on an investigational basis and may be used in those patients who require rifampin and are unable to take the oral form.

Adverse Reactions

Approximately 10% of patients taking rifampin will develop mild elevations in liver function tests.[28] It is rare to develop clinical hepatitis unless rifampin is given in combination with isoniazid or other hepatotoxic agents.

Rashes and gastrointestinal complaints may also occur but rarely require discontinuation of therapy. Various hematologic and immunologic reactions such as mild anemia and thrombocytopenia, a mild suppression of humoral and cell-mediated immunity, and a flulike illness when used intermittently, have all been reported infrequently.

Multiple drug interactions secondary to the effects of rifampin on hepatic metabolic pathways may decrease the therapeutic efficacy of other medications such as oral anticoagulants, hypoglycemics, oral contraceptives, digitoxin, methadone, and barbiturates.

ANTIFUNGAL AGENTS

Amphotericin B

Amphotericin B is a polyene, macrolide antifungal antibiotic that combines with ergosterol and other membrane sterols in the fungus and causes an increased porosity of the membrane and the eventual death of the organism.

Amphotericin B has a broad spectrum of antifungal activity and is the most effective and commonly used antifungal agent for severe infections.[87,36] Most yeast, including *Candida* spp, *Histoplasma capsulatum, Coccidioides immitis, Blastomyces dermatitidis, Cryptococcus neoformans,* and *Paracoccidioides braziliensis,* are sensitive. Other fungi such as *Aspergillus* spp, mucormycosis, and sporotrichosis are also susceptible to amphotericin B.

Amphotericin B is only available as a parenteral preparation and must be slowly administered intravenously in large volumes of dextrose solution. It cannot be mixed with saline. It achieves adequate levels in most tissues except CSF and vitreous fluids and is stored in the liver. It is only minimally excreted by the kidneys and, therefore, it does not have to be adjusted for renal insufficiency.[19] However, most infectious disease specialists do reduce the daily dose by about one half in the setting of severe renal insufficiency. The normal daily dose is 0.25 to 0.75 mg/kg/day, but may be increased to 1 mg/kg/day in severely ill patients. The drug is administered to a total accumulated dose of 200 to 2000 mg depending on the specific infection and underlying disease. There are no studies that clarify the optimum total accumulated dose for any specific infection, however. Amphotericin B has been administered as bladder irrigation solutions at a concentration of 5 μg/ml. It has also been directly instilled into joints (5 to 15 mg) and CSF in small doses (0.05 to 0.5 mg).

Toxicities with amphotericin B are frequent and severe.[116] High fevers, shaking chills, and, occasionally, hypotension may occur. To prevent these, a small test dose of 1 mg can be infused over 20 minutes to several hours to observe for these side-effects. If they occur, acetaminophen, diphenhydramine, and even hydrocortisone can be given as premedication for each successive dose. The daily dose can be slowly increased over several days to also minimize the side-effects.

Amphotericin B may be phlebitic, but this can be reduced by slowing the infusion. Some add 1000 units of heparin to the infusion to help alleviate this problem.

Nephrotoxicity occurs in most patients who receive a full course of therapy.[13] Usually, the creatinine only reaches 2.0 to 4.0 mg/dl, but occasionally can cause more severe renal problems. The renal insufficiency usually resolves over weeks or months after therapy is stopped. Renal tubular acidosis and hypokalemia from urinary loss may also occur. Every effort should be made to maintain adequate hydration and preserve normal sodium and potassium levels.[40] This has been shown to reduce the nephrotoxic potential of amphotericin B. Other infrequent side-effects include anemia, thrombocytopenia, and only rarely acute respiratory decompensation, particularly when administered during or after leukocyte or blood transfusions.

Nystatin

Nystatin is a polyene antifungal agent related to amphotericin B. It is used as a topical or oral preparation and is directed primarily against superficial skin or mucosal (oral and vaginal) candidiasis. It is available in ointments and creams, as well as suspensions. Side-effects and toxicities are minimal.

5-Fluorocytosine (5-FC)

5-FC is a fluorinated cytosine analog, which is deaminated to 5-fluorouracil (5-FU) and then 5-fluorodeoxyuridylic acid monophosphate and acts as a noncompetitive inhibitor of thymidilate synthetase leading to inhibition of DNA synthesis.[7]

This agent is the drug of choice for chromomycosis only. It, however, is also active against *Candida* spp and *Cryptococcus neoformans.* It cannot be used alone to treat a serious infection other than chromomycosis because of rapid emergence of resistance.[87] It is usually combined with amphotericin B, and this combination has become the treatment of choice for cryptococcal meningitis.

5-fluorocytosine is only available as an oral preparation. It is well absorbed and achieves good tissue levels including the CSF. It is excreted by the kidney and must be carefully adjusted in renal insufficiency.[7]

Toxicity is primarily due to bone marrow suppression, perhaps from accumulation of 5-FU, a metabolic by-product. Anemia, thrombocytopenia, and leukopenia may occur by this mechanism and may be more common when given in combination with amphotericin B because of the associated nephrotoxicity of the amphotericin B. Mild elevations in liver function tests, rash, gastrointestinal upset, and diarrhea may also occur.[49]

Ketoconazole

Ketoconazole is an oral imidazole that interferes with the formation of membrane sterols and lipids. It has excellent activity against *Candida* spp and is used to treat mucocutaneous and mucosal *Candida* infections.[117] It should not be used to treat serious systemic *Candida* infections. Recent studies have also shown some beneficial effects in the therapy of histoplasmosis, coccidiomycosis, and occasionally cryptococcosis.[23]

The agent is available in the oral form and is well-absorbed from the GI tract if gastric *p*H is acidic. It cannot be given, therefore, with antacids or H_2 blockers. It does not achieve good CSF levels and cannot be used to treat fungal infections of the CNS.

Ketoconazole may cause nausea and vomiting, which can be reduced if the agent is administered with food. Elevated liver function tests occur in 5% of patients, but only very rarely has fatal hepatitis been reported. Nevertheless, monitoring of liver function tests, particularly within the first 3 months of therapy, is necessary. Various endocrine abnormalities have also been reported, including gynecomastia, but these have not usually been clinically important.[119]

Clotrimazole is also an imidazole and is used for cutaneous and vaginal infections. Miconazole is an intravenous preparation, which is rarely used now for fungal infections, but remains the treatment of choice for the very rare *Pseudoallescheria boydii* infection.[99] Investigational imidazoles, such as fluconazole and itraconozole, show promise for the treatment of yeast infections such as candidiasis and cryptococcosis. It is hoped that these new investigational agents will be very effective, yet safer and easier to use than amphotericin B.

REFERENCES

1. Appel GB, Neu HC. The nephrotoxicity of antimicrobial agents. N Engl J Med 1977;296:663.
2. Araujo OE, Flowers FP. Stevens-Johnson syndrome. J Emerg Med 1984;2:129.
3. Bach MC, Finland M, Gold W. Susceptibility of recently isolated pathogenic bacteria to trimethoprim and sulfamethoxazole separately and combined. J Infect Dis 1973;128:S508.
4. Bartlett JG. Chloramphenicol. Med Clin North Am 1982;66:91.
5. Barza M. Imipenem: first of a new class of beta-lactam antibiotics. Ann Intern Med 1985;103:552.
6. Barza M, Weinstein L. Pharmacokinetics of penicillins in man. Clin Pharmacokinet 1976;1:297.
7. Bennett JE. Flucytosine. Ann Intern Med 1977;86:319.
8. Bloomer HA, Barton LJ, Maddock RJ Jr. Penicillin-induced encephalopathy in uremic patients. JAMA 1967;200:121.
9. Braun P. Hepatotoxicity of erythromycin. J Infect Dis 1969;119:300.
10. Brearley LJ, Storey E. Tetracycline-induced tooth changes. Part 2: Prevalence, localization and nature of staining in extracted deciduous teeth. Med J Aust 1968;2:714.
11. Brogden RN, Carmine A, Heel RC, et al. Cefoperazone: review of *in vitro* antimicrobial activity, pharmacological properties and therapeutic efficacy. Drugs 1981;22:423.
12. Brown CH, Natelson EA, Bradshaw W, et al. The hemostatic defect produced by carbenicillin. N Engl J Med 1974;291:265.
13. Burgess JL, Birchall R. Nephrotoxicity of amphotericin B, with emphasis on changes in tubular function. Am J Med 1972;53:77.
14. Calandra GB. Review of adverse experiences and tolerability in the first 2,516 patients treated with impipenem/celastatin. Am J Med 1985;78(suppl. 6A):73.
15. Carrizosa J, Kaye D. Antibiotic concentrations in serum, serum bactericidal activity, and results of therapy of streptococcal endocarditis in rabbits. Antimicrob Agents Chemother 1977;12:479.
15a. Christ W, Lehnert T, Ulbrich B. Specific toxicologic aspects of the quinolones. Rev Infect Dis 1988;10(suppl.1):s141.
16. Cohan S, Bevelander G, Tiamsic T. Growth inhibition of prematures receiving tetracycline. Am J Dis Child 1963;105:453.
17. Craft AW, Brocklebank JT, Hey EN, et al. The "grey toddler": Chloramphenicol toxicity. Arch Dis Child 1974;49:235.
18. Craig WA, Kunin CM. Trimethoprim-sulfamethoxazole: pharmacodynamics effects of urinary pH and impaired renal function. Ann Intern Med 1973;78:491.
19. Cravens PC, Ludden TM, Drutz DJ, et al. Excretion pathways of amphotericin B. J Infect Dis 1979;140:329.
20. Cunha BA, Comer JB, Jonas M. Tetracyclines. Med Clin North Am 1982;66:293.
21. Davies J. General mechanisms of animicrobial resistance. Rev Infect Dis 1979;1:23.
22. Dehaan RM, Metzler CM, Schellenberg D, et al. Pharmacokinetic studies of clindamycin phosphate. J Clin Pharmacol 1973;13:190.
23. Dismukes WE, Stamm AM, Graybill JR, et al. Treatment of systemic mycoses with ketoconazole: emphasis on toxicity and clinical response in 52 patients. Ann Intern Med 1983;98:13.
24. Edelstein PM, Mayer RD. Susceptibility of *Legionella pneumophila* to twenty antimicrobial agents. Antimicrob Agents Chemother 1980;18:403.

206

25. Eliopoulos GM, Moellering RC Jr. Azlocillin, mezlocillin, and piperacillin: new broad-spectrum penicillins. Ann Intern Med 1982;97:755.
26. Eliopoulos GM, Moellering RC Jr. Principles of antibiotic therapy. Med Clin North Am 1982;66:3.
27. Farber BF, Moellering RC. Retrospective study of the toxicity of preparations of Vancomycin from 1974 to 1981. Antimicrob Agents Chemother 1983;23:138.
28. Farr B, Mandell GL. Rifampin. Med Clin North Am 1982;66:157.
29. Fass RJ. Comparative *in vitro* activities of third-generation cephalosporins. Arch Intern Med 1983;143:1743.
30. Fass RJ. The quinolones. Ann Intern Med 1985;102:400.
31. Feingold SM. Metronidazole. Ann Intern Med 1980;93:585.
32. Finland M. Changing patterns of susceptibility of common bacterial pathogens to antimicrobial agents. Ann Intern Med 1972;76:1009.
33. Garrod LP: The erythromycin group of antibiotics. Br J Med 1957;2:57.
34. Geraci JE, Hermans PE. Vancomycin. Mayo Clin Proc 1983;58:88.
35. Gibson TP, Demetriades JL, Bland JA. Imipenem/cilastatin: pharmacokinetic profile in renal insufficiency. Am J Med 1985;78(suppl. 6A):54.
36. Graybill JR, Craven PC. Antifungal agents used in systemic mycoses: activity and therapeutic use. Drugs 1983;25:41.
37. Gutman LT. The use of trimethoprim-sulfamethoxazole in children: a review of adverse reactions and indications. Pediatr Infect Dis 1984;3:349.
38. Handwerger S, Tomasz A. Antibiotic tolerance among clinical isolates of bacteria. Rev Infect Dis 1985;7:368.
39. Haydon RC, Thelin JW, Davis WE. Erythromycin ototoxicity: analyses and conclusions based on 22 case reports. Otolaryngol Head Neck Surg 1984;92:678.
40. Heidemann HT, Gerkens JF, Spickard WA, et al. Amphotericin B nephrotoxicity in humans decreased by salt repletion. Am J Med 1983;75:475.
41. Henry SA, Bendush CB. Aztreonam: worldwide overview of the treatment of patients with gram-negative infections. Am J Med 1985;78(suppl 2A):57.
42. Holmes B, Brogden RN, Richards DM. Norfloxacin: review of its antibacterial activity, pharmacokinetic properties, and therapeutic use. Drugs 1985;30:482.
43. Hook EW III, Holmes KK. Gonococcal infections. Ann Intern Med 1985;102:229.
44. Horne D, Tomasz A. Tolerant response of *Streptococcus sanguis* to beta-lactams and other cell wall antibiotics. Antimicrob Agents Chemother 1977;11:888.
45. Jackson GG. Aminoglycoside antibiotics: resistance and toxicity—A summary. Rev Infect Dis 1983;5(suppl 2):S314.
46. Jones RN. Review of *in vitro* spectrum of activity of imipenem. Am J Med 1985;78(suppl 6A):22.
47. Kahlmeter G, Dahlager JI. Aminoglycoside toxicity: review of clinical studies published between 1975 and 1982. J Antimicrob Chemother 1984;13(suppl A):9.
48. Karchmer AW, Archer GL, Dismukes WE. *Staphylococcus epidermidis* causing prosthetic-valve endocarditis: microbiological and clinical observations as guides to therapy. Ann Intern Med 1983;98:447.
49. Kerkering TM. Present status of flucytosine therapy. Drug Therapy 1982;12:75.
50. Kerr RO, Cardamone J, Dalmasso AP, et al. Two mechanisms of erythrocyte destruction in penicillin-induced hemolytic anemia. N Engl J Med 1972;287:1322.
51. Klastersky J. Emperic treatment of infections in neutropenic patients with cancer. Rev Infect Dis 1983;5(suppl):S21.
52. Kramer WG, et al. Comparative bioavailability of intravenous and oral chloramphenicol in adults. J Clin Pharmacol, 1984;24:181.
53. Lambert TE, Jaupitre A. Norfloxacin concentrations in human prostate tissue. Twenty-fourth Interscience Conference on Antimicrobial Agents and Chemotherapy, Washington, DC, 1984.
54. Lawson DH, Paice BJ. Adverse reactions to trimethoprim-sulfamethoxazole. Rev Infect Dis 1982;4:429.
55. Leitman PS, Smith CR. Aminoglycoside nephrotoxicity in humans. Rev Infect Dis 1983;5(suppl 2):S284.
56. McGehee RF Jr, Smith CB, Wilcox C, et al. Comparative studies of antibacterial activity in vitro and absorption and excretion of lincomycin and clindamycin. Am J Med Sci 1968;256:279.
57. McHenry MC, Gavan TL. Vancomycin. Pediatr Clin North Am 1983;30:31.
58. Meares EM Jr. Prostatitis: review of pharmacokinetics and therapy. Rev Infect Dis 1982;4:475.
59. Meyers BR, Hirschman SZ. Antibacterial activity of cefamandole in vitro. J Infect Dis 1978;137(suppl):S25.

60. Miller RM. Mode of action of metronidazole on anaerobic bacteria and protozoa. In: Rhone-Poulenc Pharma, Inc, Montreal. Proc. North Amer. Metronidazole Symposium, Anaerobic Infection, Scottsdale, Arizona, Oct 1981. Surgery 1983;93:165.

60a. Mitsuhashi S. Comparative antibacterial activity of new quinolone-carboxylic acid derivatives. Rev Infect Dis 1988;10(suppl.1):s27.

61. Moellering RC Jr. In vitro antibacterial activity of aminoglycoside antibiotics. Rev Infect Dis 1983;5(suppl 2):S212.

62. Moellering RC, Krogstad DJ, Greenblatt DJ. Vancomycin therapy in patients with impaired renal function: a nomogram for dosage. Ann Intern Med 1981;94:343.

63. Moore RD, Smith CR, Lietman PS. Risk factors for development of auditory toxicity in patients receiving aminoglycosides. J Infect Dis 1984B;149:23.

64. Moore RD, Smith CR, Lipsky JJ, et al. Risk factors for nephrotoxicity in patients treated with aminoglycosides. Ann Intern Med 1984A;100:352.

65. Murray BE, Moellering RC Jr. Patterns and mechanisms of antibiotic resistance. Med Clin North Am 1978;62:899.

66. Nair SS, Kanlan JM, Levine LH, et al. Trimethoprim-sulfamethoxazole induced intrahepatic cholestasis. Ann Intern Med 1980;92:511.

67. Nelson JD (Chairman). Evolving role of erythromycin in medicine: proceedings of symposium. Pediatr Infect Dis 1986;5:118.

68. Neu HC. Antistaphylococcal penicillins. Med Clin North Am 1982B;66:51.

69. Neu HC, ed. Beta-lactamase inhibition: therapeutic advances. Am J Med 1985;79(suppl 5B):1.

70. Newfield P, Roczen MF. Hazards of rapid administration of vancomycin. Ann Intern Med 1979;91:581.

71. Nicholas P. Erythromycin: clinical review. I. Clinical pharmacology. NY State J Med 1977;77:2088.

72. Nicholas P, Meyers BR, Levy RN. Concentration of clindamycin in human bone. Antimicrob Agents Chemother 1975;8:220.

73. Norrby SR. Role of cephalosporins in the treatment of bacterial meningitis in adults: overview with special emphasis on ceftazidime. Am J Med 1985;79(suppl 2A):56.

74. Ogaroara H. Antibiotic resistance in pathogenic and producing bacteria, with special reference to beta-lactam antibiotics. Microbiol Rev 1981;45:591.

75. Parry MF, Neu HC. The safety and tolerance of mezlocillin. J Antimicrob Chemother 1982;9(suppl A):273.

76. Pearson RD, Steigbigel RT, Davis HT, et al. Method for reliable determination of minimal lethal concentrations. Antimicrob Agents Chemother 1980;18:699.

77. Petz LD. Immunologic cross-reactivity between penicillins and cephalosporins: a review. J Infect Dis 1978;137(suppl):S74.

78. Quintiliani R, ed. Symposium on cefotetan. Am J Obstet Gynecol 1986;154:945.

79. Rahal JJ Jr, Simberkof MS. Bactericidal and bacteriostatic action of chloramphenicol against meningeal pathogens. Antimicrob Agents Chemother 1979;16:13.

80. Reese RE, Betts RF. Antibiotic use. In: Reese RE, Douglas RG Jr, eds. A practical approach to infectious diseases. 2nd ed. Boston: Little, Brown & Co, 1986;559.

81. Roselle GA, Bode R, Hamilton B, Bibler M, et al. Clinical trial of the efficacy and safety of ticarcillin and clavulanic acid. Antimicrob Agents Chemother 1985;27:291.

82. Rubin RH, Schwartz MN. Trimethoprim-sulfamethoxazole. N Engl J Med 1980;303:426.

83. Sabath LD, Wilcox C, Garner C, et al. In vitro activity of cefazolin against recent clinical bacterial isolates. J Infect Dis, 1973;128(suppl):S320.

84. Sahm DF, et al. Beta-lactam antibiotics: First and second-generation cephalosporins. Antimicrobial Newsletter 1985A;2:25.

85. Sanders CV, Greenberg RN, Marier RL. Cefamandole and cefoxitin. Ann Intern Med 1985;103:70.

86. Sanders WE Jr. Rifampin. Ann Intern Med 1976;85:82.

87. Sarosi GA, Armstrong D, Barhee RA, et al. Treatment of fungal diseases. Am Rev Respir Dis 1979;120:1393.

88. Sattler FR, Weitekamp MR, Ballard JO. Potential for bleeding with the new beta-lactam antibiotics. Ann Intern Med 1986;105:924.

89. Saxon A. Immediate hypersensitivity reactions to beta-lactam antibiotics. Rev Infect Dis 1983;5(suppl 2):368.

90. Saxon A, Saxon CV, Swabb EA, and Adkinson NF. Investigation into immunologic cross-reactivity of aztreonam with other beta-lactam antibiotics. Am J Med 1985;78(suppl 2A):19.

91. Schlicter JG, Maclean H. A method of determining the effective therapeutic level in the treatment of subacute bacterial endocarditis with penicillin. Am Heart J 1947;34:209.

92. Schwalbe RS, Stapleton JT, Gilligan PH. Emergence of vancomycin resistance in coagulose-negative staphylococci. N Engl J Med 1987;316:927.

93. Schwartzberg JE, Maresca RM, Remington JS. Clinical study of gastrointestingal complications associated with clindamycin therapy. J Infect Dis 1977;135(suppl):99.

94. Sher TH. Penicillin hypersensitivity: review. Pediatric Clin North Am 1983;30:161.

95. Silva J, Batts DH, Fekety R, et al. Treatment of *Clostridium difficile* colitis and diarrhea with vancomycin. Am J Med 1981;71:815.

96. Smith AL, Weber A. Pharmacology of chloramphenicol. Pediatr Clin North Am 1983;30:209.

97. Sorrell TC, Rackhan DR, Shanker S, et al. Vancomycin therapy for methicillin-resistant *Staphylococcus aureus*. Ann Intern Med 1982;97:344.

98. Steere AC, Hutchinson GJ, Rahn DW, et al. Treatment of early manifestation of Lyme disease. Ann Intern Med 1983;99:22.

99. Stevens DA. Current perspectives on miconazole. Drug Ther 1982;12:85.

100. Sutter VL. *In vitro* susceptibility of anaerobes: comparison of clindamycin and other antimicrobial agents. J Infect Dis 1977;135(suppl):S7.

101. Swabb EA. A review of the clinical pharmacology of the monobactan aztreonam. Am J Med 1985;78(suppl 2A):11.

102. Sykes RB, Bonna DP. Aztreonam: first monobactam. Am J Med 1985;78(suppl 2A):2.

103. Sykes RB, Matthews M. The beta-lactamases of gram-negative bacteria and their role in resistance to beta-lactam antibiotics. J Antimicrob Chemother 1976;2:115.

104. Tally RP, et al. Nationwide study of susceptibility of *Bacteriodes fragilis* group in United States. Antimicrob Agents Chemother 1985;28:675.

105. Tally RP, Sullivan CE. Metronidazole: *in vitro* activity, pharmacology and efficacy in anaerobic bacterial infections. Pharmacotherapy 1981;1:28.

106. Teasley DG, Olsen MM, Gebhard RL, et al. Prospective randomized trial of metronidazole versus vancomycin for *Clostridium difficile*-associated diarrhea and colitis. Lancet 1983;2:1043.

107. Tedesco FJ. Clindamycin and colitis: review. J Infect Dis 1977;135(suppl):95.

108. Tedesco FJ. Pseudomembranous colitis: Pathogenic therapy. Med Clin North Am 1982A;66:655.

109. Tetracycline-resistant *Neisseria gonorrheae*—Georgia, Pennsylvania, New Hampshire. MMWR 1985;34:563.

110. Then RL. Mechanisms of resistance to trimethoprim, the sulfonamides, and trimethoprim-sulfamethoxazole. Rev Infect Dis 1982;4:261.

111. Thornsberry C, Hill BC, Swenson JM, et al. Rifampin: spectrum of antibacterial activity. Rev Infect Dis 1983;5(suppl 3):S412.

112. Timbrell JA. Drug hepatotoxicity. Br J Clin Pharmacol 1983;15:3.

113. Tomasz A. From penicillin-binding proteins to the lysis and death of bacteria: a 1979 view. Rev Infect Dis 1979;1:434.

114. Tomasz A. Mechanism of irreversible antimicrobial effects of penicillin: how beta-lactam antibiotics kill & lyse bacteria. Annu Rev Microbiol 1979;33:113.

115. Tomasz A. Penicillin-binding proteins in bacteria. Ann Intern Med 1982;96:502.

116. Utz JP, Bennett JE, Brandries MW, et al. Amphotericin B toxicity. Ann Intern Med 1964;61:334.

117. Van Tyle JH. Ketoconazole: mechanism of action, spectrum of activity, pharmacokinetics, drug interactions, adverse reactions and therapeutic use. Pharmacotherapy 1984;4:343.

118. Washington JA II, Wilson WR. Erythromycin: microbial and clinical perspective after 30 years of clinical use, Parts 1 and 2, Mayo Clin Proc 1985;60:189.

119. Watanakunakorn C, Guerriero JC. Interactions between vancomycin and rifampin against *Staphylococcus aureus*. Antimicrob Agents Chemother 1981;19:1089.

120. Welling PG, Craig WA, Amidon GL, et al. Pharmacokinetics of trimethoprim and sulfamethoxazole in normal subjects and in patients with renal failure. J Infect Dis 1973;128(suppl):556.

121. Wheat LJ, Kohler RB, Luft FC, et al. Long term studies of the effect of rifampin on nasal carriage of coagulase-positive staphylococci. Rev Infect Dis 1983;5(suppl 3):S459.

122. Whelton A. Tetracyclines in renal insufficiency: resolution of a therapeutic dilemma. Bull NY Acad Med 1978;54:223.

123. Williams JD, Casewell MW, eds. Ceftazidime. J Antimicrob Chemother 1981;8(suppl B):1.

124. Wise R, et al. In vitro study of clavulanic acid in combination with penicillin, amoxicillin, and carbenicillin. Antimicrob Agents Chemother 1978;13:389.

125. Wise RA, Kory M, eds. Reassessment of vancomycin, a potentially useful antibiotic. Rev Infect Dis 1981;3:S199.

126. Wright AJ, Wilkowske CJ. The penicillins. Mayo Clin Proc 1983;58:21.

127. Yogev R. Cerebrospinal fluid shunt infections: a personal view. Pediatr Infect Dis 1985;4:113.

128. Yunis AA. Chloramphenicol-induced bone marrow suppression. Semin Hematol 1973;10:225.

BIBLIOGRAPHY

Drug evaluations. 6th ed. Chicago:American Medical Association, 1986.

Drug information 86. Bethseda, MD:American Society of Hospital Pharmacists, 1986.

Handbook of antibiotic therapy. New Rochelle, NY:The Medical Letter, 1986.

Mandel GL, Douglas RG Jr, Bennett JE, eds. Principles and practice of infectious diseases. New York:John Wiley & Sons, 1985.

Reese RE, Douglas RG Jr, eds. A practical approach to infectious diseases. Boston/Toronto:Little, Brown & Co, 1986.

Roberts RB, ed. Infectious diseases. Pathogenesis, diagnosis and therapy. Chicago:Year Book Medical Publishers, 1986.

Sanford JP. Guide to antimicrobial therapy 1986. San Antonio, TX:Antimicrobial Therapy, 1986.

Appendix 8-A
Frequent Pathogens for Specific Surgical Infections

INFECTIONS	PATHOGENS
Arteriovenous shunts	*S. aureus; S. epidermidis*
Biliary tract	*E. coli; Klebsiella;* enterococci
Burns	*S. aureus;* gram-negative bacilli; *Candida*
Cellulitis/soft tissues	Streptococci; *S. aureus; Clostridium*
Intra-abdominal	*E. coli; Bacteroides fragilis;* other gram-negative bacilli; enterococci
Intravenous catheter-related sepsis	*S. aureus; S. epidermidis;* gram-negative bacilli; *Candida*
Osteomyelitis	*S. aureus; H. influenzae;* gram-negative bacilli
Pelvic	*B. fragilis, E. coli; N. gonorrheae; Clostridium* spp.; enterococci; other streptococci
Prostatitis	*E. coli;* other gram-negative bacilli
Septic arthritis	*S. aureus; N. gonorrheae;* gram-negative bacilli
Urinary tract	*E. coli;* other gram-negative bacilli; enterococci

Appendix 8-B
Antibiotic Therapy for Specific Pathogens

PATHOGEN	FIRST CHOICE	ALTERNATIVES
Aerobes		
Gram-positive Cocci		
S. aureus* or *S. epidermidis		
Non-penicillinase producing	Penicillin	Cefazolin; vancomycin; erythromycin; clindamycin
Penicillinase producing	Penicillinase-resistant penicillin	Cefazolin; vancomycin; erythromycin; clindamycin
Methicillin-resistant (intrinsically resistant)	Vancomycin (± gentamicin; ± rifampin)	Trimethoprim/sulfamethoxazole, ciprofloxacin
Streptococci		
Group A (*S. pyogenes*)	Penicillin	Erythromycin; cefazolin
Group B (*S. agalactiae*)	Penicillin	Ampicillin; cefazolin; erythromycin
Group D (enterococci)	Ampicillin (or penicillin ± gentamicin)	Vancomycin ± gentamicin
S. pneumoniae	Penicillin	Cefazolin; erythromycin chloramphenicol; vancomycin
Viriden streptococci	Penicillin ± streptomycin (or ± gentamicin)	Cefazolin; vancomycin
Gram-negative Cocci		
Branhamella catarrhalis	Trimethoprim/sulfamethoxazole	Erythromycin; tetracycline, a cephalosporin
Neisseria gonorrheae	Penicillin (or amoxicillin)	Ampicillin; ceftriaxone; spectinomycin; cefoxitin
Neisseria meningitidis;	Penicillin (or ampicillin)	Chloramphenicol; third-generation cephalosporins; sulfonamides; rifampin
Gram-positive Bacilli		
Corynebacterium (JK strain)	Vancomycin	
Erysipelothrix rhysiopathiae	Penicillin	Cefazolin; erythromycin; tetracycline
Listeria monocytogenes	Ampicillin (or penicillin) ± gentamicin	Trimethoprim/sulfamethoxazole; erythromycin; tetracyclline

Gram-negative Bacilli

Organism	Drug of choice	Alternatives
Acinetobacter calcoaceticus	Gentamycin (tobramycin) ± ticarcillin	Amikacin; piperacillin; mezlocillin; imipenem
Actinobacillus actinomycetemcomitans	Ampicillin ± gentamicin	
Brucella spp.	Tetracycline + streptomycin	Ceftriaxone; trimethoprim/sulfamethoxazole
Calymmatobacterium granulomatis (granuloma inguinale)	Tetracycline	Trimethoprim/sulfamethoxazole; chloramphenicol
Campylobacter		Streptomycin; gentamicin
jejeuni	Erythromycin	
fetus	Gentamicin	Tetracycline; gentamicin
Eikenella corrodens	Penicillin	Erythromycin
Enterobacter spp.	Gentamicin (tobramycin)	Trimethoprim/sulfamethoxazole
Escherichia coli	Gentamicin (tobramycin)	Cefuroxime; third-generation cephalosporins; imipenem; aztreonam
		Ampicillin; cephalosporins; amikacin; trimethoprim/sulfamethoxazole; aztreonam
Francisella tularensis (tularemia)	Streptomycin	Gentamicin, tetracycline; chloramphenicol; aztreonam
Gardnerella vaginale (nonspecific vaginitis)	Metronidazole	Ampicillin
Hemophilus ducreye (chancroid)	Erythromycin	Ceftriaxone; trimethoprim/sulfamethoxazole; ciprofloxacin
Hemophilus influenzae	Ampicillin	Cefuroxime; third-generation cephalosporins; chloramphenicol; trimethoprim/sulfamethoxazole
Hemophilus spp.	Ampicillin	Ceftriaxone; cefuroxime; trimethoprim/sulfamethoxazole; chloramphenicol
Klebsiella spp.	Gentamicin (tobramycin)	Cephalosporin; trimethoprim/sulfamethoxazole; aztreonam
Pasteurella multocida	Penicillin	Tetracycline; cefuroxime
Proteus mirabilis	Ampicillin	Gentamicin; cephalosporin; trimethoprim/sulfamethoxazole
Proteus spp.	Gentamicin (tobramycin)	Amikacin; cephalosporin; trimethoprim/sulfamethoxazole; aztreonam
Pseudomonas aeruginosa	Tobramycin ± ticarcillin	Azlocillin; mezlocillin; piperacillin; ceftazidime; cefoperazone; imipenem; amikacin; ciprofloxacin; aztreonam
Pseudomonas spp.	Sulfamethoxazole/trimethoprim	Chloramphenicol; amikacin; ceftazidime; aztreonam
Salmonella spp.	Chloramphenicol; ampicillin	Trimethoprim/sulfamethoxazole; third-generation cephalosporin

(continued)

211

Appendix 8-B (continued)

PATHOGEN	FIRST CHOICE	ALTERNATIVES
Serratia marcescens	Gentamicin	Amikacin; third-generation cephalosporin; imipenem; aztreonam; trimethoprim/sulfamethoxazole
Shigella spp.	Trimethoprim/sulfamethoxazole	Ampicillin; chloramphenicol; ciprofloxacin
Vibrio cholera	Trimethoprim/sulfamethoxazole	Tetracycline
Yersinia enterocolitica	Trimethoprim/sulfamethoxazole	Tetracycline; third-generation cephalosporin; gentamicin
Yersinia pestis (plague)	Streptomycin	Tetracycline; gentamicin; chloramphenicol
Anaerobes		
Gram-positive Cocci (Peptococci, peptostreptococci)	Penicillin	Clindamycin; chloramphenicol; metronidazole; tetracycline
Gram-positive Bacilli		
Clostridium botulinum	Penicillin	
Clostridium difficile	Vancomycin (oral)	Metronidazole (oral)
Clostridium perfringens	Penicillin	Chloramphenicol; metronidazole; clindamycin
Clostridium tetani	Penicillin	Chloramphenicol; clindamycin
Proprionobacterium acnes	Penicillin	Clindamycin; chloramphenicol; tetracycline
Gram-negative Bacilli		
Bacteroides fragilis	Metronidazole; clindamycin	Chloramphenicol; cefoxitin; mezlocillin; piperacillin; imipenem
Bacteroides spp.	Penicillin	Clindamycin; chloramphenicol; metronidazole; tetracycline
Chlamydia		
Chlamydia psittaci	Tetracycline	Chloramphenicol
Chlamydia trachomatis	Tetracycline	Erythromycin; sulfonamides
Mycoplasma		
Mycoplasma pneumoniae	Erythromycin; tetracycline	
Ureaplasma urealyticum	Tetracycline	Erythromycin
***Rickettsia* spp.**	Tetracycline	Chloramphenicol

Spirochetes

Organism	Drug of Choice	Alternatives
Borrelia Burgdorferei (Lyme disease)	Tetracycline	Penicillin; ceftriaxone; erythromycin
Borrelia recurrentis (Relapsing fever)	Tetracycline	Penicillin
Leptospira interrogans (Leptospirosis)	Penicillin	Tetracycline
Treponema pallidum (syphilis)	Penicillin	Tetracycline; erythromycin

Miscellaneous Bacteria

Organism	Drug of Choice	Alternatives
Actinomyces spp.	Penicillin	Tetracycline
Nocardia spp.	Sulfadiazine	Trimethoprim/sulfamethoxazole; ampicillin; amikacin; minocycline

Fungi

Organism	Drug of Choice	Alternatives
Aspergillus spp.	Amphotericin-B	
Blastomyces dermatitidis	Amphotericin-B	Ketoconazole; hydroxystilbamidine
Candida spp.	Amphotericin-B ± 5-fluorocytosine	Nystatin; ketoconazole; fluconazole*; miconazole
Chromomycoses	5-fluorocytosine	
Coccidioides immitis	Amphotericin-B	Ketoconazole
Cryptococcus neoformans	Amphotericin-B ± 5-fluorocytosine	Fluconazole*
Histoplasma capsulatum	Amphotericin-B	Ketoconazole; itraconazole*
Mucormycosis	Amphotericin-B	
Paracoccidiomycosis	Amphotericin-B	Sulfadiazine; ketoconazole
Pseudoallescheria boydii	Miconazole	
Sporothrix schenkii	Iodides	Amphotericin-B; itraconazole*

* Indicates investigational agent.

213

Appendix 8-C
Characteristics of Specific Antimicrobial Agents

GENERIC	TRADE NAME	SERUM HALF-LIFE (h)	ROUTE	DAILY ADULT DOSE	DAILY PEDIATRIC DOSE
Aminoglycosides					
Amikacin	Amikin	2.0–3.0	IM, IV	15 mg/kg	15 mg/kg
Gentamicin	Garamycin	2.0–3.0	IM, IV	3.0–5.0 mg/kg	6.0–7.5 mg/kg
Kanamycin	Kantrex Klebcil	2.0–3.0	p.o. IM, IV	4–8 g 15 mg/kg	150–250 mg/kg 15 mg/kg
Neomycin	Mycifradin Neobiotic		p.o. topical	50 mg/kg	50–100 mg/kg
Netilmicin	Netromycin	2.0–3.0	IM, IV	4.0–6.5 mg/kg	5.5–8.0 mg/kg
Streptomycin		2.0–3.0	IM	15–25 mg/kg	20–40 mg/kg
Tobramycin	Nebcin	2.0–3.0	IM, IV	3.0–5.0 mg/kg	6.0–7.5 mg/kg
Beta-Lactams, Miscellaneous					
Aztreonam	Azactam	1.6–2.1	IM, IV	1.0–8.0 g	NA
Imipenem/ Cilastatin	Primaxin	1.0	IV	2.0–4.0 g	NA
Moxalactam	Moxam	1.0	IM, IV	2.0–12.0 g	100–200 mg/kg
Cephalosporins					
Cefaclor	Ceclor	0.5–1.0	p.o.	0.75–4.0 g	20–40 mg/kg
Cefadroxil	Duracef Ultracef	1.1–2.0	p.o.	1.0–2.0 g	30 mg/kg
Cefamandole	Mandol	0.5–2.1	IM, IV	4.0–12.0 g	50–150 mg/kg
Cefazolin	Ancef Kefzol	1.2–2.2	IM, IV	2.0–6.0 g	25–100 mg/kg
Cefonicid	Monocid	3.5–5.8	IM, IV	0.5–4.0 g	NA
Cefoperazone	Cefobid	1.6–2.6	IM, IV	4.0–12.0 g	NA
Ceforanide	Precef	2.6–3.3	IM, IV	1.0–4.0 g	20–40 mg/kg
Cefotaxime	Claforan	0.9–1.7	IM, IV	4.0–12.0 g	50–180 mg/kg
Cefotetan	Cefotan	3.0–4.6	IM, IV	1.0–6.0 g	NA
Cefoxitin	Mefoxin	0.8	IM, IV	4.0–12.0 g	80–160 mg/kg

DOSING INTERVAL (h)	PEAK LEVEL (µg/ml)	ADULT DOSAGE IN RENAL FAILURE		
		80–50 ml/min	50–10 ml/min	<10 ml/min
q 8–12 h	17–38	7.5 mg/kg q 12–18 h	7.5 mg/kg q 24–36 h	7.5 mg/kg q 36–48 h
q 8–12 h	4–8	1–1.5 mg/kg q 8–12 h	1–1.5 mg/kg q 12–24 h	1–1.5 mg/kg q 24–48 h
q 1–6 h q 12 h	20–25	7.5 mg/kg q 24 h	7.5 mg/kg q 24–72 h	7.5 mg/kg q 72–96 h
q 6 h q 8 h	—	12.5 mg/kg q 6 h	12.5 mg/kg q 12–18 h	12.5 mg/kg q 18–24 h
q 8–12 h	7	1–2 mg/kg q 8–12 h	1–2 mg/kg 12–24 h	1–2 mg/kg q 24–48 h
q 12	15–40	7.5 mg/kg q 24 h	7.5 mg/kg q 24–72 h	7.5 mg/kg 72–96 h
q 8 h	4–8	1–1.5 mg/kg q 8–12 h	1–1.5 mg/kg q 12–24 h	1–1.5 mg/kg q 24–48 h
q 6–12 h	46–164	1–2 g q 12–16 h	1–2 g q 16–24 h	1–2 g q 24–36 h
q 6 h	52	0.5 g q 6–8 h	0.5 g q 8–12 h	0.25–0.5 g q 12 h
q 4–12 h	70–150	0.5–3 g q 8 h	0.25–2 g q 8 h	0.25–1 g q 8–12 h
q 6–8 h	5–34	No change	No change	No change
q 12 h	16	No change	0.5 g q 12–24 h	0.5 g q 36 h
q 4–6 h	88–165	0.75–2 g q 6 h	0.75–1.25 g q 8 h	0.5–0.75 g q 12 h
q 6–8 h	38–188	0.5–2 g q 6–8 h	0.5–2 g q 8–12 h	0.5–2 g q 12–24 lh
q 12–24 h	220	10–20 mg/kg q 24 h	4–15 mg/kg q 24–48 h	4 mg/kg q 3–5 day
q 6–12 h	100–200	No change	No change	No change
q 12 h	125	No change	1–2 g q 24 h	1–2 g q 2–3 day
q 4–6 h	100–200	No change	1–2 g q 6–12 h	1–2 g q 12 h
q 12–24 h	24–110	No change	1–2 g q 24 h	1–2 g q 48 h
q 4–6 h	60–129	1–2 g q 8–12 h	1–2 g q 12–24 h	0.5–1 g q 12–48 h

(continued)

Appendix 8-C **(continued)**

GENERIC	TRADE NAME	SERUM HALF-LIFE (h)	ROUTE	DAILY ADULT DOSE	DAILY PEDIATRIC DOSE
Ceftazidime	Fortaz Tazicef Tazidime	4.4	IM, IV	2.0–6.0 g	90–150 mg/kg
Ceftizoxime	Cefizox	1.4–1.9	IM, IV	4.0–12.0 g	50–200 mg/kg
Ceftriaxone	Rocephin	5.4–10.9	IM, IV	0.125–4 g	50–100 mg/kg
Cefuroxime	Zinacef	1.0–2.0	IM, IV	0.75–4.0 g	50–240 mg/kg
Cephalexin	Keflex	0.5–1.2	p.o.	1.0–2.0 g	80–160 mg/kg
Cephaloridine	Loridine	1.3	IM	2.0–6.0 g	NA
Cephalothin	Keflin	0.5–1.0	IV	4.0–12.0 g	75–125 mg/kg
Cephapirin	Cefadyl	0.4–0.8	IM, IV	4.0–12.0 g	40–80 mg/kg
Cephradine	Anspor Velasef	0.7–2.0	p.o. IM, IV	1.0–2.0 g 2.0–8.0 g	25–100 mg/kg 50–100 mg/kg
Chloramphenicol	Chloromycetin Mychel	4.0	p.o. IM, IV	1.0–2.0 g 2.0–4.0 g	50–100 mg/kg 50–100 mg/kg
Clindamycin	Cleocin	3.0	p.o. IM, IV	0.6–1.8 g 1.2–4.8 g	8–20 mg/kg 15–40 mg/kg
Erythromycin	Many	1.0–3.0	p.o. IV	1.0–2.0 g 1.0–4.0 g	— 30–50 mg/kg
Lincomycin	Lincocin	—	p.o. IM, IV	2.0 g 0.6–8.0 g	— 10–20 mg/kg
Methenamine	Hiprex Mandelamine	3.0–6.0	p.o.	2–4 g	50 mg/kg
Metronidazole	Flagyl	8	p.o. IV	30 mg/kg 30 mg/kg	30 mg/kg 30 mg/kg
Naladixic Acid	NegGram Furadantin	1.5	p.o.	4 g	Not recommended
Nitrofurantoin	Macrodantin	0.3	p.o.	200–400 mg	5–7 mg/kg
Penicillins					
Natural					
Aqueous cryp-talline Pen G	Many	0.5	IV	0.6–20 mil units	100,000–250,000 unit/kg
Benzathine Pen G	Bicillin	—	IM	0.6–2.4 mil units	—
Phenoxyethl Pen G	Many	0.5	p.o.	1.0–4.0 g	25–50 mg/kg

DOSING INTERVAL (h)	PEAK LEVEL (μg/ml)	ADULT DOSAGE IN RENAL FAILURE		
		80–50 ml/min	50–10 ml/min	<10 ml/min
q 8–12 h	13–132	No change	1 g q 12–24 h	0.5 g q 24–48 h
q 6–12 h	150–250	0.5–1.5 g q 12 h	0.25–1 g q 12 h	0.5–1 g q 48 h
q 12–24 h	27–100	No change	No change	1–2 g q 24 h
q 6–8 h	8–32	No change	No change	0.75 g q 12–24 h
q 6 h	9–32	No change	0.5 g q 8–12 h	0.5 g q 24–48 h
q 6 h	—	Not recommended		
q 4–6 h	14–100	2.5 g q 6 h	1–1.5 g q 6 h	0.5 g q 6–8 h
q 4–6 h	70	0.5–2 g q 6 h	0.5–2 g q 8 h	0.5–2 g q 12 h
q 6 h q 4–6 h	16–86	No change	0.5 g q 6 h 0.5 g q 12–24 h	0.25 g q 12–2 h 0.5 g q 40–70 h
q 6 h	11.2–18.4	No change	No change	No change
q 6 h	4.9–12	No change	No change	No change
q 6 h	1.8—5.3	No change	No change	No change
q 6–8 h	7–14	No change	No change	No change
q 6 h	0.3–1.9	No change	No change	No change
q 6 h	3.5–9.9	No change	No change	No change
q 6 h q 8–12 h		Not recommended		
q 6–12 h	<1.0	Not recommended		
q 6 h	6–40	No change	No change	No change
q 6 h	25	No change	No change	No change
q 6 h	20–50	Not recommended		
q 6 h	<2.0	Not recommended		

Penicillins

Natural

q 2–6 h	6–12	No change	No change	10 mil units daily
q 1–4 wks	0.1	No change	No change	No change
q 6 h	1.5–2.5	No change	No change	No change

(continued)

Appendix 8-C (continued)

GENERIC	TRADE NAME	SERUM HALF-LIFE (h)	ROUTE	DAILY ADULT DOSE	DAILY PEDIATRIC DOSE
Phenoxymethyl Pen V	Many	0.5–1.0	p.o.	1.0–4.0 g	25–50 mg/kg
Procaine Pen G	Many	—	IM	0.6–4.8 mil units	25–50 mg/kg
Penicillinase-resistant					
Cloxacillin	Cloxapen Tegopen	0.5	p.o.	1.0–4.0 g	50–100 mg/kg
Dicloxacillin	Dycill/ Dynapen Pathocil	0.5	p.o.	1.0–4.0 g	12.5–25 mg/kg
Methicillin	Staphcillin	0.5	IM, IV	6.0–12.0 g	100–200 mg/kg
Nafcillin	Nafcil/Nallpen Unipen	0.5	p.o. IM, IV	1.0–4.0 g 4.0–12.0 g	— 100–200 mg/kg
Oxacillin	Bactocill Prostaphin	0.5	p.o. IM, IV	1.0–4.0 g 4.0–12.0 g	— 100–200 mg/kg
Aminopenicillins					
Amoxicillin	Amoxil/Larotic Polymox/ Trimox	1.0	p.o.	0.75–1.5 g	20–40 mg/kg
Amoxicillin/ Clavulanic Acid	Augmentin	1.0	p.o.	0.75–1.5 g	20–40 mg/kg
Ampicillin	Many	1.0	p.o. IM, IV	1.0–4.0 g 4.0–12.0 g	— 100–200 mg/kg
Ampicillin/ Sulbactam	Unasyn	1.0	IM, IV	4.0–12.0 g	—
Bacampicillin	Spectrobid	1.0	p.o.	0.8–1.6 g	25–50 mg/kg
Cyclacillin	Cyclapen	0.7–0.75	p.o.	1.0–2.0 g	50–100 mg/kg
Antipseudominonal Penicillins					
Azlocillin	Azlin	0.8–1.0	IM, IV	12–24 g	450 mg/kg
Carbenicillin	Geopen/ Pyopen	1.1	IM, IV	4.0–40 g	400 mg/kg
Carbenicillin Indanyl	Geocillin	1.1	p.o.	1.528–3.056 g	NA
Mezlocillin	Mezlin	0.8–1.2	IM, IV	6.0–18.0 g	300 mg/kg
Piperacillin	Pipracil	1.0–1.3	IM, IV	12.0–24.0 g	200–300 mg/kg
Ticarcillin	Ticar	1.2	IM, IV	4.0–18.0 g	200–300 mg/kg
Ticarcillin/ Clavalanic Acid	Timentin	1.2	IM, IV	4.0–18.0 g	200–300 mg/kg

DOSING INTERVAL (h)	PEAK LEVEL (μg/ml)	ADULT DOSAGE IN RENAL FAILURE		
		80–50 ml/min	50–10 ml/min	<10 ml/min
q 6 h	3–5	0.5 g q 6h	0.5 g q 8h	0.5 g q 12h
q 12 h	3	No change	No change	No change
Penicillinase-resistant				
q 6 h	10	No change	No change	No change
q 6 h	15	No change	No change	No change
q 4–6 h	12–40	2 g q 6h	2 g q 8h	2 g q 12h
q 6 h	—	No change	No change	No change
q 4–6 h	5–40	No change	No change	No change
q 8 h	4–6	No change	No change	No change
q 4–6 h	14–40	No change	No change	No change
Aminopenicillins				
q 8 h	6–8	No change	0.75–1.5 g q 12 h	0.75–1.5 g q 12–24 h
q 8 h	4.4–7.6 (Amox) 2.3 (Clav Acid)	No change	0.75–1.5 g q 12 h	0.75–1.5 g q 12–24 h
q 6 h	2.5–5.0	No change	No change	No change
q 4–6 h	40	No change	No change	2 g q 12 h
q 4–6 h	40 (Ampi)	No change	No change	2 g q 12 h
q 12 h	8–20	No change	No change	0.8–1.6 q 24 h
q 6 h	11–12	No change	1–2 g q 12–24 h	1–2 g q 24 h
Antipseudominonal Penicillins				
q 4–6	165–500	No change	2–3 g q 8 h	2–3 g a 12 h
q 4 h	20–150 (500)	No change	2–3 g q 6 h	2 g a 12 h
q 6 h	10	No change	No change	Not recommended
q 4–6 h	250–400	No change	2–3 g q 6–8 h	2–3 g q 8–12 h
q 4–6 h	30–350	No change	3 g q 6–12 h	3 g q 12 h
q 4–6 h	20–300	No change	2–3 g q 6–8 h	2 g q 12–24 h
q 4–6 h	330 (Ticar.) 8 (Clav. A.)	No change	2 g q 4–8 h	2 g q 12–24 h

(continued)

Appendix 8-C (continued)

GENERIC	TRADE NAME	SERUM HALF-LIFE (h)	ROUTE	DAILY ADULT DOSE	DAILY PEDIATRIC DOSE
Miscellaneous Penicillins					
Amdinocillin	Coactin	0.8–1.0	IM, IV	40–60 mg/kg	NA
Polymixins					
Colistimethate	Coly-mycins	2–4.5	IM, IV	2.5–5.0 mg/kg	2.5–5.0 mg/kg
Polymixin B	Aerosporin	6–7	IV	1.5–2.5 mg/kg	1.5–2.5 mg/kg
Quinolones					
Ciprofloxacin	—	3.9	p.o. IM, IV	1.0 g	Not recommended
Norfloxacin	Noroxin	3.5	p.o.	800 mg	Not recommended
Rifampin	Rifadin Rimactane	1.5–5.0	p.o. IV	600–1200 mg 600–1200 mg	10–20 mg/kg 10–20 mg/kg
Spectinomycin	Trobicin	1.0–3.0	IM	2 g (4 g)	40 mg/kg
Sulfonamides					
Sulfadiazine	—	17	p.o.	2–4 g	75–150 mg/kg
Sulfasoxazole	Gantrisin	5–6	p.o. SC, IV	2–8 g 50–100 mg/kg	75–100 mg/kg 50–100 mg/kg
Sulfamethox- azole/ trimethoprim	Bactrim Septra	10–12 9–11	p.o. IV	4 tabs (400/80) 2 DS(800/160) 4–12 amps	8 mg/kg TMP/40 mg/kg sulfa 10 mg/kg TMP/40 mg/kg sulfa
Tetracyclines					
Doxycycline	Vibramycin	18	p.o. IV	0.2–0.4 g 0.1–0.2 g	2.2–4.4 mg/kg
Minocycline	Minocin	16	p.o. IV	0.1–0.2 g 0.2–0.4 g	2.0–4.0 mg/kg 2.0–4.0 mg/kg
Other tetracyclines	Many	8–14	p.o. IM, IV	1.0–2.0 g 0.5–1.0 g	25–50 mg/kg (over 8 yrs old) 15–25 mg/kg (over 8 yrs old)
Trimethoprim	Proloprim Trimpex	11	p.o.	100–400 mg	N/R
Vancomycin	Vancocin	5–11	IV p.o.	2 g 0.5–2.0 g	40–60 mg/kg 50 mg/kg

DOSING INTERVAL (h)	PEAK LEVEL (μg/ml)	ADULT DOSAGE IN RENAL FAILURE		
		80–50 ml/min	50–10 ml/min	<10 ml/min
Miscellaneous Penicillins				
q 4 h	26–60	No change	10 mg/kg q 6–8 h	10 mg/kg q 6–8 h
Polymixins				
q 8–12 h	5–6	2.5–3.8 mg/kg daily	2.5 mg/kg q 2–3 d	1.5 mg/kg q 5–7 d
q 12 h	5	1–1.5 mg/kg daily	1–1.5 mg/kg q 2–3 d	1 mg/kg q 5–7 d
Quinolones				
q 12 h	0.75		Not available	
q 12 h	1.58	No change	400 mg/day	400 mg/day
q 12–24 h	150–600	No change	No change	No change
q 12–24 h	150–600	No change	No change	No change
single doses	100	No change	No change	No change
Sulfonamides				
q 4–6 h	30–60	No change	?	?
q 4–6 h	11–25	0.5–2 g q6h	0.5–2 g q8–12h	0.5–2 g q8–12h
q 6–8 h	16.7	0.5–2 g q6h	0.5–2 g q8–12h	0.5–2 g q8–12h
q 12 h	1–2 Trimeth/ 20–40 sulfa	No change	one tab a 12 h 1–3 amps	Not recommended
q6–12 h	8.8 Trimeth/ 160 sulfa	No change	q 12 h	Not recommended
Tetracyclines				
q 12 h	2.5	No change	No change	No change
	4	No change	No change	No change
q 12 h	2.5	No change	Not recommended	
	4	No change		
q 6 h	4	No change	Not recommended	
q 6–1 h	8	No change		
q 12 h	1–2	No change	50 mg q12h	Not recommended
q 6–12 h	20–40	1 g q1–3d	1 g q3–7d	1 g q5–10d
q 6 h		No change	No change	No change

9

○　○　○　◉　●　◉

SEPSIS IN
BURN PATIENTS

William G. Jones
William F. McManus
Cleon W. Goodwin

In no other surgical patient is the problem of infection as great as in the burned patient. Despite the numerous advances over the past two decades that have occurred in fluid resuscitation, metabolic and nutritional support, and topical and systemic antibiotic therapy, infection remains the leading cause of morbidity and mortality in victims of thermal injuries.[92] Sepsis in severe burns still carries a mortality of greater than 75%, a rate that has remained relatively unchanged.[107] Approximately 75% of deaths in burned patients are the result of infection[1] (Fig. 9-1). In the vast majority of patients who survive the initial injury and subsequent resuscitation, sepsis appears to be the final common pathway leading to death (Fig. 9-2).

FACTORS PREDISPOSING TO SEPSIS IN BURNED PATIENTS

Patients with thermal injuries have an increased susceptibility to infection, and this increase is related to the extent of the burn.[122] The larger and deeper the burn wound, the more prone to infection the patient becomes. The precise nature of this predisposition is complex and multifactorial and, thus, difficult to define. Sepsis occurs when the balance of interactions between host and opportunistic organisms is unfavorably altered.[91] Such factors as the creation of new portals of entry, altered host defenses, and exposure to potentially pathogenic and opportunistic organisms are important determinants of sepsis in burned patients.

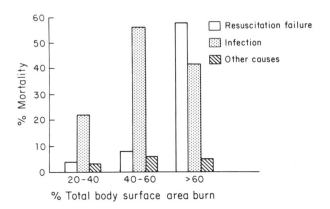

Figure 9–1.
Causes of mortality among 200 consecutive adult admissions to the New York Hospital Burn Center, 1982.

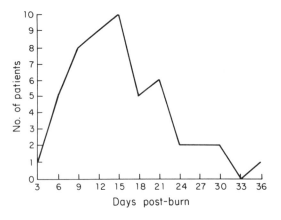

Figure 9–2.
The appearance of sepsis-related deaths following burn injury in 200 consecutive adult admissions to the New York Hospital Burn Center, 1982.

Creation of New Portals of Entry

Burn injury creates a new potential portal of entry for organisms into the patient by destruction of the mechanical barrier of the skin and the presence of a large open wound. Diminished blood supply, denatured proteins, and devitalized tissue at the wound provide an excellent culture media for bacterial growth and subsequent invasions.[93] Additionally, the presence of intravascular foreign bodies necessitated by monitoring and therapy not only may allow access of organisms to previously sterile body compartments but also act to propagate the infections. These include intravenous and intra-arterial cannulae, endotracheal tubes, and urethral catheters. Associated wounds from nonthermal trauma and decubitus ulcers developing from prolonged immobilization may also allow entry of organisms and subsequent sepsis.[92]

Alteration of Host Defenses

Burn injuries induce a series of profound alterations of host defenses. Numerous studies in both burned patients and a variety of animal models have demonstrated effects of thermal injuries on virtually every mechanism of host defense.[3, 4, 46, 58, 75] However, most of these studies have been directed toward isolated defense mechanisms rather than toward the host reaction as a whole. As a consequence, it is often difficult to determine whether specific abnormalities are the direct result of the burn injury itself, or the secondary result of altered metabolic responses, infection, or other alterations of host defenses.

Host defenses can be divided into nonspecific reactions, including the mechanical barrier of the skin, circulating phagocytes, the reticuloendothelial (RE) system, serum components, such as the complement system; and specific immune reactions, consisting of cell mediated and humoral immunity[34] (Table 9-1). Interaction between

Table 9–1
Alterations in Host Defenses in Burned Patients

Nonspecific Reactions	Specific Reactions
Mechanical barrier loss	Changes in cell-mediated immunity
Changes in circulating phagocytes	Prolonged graft survival
Neutrophils	Cutaneous anergy
Decreased chemotaxis	Diminished lymphroproliferative response
Decreased intracellular killing	Decreased lymphokine levels
Degranulation, decreased lysozyme content	Change in OKT-4/OKT-8 ratio
Macrophages	Decreased helper function
Decreased phagocytic activity	Increase suppressor function
Increased inhibitory function	Changes in humoral immunity
Changes in fixed phagocytes (RES)	Transient immunoglobulin depression
Defective clearance	Altered antigen responsiveness
Diminished fibronectin levels	
Activation of complement	

specific and nonspecific defenses results in a complex but highly coordinated reaction of the host toward the potential pathogen. Burn injuries result in skin tissue loss, and this robs the host of a mechanical barrier to infection. Loss of blood supply within the burned tissues due to coagulation and thrombosis undermines the ability of the host to mount an effective local response.[93] The skin harbors other defense mechanisms such as Langerhans cells, which act to contain local infection and recognize foreign antigens for processing, and these, too, are lost as a result of burn injury.[24]

Circulating phagocytes, consisting primarily of neutrophils and macrophages, have been studied extensively in burned patients. Decreased granulocyte hemotaxis has been well documented and correlates in a linear fashion with extent of the injury.[14,33,114,115] Neutrophil phagocytosis appears to be essentially normal, but intracellular killing, especially of certain organisms such as staphylococci, is decreased.[5] Nitroblue tetrazolium reduction by neutrophils, reflecting the bacteriocidal property of peroxidase is diminished and correlates with the appearance of wound infection and sepsis.[21] Neutrophil lysozyme content is decreased and is associated with increased serum lysozyme concentrations leading to postulation of selective degranulation.[23] A linear correlation exists between the decrease in intracellular lysozyme content and the degree of impairment of chemotaxis. Neutrophil glucose utilization is also abnormal.[92] Similarly, functional changes in macrophages, particularly in the pulmonary alveolae, have also been demonstrated.[44,57] Phagocytosis by macrophages is decreased, but intracellular microbial killing appears increased over controls. These changes in macrophage function are associated with increased prostaglandin synthesis.[34]

The RE system, representing a fixed pool of phagocytes lying in close proximity to vascular beds throughout the body, has been studied extensively by Saba and associates.[53] Burn injury markedly depresses the function of the RE system, as evidenced by defective clearance of particulate matter and[51]Cr-labeled red blood cells,[104] and a decreased resistance to shock and infection has been postulated to result.[52] This may represent an "overload" of the system created by the release of particulates from the burn or other sources and correlates closely with a depletion of fibronectin.[53] Fibronectin is an glycoprotein opsonin present in the serum that binds to a variety of materials leading to their phagocytosis. Fibronectin is initially reduced in burn patients but returns to normal with recovery. Subsequent reductions in fibronectin levels have been noted in burned patients 1 to 2 days prior to the onset of sepsis and has led to controversy over whether this observation represents a cause or effect of infection.[31] Fibronectin replacement therapy can restore serum opsonin levels in animal models but fails to correct completely functional deficits of the RE system, leading to the conclusion that other factors are involved as well.[51]

The complement system acts as an important nonspecific mediator of host defense, and burn injury has been shown to be associated with abnormal activation of both the alternate and classical complement pathways.[15,38] Tissue damage can also activate the intrinsic coagulation and fibrinolytic systems, which, in turn, leads to complement activation. This results in production of highly reactive complement components, which can circulate and have far-reaching local and systemic effects. Complement activation leads to the release of vasoactive substances such as serotonin and histamine, which can alter local tissue perfusion.[34] Complement activation products also increase granulocyte aggregation and adhesiveness.[108] This latter effect can cause a relative circulating granulocytopenia and may lead to sequestration of granulocytes within the pulmonary microvasculature, which has been implicated in the pathophysiology of the adult respiratory distress syndrome.[34]

Defects in specific immunity are most profound in cell-mediated responses, which are under the control of T cells.[16] This is evidenced by the prolonged survival of allografts and xenografts in burned patients.[87] Cutaneous energy has also been noted.[45, 119] Other evidence of depressed cell-mediated immunity includes diminished lymphoproliferative responses to mitogens, decreased *in vitro* cell cytotoxicity, and decreased production of lymphokines.[61, 69, 70, 80]

Lymphopenia, common in severe burn injuries, has been found to be primarily a deficiency of T cells.[85] Further analysis of T-cell subsets has revealed a greater depression of helper/inducer OKT-4 cells than in suppressor/cytotoxic OKT-8 cells.[7] The resultant decrease in OKT-4 to OKT-8 ratio changes the balance of T-cell activity in favor of suppression and appears to be predictive of septic death.[8]

Changes in immunoglobulin levels can be minimal but are most pronounced in young children.[13] Transient depressions in IgG, IgA, and IgM have been noted, but this does not appear to be invariable.[9, 79, 102] Possible etiologies of immunoglobulin depression may relate to decreased production, increased catabolism, protein leakage, or dilution by resuscitation fluids.[32] Further studies of antibody production have demonstrated a depressed primary humoral response and an enhanced secondary anamnestic response.[2, 48] This, however, may be related to dysfunctional antigen processing helper T cells and macrophages, rather than a B-cell defect.

Postulated mechanisms of host defense depression are as varied as the alterations themselves (Table 9-2). As discussed above, alterations in T-cell subsets upset the balance between helper and suppressor function. Many researchers believe this excessive suppressor function to be primarily responsible for burn injury-induced immunosuppression.[63, 76, 118] Altered levels of the cytokin interleukin-2 may play an additional role.[8, 120] Interleukin-2 is a humoral factor produced by helper T cells that appears to promote T-cell development and proliferation and both specific and nonspecific cytotoxicity. Decreased serum IL-2 may mediate the diminished lympho-

Table 9–2
Postulated Mechanisms of Host Defense Depression

Excessive suppressor function
Decreased interleukin-2 levels
Excessive prostaglandin production
Excessive serum cortisol
Other serum inhibitory factors
   Endotoxin
   "Burn toxins"
   Immunoregulatory proteins
   Immune complexes and autoantibodies
Iatrogenic factors

proliferation and cytotoxicity observed in burn patients. Such decrease in IL-2 may be due to either diminished production or impaired release.[8] The recent finding that numbers of circulating OKT-4 helper cells return to normal before restoration of levels of IL-2 and a failure to establish a correlation between absolute helper cell numbers and IL-2 levels suggests the presence of a defect in function beyond just diminished numbers of producing cell.[120] Serum levels of interleukin-1, a macrophage-derived stimulator of IL-2 production, remain normal following thermal injury.

Macrophages have known inhibitory functions, and arachidonic acid metabolites, including prostaglandins and leukotrienes, have been implicated in this activity.[55] Altered arachidonic acid metabolism in burned patients is reflected by elevated concentrations of prostaglandins, which may mediate macrophage-induced suppression.[88] Elevated serum cortisol, a normal hormonal response to trauma and burns, may also be involved.[92]

Multiple investigators have demonstrated the suppressive action of serum from burned patients on granulocytes and lymphocytes from normal donors.[86,118,119] A number of possible serum inhibitory factors have been investigated. Endotoxin, produced by gram-negative bacilli, has been shown to cause many immunosuppressive effects. Some may be mediated by stimulation of prostaglandin synthesis.[88] The presence of endotoxin within the serum of burned patients may be the result of either gram-negative infection or of translocation from the gastrointestinal tract, a known reservoir of endotoxin. This translocation, normally prevented by intact cell-mediated immunity, has been demonstrated in animal models following experimental burns.[25] Another high molecular weight substance, a so-called burn toxin, has been shown by several authors to have immunosuppressive properties.[64,86] The nature of this substance has yet to be elucidated, but it may be a product of burned cutaneous tissues. Additionally, numerous serum proteins have been implicated, including alpha-1 immunoregulatory globulin (IRA), circulating immune complexes and autoantibodies, and transferrin.[19,34]

Finally, iatrogenic factors relating to treatment of the burned patient may themselves by immunosuppressive. The failure to recognize the hypermetabolic state of the burned patient and to correct malnutrition can have far-reaching effects.[27] Topical agents used to prevent burn wound infection, such as silver sulfadiazine, have been shown to produce granulocytopenia.[18] Likewise, anesthetic agents and other medications can have immunosuppressive side-effects.[46] The administration of fluids and blood products during initial resuscitation not only may produce dilutional effects but also may directly depress circulating immune competent cells.

Many innovative attempts have been made to treat these abnormalities of host defense. Complete closure of the burn wound appears to correct the immunodeficiency and has led some to advocate early excision.[30] Active immunization byu administration of gamma globulin is under study and may be an effective means of providing some protection.[92,97] Clinical evidence of its efficacy on incidence of infection and mortality, however, is lacking. The development and use of specific monoclonal antibodies have been shown to decrease significantly mortality from lethal bacterial challenges in animal models.[6] Their major drawback is that these antibodies are strain specific and, thus, must be developed for each strain of potentially pathogenic organisms to obtain complete coverage. The use of immunomodulators, which improve immunoresponsiveness in a less specific manner, may be more effective. Several substances are currently being investigated in both animal and clinical models.[28,109,116] Finally, plasmapheresis to remove inhibitory serum factors has produced beneficial effects on immune function in early clinical trials.[66]

Exposure to New Potential Pathogens

The microbial flora of the burn patient and his environment is constantly changing and provides a source of multiple microorganisms, each containing various factors that promote their virulence.[97] Important among these factors are motility and the production of collagenase.[65] The creation of specialized units for the care of burned patients has undoubtedly contributed to their improved overall survival.[106] However, such units harbor organisms such as *Pseudomonas, Serratia,* and *Providencia,* which are highly pathogenic in these severely compromised patients. Cyclic variations in the offending organisms are known to occur.[40] Inappropriate use of antibiotics can select for resistant organisms, and the use of prophylactic systemic antibiotics in hospitalized burned patients has been known to increase nosocomial infections.[43] As a consequence of altered host defenses, "opportunistic" organisms, such as fungi and enterococci, which are usually considered nonpathogenic, may produce clinical infections and sepsis.[17,49]

MANIFESTATIONS OF SEPSIS IN BURNED PATIENTS

The clinical manifestations of sepsis in the burned patient are often nonspecific, and diagnosis requires a high degree of suspicion on the part of the clinician. Many of the generally accepted signs of infection, such a leukocytosis or fever, are unreliable following burn injury because they also reflect tissue injury and the associated hypermetabolic state in absence of infection. However, any deterioration of a previously stable clinical situation must always prompt consideration of a septic etiology.

Pruitt has described the systemic signs associated with invasive infection in burned patients[92] (Table 9-3). Alterations in body temperature, mental status, glucose

Table 9–3
Systemic Manifestations of Sepsis in Burned Patients

Altered body temperature control
Altered mental status
Altered glucose metabolism
Altered fluid requirements and hypotension
Altered organ function
    Ileus
    Adult respiratory distress syndrome
    Oliguria
    Thrombocytopenia, leukocytopenia

tolerance, or evidence of organ failure must be assumed to represent sepsis until proven otherwise. Manifestations of organ failure include ileus, respiratory failure requiring mechanical ventilatory support, oliguria, hypotension with increased fluid requirement, leukopenia and thrombocytopenia.

SOURCES OF SEPSIS IN BURNED PATIENTS

Burn Wound Infection

The burn wound, although initially sterilized by the heat of the injury, becomes colonized with a wide variety of microbial organisms soon after the injury occurs.[42] The sources of these organisms include not only the patient's environment, but his own flora as well. The numbers and types of organisms change over time following the injury. Gram-positive organisms, such as *Streptococcus* and *Staphylococcus* species, were once the most common cause of clinical burn wound infections and are the predominate colonizers in the early post-burn period.[97] Probably arising from the depths of the sweat glands and hair follicles, these gram-positive organisms are largely controlled by current topical therapy and are soon supplanted by gram-negative and, later, fungal species (Table 9-4). The wide variety of these organisms ranges from *Pseudomonas, Providencia,* and *Enterobacter* species to opportunists such as *Candida, Phycomycetes,* and enterococci.[68] Herpetic viral infections of the burn wound have also been reported.[35] This microbial milieu provides the organisms not only for burn wound infections of importance in burned patients as well (Table 9-5).

Colonization of the burn wound arises from the proliferation of microbial organisms in the avascular and nonviable burned tissues and eschar and is not itself a true infection.[97] Burn wound infection requires the spread and growth of bacteria into viable adjacent and subeschar unburned tissues.[68] The spectrum of burn wound

Table 9–4
Microorganisms Colonizing the Burn Wound*

Enterbacter cloacae	27%
Staphylococcus aureus	19%
Candida species	12%
Streptococcus fecalis	10%
Pseudomonas aeruginosa	9%
Klebsiella pneumoniae	9%
Staphylococcus epidermidis	5%
Escherichia coli	3%
Other	5%

* Percentages of total isolates present in burn wound biopsies at The New York Hospital Burn Center, 1983.

Table 9–5
Infections in Burned Patients

Burn wound infections
Pneumonia—airborne, hematogenous, aspiration
Tracheobronchitis
Suppurative thrombophlebitis
Endocarditis
Genitourinary—periurethritis, prostatitis, cystitis, pyelonephritis
Intra-abdominal—perforated Curling's ulcers, acalculous, cholecystitis, necrotizing
  enterocolitis, colonic pseudo-obstruction with perforation

---

infection ranges from well localized cellulitis to often lethal invasive infections with generalized sepsis. The risk of development of burn wound infection remains until the nonviable tissues are excised and the wound is definitively closed, leading some to advocate early excision.[26,59]

Prevention of burn wound infection prior to closure requires control of the colonizing organisms through the use of topical antimicrobial therapy.[99] The effectiveness of this therapy is monitored by physical examination of the wound through burn wound biopsy techniques. Surface cultures, including swab and touch plate techniques, can identify the organisms colonizing the top of the burn wound but fail to address the microbial status of the underlying viable tissues.[96] Furthermore, technical problems, such as delayed processing or the inclusion of pooled secretions or topical agents within the cultured material, further reduce the reliability of surface cultures.[97]

Burn wound biopsies, similar to the techniques described by Loebl and others, should be performed serially until the burn is closed and the risk of infection is abated[56,96] (Fig. 9-3). The number of biopsies performed depends on the size of the burn and its appearance. At the New York Hospital Burn Center, one specimen is taken per 18% surface area of burn as a minimum, with additional biopsies taken as clinically indicated. Biopsy surveillance is carried out two to three times each week. Quantitative cultures are then prepared from the specimens. The presence of more than 10^5 organisms per gram of tissue has been shown to correlate with bacterial growth into viable subeschar tissues and burn wound infection and is thus helpful in differentiating mere colonization from true wound infection.

The reliability of quantitative burn wound biopsies alone in determination of infection and invasive wound sepsis has been questioned.[121] Thus, a portion of the biopsy specimen should be submitted for histology. The microscopic finding of organisms in viable subeschar or adjacent tissue appears to be the most definitive means of diagnosing burn wound infection[92] (Fig. 9-4). Pruitt and Foley[96] have described a graded scheme of histologic classification ranging from surface contamination to the growth of organisms in viable unburned tissues that defines burn wound invasion. Further, results of histologic examination can be readily obtained following procure-

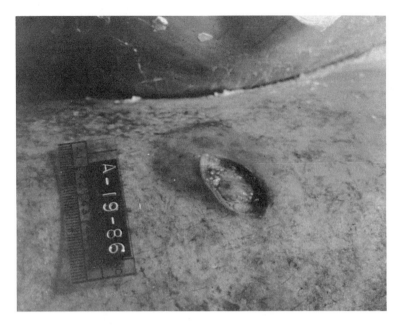

Figure 9–3.
Biopsy of *Pseudomonas* ecthyma gangrenosum in a patient with burn wound sepsis. The 500-mg, lenticular-shaped biopsy includes adjacent normal skin and underlying viable tissue.

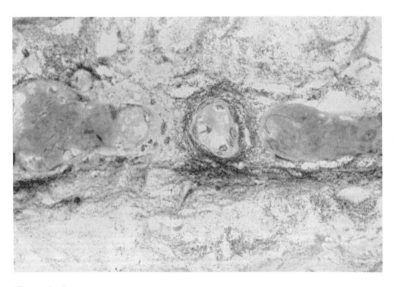

Figure 9–4.
Gram's stain of burn with invasive wound infection. *Pseudomonas aeruginosa* are clustered around the thrombosed blood vessel and also can be seen in viable subcutaneous fat.

ment of the specimen using frozen section or permanent techniques, giving information regarding not only the depth of invasion but the type of organisms involved as well.

Burn wound infections may be viewed as a loss of local control. This is suggested by the presence of greater than 10^5 organisms per gram of tissue in quantitative burn wound biopsies or by a 100-fold increase in the bacterial counts over two serial biopsies. Biopsy results, however, must always be interpreted in the light of the patient's clinical condition. A negative biopsy in the setting of a deteriorating clinical course should prompt repeat and perhaps more extensive biopsies, as well as an examination of other potential sources.

Locally, burn wound infection is manifested by (1) the appearance of dark, violaceous discolorations in the wound or its margins (Fig. 9-5); (2) conversion of a partial thickness to a full thickness injury; (3) rapid separation of the eschar; (4) the appearance of erythematous nodules (erythema gangrenosa) in unburned skin; and (5) hemorrhagic discoloration of subeschar tissues[92] (Fig. 9-6). Identifying the presence of these signs requires that the burn wound be examined in its entirety and that a high index of suspicion be maintained.

The presence of increasing bacterial density in the burn wound represents loss of local control, and treatment requires a change in topical therapy before invasive sepsis occurs.[40] The topical antimicrobial agent should be changed to an agent with increased eschar penetration or better microbial coverage. Mafenide acetate is the most effective topical therapy for a deteriorating wound. When appropriate, the wound is excised and grafted.[92]

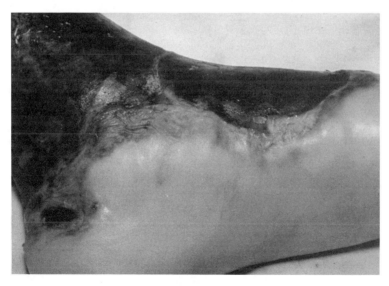

Figure 9–5.
Pseudomonas burn wound infection of a lower extremity eschar. The heaped-up margins around the eschar on the ankle represent invasion into adjacent uninjured tissue.

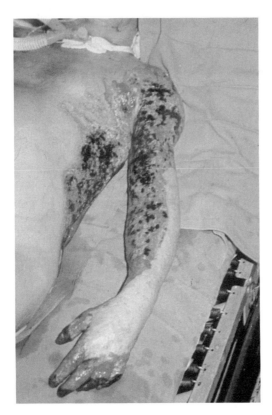

Figure 9–6.
Focal invasion of a chronic burn wound by
Aspergillus. This fungus characteristically
appears as well circumscribed lesions,
which eventually coalesce if excision of the
wound is delayed.

Cellulitis of the burn wound may also develop and is usually manifested by an expanding margin of erythema and edema in surrounding unburned skin (Fig. 9-7). As with other infections in the burned patient, fever may not be an accompanying sign. Gram-positive organisms, predominately streptococci and staphylococci, are the usual causative organisms and, in the case of the latter, may be associated with cutaneous microabscesses. Treatment of burn wound cellulitis requires parenteral antibiotics with good gram-positive coverage. Cellulitis may also develop in skin graft donor sites and responds well to similar therapy.

Invasive burn wound infections, ultimately leading to bacteremias and generalized sepsis, were previously the most common causes of death in burned patients.[68] The development of topical antimicrobial therapy has led to a decreased incidence of this complication and, thus, an improvement in survival, but invasive burn wound infections remain a major cause of morbidity and mortality.[99] Invasive burn wound infections rarely occur in injuries of less than 30% total body surface area and most commonly arise in children and elderly patients.[92] The appearance of systemic sepsis resulting from hematogenous dissemination of organisms from invasive burn wound infection, so-called burn wound sepsis, is a late sign and if uncontrolled is rapidly followed by the death of the patient. There is evidence to suggest that bacteremias

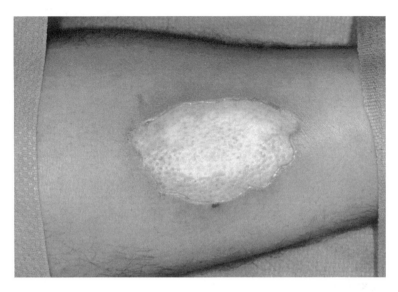

Figure 9–7.
Cellulitis surrounding a small burn. Cellulitis usually occurs within the first week of injury and presents as erythema extending more than 1 cm beyond the margin of the burn.

from burn wound sources, especially of opportunistic organisms, may be associated with higher mortality than bacteremias in burned patients arising from other sources[49] (Fig. 9-8).

In the 1960s, burn wound sepsis caused by *Pseudomonas aerugenosa* was identified, and its pathogenesis was defined by Teplitz.[101, 113] It has been shown that this organism proliferates within the burn eschar and subsequently invades underlying or adjacent viable tissues.[111] This is followed by an invasion of blood vessels with hematogenous spread and resultant septicemia.[112] *Pseudomonas* has been considered the prototype for invasion, and it was on the basis of these studies that effective topical chemotherapy was developed.[73] Other infecting agents with different virulence factors may manifest a different but as yet unelucidated pathophysiology. Sepsis resulting from the absorption of endotoxin and exotoxin from the burn wound without actual hematogenous spread of organisms has been postulated to explain frequently negative blood cultures in patients with invasive burn wound infections.[26]

Once the diagnosis of invasive burn wound infection is made and confirmed by histology, therapy is dictated by the infecting organisms, depth of penetration, and extent of injury. Broad-spectrum systemic antibacterial and antifungal agents should be administered. However, antibiotic therapy alone is inadequate treatment for the infected burn wound. Small localized and even some multifocal areas of burn wound infection can be controlled effectively by clysis techniques involving the subeschar infusion of antibiotic solution[12, 67] (Fig. 9-9). However, invasive burn wound sepsis involving greater than 1% to 2% of total body surface area is best treated by excision,

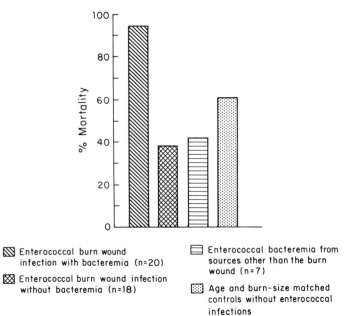

Figure 9–8.
Mortality associated with enterococcal infection in burned patients.

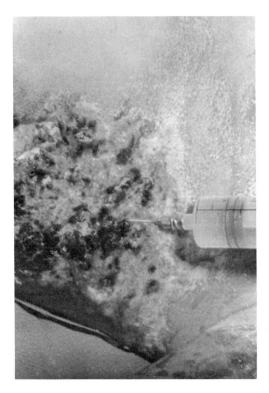

Figure 9–9.
Subeschar clysis of an invaded burn. Spinal needle is inserted serially in a fan-shaped pattern until the subeschar space of the entire wound is infiltrated.

with clysis and adjuvant therapy only.[42] Once the infection is controlled, definitive closure using autograft can be carried out.

The relative vascularity of the burn wound limits the delivery and, thus, the usefulness of systemic antibiotics in burn wound infections. The development of topical antibiotic therapy has been one of the greatest advancements in controlling burn wound infection[71] (Fig. 9-10). These agents do not prevent the colonization of the burn wound but maintain bacterial counts at a level low enough to be controlled by even the compromised host.[99] Currently three preparations enjoy widespread use (Table 9-6). Manfenide acetate (Sulfamylon) cream, introduced by Moncrief and co-workers in 1964,[72] has a wide spectrum of activity, especially against gram-negative organisms. It is suspended in a water-dispersible base and, thus, diffuses through the eschar to achieve concentrations at the interface between viable and nonviable tissues. Its side-effects include pain on application to partial thickness burns, hyper-sensitivity reactions in 5% to 7% of patients, and carbonic anhydrase inhibition resulting in loss of bicarbonate and secondary acidosis.[10]

Silver nitrate soaked dressings, introduced by Moyer and co-workers in 1964,[74] maintains a broad spectrum of antibiotic activity and is painless on application. However, it requires occlusive dressings, which must be kept constantly moist to prevent concentration of the potentially toxic silver nitrate by evaporation. The combination of absorption of water from the dressings and the leeching of electrolytes by the silver compound can lead to hyponatremia and free water overload. Staining of the patient, his environment, and his care providers by the silver nitrate is a less serious but bothersome problem.

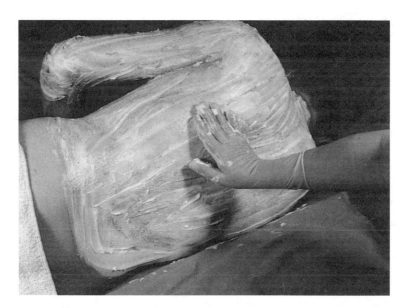

Figure 9–10.
Application of mafenide acetate to burn wound. Topical antimicrobial agent is spread over the entire wound by sterilely gloved hand and maintained by repeated applications if necessary.

Table 9–6
Topical Antibiotic Preparations for Use on Burn Wounds

	MAFENIDE	SILVER NITRATE	SILVER SULFADIAZINE
Spectrum of activity*	Gr(−)	Gr(+), fungi, most Gr(−)	Gr(+), Gr(−) *Candida*
Eschar penetration	Deep	Poor	Little
Development of resistance	No	No	Some Gr(−)
Toxicity	Carbonic anhydrase inhibition	Electrolyte losses	Leukopenia
Bacteriostatic	Yes	Yes	Yes
Hypersensitivity reactions	Yes	No	Yes
Other	Painful	Requires occlusive dressings	

* Gr(−) = gram-negative; Gr(+) = gram-positive.

Silver sulfadiazine cream, introduced by Fox and co-workers in 1968,[36] also has broad-spectrum activity but without the electrolyte or acid–base disturbances of its predecessors. It is painless on application but can be associated with rare hypersensitivity reactions and neutropenia, which resolves when the drug is discontinued. Ineffectiveness against certain *Pseudomonas* and *Enterobacter* strains due to resistance has been reported, however, and its water-miscible base allows very little diffusion into the eschar.

Each of these agents is effective, and considerable experience with their use has accumulated. The initial choice of an agent must be based on application of the advantages and disadvantages of the agent against the clinical situation. A change in that clinical situation, such as the development of signs of burn wound infection, then mandates reappraisal and change to a more appropriate drug.

Respiratory Infections

Largely because of the development of topical antibiotic therapy, respiratory infections have replaced the burn wound as the most frequent primary source of sepsis in the burn patient.[26] Pneumonia may result from either bloodborne or airborne organisms, but in either case the infecting organisms are usually among those present in the flora of the burn wound.[92] Bronchopneumonia accounts for approximately 65% of respiratory infections in the burn patient.[95] The process begins as organisms migrate down the airway resulting in a bronchiolitis that spreads into the alveoli. Endotracheal tubes or tracheotomies facilitate the passage of organisms into the pulmonary tree while the presence of inhalation injury and atelectasis appear to be further predisposing factors. Bronchopneumonia usually presents in the second post-burn week, arising initially as an infiltrate in dependent portions of the lungs on roentgenograms (Fig. 9-11).

In contrast, hematogenous pneumonia results from embolization of organisms to the pulmonary capillaries from a primary source, such as the burn wound, infected veins, endocarditis, or abscesses. This causes inflammation of the microvasculature, which then spreads to involve the alveoli. As the incidence of burn wound sepsis has decreased, hematogenous pneumonia has become less common. Almost half of cases of hematogenous pneumonia are now secondary to suppurative thrombi from a peripheral vessel.[94] Hematogenous pneumonia tends to occur during the third post-burn week. The initial radiographic picture is of a solitary nodular infiltrate, and its appearance should prompt investigation of all likely primary sites (Fig. 9-12). If the pulmonary source remains unchecked, multiple areas may appear in a random distribution, ultimately coalescing to form a picture similar to that of bronchopneumonia.

The treatment of pneumonia requires the use of systemic antibiotics chosen on the basis of sputum Gram's stains and culture results. Culture specimens are best obtained by transtracheal aspiration or by way of bronchoscopy. In the case of hematogenous pneumonia, the primary source must also be identified and treated. Vigorous attention to chest physiotherapy and pulmonary toilet, judicious use of bronchoscopy, and avoidance of tracheal intubation are all effective preventive measures. For patients on mechanical ventilators, daily chest roentgenograms should also be monitored, as well as routine sputum Gram's stains and cultures to follow changing patterns of respiratory colonization and facilitate early diagnosis.

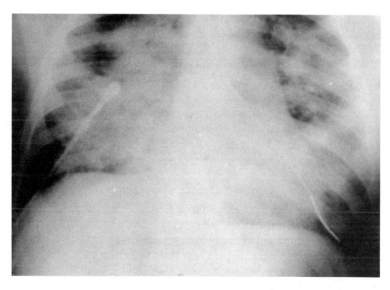

Figure 9–11.
Bronchopneumonia in a burned patient with inhalation injury. Infiltrates often begin centrally and spread to the peripheral margins of the lung.

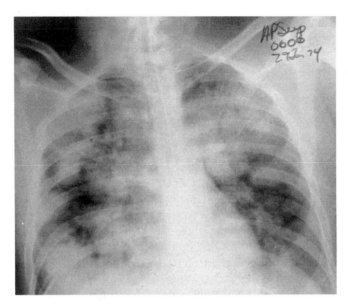

Figure 9–12.
Hematogenous pneumonia in a patient with suppurative thrombophlebitis. This form of pneumonia characteristically appears as discreet, randomly distributed infiltrates that are well demarcated. Later, these densities coalesce to form a pattern resembling diffuse bronchopneumonia.

Aspiration pneumonia may occur in burn patients due to the debilitating nature of the injury and the presence of post-burn gastric dilation and ileus. The initial lesion is a chemical bronchitis, especially with the aspiration of gastric contents with pH less than 4.[40] This may then progress to secondary bacterial infection and pneumonia. Early placement of nasogastric tubes for decompression and drainage following injury has greatly decreased the incidence of this complication and is the key to its prevention. Antibiotics are administered when the presence of infection is verified by Gram's stains of sputum, and their use is guided by microbial surveillance data. There is no role for steroid therapy in aspiration pneumonia in the burned patient.[92]

Tracheitis and tracheobronchitis are frequent complications associated with the inhalation of products of incomplete combustion present in smoke. The initial reaction is a chemical irritation that is often complicated by further irritation produced by the presence of endotracheal and tracheostomy tubes.[20] This may progress to the complete syndrome of destruction of the respiratory epithelium with loss of ciliary action and accumulation of cellular debris. Rapid colonization with organisms occurs, largely reflecting the flora of the burn wound. Invasive infection even though the chest roentgenogram may remain normal. Secondary bronchospasm may also occur.

Gram-negative organisms, especially *Pseudomonas*, frequently cause the suppurative infection. *Candida* may also colonize, but is only rarely associated with invasive infection.[20] Therapy consists of early vigorous pulmonary toilet to maintain airway patency and remove debris and mucous plugs. Judicious use of endotracheal tubes and mechanical ventilation must be employed. The progression to suppuration and systemic sepsis requires the use of broad-spectrum parenteral antibiotics. Choice of antibiotic therapy should be based on the results of sputum Gram's stains and later adjusted on the basis of culture and sensitivity testing. Aerosolized antimicrobial therapy, primarily with aminoglycosides, has also been employed.

Infection Related to Intravenous Catheters

The requirements of large volume fluid resuscitation, monitoring devices, and parenteral medications and alimentation make the presence of intravenous catheters in the burned patient a necessity. Not surprisingly, these devices represent a major source of infection and are the cause of sepsis in approximately 5% of critically ill patients in some reports.[89] The pathophysiology of these infections apparently is related to damage of the vessel endothelium by the catheter tip.[40] This leads to formation of a fibrin clot that may either be infected by entrance of organisms in the administered fluids or seeded by bacteremia from other sources. The infected clot may then serve as nidus of further bacteremia and so-called line sepsis.

The diagnosis of line sepsis requires recovery of the same organisms from blood and from semiquantitative culture of the catheter tip.[60] Because of the possibility of secondary hematogenous seeding of the catheter site, other potential septic sources must be ruled out. Once the diagnosis of the line sepsis is made or highly suspected, the offending catheter should be removed, and appropriate antibiotics should be administered. Gram-positive organisms, particularly *Staphylococcus aureus*, are the usual causative organisms, although *Candida* has also been demonstrated, especially in conjunction with hyperaliamentation infusions.[20]

Thrombophlebitis of the cannulated vein is a common occurrence and is related to the type of fluid infused, the size and composition of cannula employed, and duration of cannulization. Simple, sterile thrombophlebitis usually responds to removal of the catheter and the local application of moist heat. However, the thrombotic vein may become infected by way of extension of skin organisms or by seeding from other bacteremia. Suppuration may then occur, and the infected thrombus then serves as a hematogenous source of infectious emboli and distant abscesses[100] (Fig. 9-13). This syndrome of suppurative thrombophlebitis is particularly prevalent in peripheral "cut down" sites.

The diagnosis of suppurative thrombophlebitis is often difficult to make, because as many as half of affected patients will display no sign or symptom of venous disease prior to the onset of bacteremia.[92] Extrusion of pus from the vein confirms the diagnosis and may be present as long as 3 weeks after the catheter has been removed.[40] *Staphylococcus aureus* is by far the most common organism involved, and proper treatment requires that the infected vein be ligated and excised, in addition to the administration of parenteral antibiotics.[92] Preventive measures are probably more successful in decreasing the incidence of this complication than any other infection associated with burn injury.[40] Avoidance of cutdown venotomies, use of central veins for catheterization, careful attention to aseptic techniques of insertion, and frequent

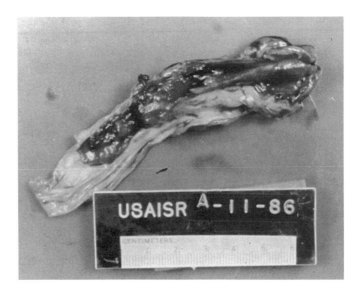

Figure 9–13.
Infected thrombus in a subclavian vein.

catheter and site changes with associated surveillance cultures can all contribute to a lowered incidence of suppurative thrombophlebitis.

Bacterial Endocarditis

Intimately associated with the use of intravenous catheters and pulmonary artery monitoring devices, acute bacterial endocarditis is an uncommon but often insidious cause of sepsis in the burn patient.[11] Most lesions occur in the valves or endothelium of the right heart and are only rarely associated with preexisting valvular disease[40] (Fig. 9-14). The diagnosis is difficult to make but is suggested by multiple unexplained blood cultures growing known causative organisms such as staphylococci and can be confirmed by echocardiography. Long-term courses of antibiotics, often 6 weeks or more, are required, and valve replacement surgery must be considered in those patients who fail to respond to medical therapy. When possible, catheters should not be placed within cardiac chambers but should remain within the large central veins in an effort to prevent this devastating complication.

Genitourinary Infections

The use of urethral catheters in burned patients is required for monitoring of urinary output and assessment of volume status. Subsequent infection of the lower urinary tract is not uncommon, and prolonged catheter use may lead to prostatic or periurethral abscesses. These usually are palpable on rectal examination. Aseptic

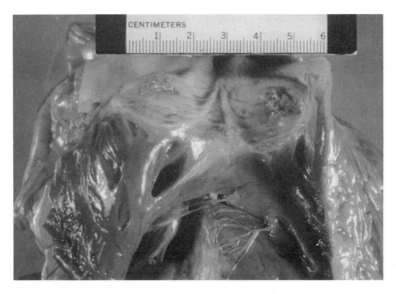

Figure 9–14.
Vegetation on the leaflets of an infected aortic valve of a patient with burn wound sepsis.

technique of insertion and catheter care, the use of closed drainage systems, and the removal of the catheter at the earliest clinically indicated time are effective preventive measures. Pyelonephritis may also occur, either as an ascending infection from a concurrent cystitis or by way of hematogenous spread of infection. Hematogenous infections may result in renal abscesses as well. Again, causative organisms reflect the flora of the burn wound, with *Pseudomonas* and other gram-negative organisms most common. Therapy consists of appropriate parenteral antibiotics and drainage of collections.

Intra-abdominal Infections

Unrecognized associated intra-abdominal injury, such as a perforated viscus, can result in sepsis in the burned patient,[41] as may complications of the repairs of such injuries. In addition, it must always be remembered that burned patients may also still suffer from any of the causes of an acute abdomen in the unburned patient, such as appendicitis or diverticulitis. In light of the debilitated and immobilized condition of the severely burned patient, colonic volvulus may also occur.

The diagnosis of the acute abdomen in the burned patient may present quite a clinical challenge. Burn injury is often accompanied by ileus requiring nasogastric decompression. Obtundation produced by injury or sedation may mask symptoms and make the examination of the abdomen unreliable. Burn injury to the abdominal wall and tissue edema further complicate the exam. Finally, circulating levels of corticosteroids may suppress development of peritoneal signs. A high index of suspicion coupled with a low threshold for performing appropriate diagnostic studies is of extreme importance.

Burned patients have a predisposition for the development of certain intra-abdominal complications and infections. Curling's ulcers, the acute stress mucosal ulcerations of the stomach and duodenum arising in burned patients, appear to be related to sepsis.[90] They are often multiple and usually occur after the first post-burn week. These ulcers may lead to perforation with pneumoperitoneum and peritoneal soiling. Vigorous medical therapy with antacids has largely eliminated this complication.[92]

Acute acalculous cholecystitis may result either from hematogenous seeding of the gallbladder from systemic sepsis or from the effects of hemolysis, dehydration, and biliary stasis.[78] The presence of jaundice and right upper quadrant fullness or a mass often associated with prolonged periods of hypovolemia and nasogastric suction should suggest the diagnosis. Symptoms usually develop after the first post-burn week. Ultrasonography probably represents the most useful diagnostic test, and, if the patient is in an appropriate clinical setting, cholecystectomy or cholecystostomy should be performed.

Ischemic enterocolitis may result from acute occlusion of mesenteric arteries, venous thrombosis, or secondary to prolonged hypotension with poor perfusion and disseminated intravascular coagulopathy. This latter entity, termed nonocclusive ischemic enterocolitis, occasionally occurs in burned patients and is characterized by progressive mucosal necrosis and often pseudomembrane formation.[90] Perforation may occur, leading to generalized peritonitis. Diagnosis of necrotizing enterocolitis can be very difficult, although colonoscopy may be helpful in identifying suspicious mucosal changes.

Marked dilation of the colon without apparent obstruction will develop in approximately 1% of burned patients and has been termed colonic pseudo-obstruction.[54] It is accompanied by abdominal distention, pain, and obstipation. Perforation is most likely to occur at the cecum and is a significant risk once the cecal diameter reaches 12 cm or greater. Diagnosis is usually made on plain abdominal films. Decompression may be accomplished by endoscopy, although occasionally tube cecostomy is required. The etiology is unclear but may be related to ischemia, metabolic, or hormonal responses to the injury, or analgesic use.

Other Infections

Both thermal injury and external pressure on the ear may lead to necrosis of the auricular cartilage, which may then become secondarily infected.[29] Localized areas of auricular chondritis may be drained, but the presence of generalized chondritis mandates removal of all affected cartilage. *Pseudomonas* is almost always the infecting organism, and the use of Sulfamylon in burns of cartilaginous structures is effective in preventing this complication.

Herpetic infections may occur in the burn wound, and they primarily affect healing or healed second-degree burns, especially of the face[35] (Figs. 9-15 and 9-16).

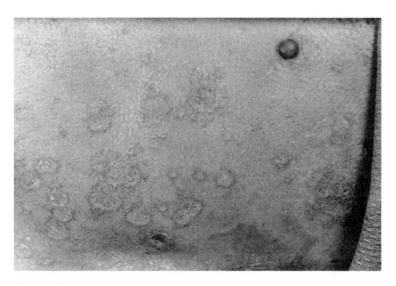

Figure 9–15.
Herpetic lesions in a healing partial thickness burn. Such infections may cause progression of injury to involve the full thickness of the skin.

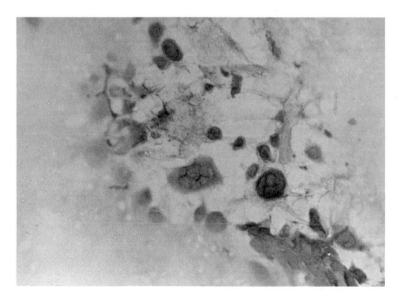

Figure 9–16.
Biopsy of herpetic wound lesion. The intranuclear inclusion bodies are characteristic of invasive herpetic infection.

Herpetic infections of the upper gastrointestinal tract, liver, and lungs occur rarely and can result in perforation and systemic viremia.[81] Treatment requires the use of systemic antiviral agents such as acyclovir. Infections with varicella and cytomegalovirus have also been reported.[81] Clostridial infections in burned patients are rare but have been reported.[22] Every burned patient should be treated with appropriate tetanus prophylaxis at the initial examination.

WORKUP OF SUSPECTED SEPSIS IN THE BURNED PATIENT

The presence of clinical signs of sepsis or a deteriorating clinical condition should mandate a septic workup in the burned patient. The most important step is a complete physical examination of the patient to detect signs of an acute abdomen, endocarditis, or other causes. The burn wound must be examined in its entirety out of topical agent, and special attention should be paid to sites of intravenous catheters.

Routine surveillance culture results should be reviewed to detect any trends such as progressive increases in quantitative bacterial counts on burn wound biopsies. Serial blood cultures should be performed after careful preparation of the skin, with different sites employed to minimize the risk of contamination.[62] Transtracheal aspiration or deep nasotracheal suction for sputum as well as urine and stool specimens for Gram's stain and culture should be obtained. Intravenous catheters should be removed and placed in new sites with the tips sent for semiquantitative culture.[29] Suspicious areas of the burn wound should also be biopsied for quantitative culture and histology.

Sputum and other suspicious materials, such as drainage from catheter sites, should be Gram-stained, and the initial selection of antibiotics should be based on these studies and on surveillance cultures. Radiographs of the chest should be obtained as well as abdominal studies if clinically indicated. Special studies such as echocardiograms and lumbar puncture should be performed based on suspicion and examination. Because of the particularly serious nature of sepsis in the burned patient, these measures should be undertaken quickly, and presumptive therapy should be begun as early as possible.

USE OF ANTIBIOTICS IN THE BURNED PATIENT

The presence of systemic signs and symptoms of sepsis associated with an infection in the burned patient requires treatment with systemic antibiotics. Systemic antibiotics are also important adjuvant therapy in localized infections where the potential for septicemia is great, even prior to the development of systemic manifestations, or when the intravascular route provides adequate delivery to the primary source.

The choice of systemic antibiotic regimens for infections in burned patients from the myriad of available drugs depends on the suspected organism, its likely patterns of sensitivity and resistance, and the location of the primary source. Ideal therapy would involve maximal delivery of the drug to the site of infection, effective bacteriocidal action against the causative organisms, and minimal patient toxicity.[43] Resistance to antibiotics is frequently the result of plasmid acquisitions, which may be transferred among organisms of the same or different species, or through the induction of degrading enzymes.[47] These may be particular problems among strains of *Pseudomonas*, *Klebsiella*, and *Enterobacter*. At present, no means exist to combat acquired resistance, and a knowledge of previous resistance patterns within the burn unit is necessary to select those drugs most likely to be effective.

Numerous studies have demonstrated altered pharmacokinetics of antibiotics in burned patients resulting in lowered serum drug levels when the usual recommended dosage is employed.[39, 123, 124] In many cases such dosages are subtherapeutic in the burned patient, especially among antibiotics that are predominately renally excreted. Thus, the initial loading and maintenance dosages should probably be increased by approximately 50% in patients with large burns, and serum levels should be monitored frequently and early in the course of therapy.[43] Incorrect peak levels should prompt alteration in the dosage, while inadequate trough levels should prompt shortening of the dosage interval.[103] The presence of renal insufficiency should not be considered a contraindication to the use of any drug in the case of life-threatening sepsis in the burned patient, but the toxic effects should be avoided or minimized by the use of serum level monitoring.

Because the results of cultures taken at the onset of clinical signs of infection may not be available for 48 to 72 hr, initial presumptive antimicrobial therapy must be based on the organisms most likely to cause the primary infection or, ideally, on the results of appropriate Gram's stains. The presumptive choice is then altered when culture and sensitivity results are available to a more appropriate or less toxic regimen. Therapy is generally continued for 10 to 14 days for most infections. However, deterioration of clinical condition during the course of antibiotic therapy, especially following an initial response, may require that the antibiotic regimen be discontinued and the patient recultured.

Table 9-7 lists the most likely organisms to be encountered based on the site or type of infection, as well as the most likely primary sources when a bacteremia of unclear etiology is identified. Based on this information, and more importantly on the results of appropriate Gram's stains, an initial antibiotic choice can be made. Single agents should be employed whenever possible, because the indiscriminate use of multiple agents promotes overgrowth of opportunistic and resistant species.

Gram-positive organisms most frequently encountered include streptococci and staphylococci. The former have remained extremely sensitive to penicillin, while *Staphylococcus* species have become increasingly resistant. A penicillinase-resistant drug, such as naficillin, is an appropriate choice to cover both groups, especially for infections such as cellulitis. Resistance to penicillinase-resistant drugs by staphylococci may be a problem in hospital-acquired infections, however, and more serious gram-positive infections in the burned patient probably warrant the use of vancomycin. Enterococci, or group D streptococci, have developed widespread resistance

Table 9–7
Sources of Sepsis in Burned Patients

GRAM-POSITIVE ORGANISMS	GRAM-NEGATIVE ORGANISMS	FUNGAL ORGANISMS
Burn wound	Burn wound	Burn wound
Airborne pneumonia	Airborne pneumonia	Airborne pneumonia
	Hematogenous pneumonia	
	Tracheobronchitis	?Tracheobronchitis
Line sepsis		Line sepsis
Suppurative thrombophlebitis		
Endocarditis		
Lower genitourinary tract*	Intra-abdominal sources	?Intra-abdominal sources
	Lower genitourinary tract	Lower genitourinary tract
	Hematogenous pyelonephritis	

* *Enterococci.*

to penicillin and, although the role of enterococci in infections remains controversial, should be treated with ampicillin, pipercillin, or vancomycin, alone or in combination with aminoglycosides.

Gram-negative infections remain the most troublesome in the burned patient. In addition to *Pseudomonas* species, *Enterobacter cloacae, Providencia stuartii, Serratia marcesans,* and *Klebsiella pneumoniae* are important causes of gram-negative infections. Aminoglycosides, including gentamicin, tobramycin, and amikacin, have been the mainstay of therapy in burned patients. Thienamycin compounds, offering the broadest spectrum of antimicrobial activity in a single drug, also have great potential for use in gram-negative infections in this population.[50] Because of the demonstrated potential for overgrowth of resistant and opportunistic organisms, third-generation cephalosporins should be avoided for at least initial therapy. Anaerobic infections, rarely a problem in the burned patient except in intra-abdominal infections,[92] respond well to appropriate drainage and parenteral clindamycin or metronidazole.

The presence of signs and symptoms of generalized sepsis without a clear etiology presents a challenging clinical problem with poor prognosis unless a primary source can be identified and treated. Following complete investigation as described above, if no clear source is determined, empiric broad-spectrum parenteral antibiotics providing both gram-positive and negative coverage should be administered. Even after antibiotics are begun, however, the search for the primary infection must continue, because the treatment of the bacteremia alone is too often inadequate therapy. Failure to improve after the addition of antibiotics, especially without an identified source or causative organism, should raise the question of a fungal infection.

Prolonged use of broad-spectrum systemic antibiotics as described above can result in fungal superinfection in these compromised hosts.[83] This complication may be heralded by a change in clinical condition midway through the course of antibiotic therapy. *Phycomycetes* and *Aspergillus* have been demonstrated to cause invasive burn wound sepsis,[16] but burn wound infections are rarely the cause of systemic candidiasis.[84] Candidemia is more likely the result of infections of the lung, urinary tract, or intravenous catheters.[110] The isolation of fungi from the blood requires aggressive therapy with systemic amphotericin B.[37] As with bacterial infections, attention should also be directed toward local control and eradication of the primary source as well. Systemic viral infections are rarely demonstrated as causes of morbidity except at autopsy. If discovered, however, appropriate systemic therapy, such as with parenteral acyclovir, should be administered.

REFERENCES

1. Alexander JW. Control of infection following burn injury. Arch Surg 1971;103:435.
2. Alexander JW, Moncrief JA. Immunologic phenomenon in burn injuries. JAMA 1967;199:257.
3. Alexander JW, Ogle CK, Stinnett JD, et al. A sequential, prospective analysis of immunologic abnormalities and infection following severe thermal injury. Ann Surg 1978;188:809.
4. Alexander JW, Stinnet JD, Ogle CK, et al. A comparison of immunologic profiles and their influences on bacteremia in surgical patients with a high risk of infection. Surgery 1979;86:94.
5. Alexander JW, Wixson D. Neutrophil dysfunction and sepsis in burn injury. SG&O 1971;130:435.
6. Antonacci AC, Chiao J, Calvano SE, et al. Development of monoclonal antibodies against virulent gram-negative bacteria: efficacy in a septic mouse model. Surg Forum 1984;35:116.
7. Antonacci AC, Good RA, Gupta S. T-cell subpopulationa following thermal injury. SG&O 1982;155:1.
8. Antonacci AC, Reaves LE, Calvano SE, et al. Flow cytometric analysis of lymphocytes subpopulations after thermal injury in human beings. SG&O 1984;159:1.
9. Artuson G, Johansson SGO, Hagman CF, et al. Changes in immunoglobulin levels in severely burned patients. Lancet 1969(1):546.
10. Asch MJ, White MG, Pruitt BA. Acid−base changes associated with topical Sulfamylon therapy: retrospective study of 100 burn patients. Ann Surg 1970;172:946.
11. Baskin TW, Rosenthal A, Pruitt BA. Acute bacterial endocarditis: a silent source of sepsis in the burn patient. Ann Surg 1976;185:618.
12. Baxter CR, Curreri PW, Marvin JA. The control of burn wound sepsis by the use of quantitative bacteriologic studies and subeschar chlysis with antibiotics, Surg Clin North Am 1973;53:1509.
13. Bjornson AB, Altemeier WA, Bjorson HS. Changes in humoral components of host defense following burn trauma. Ann Surg 1977;186:88.
14. Bjorson AB, Bjorson HS, Altemeier WA. Serum mediated inhibition of polymorphonuclear leukocyte function following burn injury. Ann Surg 1981;194:568.
15. Bjorson AB, Bjorson HS, Lincoln NA, et al. Relative roles of burn injury, wound colonization, and wound infection in induction of alterations of complement function in a guinea pig model of burn injury. J Trauma 1984;24:106.
16. Bruck HM, Nash G, Foley FD, et al. Opportunistic fungal infections of the burn with *Phycomycetes* and *Aspergillus:* a clinical−pathologic review. Arch Surg 1971;102:476.
17. Bruck HM, Nash G, Stein JM. Studies in the occurrence and significance of yeast and fungi in the burn wound. Ann Surg 1972;176:108.
18. Caffee HH, Bingham HG. Leukopenia and silver sulfadiazene. J Trauma 1982;22:586.
19. Cooperband SR, Nimberg R, Schmid K. Humoral immunosuppressive factors. Transplant Proc 1972;8:225.
20. Curreri PW. Burns. In: Simmons RL, Howard RJ, eds. Surgical infectious disease. New York: Appleton-Century-Crofts, 1982:1125.
21. Curreri PW, Heck EL, Browne L, et al. Stimulated nitroblue tetrazolium test to assess neutrophil antibacterial function: prediction of wound sepsis in burned patients. Surgery 1973;74:6.
22. Davis DM. Gas gangrene as a complication of burns. Scand J Reconstr Surg 1979;13:73.
23. Davis JM, Dineen P, Gallin JI. Neutrophil degranulation and abnormal chemotaxis after thermal injury. J Immunol 1980;124:1467.

24. Daynes RA. What is the relationship between the status of a patient's host defense mechanisms, his metabolic response, and his ability to respond to injury? J Trauma 1984;24(S):84.

25. Deitch EA, Winterton J, Berg R. Thermal injury promotes bacterial translocation from the gastrointestinal tract in mice with impaired T-cell mediated immunity. Arch Surg 1986;21:97.

26. Demling RH. Burns. N Engl J Med 1985;313:1389.

27. Dionigi RD, Zonta A, Dominioni L, et al. The effects of total parenteral nutrition on immunodepression due to malnutrition. Ann Surg 1977;185:467.

28. Donati L, Lazzarin A, Signorini M, et al. Preliminary clinical experiences with the use of immunomodulators in burns. J Trauma 1983;23:816.

29. Dowling JA, Foley FD, Moncrief JA. Chondritis in the burns ear. Plast Reconstr Surg 1968;42:115.

30. Echinard CE, Sajdel-Sulkowska E, Burke PA, et al. The beneficial effect of early excision on clinical response and thymic activity after burn injury. J Trauma 1982;22:560.

31. Ekindjian OG, Marien M, Wasserman D, et al. Plasma fibronectin time course in burned patients: influence of sepsis. J Trauma 1984;24:214.

32. Faillace DF, Ledgerwood AM, Lucas CE, et al. Immunoglobulin changes after varied resuscitative regimens. J Trauma 1982;22:1.

33. Fikrig SM, Karl SC, Suntharalingram K. Neutrophil chemotaxis in patients with burns. Ann Surg 1977;186:746.

34. Finkelstein AL. What are the immunological alterations induced by burn injury? J Trauma 1984;24(S):72.

35. Foley FD, Greenawald KA, Nash G, et al. Herpes virus infection in burned patients. N Engl J Med 1980;282:652. 1980 1969.

36. Fox CL, Rappale BW, Stanford W. Control of *Pseudomonas* infection in burns by silver sulfadiazine. SG&O 1969;128;1021.

37. Gauto A, Law EJ, Holder IA. Experience with amphotericin B in the treatment of systemic candidiasis in burn patients. Am J Surg 1977;133:174.

38. Gelfand JA, Donelan M, Burke JF. Preferential activation and depletion of the alternate complement pathway by burn injury. Ann Surg 1983;198:58.

39. Glew RH, Moellering RC, Burke JF. Gentamicin dosage in children with extensive burns. J Trauma 1976;16:819.

40. Goodwin CW. Current burn treatment. In: Shires GT, ed. Advances in surgery. Vol 18. Chicago: Year Book Medical Publishers, 1984:15.

41. Goodwin CW, McManus WF, Mason AD, et al. Management of abdominal wounds in thermally injured patients. J Trauma 1982;22:92.

42. Goodwin CW, Pruitt BA. Burns. In: Kagan BM, ed. Antimicrobial therapy. 3rd ed. Philadelphia: WB Saunders, 1980:397.

43. Haburchak DR, Pruitt BA. Use of systemic antibiotics in the burned patient. Surg Clin North Am 1978;58:1119.

44. Hansbrough JF, Peterson V, Kortz E, et al. Postburn immunosuppression in an animal model. Monocyte dysfunction induced by burned tissue. Surgery 1983;93:415.

45. Hiebert JM, McGough M, Rodeheaver G. The influence of catabolism on immunocompetance in burned patients. Surgery 1979;86:242.

46. Howard RJ. Effect of burn injury, mechanical trauma, and operation on immune defenses. Surg Clin North Am 1979;59:199.

47. Hummel RP, Miskell PW, Altemeier WA. Antibiotic resistance transfer from nonpathogenic to pathogenic bacteria. Surgery 1977;82:382.

48. Jones RL, Lowburg EJL. Staphlycoocellabtibodies in burned patients. Br J Exp Pathol 1963;44:576.

49. Jones WG, Barrie PS, Yurt RW, et al. Enterococcal burn sepsis: a highly lethal complication of severe thermal injury. Arch Surg 1986;121:649.

50. Kropp R. Thienamycins. Rev Infect Dis 1985;7(3):389.

51. Lanser ME, Saba TM. Correction of serum opsonic defects after burn and sepsis by opsonic fibronectin administration. Arch Surg 1983;118:338.

52. Lanser ME, Saba TM. Opsonic fibronectin deficiency and sepsis. Ann Surg 1982;195:340.

53. Lanser ME, Saba TM, Scovill WA. Opsonic glycoprotein (plasma fibronectin) levels after burn injury. Ann Surg 1980;192:776.

54. Lescher TJ, Teegarden OK, Pruitt BA. Acute pseudo-obstruction of the colon in thermally injured patients. Dis Colon Rectum 1978;21:618.

55. Lewis RA. How are prostaglandins and leukotrienes involved in immunological alterations? J Trauma 1984;24(S):125.

56. Loebl EC, Marvin JA, Heck EL, et al. The method of quantitative burn wound biopsy culture and its routine use in the care of the burned patient. Am J Clin Pathol 1984;61:20.

57. Loose LD, Turinsky J. Macrophage dysfunction after burn injury. Infect Immun 1979;26:157.

58. Lundy J, Ford CM. Surgery, trauma and immune suppression: evolving the mechanism. Ann Surg 1983;197:434.

59. MacMillan BG. Indications for early excision. Surg Clin North Am 1970;50:1337.

60. Maki DG, Weise CE, Sarafin HW. A semiquantitative culture method for identifying intravenous catheter related infection. N Engl J Med 1977;296:1305.

61. Markley K, Smallman ET. Effect of burn trauma in mice on the generation of cytotoxic lymphocytes. Proc Soc Exp Biol Med 1979;160:468.

62. Marvin JA, Heck EL, Loebl EC, et al. Usefulness of blood cultures in confirming sepsis complications in burned patients: evaluation of a new culture method. J Trauma 1975;15:657.

63. McIrvine AJ, O'Mahoney JB, Saporoschetz I, et al. Depressed immune response in burn patients: use of monoclonal antibodies and functional essays to define the role of suppressor cells. Ann Surg 1982;196:297.

64. McLoughlin GA, Wu AV, Saporoschetz I, et al. Correlation between anergy and a circulating immunosuppressive factor following major surgical trauma. Ann Surg 1979;190:297.

65. McManus AT, Mason AD. Bacterial mobility: a component in experimental *Pseudomonas aeruginosa* burn wound sepsis. In: Annual Research Progress Report. Fort Sam Houston:US Army Institute of Surgical Research, Brooke Army Medical Center, 1978:57

66. McManus WF. Is there a role for plasmaphoresis (exchange transfusions) in the treatment of the septic burned patient? J Trauma 1984;24(S):137.

67. McManus WF, Goodwin CW, Pruitt BA. Subeschar treatment of burn wound infection. Arch Surg 1983;118:291.

68. McManus WF, Goodwin CW, Pruitt BA. Burn wound infection. J Trauma 1981;21:753.

69. Menon T, Sundararaj T, Subramanian S, et al. Kinetics of peripheral blood T cell numbers and functions in patients with burns. J Trauma 1984;24:220.

70. Miller CL, Baker CC. Changes in lymphocyte activity after thermal injury: the role of suppressor cells. J Clin Invest 1979;63:202.

71. Moncrief JA. Topical therapy for control of bacteria in the burn wound. World J Surg 1978;2:151.

72. Moncrief JA, Lindberg RB, Switzer WE. The use of topical sulfonamide in the control of burn wound sepsis. J Trauma 1966;6:407.

73. Moncreif JA, Teplitz C. Changing concepts in burn sepsis. J Trauma 1964;4:233.

74. Moyer CA, Brentano L, Gravens DL. Treatment of large human burns with 0.5 percent silver nitrate solution. Arch Surg 1965;90:812.

75. Munster AM. Immunologic responses of trauma and burns: an overview. Am J Med 1984;76:142.

76. Munster AM. Post-traumatic immunosuppression is due to activation of suppressor T-cells. Lancet 1976(1):1329.

77. Munster AM, Eurenious K, Katz RM, et al. Cell-mediated immunity after thermal injury, Ann Surg 1973;177:139.

78. Munster AM, Goodwin MN, Pruitt BA. Acalculous cholecystitis in burn patients. Am J Surg 1971;122:591.

79. Munster AM, Hoagland HC, Pruitt BA. The effect of thermal injury on serum immunoglobulins. Ann Surg 1970;172:965.

80. Munster AM, Winchurch RA, Birmingham WJ, et al. Longitudinal assay of lymphocyte responsiveness in patients with major burns. Ann Surg 1980;192:772.

81. Nash G, Asch MJ, Foley FD, et al. Disseminated cytomegalic inclusion disease in a burned adult. JAMA 1970;214:587.

82. Nash G, Foley FD. Herpetic infection of the middle and lower respiratory tract. Am J Clin Pathol 1970;54:857.

83. Nash G, Foley FD, Goodwin MN, et al. Fungal burn wound infection. JAMA 1977;215:1664.

84. Nash G, Foley FD, Pruitt BA. *Candida* burn wound invasion: a cause of systematic candidiasis. Arch Pathol 1970;90:75.

85. Neilan BA, Toddeini L, Strate RG. T-lymphocyte rosette formation after major burns. JAMA 1977;238:493.

86. Ninnemann JL, Condie JD, Davis SE, et al. Isolation of immunosuppressive serum components following thermal injury. J Trauma 1982;22:837.

87. Ninnemann JL, Fisher JC, Frank HA. Prolonged survival of human skin allografts following thermal injury. Transplantation 1978;25:69.

88. Ninnemann JL, Stockland AE, Condie JT. Induction of prostaglandin synthesis-dependent suppressor cells with endotoxin: occurrence in patients with thermal injuries. J Clin Immun 1983;3:142.

89. O'Neill JA, Pruitt BA, Foley FD, et al. Suppurative thrombophlebitis—a lethal complication of intravenous therapy. J Trauma 1968;8:256.

90. Panke TW, McLeod CG. Pathology of thermal injury: a practical approach. Orlando, FL: Grune & Stratton, 1985.

91. Pruitt BA. Host–opportunist interactions in surgical infection. Presidential address. Arch Surg 1986;121:13.

92. Pruitt BA. The burn patient. II. Later care and complications of thermal injury. Curr Probl Surg 1979;16:4.

93. Pruitt BA, Curreri PW. The burn wound and its care. Arch Surg 1971;103:461.

94. Pruitt BA, DiVincenty FC, Mason AD, et al. The occurrence and significance of pneumonia and other pulmonary complications in burned patients: comparison of conventional and topical treatments. J Trauma 1970;10:519.

95. Pruitt BA, Flemma RJ, DiVincenty FC. Pulmonary complications in burn patients: a comparative study of 697 patients. J Thorac Cardiovasc Surg 1970;59:7.

96. Pruitt BA, Foley FD. The use of biopsies in burn patient care. Surgery 1973;73:887.

97. Pruitt BA, McManus AP. Opportunistic infections in severely burned patients. AM J Med 1984;76:146.

98. Pruitt BA, McManus WF, Kim SH, et al. Diagnosis and treatment of cannula-related intravenous sepsis in burn patients. Ann Surg 1980;191:546.

99. Pruitt BA, O'Neill JA, Moncrief JA. Successful control of burn wounds sepsis. JAMA 1968;203:1054.

100. Pruitt BA, Stein JM, Foley ED, et al. Intravenous therapy in burn patients. Suppurative thrombophlebitis and other life threatening complications. Arch Surg 1970;100:399.

101. Rabin ER, Graber CD, Vogel EH, et al. Fatal *Pseudomonas* infection in burned patients: a clinical bacteriologic and anatomic study. N Engl J Med 1961;265:1225.

102. Ritzman SE, McClung C, Falls D, et al. Immunoglobulin levels in burned patients. Lancet 1969(1):1152.

103. Sabath LD, Casey JI, Ruch PA. Rapid microassay of entamicin, kanamycin, neomycin, streptomycin, and vancomycin in serum or plasma. J Lab Clin Med 1970;78:457.

104. Schildt BE. Function of the RES after thermal and mechanical trauma in mice. Acta Chir Scand 1970;136:359.

105. Seldinger SI. Catheter replacement of a needle in percutaneous arteriography. New technique. Acta Radiol 1953;39:368.

106. Shirani KZ, McManus AT, Vaughn GM, et al. Effects of environment on infection in burn patients. Arch Surg 1986;121:31.

107. Shires GT, Dineen P. Sepsis following burns, trauma and intra-abdominal infections. Arch Intern Med 1982;142:2012.

108. Solomkin JS, Nelson RD, Chenoweth DE, et al. Regulation of neutrophil migratory function in burn injury by complement activation products. Am Surg 1984;200:742.

109. Stinnett JD, Loose LD, Miskell P, et al. Synthetic immunomodulators for prevention of total infections in a burned guinea pig model. Ann Surg 1983;198:53.

110. Stone HH, Colb LD, Currie CA, et al. *Candida* sepsis: pathogenesis and principles of treatment. Ann Surg 1974;179:697.

111. Teplitz C, Davis D, Mason AD. *Pseudomonas* burn wound sepsis. I. Pathogenesis of experimental *Pseudomonas* burn wound sepsis. J Surg Res 1964;4:210.

112. Teplitz C, Davis D, Walker HL. *Pseudomonas* burn wound sepsis. II. Hematogenous infection at the junction of the burn wound and unburned hypodermis. J Surg Res 1976;4:217.

113. Teplitz C, Davis D, Walker HL. *Pseudomonas* burn wound sepsis. J Surg Res 1964;4:200.

114. Warden GD, Mason AD, Pruitt BA. Suppression of leukocyte chemotaxis *in vitro* by chemotherapeutic agents used in the management of thermal injuries. Ann Surg 1975;181:363.

115. Warden GD, Mason AD, Pruitt BA. Evaluation of leukocyte chemotaxis *in vitro* in thermally injured patients. J Clin Invest 1974;54:1001.

116. Waymack JP, Miskell P, Gonce SJ, et al. Immunomodulators in the treatment of peritonitis in burned and malnourished animals. Surgery 1984;96:308.

117. Waymack JP, Rapien J, Garnett D, et al. Effect of transfusion on immune function in a traumatized animal model. Arch Surg 1986;121:50.

118. Wolfe JHN, Saporoschetz I, Yound AE, et al. Suppressive serum, suppressor lymphocytes, and deaths from burns. Abb Surg 1981;193L:513.

119. Wolfe JHN, Wu A, O'Connor NE, et al. Allergy, immunosuppressive serum and impaired lymphocyte blastogenesis in burned patients. Arch Surg 1982;117:1266.
120. Wood J, Rodrick ML, O'Mahony JB, et al. Inadequate interleukin 2 production. Ann Surg 1984;200:311.
121. Woolfrey BF, Fox JM, Quall CO. An evaluation of burn wound quantitative microbiology. I. Quantitative cultures. Am J Clin Pathol 1981;75:532.
122. Yurt RW, McManus AT, Mason AD, et al. Increased susceptibility to infection related to extent of burn injury. Arch Surg 1984;119:183.
123. Zaske DE, Sawchuk RJ, Gerding DN, et al. Increased dosage requirements of gentamicin in burn patients. J Trauma 1976;16:824.
124. Zaske DE, Sawchuk RJ, Strate RG. The necessity of increased doses of amikacin in burned patients. Surgery 1978;84:603.

10

○   ○   ○   ●   ●   ●

NUTRITIONAL RESPONSE IN SEPSIS

Kevin J. Tracey
Stephen F. Lowry

Serious infection in humans frequently elicits profound derangements of metabolic and nutritional homeostasis, which, if unresolved, may progress to wasting of vital protein stores, organ failure, and death. Therapeutic intervention must be directed toward both eradication of the underlying infectious process and abrogation of the catabolic nutrient losses. Failure to reverse the consequences of malnutrition will worsen the complications of infection. Current nutritional therapy is based on a rational assessment of energy requirements and the safe provision of enteral or parenteral feeding regimens. The formulation of this treatment approach is facilitated by an understanding of the characteristic nutritional responses in sepsis.

In this chapter we will review the principles of energy utilization during unstressed starvation as it contrasts to the metabolic sequelae of starvation occurring in the presence of sepsis. The humoral mediators of these responses will be discussed to provide a basis for a rational formulation of nutritional therapy. A method of nutritional assessment for the septic patient and the selection of an appropriate nutritional support technique will be discussed. Finally, the application of enteral and parenteral feeding to the septic patient will be outlined as a practical guide to clinical practice.

NUTRITIONAL RESPONSES IN UNSTRESSED STARVATION

Normal nutritional homeostasis provides a continuous source of metabolic fuel (substrate) to vital organs and tissues for maintenance of cellular regeneration and function. Latent molecular energy is stored in the hydrogen–carbon bond and can be transduced (usually through ATP) into a form usable for protein synthesis, muscular contraction, or maintenance of cellular membrane function. There are three principal storage depots of body fuel: (1) Fat is stored in adipocytes, has a high caloric density (9 kcal/g), and comprises the largest reservoir of available substrate that can be mobilized efficiently over a period of 4 to 6 weeks; (2) Glycogen stores (1 to 1.5 kcal/g) are primarily located in hepatic and muscle tissues in quantities sufficient to maintain normal blood glucose levels for only about 12 hr; (3) Protein is oxidized at a relatively low caloric value (4 kcal/g) but fulfills enzymatic and structural roles necessary for cellular activity. The maintenance of nutritional homeostasis during normal activity depends on an integrated metabolic system that regulates the continuous provision of substrate for tissue utilization.

The survival of a species during nutritional shortage in nature depends on the preservation of host mobility and function. Evolutionary pressures have therefore selected a nutritional response to unstressed starvation that reduces resting energy expenditure (REE), minimizes protein turnover, and conserves amino acids. After an early depletion of carbohydrate reserves there is a shift toward fat oxidation, and free fatty acids are subsequently used as the primary whole-body substrate. The initial response to exogenous nutritional shortage includes decreased insulin levels, increased glucagon levels, and activation of catecholamine-dependent lipases with a resultant mobilization of triglycerides from adipose stores to meet energy requirements.[23–25] The breakdown of functional, lean tissue protein is reduced to that rate necessary to maintain the conversion of amino acids into glucose for utilization by glucose-dependent tissue (red blood cells, renal medulla, nervous tissue). Circulating lipids are oxidized to produce acetyl-CoA, which is converted to ketone bodies in the liver. As circulating levels of ketone bodies increase, critical organs increasingly use ketones as the primary energy source, thereby limiting irreversible losses of amino acids from the system. Nitrogen excretion is reduced to a minimal level (50 mg/kg-day), and thus significant depletion of lean body mass and protein during unstressed starvation does not occur until after approximately 2 weeks.

The mechanisms that regulate whole-body protein kinetics during unstressed starvation have been characterized by a variety of methods including isotopic tracer techniques and measurements of 3-methylhistidine (3MH) excretion. Because 3MH is a nonreusable amino acid produced during the degradation of myofibrillar protein, urinary excretion of 3MH depends on the rate of whole-body protein breakdown from all 3MH-containing tissues (muscle, splanchnic bed, dermis).[7,110] During unstressed starvation in normal humans, whole-body protein breakdown, as determined by urinary 3MH excretion or [^{15}N]glycine turnover, is increased slightly, reflecting the mobilization of substrate necessary for cellular oxidation and synthetic requirements.[69,97] However, skeletal muscle protein breakdown is relatively spared, because during starvation muscle protein is conserved and extremity 3MH efflux and total amino acid efflux are reduced.[2,97] Whole-body protein synthesis as determined by [^{15}N]glycine is decreased during protein-calorie fasting.[97] Energy expenditure correlates closely to whole-body protein turnover and is reduced during unstressed starvation.[24,97] Thus, the normal sequence of metabolic events during unstressed starvation results in the preservation of vital tissue protein.

SEPSIS-MEDIATED ALTERATIONS OF THE STARVATION RESPONSE

The metabolic response to sepsis depends on many factors including the severity of the infectious process, the antecedent nutritional status of the host, and the coexistence of any underlying disease.[10] During gram-negative bacteremia and resuscitation there may be a generalized lowering of metabolic rate, a condition that has been termed the "ebb phase" response.[73] Following this early response, the "flow phase" is typically characterized by an increase in REE, acceleration of whole-body protein breakdown, and peripheral tissue glucose intolerance.[73] The flow phase alterations in metabolic energy utilization may persist for days to weeks, and during this "catabolic" period, whole-body substrate requirements often outstrip the supply of exogenous nutrients. Although the provision of hypocaloric dextrose intravenously in normal subjects will reduce nitrogen wasting,[23] during sepsis the nitrogen losses from lean body tissue are not significantly abrogated by hypocaloric dextrose.[76,102]

In general, the adaptive (protein-sparing) responses induced by unstressed starvation do not occur during the flow phase response to sepsis. Cuthberson first characterized this catabolic process in the 1930s following his studies of patients with multiple trauma.[34] He observed a paradoxical increase of nitrogen excretion during the semistarvation period of hospitalized recovery. This persistent degradation of protein stores and increased rate of amino acid oxidation are characteristically associated with increased REE, negative nitrogen balance, weight loss, and retention of body sodium and water.[10,31,34,37,58] Loss of lean body tissue becomes clinically evident within 7 to 10 days, and this type of protein-calorie malnutrition adversely impacts both survival and recovery of function.[66]

The increased REE occurring during the flow phase is the result of the accelerated rates of oxygen consumption and carbon dioxide production necessary for cellular membrane function. While protein-calorie starvation may occur during the flow phase, tachycardia, fever, elevated cardiac output, and release of endogenous mediators all contribute to accelerated protein turnover and increased REE.[11,38,49,88] In addition to these increased energy demands, during the diagnostic and operative evaluation of the patient with surgical sepsis there frequently has been some period (from 3 to 14 days) of protein-calorie depletion prior to the onset of flow phase catabolism. Thus, accelerated protein and substrate turnover may be superimposed on depleted protein-calorie reserves. The magnitude of increased REE is multifactorial, but the response to sepsis may enhance caloric requirements to greater than 60% above basal levels (Fig. 10-1).

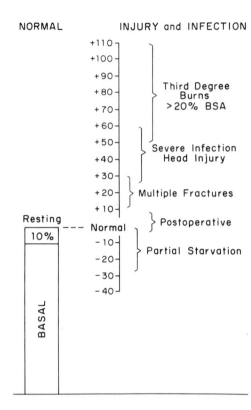

NORMAL INJURY and INFECTION

Figure 10–1.
Resting energy expenditure (REE) is decreased during partial starvation but increased during the flow phase responses to trauma, burn injury, or sepsis. The percentage of increased REE above basal conditions is used to estimate total caloric requirements during the relatively hypermetabolic responses. (Kinney JM. The application of indirect calorimetry to clinical studies. In: Kinney JM, ed. Assessment of energy metabolism in health and disease. Columbus, OH: Ross Laboratories, 1980)

SUBSTRATE UTILIZATION DURING SEPSIS

During the study of hypermetabolism associated with sepsis, investigators have used respiratory gas analysis by indirect calorimetry to estimate the relative contribution of endogenous substrate oxidation to net energy expenditure. The principles of indirect calorimetry are based in part on the relationship of oxygen consumed (VO_2) and carbon dioxide produced (VCO_2) during the complete oxidation of a given substrate. For example, the oxidation of 1 mole of glucose consumes 6 moles of oxygen and produces 6 moles of carbon dioxide. Thus, the ratio of whole-body carbon dioxide output to oxygen consumption (respiratory quotient, RQ) measured during the utilization of carbohydrate is 1.0. This technique can also be used to estimate the relative contribution of nonprotein substrate (carbohydrate or lipid) to whole-body energy utilization. The RQ of normal subjects after an overnight fast (postabsorptive) is approximately 0.85, indicative of mixed fuel oxidation, but during the flow phase response in sepsis the decreased RQ (0.71) suggests an increased rate of lipid utilization.[4,38,50,95,104]

The extent of lipid utilization during sepsis depends on the severity, duration, and nature of the infection. Whereas serum free fatty acid levels or triglycerides may be increased or decreased, hypertriglyceridemia has been considered a hallmark of gram-negative bacteremia and sepsis.[20] Suppression of systemic lipoprotein lipase activity during the flow phase response results in a decreased clearance of triglycerides from the plasma compartment.[53] Catecholamine-dependent lipases in adipose tissue are activated, and lipolytic enzyme activity is increased, resulting in enhanced hydrolysis of triglycerides to fatty acids and glycerol.[91] Isotopic tracer studies demonstrate increased whole-body turnover of both glycerol and free fatty acids, again suggesting accelerated mobilization of peripheral fat stores.[26,75] While the rate of whole-body lipid oxidation may be increased, the metabolic efficiency of lipid utilization during sepsis may actually be decreased as evidenced by a diminished rate of production of ketone bodies.[12,45] Analysis of ^{14}C-palmitate turnover in patients receiving total parenteral nutrition (TPN) with exogenous lipid, fails to demonstrate any significant oxidation of the infused lipid emulsions during sepsis.[76] One consequence of the failure to use lipid energy efficiently is an ongoing requirement for glucose as an energy source, resulting in a depletion of amino acid carbon skeletons that are persistently catabolized from muscle and utilized for glucogenesis.[12,80]

Insulin is the primary storage hormone of the body. It is released from pancreatic beta cells in response to hyperglycemia as well as other endocrine stimulae and mediates cellular glucose uptake, lipogenesis, and protein synthesis.[24,101] However, significant alterations of insulin metabolism occur during the flow phase response in sepsis. Peripheral tissue responses to insulin are blunted, leading to increased levels of both insulin and glucose.[32,77] The glucose tolerance curve during this period resembles that of a diabetic patient and has been termed "stress diabetes."[30,47,48,64] The molar ratio of insulin to glucagon is frequently decreased[101] and, when coupled with the increased whole-body energy requirements, stimulates a rapid depletion of hepatic and muscle glycogen stores. This further necessitates the shift toward splanchnic glucose production in a cycle that requires the constant delivery of amino acids from the peripheral tissues to maintain blood glucose levels.[106]

The alterations of carbohydrate metabolism during sepsis have been characterized by tissue-specific and whole-body methodologies. In general, hepatic glucose "overproduction" and hepatic resistance to insulin suppression of gluconeogenesis have been observed.[106,109] Skeletal muscle insulin resistance participates in a diminished rate of cellular glucose uptake and oxidation through as yet uncharacterized postreceptor mechanisms.[48] Glucogenic amino acids and lactate are released from the skeletal muscle tissues for incorporation into glucose in the splanchnic tissues.[42,63] As splanchnic gluconeogenesis increases, the nitrogen released during the deamination of the glucogenic amino acids is largely incorporated into urea and excreted. By this route, nitrogen is irreversibly lost from the catabolic patient.

Flow phase protein metabolism is characterized by a net wasting of skeletal muscle protein and whole-body nitrogen. Whereas whole-body protein synthesis may be increased during sepsis, whole-body protein breakdown occurs at a greater rate, and causes accelerated net losses of body protein.[18,62,106] This erosion of lean body mass is manifested by increased urinary nitrogen losses which can exceed 350 to 400 mg N/kg-day. Extremity amino acid and 3MH efflux is increased significantly, suggest-

260

ing that a progressive stimulus to muscle protein breakdown occurs even in tissues distant from the site of infection.[5,29,79] Studies using ^{14}C-alanine turnover during sepsis demonstrate increased rates of conversion of alanine to glucose and support the hypothesis that peripheral amino acid carbon-skeletons are used for splanchnic and/or renal gluconeogenesis and protein synthesis.[42,63]

Circulating levels of several trace elements, minerals, and acute phase proteins also change significantly during the flow phase response. Decreased levels of zinc appear to be related to increased biosynthesis of metallothionine, an acute phase protein that binds circulating zinc.[89] Serum copper levels rise and ceruloplasmin synthesis is increased. Iron is sequestered out of the plasma compartment in part through the release of neutrophil lactoferrin, which mediates the deposition of hemosiderin as an iron storage compound.[103] These alterations of micronutrient metabolism reflect both the mobilization of specific immune protective mechanisms and the shift of protein synthesis toward the production of nonstructural, acute phase proteins.

HUMORAL MEDIATORS OF THE CATABOLIC STRESS RESPONSE

The search for the mediators that initiate and propagate host catabolism has focused on the isolation and characterization of endogenous factors that trigger and propagate the pathophysiological responses. It is clear that if endogenous mediators direct the catabolism during persisting sepsis, a life-threatening erosion of protein and energy reserves will result. Recent advances in understanding the role of such mediators may lead to the development of therapeutic methods that attenuate the protein wasting without compromising the necessary, beneficial responses of the flow-phase, hormone milieu.

Neuroendocrine Mediators

A large body of literature has implicated neuroendocrine hormones as the primary, dominant metabolic signals during the flow phase (for review see References 65 and 105). Afferent pathways stimulated by pain, fear, and dehydration have been shown to stimulate the discharge of the sympathetic, adrenergic neuropeptides and hormones. Elevated levels of serum catecholamines, corticosteroids, thyroid hormones, adrenocorticotropic hormone, prolactin, antidiuretic hormone, and growth hormone have been invariably reported and are the subject of several comprehensive reviews.[65,73,105,107]

Many workers have attempted to reproduce the flow phase catabolic response through combined "catabolic" (glucose counterregulatory) hormone infusions to identify the role of such hormones in mediating the flow phase responses. Observations in our laboratory and elsewhere suggest that cortisol exerts a permissive effect on skeletal muscle protein breakdown whereas epinephrine stimulates the acute uptake of amino acids into peripheral tissues.[3,61] Epinephrine also appears to participate in many of the metabolic alterations during sepsis by increasing REE,[14,108] stimulating hyperglycemia by enhancement of both glycogenolysis and gluconeogenesis,[83] and inducing skeletal muscle insulin resistance.[13,108] However, treatment of severely catabolic burn patients with adrenergic antagonists fails to inhibit accelerated proteolysis[108] suggesting the importance of other hormones in the development of net protein catabolism. The combined infusion of epinephrine, glucagon, and cortisol[14] stimulated whole-body glucose turnover and nitrogen excretion, but these infusions stimulate only minimal increases of REE, whole-body protein turnover, and urinary excretion of 3MH. Thus, although the elevated levels of epinephrine, glucagon, and cortisol were similar to the levels observed during flow phase, they are not sufficient to initiate the characteristic protein metabolic responses to sepsis. While the release of the "classical" catabolic hormones is necessary for the modulation of carbohydrate and lipid metabolism during the flow phase, they are not sufficient to stimulate the whole spectrum of protein-metabolic alterations. It appears that other humoral factors are critical to the pathophysiologic responses during sepsis.

Immunopeptide Mediators

Several cytokines released by the immune system in response to bacterial endotoxin (lipopolysaccharide; LPS), including cachectin (tumor necrosis factor; TNF), interleukin-1 (IL-1), and the interferons, appear to occupy a central role in the regulation of host metabolic derangements. While it has long been appreciated that many of the products of LPS-stimulated macrophages can act directly on the hypothalamus to cause fever, recent investigation has focused on other metabolic and physiologic responses of normal tissue to the hormonal actions of cytokines.

The immunomodulatory and physiologic responses to IL-1 have been extensively reviewed.[35,56] A potent pyrogen, IL-1 mediates the synthesis of PGE_2 in the hypothalamus and contributes to the increased energy expenditure of flow phase. A direct effect of IL-1 on the transcription and translation of acute phase proteins in an isolated hepatocyte system has been reported.[78] This peptide also appears to participate in stimulating the release of pancreatic insulin and glucagon through a glucose-independent mechanism.[44] Using a nonrecombinant preparation of IL-1, enhanced protein breakdown was observed in skeletal muscle *in vitro.*[8] In addition, a factor in the plasma of some patients with sepsis, purported to be a cleavage product of IL-1, has been observed to stimulate skeletal muscle protein breakdown *in vitro.*[36] The proteolysis-inducing effects have not been confirmed using recombinant IL-1, and the role of IL-1 as a mediator of muscle protein breakdown remains uncertain.

Another important cytokine is cachectin, which was discovered during the search for a factor mediating cachexia of chronic parasite infection.[81] The wasting diathesis of cachectic rabbits infected with *Trypanasoma brucei* causes a preterminal depletion of up to 50% of lean body mass in association with a paradoxical increase of serum triglycerides. The elevated triglyceride levels were found to be secondary to the suppression of LPL activity in the infected animals, since LPL normally removes circulating lipids from the serum compartment.[54] The suppression of LPL was dependent on the release of a macrophage product (released in response to infection), which was isolated and named cachectin because of its presumed role in the development of cachexia.[55]

Recombinant cachectin and recombinant TNF were subsequently shown to be identical.[15] The presence of LPS or bacteria in the blood stimulates cachectin release from macrophages and the reticuloendothelial system.[16] Cachectin appears to occupy a pivotal, early role as a signal capable of initiating many of the pathophysiologic responses to endotoxemia or bacteremia. Passive immunization of mice with antibodies against cachectin significantly abrogates mortality during subsequent exposure to LPS.[17] Moreover, anticachectin antibodies prevent septic shock syndrome and death in primates given lethal doses of live gram-negative bacteria.[96] The acute metabolic response to lethal doses of cachectin is characterized by significant elevations of circulating catecholamines, glucagon, and cortisol.[100] Thus, it appears that the release of this single host factor is capable of initiating many of the acute pathophysiologic responses to endotoxin.

Further evidence implicates cachectin as an important mediator of cellular energy metabolism. Exposure of the lipid-laden 3T3-L1 adipocytes to cachectin (at doses in the range of 10^{-12} molar) results in a depletion of stored lipid with a reversion of cellular morphology to that of normal fibroblasts *in vitro.*[94] In addition to the suppression of LPL activity, lipid energy stores were mobilized by inhibition of the transcription of the lipogenic enzymes necessary to convert glucose into fat. Cachectin also appears to mediate catabolic responses in skeletal muscle related to energy metabolism and substrate utilization. Incubation of L-6 myotubules with cachectin stimulated marked acceleration of glucose uptake, glycogenolysis, lactate efflux, and enhanced expression of hexose transporters.[60] We have reported that cachectin mediated a dose-dependent reduction of resting transmembrane potential difference in skeletal muscle organ culture, which may also be related to cellular energy responses as well.[98] In addition, cachectin stimulates IL-1 release, which may amplify the pathophysiologic flow phase responses in a variety of normal host tissues.[99]

Theoretically, the combined hormonal activity of several endogenous mediators could account for many of the early flow phase responses observed after sepsis (Fig. 10-2). A direct effect on the hypothalamus by IL-1 and cachectin mediates fever and adrenergic discharge, which contribute to increased energy expenditure. The elevated levels of stress hormones might, in turn, modulate many of the peripheral tissue responses with stimulation of pancreatic insulin and glucagon secretion, and altered peripheral tissue sensitivity to substrate background and hormonal feedback control. Lipoprotein lipase is suppressed and circulating triglycerides levels increase secondary to enhancement of the catecholamine-dependent lipases and cachectin-mediated suppression of lipogenic enzymes synthesis. Acute phase proteins are transcribed and released, protein breakdown is stimulated, and energy stores are mobilized in response to the biologic activity of the circulating immunopeptide and neuroendocrine mediators. Although the investigation of these pathophysiologic mediators is in its

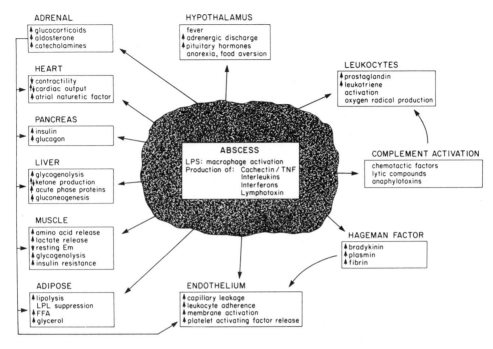

Figure 10-2.
Graphic representation of the complex relationship between circulating neuroendocrine hormones as mediators of the multiple responses during flow phase. The progression of these responses in a variety of tissues may lead to lipid and carbohydrate catabolism, protein wasting, and altered energy utilization. If not reversed, the progression of these responses frequently leads to multiple organ system failure, shock, and death.

infancy, the potential for developing a clinically useful inhibitor of the deleterious consequences of accelerated catabolism is being actively pursued.

COMPLICATIONS OF NUTRITIONAL DEPLETION

Malnutrition in hospitalized patients is frequent even among those patients not afflicted with the additional nutritional demands of sepsis. Morbidity and mortality increase with the degree of protein-calorie deficiency and may adversely affect both immunologic and critical organ function. Pneumonia represents the most common serious complication of hospitalized starvation and is associated with respiratory failure and progressive sepsis.[57] Dysfunction of the respiratory musculature and prolonged bedrest contribute to the marked reduction of vital capacity and minute ventilation that promote inspissation of mucous and bronchiolar obstruction. In the absence of trophic stimulation from an enteral diet, the gastrointestinal tract undergoes marked atrophy with loss of absorptive surface integrity. In addition to the symptomatic, paralytic ileus, which frequently accompanies sepsis, impaired motility or diarrhea may lead to bacterial overgrowth and the absorption of endotoxin into the portal circulation.[92]

Malnutrition associated with the loss of even 10% of protein mass may lead to suppression of immune function. The alterations of immune status occur by way of both impaired cell-mediated and diminished humoral antibody responses,[39] total lymphocyte count, increased ratio of suppressor T cells to helper T cells, impaired polymorphonuclear leukocyte chemotaxis and intracellular killing, and diminished synthesis of peptide modulators.[46] Depressed immune function increases the risk of both recurrent and opportunistic infections.

Malnutrition during sepsis tends to worsen cardiopulmonary function and reserve.[86] While a decrease in maximal oxygen capacity will occur after prolonged bedrest, the additional stress of protein-calorie depletion accelerates the loss of functional capacity.[1] The resultant decrease of cardiac reserve can be associated with measurable decreases of cardiac index, contractility, and amplitude of the QRS complex.[59] The presence of a circulating myocardial depressant factor during sepsis can worsen the intolerance to volume loading and cardiotonic agents that occur in malnutrition. While such changes can be readily identified, the extent to which nutritional support alone can reverse these processes remains controversial.[1,86]

Abnormal collagen synthesis may occur during malnutrition and serves to compromise dermal and mucous membrane integrity. Diminished mucous secretion and enhanced epithelial cell breakdown provide a portal of entry for secondary infection by way of the dermis and underlying tissue. Normal wound healing is depressed, fibroplasia is delayed, and the risk of wound disruption is increased unless nutritional depletion is corrected.[19]

NUTRITIONAL ASSESSMENT

The preliminary nutritional assessment of the septic patient should provide an estimation of (1) *the extent of antecedent protein-calorie depletion* and (2) *the current protein-calorie requirements*. A variety of parameters have been investigated and used during nutritional assessment; the most commonly referenced are body weight and history of weight loss, anthropometry of tissue masses, urinary excretion of nitrogen (reflecting net protein losses), creatinine excretion (reflecting lean tissue), delayed hypersensitivity to intradermal antigens, and measurement of serum proteins levels (as indicators of visceral protein synthesis). However, each of these indices can be obscured during sepsis or following injury.

The septic patient invariably develops a syndrome of extravascular fluid sequestration, which confounds the interpretation of body weight from a nutritional perspective. Edema in peripheral tissue significantly obscures anthropometric measurements, and a significant redistribution of plasma volume can similarly confound the interpretation of circulating serum proteins levels. The presence of sepsis can delay the cutaneous hypersensitivity responses without implicating antecedent or current nutritional depletion. Therefore, the prudent approach to nutritional assessment is based on a careful dietary history, including both an estimation of the duration of nutritional shortages and the anticipated period of subsequent decreased intake. In general, any septic patient in the hypermetabolic flow phase who has experienced greater than 5 days of diminished nutritional intake or is facing any prolonged period (>5 to 7 days) until the return of "normal" dietary intake will require some type of nutritional support. The nutritional support should be tailored to meet the total calorie and nitrogen requirements for the individual patient.

Total Caloric Requirements

The estimation of caloric requirements for septic patients can be based on either a calculation using available equations,[66] or a direct measurement of nitrogen losses and energy expenditure. Due to the wide variation in energy expenditure during sepsis (Table 10-1), the importance of accurately determining caloric requirements warrants measurement of REE by one of the following methods whenever possible. Indirect calorimetry is the most accurate readily available method for estimation of energy requirements for the hospitalized patient. The respiratory gas is collected, whole-body oxygen consumption (VO_2) and carbon dioxide production (VCO2) are measured, and REE is calculated by the following:

$$REE (kcal/day) = (3.9 \text{ kcal/L} \times VO_2 \text{ L/day}) + (1.1 \text{ kcal/L} \times VCO_2 \text{ L/day})$$

If an indirect calorimeter is not available, a reasonable estimation of VO_2 can be obtained in any patient with an indwelling Swan-Ganz catheter. Oxygen consumption is estimated from the difference between arterial and mixed venous oxygen saturation

Table 10-1
Resting Energy Expenditure in Normal and Septic Hospitalized Humans During Various Nutritional Conditions

STUDY CONDITION	STUDY METHOD	REE (KCAL/DAY)	REFERENCE
Unstressed, postabsorptive	Harris-Benedict*	1688 ± 94	Tracey et al[97]
	Indirect calorimetry	1644 ± 102	Tracey et al[97]
Unstressed, starvation	Indirect calorimetry	1301 ± 57	Tracey et al[97]
Sepsis	Indirect calorimetry	2018 ± 85	Weissman et al[104]
	Indirect calorimetry	1545 ± 102	Smith et al[88]
	Indirect calorimetry	1554 ± 95	Baker et al[6]
	Indirect calorimetry	1853 ± 109†	Gump et al[49]
	Indirect calorimetry	1420 ± 79	Tracey et al[95]

* Harris-Benedict Formula:
males: 66.423 + (13.7516)Wt + (5.0033)Ht − (6.7750)A
females: 655.0955 + (9.6534)Wt + (1.8496)Ht − 4.6756A
where Wt is weight in kg, Ht is height in cm, and A is age in years.
† Reported as VO_2, corrected to REE by multiplication by 4.83 as per text.

(arterial-mixed venous difference, volume %), blood hemoglobin concentration (Hgb g/dL), and cardiac output (C.O. liter/min) by:

$$VO_2 \ (L/min) = (O_2 \ \text{Arterial-Mix. Venous Diff.})([Hgb])(1.34)(C.O.)$$

where arterial-mix. venous diff. is obtained from measured oxygen saturation obtained from arterial and mixed venous blood, respectively, and 1.34 (liter/g) represents the O_2 carrying capacity of hemoglobin. In our laboratory, calculation of VO_2 by this method correlates well with indirect calorimetric determination. More than 95% of whole-body energy expenditure is derived from the reaction of oxygen with substrate, and the quantity of energy liberated per liter of O_2 is 4.83 ± 0.10 kcal. Therefore, caloric expenditure can then be estimated by:

$$REE \ (kcal/day) = (4.83 \ kcal/L) \times (VO_2 \ L/day)$$

If the facilities for the physiologic gas exchange measurements are unavailable, however, the Harris-Benedict equation for estimated basal energy expenditure in the unstressed state can be used and then corrected for hypermetabolic requirements with appropriate stress factors (Fig. 10-1 and Table 10-1). These estimations provide a target rate for daily total calorie intake that should be delivered as non-nitrogen nutritional sources. In our experience, positive caloric balance is usually achieved in most septic patients with a nonprotein caloric intake of 26 to 34 kcal/kg-day.[95]

Nitrogen Requirements

The average ratio of total energy calories to nitrogen intake is approximately 300 to 350:1 (kcal:g N) in healthy, unstressed subjects. Nitrogen balance equals the nitrogen intake minus the nitrogen losses. The variable alterations of protein metabolism during sepsis warrant measurement of nitrogen losses on an individual basis whenever feasible. Protein or amino acids may then be delivered at a rate calculated to achieve a positive net nitrogen balance without delivering excessive nitrogen.

When circumstances preclude obtaining precise measurements of total nitrogen losses, urinary urea nitrogen (UUN) is readily measured and can generally be assumed to represent 80% of total urinary nitrogen loss during unstressed starvation or hospitalized TPN. Thus, total nitrogen losses (N_{out}) are estimated with correction for fecal and skin losses (approximately 2 g/day) by:

$$N_{out} \ gm/day = (UUN) + (UUN \times 0.2) + 2$$

A reasonable estimate of net nitrogen balance can therefore be obtained after subtraction of nitrogen losses from the nitrogen intake.

Most current nutritional support regimens have a fixed ratio of calories to nitrogen. If the targeted level of nonprotein calories is within the typical range (26–34 kcal/kg-day), this will result in a nitrogen intake of 0.25 to 0.35 g N/kg-day. In septic patients not manifesting excessive nitrogen losses from diarrhea or fistulae, we have found this level of intake sufficient to achieve positive nitrogen balance. These formulations generally provide a mixture of essential and nonessential amino acids and prevent the development of amino acid deficiencies.

Vitamin and Mineral Requirements

The precise requirements for many trace elements during nutritional support in sepsis have not been adequately defined. The evolution of trace mineral deficiencies may occur over several months but is prevented by the provision of these elements in commercially available enteral feeding regimens or by addition to parenteral solutions (discussed below). The clinical presentation of the deficiency syndromes (Table 10-2) occurs more frequently in the neonate or elderly patient with sepsis, and the clinician must be alert to these signs and symptoms during nutritional support.[68,70]

Hypophosphatemia frequently complicates nutritional therapy during sepsis because phosphorus requirements increase with glucose infusions.[85,87] Approximately 25 mEq of elemental phosphorus are required for each 1000 kcal of glucose administered. Similarly, depletion of intracellular stores of magnesium may precipitate cardiac arrythmias and seizures.[52] The serum level of magnesium does not reflect the intracellular stores, which may become depleted during nutritional therapy.[93] Hypomagnesemia is usually prevented with the provision of 10 mEq/day during nutritional support.

The supplementation requirements for vitamins during nutritional support regimens are incompletely understood, but deficiencies are frequently identified in critically ill patients.[67] Because the fat-soluble vitamins (A, D, E, and K) have relatively large reservoirs in previously well-fed patients, acute deficiencies are rare. However, the water-soluble vitamins have negligible stores and may be rapidly depleted. Therefore, water-soluble vitamins should be administered throughout the nutritional support period at 1.5 to 2 times the recommended daily allowance.

DELIVERY OF NUTRITIONAL SUPPORT

Hemodynamic stabilization, antimicrobial therapy, and abscess drainage should all occur as needed in the early management of sepsis. Once the patient is stabilized, the selection of a nutritional regimen should be based on the primary objective of nutritional therapy which is: *the delivery of nutrients of sufficient quality and quantity to maintain or replete energy and protein stores.*

Enteral Nutritional Support

The provision of nutrients by the enteral route is the preferred method of delivery, being more cost-effective and, if properly performed, associated with lesser risk.[71] The gastrointestinal tract, if it is functional, should be used (unless contraindicated by the necessity for bowel rest or other clinical circumstance). The anorexia and food aversion that accompanies sepsis invariably prevents the voluntary consumption

Table 10–2
Clinical Presentation of Selected Vitamin and Mineral Deficiencies in
Adults During Nutritional Support

VITAMIN/ MICRONUTRIENT	SIGNS/SYMPTOMS
Vitamin A	Decreased night vision Biot's spots Corneal/conjunctival xerosis Keratomalacia Follicular hyperkeratosis
Vitamin B_1 (thiamine)	Calf muscle tenderness Loss of ankle and knee jerks Hypoesthesia and paresthesia Edema Cardiac enlargement and tachycardia
Vitamin B_3 (niacin)	Pellagra Atrophic lingual papillae Diarrhea
Vitamin B_6 (pyridoxine)	Peripheral neuropathy Nasolabial seborrhea Glossitis
Vitamin C	Scurvy Spongy and bleeding gums Petechiae and ecchymosis Follicular hyperkeratosis with perifollicular hemorrhage Impaired wound healing Painful epiphyseal enlargement
Vitamin D	Frontal or parietal bossing Osteomalacia
Riboflavin	Cheilosis Lingual papillae atrophy, magneta tongue Dyssebacea Scrotal dermatosis Corneal vascularization
Vitamin K	Bleeding diathesis
Chromium	Glucose intolerance
Copper	Neutropenia, anemia Pallor
Iron	Mucous membrane pallor Lingual papillae atrophy Angular stomatitis Thin brittle nails with spooning Weakness
Zinc	Ageusia/dysgeusia Hair loss Night blindness Rash Impaired wound healing Glucose intolerance

of an adequate dietary regimen even in the alert patient. However, small caliber Silastic feeding tubes are well tolerated and readily passed with a guide wire. Rarely, enteral feeding tubes may require endoscopic guidance for proper placement. Roentgenographic confirmation of tube placement in the duodenum is recommended prior to the initiation of feeding in all cases. During enteric feeding, the patient should be maintained with the head of the bed elevated slightly. If laparotomy is necessary for the treatment of the septic focus, consideration should be given to placement of a jejunostomy feeding tube, which can be subsequently used for both nutritional and fluid support.[51,66] This method of therapy is well tolerated and provides secure and continuous nutrient delivery.

After selection of the appropriate enteric route, the daily caloric and nitrogen requirements can be estimated (discussed above), and an enteral regimen designed to achieve these requirements.

Enteral Regimens

There is a wide variety of enteral feeding formulas available for oral or enteric catheter feedings: (1) *Polymeric diets* are composed of oligosaccharides and intact or partially hydrolyzed protein. (2) *Monomeric diets* have higher osmotic concentrations of saccharide and nitrogen sources. (3) *Modular diets* are composed of individual constituents of dextrose, lipid, and nitrogen.

The selection of an enteral formula is based on the individual patient's absorptive capacity, substrate tolerances, and any specialized requirements.

The continuous infusion of enteral feedings is most safely performed by volumetric pump. The composition, target rate, and final volume to be delivered are determined as outlined in the nutritional assessment section (above). Dilute strength solutions are usually started at 30 to 50 ml/hr and advanced as tolerated until the target infusion level is achieved. Because many of the defined formula diets are hyperosmolar (450 to 800 mOsm), the patients should be monitored for glucose intolerance and hyperosmolarity. Frequently, antidiarrheal therapy such as opiates or anticholinergics will be required; these are best administered with the feeding solution. Any evidence of gastrointestinal intolerance, nausea, or abdominal pain must be carefully evaluated.

Complications of Enteral Support

Physiologic complications of gastrointestinal function are commonly observed during enteral nutritional support.[27] Diarrhea may be unresponsive to or require the use of high doses of medication. In such cases the nutrient infusion rate should be decreased, or the feeding regimen substituted for one of lower osmolarity or fat content. Metabolic complications are rarely severe but include glucose intolerance (may be enhanced by sepsis), hyperosmolar dehydration (may precipitate coma if undetected), total body sodium overload or hypernatremia, and essential fatty acid deficiencies (prevented by the provision of intravenous lipid two times per week). When renal function is normal, azotemia may occur secondary to either the administration of nitrogen in excess of body requirements or to intravascular dehydration.

The most frequent serious complication of enteric feeding is aspiration. The incidence of aspiration can be minimized by meticulous attention to proper tube position, frequent assessment of residual volumes, and maintenance of partially upright positioning.[90] However, the risk of aspiration cannot be completely eliminated by any of the above maneuvers, and the incidence varies between 1% and 15% when determined by dye or isotope recovery from pulmonary secretions. Asymptomatic aspirations appear to occur with some frequency, and any respiratory symptoms or change in mental status in the patient receiving tube feeding warrants careful consideration of this complication. Symptomatic complaints of oropharyngeal irritation should be evaluated in light of the potential for mucosal erosion, epistaxis, or, rarely, tracheoesophageal fistula formation during nasoenteric feedings. The use of soft, Silastic feeding tubes, to the exclusion of large bore nasogastric tubes for feeding, and the judicious use of topical anesthetics can usually minimize patient discomfort associated with nasoenteric feeding catheters.

Parenteral Nutritional Support

TPN was introduced for human use in 1968.[21,22] Since then, patients who previously would have been unable to receive adequate nutrition are readily maintained on complete parenteral diets consisting of various combinations of amino acids, dextrose, and lipid. Any septic patient who requires nutritional support but does not have a functional gastrointestinal tract or the ability to tolerate the required rate of enteric feeding is a potential candidate for parenteral nutrition.

Peripheral Vein Feeding

This type of intravenous nutritional support is appealing because of the presumed reduced risks of peripheral venous access as compared to those of central venous access. These solutions are near isotonic and therefore consist of lower concentrations of amino acids and glucose, which cannot usually be infused at a rate sufficient to supply total nutrient requirements during the hypermetabolic phase. When supplemented with lipid infusions (10% or 20%) or enteral feeding, peripheral vein feeding may be appropriate for a limited number of patients with sepsis.

Total Parenteral Nutrition

The solutions for TPN are hyperosmolar (>1500 mOsm), thereby necessitating delivery by way of a central venous route. These solutions contain dextrose as the major caloric source (usual dextrose concentration 25 to 45 g/100 ml) and crystalline amino acids (3 to 5 g a.a./100 ml) as the nitrogen source (Table 10-3). These solutions should always be infused continuously by volumetric pump. The target rate of daily calories to be delivered should be calculated during the nutritional assessment (above), and amino acids should be provided on the basis of measured nitrogen losses. Unless nitrogen intolerance complicates the therapy, a minimum acceptable rate of 0.25 to 0.35 g N/kg-day in general is adequate.

Table 10–3
A Method of Formulating Central-Vein Feeding Solutions

	ADULT STANDARD FORMULA	ADULT CARDIAC FORMULA	ADULT RENAL FORMULA
Amino acids, g	50	30	15.7
Dextrose, g	250	350	350
Calcium, mEq	4.7		
Magnesium, mEq	8	8	
Potassium, mEq	43	39	1.6
Sodium, mEq	52		
Acetate, mEq	92	44	31.5
Chloride, mEq	70	20	
Gluconate, mEq	4.7		
Phorphorus, mmol	12	12	
Vitamin complex, ml	5	5	5
Final volume, ml	1050	850	800
Dextrose concentration, %	25	41	44

Note: As practiced at New York Hospital–Cornell Medical Center.

Prior to beginning TPN, a sterile catheter should be inserted, and appropriate placement in the superior vena cava should be confirmed by chest x-ray. The infusion of the TPN solution can be started at a relatively slow rate (30 to 40 ml/hr) and increased over 24 to 48 hr to achieve the target rate. Glucose intolerance during TPN in septic patients occurs frequently and requires frequent monitoring of plasma glucose, as well as urinary glucose and ketones. Insulin supplementation may be administered subcutaneously during the first day of TPN, unless extreme hyperglycemia warrants intravenous insulin. Thereafter, we have found it useful to provide one half of the previous daily total insulin requirement in solution with the TPN. In general, titration of the TPN delivery rate to control glucose levels often precludes adequate delivery of substrates; hyperglycemia is best managed by careful insulin administration. Once the septic process is controlled, insulin requirements may drastically diminish, and frequent monitoring during TPN is recommended to prevent hypoglycemia. When TPN is to be discontinued, the infusion rate should be reduced gradually, allowing time for adaptation to the reduced daily glucose load.

In addition to monitoring glucose, fluid balances should be recorded, daily weights should be followed, and weekly determination of complete blood count, blood urea nitrogen, serum electrolytes, and hepatic enzymes should be performed.

The delivery of TPN as the sole nutrient source can precipitate a deficiency of essential lipids.[9,33] To prevent this syndrome, lipid emulsions of soy or safflower oil are available in 10% to 20% concentrations and provide 1.1 to 2.2 kcal/ml. The use of lipid as the major nonprotein caloric source has been widely advocated for achieving maximal caloric intake and optimal control of glucose intolerance,[4, 40, 74–76] but the efficacy of lipids during sepsis remains controversial. Although the clearance of lipid emulsions from the serum of patients with sepsis may be increased, data demonstrating efficient oxidation of this infused substrate are lacking. In addition, patients receiving adequate calories and nitrogen will synthesize endogenous lipids and require only essential lipids (at 5% to 10% of total calories) to maintain optimal substrate utilization. Finally, patients with pulmonary compromise, coagulopathy, lipoid nephrosis, or abnormalities of fat transport, which frequently accompany sepsis, should not receive excessive lipid therapy.[66]

Complications of Parenteral Nutrition

Prominent complications of TPN are related to the placement and management of the central venous catheter. The complication rate during insertion of the catheters is directly related to the experience of the physician performing the procedure.[82] Serious complications have been reported to occur in 1% to 5% of patients and include pneumothorax, which may be immediate or delayed after catheter placement; hemothorax; myocardial perforation; arterial injury; brachial, recurrent laryngeal, phrenic, or vagus nerve injury; lymphatic leak; catheter embolism; air embolism; and thrombosis of the vein. The insertion of the catheters under optimal sterile conditions by an experienced physician can reduce the potential morbidity in the septic patient requiring TPN. The administration of low doses of heparin (5000 U/day) in the feeding solution has been reported to reduce the incidence of subclinical venous thrombosis.[66]

The incidence of infectious complication has been reported to be as high as 5% to 10% in some centers. While the septic patient may be at some increased risk of catheter-related sepsis secondary to transient bacteremia or suppressed immune function, meticulous care of the catheter site and strict adherence to line sterility can dramatically reduce this risk. Experienced centers have reported the risk of infectious complications during long-term TPN (longer than 1 week) at less than 1%.[84] The catheter should be used exclusively for TPN solutions; drugs or other fluids should be administered by way of a separate line. If the patient develops signs of recurrent sepsis or evidence of clinical deterioration such as changes in fever curve or mental status, respiratory alkalosis, positive blood cultures or unexplained neutropenia or leukocytosis, the catheter should be changed and the tip should be cultured. In high-risk patients, the risk of line sepsis can also be minimized by changes of the catheter over a J-wire at frequent (3- to 7-day) intervals; the catheter tip should always be cultured with these line changes.

Abnormalities of electrolyte and metabolic parameters occur frequently during TPN in crtically ill patients. Hyperglycemia, if extreme, can stimulate persistent osmotic diuresis with dehydration and progression to hyperosmolar coma. Sepsis-mediated alterations of renal function during TPN have to be carefully monitored, because the consequences of continual infusion of potassium and phosphate in this setting can be life-threatening. Calcium and magnesium levels should be monitored, particularly during the recovery period when the circulating levels of these minerals can be rapidly diminished during the restoration of intracellular protein stores.

Abnormalities of hepatic transaminases and alkaline phosphatase levels frequently develop during the initial 10 to 14 days of TPN but rarely exceed twice the normal value. Significant elevations of bilirubin are rare and should prompt the investigation for other diagnoses. While these changes usually stabilize or decrease after 2 to 3 weeks, hepatitis or biliary tract infection should not be overlooked in the patient with any suggestive symptoms.

A careful assessment of nutritional requirements should minimize the potential complications inherent to overfeeding the patient with sepsis. The delivery of carbohydrate in excess of the whole-body nonprotein caloric requirement can lead to excess CO_2 production. Increased arterial levels of pCO_2 may initiate an increase in the work of breathing and precipitate dyspnea, thus diminishing ability to wean the patient from ventilatory assistance. Should the septic patient receiving any form of nutritional support develop an unexplained increase of pCO_2, overfeeding should be considered. This complication only rarely occurs when the calories are being provided at less than 1.2 times the REE.

NUTRITIONAL SUPPORT DURING ORGAN FAILURE

The use of nutritional support during organ system failure has been extensively reviewed[28, 41, 43, 66] and will be discussed below as it pertains to the management of the septic patient. The rational approach to nutritional support in these cases should remain focused on the assessment of daily caloric and nitrogen reuirements, interpreted in reference to the specific limitations of fluid, electrolyte, or substrate compromises resulting from organ failure.

Pulmonary Failure

Sepsis is frequently complicated by pulmonary failure with a requirement for mechanical ventilatory assistance. Adequate nutritional support is important to maximize the potential for recovery of respiratory muscle function and resumption of normal clearance of bronchiolar secretions. Excess lipid should be avoided in these patients because of an association with depressed pulmonary function from lipid accumulation. As noted above, care should be taken not to overfeed these patients as well, and indirect calorimetry may be necessary to document daily energy requirements and ensure that the RQ is ≤ 1.0 during nutritional support.

Renal Failure

The development of renal failure during sepsis is often associated with decreased clearance of nitrogen, potassium, phosphorus, and other metabolites of normal cellular metabolism. The use of hemodialysis can result in an additional nitrogen requirement of 1 to 2 g/day, and peritoneal dialysis can precipitate losses of >4 g/day.[66] Consideration of these increased nitrogen losses should accompany the assessment of such patients. It is increasingly clear that the institution of dialysis in a timely fashion and the simultaneous provision of essential and nonessential amino acids and nonprotein calories promote optimal return of renal function.

As a general rule, TPN solutions during renal failure are concentrated, electrolyte-restricted (Table 10-3), and delivered at the rate necessary to provide caloric and nitrogen requirements. Patients with severe, oliguric renal failure are most often managed with solutions containing only the essential amino acids and a more concentrated caloric source to minimize fluid administration and to optimize electrolyte replacement. The patient with nonoliguric renal failure may benefit from a balanced formula containing essential and nonessential amino acids.

Cardiac Failure

The most troublesome complication from nutritional support in the septic patient with heart disease is sodium and fluid overload. This is best addressed by restriction of sodium and increasing the concentration of nonprotein calories (Table 10-3) to minimize volume delivery. As noted above, close monitoring of magnesium, calcium, potassium, and phosphorus is critical in these patients who are frequently on inotropic agents and can manifest life-threatening rhythm abnormalities in the presence of abnormal concentrations of electrolytes. The occurrence of renal dysfunction in the patient with sepsis and heart failure may mandate the additional consideration of a reduced nitrogen density.

Hepatic Failure

Liver failure is associated with abnormalities of gluconeogenesis, lipogenesis, neutralization of circulating toxins, and utilization of micronutrients. Glucose should be monitored closely in the septic patient with advancing liver failure, particularly in the cirrhotic patient in whom severe hypoglycemia may occur.[41] Hepatic encephalopathy may develop secondary to a defect in the clearance of nitrogenous wastes leading to increased levels of ammonia and the aromatic amino acids. A solution of branched-chain amino acids has been advocated in this setting based on observations of improved mentation during this type of nutritional support.[72] While the physiologic implications are intriguing, these formulations are expensive, and prospective studies have failed to unequivocally demonstrate improvements in morbidity and mortality as compared to balanced amino acid solutions. The septic patient with liver failure requires essential amino acids, which are best delivered by way of a balanced amino acid solution.

REFERENCES

1. Albert JD, Legaspi A, Horowitz GD, et al. Preservation of functional aerobic capacity with daily submaximal exercise during intravenous feeding in hospitalized normal man. World J Surg, 1988;12:123–131.

2. Albert JD, Legaspi A, Horowitz GD, et al. Extremity amino acid metabolism during starvation and intravenous refeeding in humans. Am J Physiol 1986;251:E604.

3. Albert JD, Tracey KJ, Fahey TJ III, et al. Peripheral tissue conservation during acute elevations of plasma epinephrine in normal man. Surgical Forum 1986;37:53.

4. Askanazi J, Carpentier YA, Elwyn DH, et al. Influence of total parenteral nutrition in injury and sepsis. Ann Surg 1980;191:40.

5. Aulick L, Wilmore DW. Increased peripheral amino acid release following burn injury. Surgery 1979;85:560.

6. Baker JP, Detsky AS, Stewart S, et al. Randomized trials of total parenteral nutrition in critically ill patients: metabolic effects of varying glucose-lipid ratios as the energy source. Gastroenterology 1984;87:53.

7. Ballard FJ, Tomas PM. 3-methylhistidine as a measure of skeletal muscle protein breakdown in human subjects: the case for its continued use. Clin Sci 1983;65:209.

8. Baracos V, Rodermann HP, Dinarello CA, et al. Stimulation of muscle protein degradation and prostaglandin E_2 release by leukocytic pyrogen (interleukin-1). N Engl J Med 1983;308:553.

9. Barr LH, Dunn GD, Brennan MF. Essential fatty acid deficiency during total parenteral nutrition. Ann Surg 1987;193:304.

10. Beisel WR. Magnitude of the host nutritional responses to infection. Am J Clin Nutr 1977;30:1236.

11. Beisel WR, Goldman RF, Joy JT. Metabolic balance studies during induced hyperthermia in man. J Appl Physiol 1968;24:1.

12. Beisel WR, Wannemacher RW. Gluconeogenesis, ureagenesis, and ketogenesis during sepsis. JPEN J Parenter Enteral Nutr 1980;4:277.

13. Bessey PQ, Brooks DC, Black PR, et al. Epinephrine mediates skeletal muscle insulin resistance. Surgery 1983;94:172.

14. Bessey PQ, Walters JM, Aoki TT. Combined hormonal infusion stimulates the metabolic response to injury. Ann Surg 1984;200:264.

15. Beutler B, Greenwald D, Hulmes JD, et al. Identity of tumor necrosis factor and the macrophage-secreted factor cachectin. 1985;316:552.

16. Beutler B, Milsark IW, Cerami A. Cachectin/tumor necrosis factor: production, distribution and metabolic fate *in vivo*. J Immunol 1985;135:3972.

17. Beutler B, Milsark IW, Cerami A. Passive immunization against cachetin/tumor necrosis factor (TNF) protects mice from the lethal effect of endotoxin. Science 1985;229:869.

18. Birkhahn RH, Long CL, Fitkin D. Whole body protein metabolism due to trauma in man as estimated by L-(^{15}N)-alaine. Am J Physiol 1981;E241:64.

19. Bistrian BR, Blackburn GL, Hallowell E, et al. Protein status of general surgical patients. JAMA 1974;230:858.

20. Blackburn GL. Lipid metabolism in infection. Am J Clin Nutr 1972;30:1321.

21. Dudrick SJ, Wilmore DW, Vars HM, et al. Can intravenous feeding as the sole means of nutrition support growth in the child and restore weight loss in an adult? An affirmative answer. Ann Surg 1969;169:974.

22. Dudrick SJ, Wilmore DW, Vars HM, et al. Long term total parenteral nutrition with growth, development and positive nitrogen balance. Surgery 1968;64:134.

23. Cahill GF, Jr. Physiology of insulin in man. Diabetes 1971;20:785.

24. Cahill GF, Jr. Starvation in man. N Engl J Med 1970;282:668.

25. Cahill GF Jr, Aoki TT, Rossini AA. Metabolism in obesity and anorexia nervosa. In: Wurtman RJ, Wurtman JJ, eds. Nutrition and the brain. Vol 3. Disorders of eating and nutrients in the treatment of brain diseases, New York: Raven Press, p 1.

26. Carpenter YA, Jeevanandam M, Robini AP, et al. Measurement of glycerol turnover by infusion of nonisotopic glycerol in normal and injured subjects. Am J Physiol 1984;247:E409.

27. Cataldi-Betcher EL, Seltzer MH, Slocum BA, et al. Complications occurring during enteral nutritional support: a prospective study. JPEN J Parenter Enteral Nutr 1983;7:546.

28. Cerra FB, McMillen M, Angelico R, et al. Cirrhosis, encephalopathy and improved results with metabolic support. Surgery 1983;94:612.

29. Clowes GH Jr, Hirsch E, George BC. Survival from sepsis: the significance of altered protein metabolism regulated by proteolysis inducing factor, the circulating cleavage product of IL-1. Ann Surg 1985;202:446.

30. Clowes GH Jr, Martin H, Walji S, et al. Blood insulin responses to blood glucose levels in high output sepsis and septic shock. Am J Surg 1978;135:577.

31. Clowes GHA, O'Donnell TF, Ryan NT, et al. Energy metabolism in sepsis: treatment based on different patterns in shock and high output stage. Ann Surg 1974;179:684.

32. Clowes GHA, Randall HT, Cha C-J. Amino acid and energy metabolism in septic and traumatized patients. JPEN J Parenter Enteral Nutr 1980;4:195.
33. Connor WE. Pathogenesis and frequency of essential fatty acid deficiency during total parenteral nutrition. Ann Intern Med 1975;83:895.
34. Cuthbertson DP. Observations on the disturbance of metabolism produced by injury to the limbs. Q J Med 1932;1:233.
35. Dinarello CA. Interleukin-1. Rev Infect Dis 1984;6:51.
36. Dinarello CA, Clowes GH Jr, Gordon AH, et al. Cleavage of human interleukin-1: isolation of a peptide fragment from plasma of febrile humans and activated monocytes. J Immunol 1984;133:1332.
37. DuBois E. Basal metabolism in health and disease. New York: Lea & Febiger, 1924:1.
38. Duke JH, Jorgenson SB, Broell Jr, et al: Contribution of protein to caloric expenditure following injury. Surgery 1970;68:168.
39. Edelman R. Cell mediated immune response in protein caloric malnutrition. In: Suskind RM, ed. Malnutrition and the immune response. New York: Raven Press, 1977.
40. Elwyn DH, Kinney JM, Gump FE, et al. Some metabolic effects of fat infusions in depleted patients. Metabolism 1980;29:125.
41. Feinstein EI, Blumendrantz MJ, Heady M, et al. Clinical and metabolic responses to parenteral nutrition in acute renal failure. Medicine 1981;60:124.
42. Felig P. The glucose alanine cycle. Metabolism 1973;22:179.
43. Fischer JE, ed. Surgical nutrition. 1st ed. Boston: Little Brown & Co, 1983.
44. George DT, Abeles FB, Mopes CA. Effect of leucocyte endogenous mediators on endocrine pancrease secretory responses. Am J Physiol 1977;233:E240.
45. Grecos GP, Abbott WC, Schiller WR, et al. The effect of major thermal injury and carbohydrate-free intake on serum triglycerides, insulin and 3-methylhistidine excretion. Ann Surg 1984; 200:632.
46. Gross RL, Newberne PM. Nutrition and immunologic function. Physiol Rev 1980;60:188.
47. Gump FE, Long CL, Geiger JW. The significance of altered gluconeogenesis in surgical catabolism. J Trauma 1975;15:704.
48. Gump FE, Long CL, Killian P, et al. Studies of glucose intolerance in septic injured patients. J Trauma 1974;14:378.
49. Gump FE, Price JB, Kinney JM. Whole body and splanchnic blood flow and oxygen consumption measurements in patients with intraperitoneal infections. Ann Surg 1970;171:321.
50. Guyton AC. Textbook of medical physiology. 5th ed. Philadelphia: WB Saunders, 1976:904.
51. Hoover, HC Jr, Ryan JA, Anderson EJ, et al: Nutritional benefits of immediate postoperative jejunal feeding of an elemental diet. Am J Surg 1980;139:153.
52. Juan D. Clinical review: the clinical importance of hypomagnesemia. Surgery 1982;91:510.
53. Kaufman RL, Matson CF, Beisel WR. Hypertriglyceridemia produced by endotoxin: role of impaired triglyceride disposal mechanisms. J Infect Dis 1986;133:548.
54. Kawakami M, Cerami A. Studies of endotoxin-induced decrease in lipoprotein lipase activity. J Exp Med 1981;154:631.
55. Kawakami M, Pekala PH, Lane MD, et al. Lipoprotein lipase suppression in 3T3-L1 cells by an endotoxin-induced mediator from exudate cells. Proc Natl Acad Sci 1982;79:912.
56. Keusch GT, Farthing MJG. Nutrition and infection. Annu Rev Nutr 1986;6:131.
57. Keys A, Brosek J, Henschel A. The biology of human starvation. Minneapolis: University of Minnesota Press, 1950.
58. Kinney JM. Energy requirements in injury and sepsis. Acta Anaesthesiol Scand (Suppl) 1974;55:15.
59. Kyger ER III, Block WJ, Roach G, et al. Adverse effects of protein malnutrition on myocardial function. Surgery 1977;84:174.
60. Lee DM, Zentella A, Pekala PH, et al. Effect of endotoxin-induced monokines on glucose metabolism in the muscle cell line L-6. Proc Natl Acad Sci 1987;84:2590–2594.
61. Legaspi A, Albert JD, Calvano SE, et al. Proteolysis of skeletal muscle in response to acute elevation of plasma cortisol in man. Surgical Forum 1985;36:16.
62. Long CL, Jeevanandam M, Kim BM. Whole body protein synthesis and catabolism in septic man. Am J Clin Nutr 1977;30:1340.
63. Long CL, Kinney JM, Geiger JW. Nonsuppressability of gluconeogenesis by glucose in septic patients. Metabolism 1976;25:193.
64. Long CL, Spencer JL, Kinney JM. Carbohydrate metabolism in man: effect of elective operations and major injury. J Appl Physiol 1971;31:110.
65. Lowry SF. Host metabolic response to injury. In: Gallin JI, Fanci AS, eds. Advances in host defense mechanisms. Vol 6. New York: Raven Press, 1986.

66. Lowry SF. Nutritional support of the traumatized patient. In: Shires GT, ed. Principles of trauma care. 3rd ed. New York: McGraw-Hill, 1985.

67. Lowry SF, Goodgame JT, Maher MM, et al. Parenteral vitamin requirements during intravenous feeding. Am J Clin Nutr 1978;30:2149.

68. Lowry SF, Goodgame JT, Smith JC, et al. Abnormalities of zinc and copper during total parenteral nutrition. Ann Surg 1979;189:120.

69. Lowry SF, Horowitz GD, Jeevanandam M, et al. Whole-body protein breakdown and 3-methylhistidine excretion during brief fasting, starvation and intravenous repletion in man. Ann Surg 1985;202:21.

70. Lowry SF, Smith JC, Brennan MF. Zinc and copper replacement during total parenteral nutrition. Am J Clin Nutr 1981;34:1853.

71. McArdle AH, Palmason C, Morency I, et al. A rationale for enteral feeding as the preferable route for hyperalimentation. Surgery 1981;90:616.

72. Millikan WJ, Henderson JM, Warren WD, et al. Total parenteral nutrition with F080® in cirrhotics with subclinical encephalopathy. Ann Surg 1983;197:294.

73. Moore FD. The metabolic care of the surgical patient. Philadelphia: WB Saunders, 1959.

74. Nordenstrom J, Askanazi J, Elwyn DH, et al: Nitrogen balance during total parenteral nutrition: glucose vs fat. Ann Surg 1983;197:27.

75. Nordenstrom J, Carpentier YA, Askanazi J, et al. Metabolism and utilization of intravenous fat emulsion during total parenteral nutrition. Ann Surg 1982;196:221.

76. Nordenstrom J, Carpenter YA, Askanazi J, et al. Free fatty acid mobilization and oxidation during total parenteral nutrition in trauma and infection. Ann Surg 1983;198:725.

77. O'Donnell TF, Clowes GHA, Blackburn GL, et al. Proteolysis associated with a deficit of peripheral energy fuel substrate in septic man. Surgery 1976;80:192.

78. Perlmutter DH, Dinarello CA, Punsal PI. Cachectin/tumor necrosis factor regulates hepatic acute phase gene expression. J Clin Invest 1986;78:1349.

79. Rennie MJ, Bennegard K, Eden E, et al. Urinary excretion and efflux from the leg of 3-methylhistidine before and after major surgical operation. Metabolism 1984;33:250.

80. Rennie MH, Holloszy JO. Inhibition of glucose uptake and glycogenolysis by availability of oleate in well-oxygenated perfused skeletal muscle. Biochem J 1977;168:161.

81. Rouzer CA, Cerami A. Hypertriglyceridemia associated with *Trypanosoma brucei* infection in rabbits: role of effective triglyceride removal. Mol Biochem Parasitol 1980;2:31.

82. Ryan JA, Abel RM, Abbott WM, et al. Catheter complications in total parenteral nutrition; a prospective study of 200 consecutive patients. N Engl J Med 1974;290:755.

83. Sacca L, Vigorito C, Cicala M. Role of gluconeogenesis in epinephrine stimulated hepatic glucose production in humans. Am J Physiol 1983;245:E294.

84. Sanders RA, Sheldon GF. Septic complications of total parenteral nutrition. Am J Surg 1976;132:214.

85. Sheldon GF, Gryzyb S. Phosphate depletion and repletion: relation to parenteral nutrition and oxygen transport. Ann Surg 1975;182:683.

86. Sheldon GF, Peterson SR. Malnutrition and cardiopulmonary function. JPEN J Parenter Enteral Nutr 1980;4:376.

87. Sloan GM, White DE, Brennan MF. Calcium and phosphorous metabolism during total parenteral nutrition. Ann Surg 1983;197:1.

88. Smith RC, Birkshaw L, Hill GL. Optimal energy and nitrogen for gastrointestinal patients requiring intravenous nutrition. Gastroenterology 1982;82:445.

89. Sobocinski PZ, Canterbury WJ Jr, Mapes CA, et al. Involvement of hepatic metallothioneins in hypozincemia associated with bacterial infection. Am J Physiol 1987;234:E399.

90. Steffee WP, Krey SH. Enteral hyperalimentation for patients with head and neck cancer. Otolaryngol Clin North Am 1980;13:437.

91. Steinberg D. Hormonal regulation of lipase, phosphoorylase and glycogen synthetase in adipose tissue. Adv Cyclic Nucleotide Protein Phosphorylation Res 1975;5:549.

92. Suharjono, Gracey M, Sunoto, et al. Microbial contamination of the gut: another feature of malnutrition. Am J Clin Nutr 1973;26:1170.

93. Swenson SA Jr, Lewis JW, Sebby KR. Magnesium metabolism in man with special reference to jejunoileal bypass for obesity. Am J Surg 1974;127:250.

94. Torti FM, Dieckmann B, Beutler B, et al. A macrophage factor inhibits adipocyte gene expression: an *in vitro* model of cachexia. Science 1985;229:867.

95. Tracey KJ, Albert JD, Legaspi A, et al. Impact of intravenous feeding on peripheral tissue amino acid uptake during critical illness. Clin Nutr 1986;5(Suppl):58.

96. Tracey KJ, Fong Y, Hesse DG, et al. Anti-cachectin/TNF monoclonal antibodies prevent septic shock during lethal bacteremia. Nature 1987;330:662–664.

97. Tracey KJ, Legaspi A, Albert JD, et al. Protein and substrate metabolism during starvation and parenteral refeeding. Clin Sci 1988;74:123–132.

98. Tracey KJ, Lowry SF, Beutler B, et al. Cachectin/TNF mediates changes of skeletal muscle membrane potential. J Exp Med 1986;164:1368.

99. Tracey KJ, Vlassara H, Cerami A. Cachectin/TNF (tumour necrosis factor). Lancet 1989;1:1122–1126.

100. Tracey KJ, Lowry SF, Fahey TJ, et al. Cachectin/tumor necrosis factor induces lethal shock and stress hormone responses in the dog. Surg Gynecol Obstet 1987;164:415.

101. Unger RH. Glucagon and the insulin:glucagon ratio in diabetes and other catabolic illnesses. Diabetes 1971;20:834.

102. Vaidyamath, N, Oswald G, Treitley G. Turnover of amino acids in sepsis and starvation. J Trauma 1976;16:125.

103. Van Snick, JL, Masson PL, Hermans JF. The involvement of lactoferrin in the hyposideremia of acute inflammation. J Exp Med 1974;140:1068.

104. Weissman C, Kemper M, Askanazi J, et al. Resting metabolic rate of the critically ill patient; measured versus predicted. Anesthesiology 1986;64:673.

105. Wilmore DW, Aulick LH, Becker RA. Hormones and the control of metabolism. In: Fischer J, ed. Surgical nutrition. 1st ed. Boston: Little, Brown & Co, 1985.

106. Wilmore DW, Goodwin CW, Aulick LH, et al. Effect of injury and infection on visceral metabolism and circulation. Ann Surg 1980;192:491.

107. Wilmore DW, Long JM, Mason AD, et al. Stress in surgical patients as a neurophysiologic reflex response. Surg Gynecol Obstet 1976;142:257.

108. Wilmore DW, Long JM, Mason AD. Catecholamines: mediator of the hypermetabolic response to thermal injury. Ann Surg 1974;180:653.

109. Wolfe RR, Allsop JR, Burke JF. Glucose metabolism in man: responses to intravenous glucose infusion. Metabolism 1979;28:210.

110. Young VR, Munro HN. 3-methylhistidine and muscle protein turnover: an overview. Fed Proc 1978;37:2291.

11

○   ○   ○   •   •   ○

SURGICAL INFECTIONS IN DIABETIC PATIENTS

Claude H. Organ, Jr.

Man may be the captain of his fate but he is also the victim of his blood sugar.

——*Wilfred G. Oakley*

More than 11 million people in the United States have diabetes, one half of whom are unaware they harbor this chronic disease. Each year an additional 500,000 Americans are diagnosed with diabetes. One million have the insulin-dependent variety (type I); the remainder have non-insulin dependent diabetes (type II), which usually develops in overweight persons over 40 years of age. Three hundred thousand people die as a result of diabetes and its complications each year; 5000 lose their eyesight because of diabetic retinopathy; 10% have kidney disease; and 45% of all nontraumatic leg and foot amputations in the United States are caused by diabetes. One third of all diabetics have a positive family history of diabetes mellitus.[2]

Following the introduction of insulin, the mortality of diabetics undergoing amputation was 50%. With the availability of antibiotics, the mortality rate dropped to 33% in the 1940s and has now declined to 9%. Gangrene is 53 times more frequent in diabetic men over the age of 40 than in nondiabetics and a disturbing 71 times more frequent in diabetic women in the same age category.[6]

Are diabetic patients more prone to infection? Are diabetic infections more serious and refractory to management? The presumption that diabetics are prone to infection is unclear, poorly documented, and controversial. One fact remains clear and well documented: infection is the major cause of morbidity and mortality in diabetics and accounts for the majority of their hospital admissions. Some clinical investigators believe there is an increased frequency of infections in the diabetic, although the precise reason is not known. Others have concluded that infections are no more common in well-controlled diabetics than nondiabetics. The incidence of postoperative infections in the diabetic surgical patient has been found to be doubled or normal depending on the reference source.[3] The difficulties experienced by surgeons in the surgical management of diabetes with simple hand or foot infections (as well as moist fungal infections) suggest that infections are more serious and difficult to eradicate in this group (Fig. 11-1). Savin has postulated that organisms thrived in a high-sugar medium.[10] More recent evidence reveals that some gram-positive cocci prefer high concentrations of sugar, but the opposite effect was observed with gram-negative organisms.[10] The controversy as to whether patients with diabetes mellitus are more susceptible to infection than age- and sex-matched nondiabetic control subjects continues. Physicians have long noted the appearance of newly diagnosed insulin diabetes following acute infection.

PATHOLOGY AND PATHOPHYSIOLOGY

Acute infection alters the endocrine-metabolic status of the host organism in both the diabetic and nondiabetic, leading to difficulty in controlling blood sugar levels in diabetics and ketoacidosis. Control of blood sugar levels in diabetic patients is the

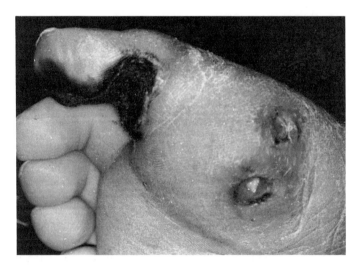

Figure 11-1.
A 61-year-old diabetic male with gangrene and a soft tissue infection of the right foot.

sine qua non in the prevention of certain infections and supports those host defense mechanisms that determine the diabetic patient's resistance and response to infection.

The following factors in diabetic patients may play a role in altering their defense mechanisms for infection: altered leukocyte function (*i.e.,* chemotaxis), phagocytosis, intracellular bactericidal activity, and serum opsonic activity. Acute infection can adversely affect carbohydrate metabolism indirectly through the antagonism of insulin action by hormones secreted in excess quantity during infection (growth hormone, glycogen, and cortisol), or directly through the destruction of islet tissue by an infectious agent such as the mumps virus (Fig. 11-2). The uncontrolled diabetic develops osmotic diuresis leading to a hyperosmolar state with accelerated fluid loss and dehydration.[3,6]

Several pathologic changes are distinguishing diabetic features (*i.e.,* neuropathies, angiopathies, and immunopathies), all predisposing the diabetic to infection.[3,6,10,12] The presence of diabetic neuropathy predisposes these patients to infection by decreasing their sensitivity to chemical, mechanical, thermal, and other injurious processes. Diabetic neuropathy results from angiopathic changes in the vasa nervorum, damage to nerve sheath synthesis, or elevated blood sugars, which lead to an increase in polyalcohol sorbitol accumulation.[6] Diabetic neuropathy leads to numbness, tingling, aching, burning, and, if of longstanding, Charcot's joint. Frequently, ulceration occurs on the plantar surfaces of the feet. The autonomic changes include anhydrosis with dryness and fissuring of the skin. Motor loss usually manifests itself as wasting of the intrinsic muscles in the extremities.

Diabetic Angiopathy

These vascular lesions appear 50 times more frequently, progress to more advanced stages, and tend to be more widespread in diabetics over the age of 40 than

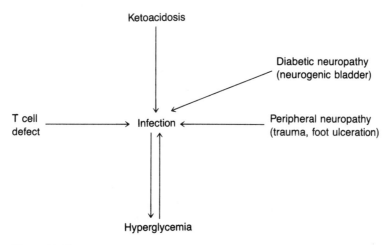

Figure 11–2.
Factors interacting in the diabetic with infection.

in nondiabetics. Diabetic angiopathy is the most common cause of morbidity and mortality in the diabetic patient. These vascular lesions, which jeopardize the viability of the skin and lead to infection, attack both the large vessels (macroangiopathy) and small vessels (microangiopathy). Diabetic angiopathic changes (1) are more diffuse, (2) show an increase in bilateral involvement (the second limb syndrome), (3) demonstrate more disease below the knee, (4) present with gangrene more often, and (5) demonstrate more extensive microangiopathy than in nondiabetics.[5, 6, 12]

The microangiopathic changes in this disease do not necessarily progress at the same rate as in the large vessels. No organ, however, is immune from the effects of diabetic microangiopathy. The cause of this microangiopathy is multifactorial (*i.e.*, capillary basement membrane thickening, increased blood viscosity, platelet aggregation, and an accelerated capillary epithelial cell aging process). The increased incidence of microvascular disease in diabetics needs better documentation through light microscopy vascular casting and physiologic studies.[6]

Diabetic Immunopathy and Host Defense Mechanisms

The host defense mechanisms in the diabetic at the cellular level are altered by hyperglycemia, peripheral vascular disease, neuropathy, impaired phagocytic activity, and a decreased response of lymphocytes to stimulation and impaired wound healing. The impaired phagocytic activity may represent a constellation of processes including a reduction of *in vitro* leukocyte chemotaxis, reduced leukocyte adherence, decreased intracellular killing of organisms, or impaired leukocyte mobilization. Once an infection is begun in a neuropathic or angiopathic diabetic foot, the mortality and morbidity increase significantly.[8]

Normal skin usually maintains a nonpenetrating barrier hostile to most pathogenic bacteria. Although skin and blood glucose levels are directly related, minimal evidence exists that diabetics with skin infections have higher blood glucose determinations. Normal nutrition, adequate tissue oxygen, and an adequate blood supply are essential factors in the delivery of humoral and cellular components to the immune system.[3] Polymorphonuclear cells and macrophages metabolize glucose by way of anaerobic glycolysis. A vast amount of information is currently available on the types and function of lymphocytes including substances elaborated by these cells when exposed to antigens. In diabetics, agglutinating antibodies to *Salmonella typhi*, *Escherichia coli*, and *Staphylococcus aureus* are decreased. There are decreased antitoxin antibodies to *Staphylococcus aureus* and *Corynebacterium diphtheriae* in diabetics when compared with nondiabetics.[6] Other studies, however, have failed to confirm these findings. Phagocytosis of bacteria occurs poorly in the absence of opsonization. Bacterial phagocytosis in some diabetics could be improved with better control of their metabolic state. Cell-mediated immunity as measured by blast transformation of peripheral blood lymphocytes has been measured and found altered in diabetic patients.[3, 5, 10]

THE DIABETIC AND INFECTION

Certain infections occur almost exclusively in diabetic patients while other infections occur no more frequently than in the general population. Fifty-four percent of type I diabetic adults are nasal carriers of *Staphylococcus aureus* compared to 34% of nondiabetics. Diabetic patients have a worse prognosis than nondiabetics with certain infections such as staphylococcal bacteremias, acute pyelonephritis, and emphysematous pyelonephritis.[3,7] A study of patients admitted to an intensive care unit with diabetic ketoacidosis revealed that 26% of these cases were caused by infections; in the next highest group, no etiology could be determined.[3] In another well-controlled study of diabetic patients admitted to an intensive care unit, infection was the precipitating cause of their ketoacidosis in 77% of these cases.[6] Presently and in the future the major cause of morbidity and mortality will be infection.

Bacteremiology

Certain bacteria appear to pose a particular threat to the diabetic patient:

Staphylococcal Bacteremia

Skin infections and intravascular catheters are common foci for infection. Both granulocyte deficiencies and impaired cell-mediated immunity may be responsible for the increased severity of staphylococcal disease among diabetic patients.

Streptococcal Bacteremia

Beta-hemolytic streptococci of the Lancefield Group B have a striking predilection for diabetics. The drug of choice for the treatment of Group B streptococcal infections is penicillin.

Gram-Negative Rod Bacteremia

This bacteremia is usually related to urinary or gastrointestinal tract infections or gallbladder disease in the hospitalized patient. In the diabetic, the synergistic gangrene and gram-negative rod pneumonias are a serious hazard. Numerous studies confirm a high prevalence of diabetes among patients with gram-negative rod bacteremias with a mortality rate almost twice the overall mortality in these cases. These infections require the use of aminoglycosides, which may be toxic to diabetic patients with compromised renal function. The dosages of aminoglycosides and the status of renal function must both be monitored carefully.

Tuberculosis and Fungal Infections

Cell-mediated immunity is the major host defense mechanism against tuberculosis. Diabetes was second only to alcoholism as a major factor in the reactivation of tuberculosis. In diabetics with tuberculosis, the incidence of the active disease is three times greater in those with severe diabetes. The treatment for tuberculosis is well established and has been most effective in avoiding the reactivation of the tuberculous process in the diabetic.

The bacteriology of the diabetic usually involves mixed flora, overlooked until recent years. With the advent of improved methods of tissue culture, obligate anaerobes are now known to play a significant role in these infections. Sapico demonstrated a mean of 4.1 species isolated from diabetic infections (2.84 aerobes and 1.97 anaerobes). The most common aerobic isolates were *Proteus mirabilis,* group D Streptococcus, *E. coli,* and *Staphylococcus aureus.* The most common anaerobes were *Bacteroides fragilis* followed by peptococcus. *Clostridium perfringens* was seldom isolated.[9]

The location from which a culture is obtained and the technique employed is important for the isolation of the infectious agent(s). Improved results are observed when a biopsy of deep tissue is performed for culture and sensitivity under aseptic conditions. Organisms in deep tissues often cannot be cultured from superficial tissues. When compared with other techniques (*i.e.,* swabbing of the ulcer, needle aspiration, and curettage of the ulcer base), the best yield consistently comes from deep cultures. The least reliable method is the superficial ulcer swab technique.[3,6]

Skin and Soft Tissue Infections

Skin infections caused by *Staphylococcus aureus* are more common among diabetic persons. Skin infections occur more frequently, are more severe, and are more intractable in diabetics than nondiabetic persons. Postoperative infections also are more common among diabetic than nondiabetic patients. Fungal infections in the diabetic patient are aggravated by obesity and prior antimicrobial therapy. *Candida* skin infections will occur in moist, warm areas around the breasts, thighs, and genitalia. These infections result in breakdown of skin and the entrance of virulent organisms into the systemic circulation.[7]

Necrotizing Infections

These infections of the skin and underlying soft tissues are serious and often life-threatening infections (Fig. 11-3). They are caused by multiple bacteria but mainly include *Staphylococcus aureus,* followed by streptococci, enterobacteria, and *Pseudomonas.* Other microorganisms involved include bacteria acting synergistically with microaerophilic or aerobic gram-positive organisms such as peptococci, peptostreptococci, or gram-negative bacteroides. Nonclostridial gas gangrene is more common in the diabetic than clostridial gas infection. This syndrome is probably related to the angiopathy and neuropathy diabetics have, leading to minor infections that become difficult to eradicate. Aerobic organisms use the already compromised oxygen supply, which symbiotically allows anaerobic organisms to thrive. The presentation of necrotizing infections may vary from that of an indolent ulcer to a fulminant infection with severe systemic toxicity and possibly death.[5,6,9]

These patients present with a high fever and are very toxic, with skin ulcers draining a serosanguinous, purulent type discharge. Subcutaneous gas may or may

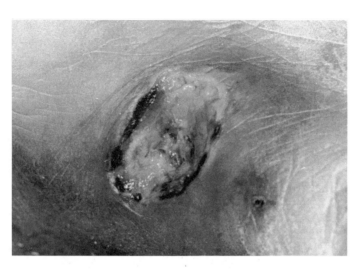

Figure 11–3.
Necrotizing enterocolitis.

not be present and can be confirmed with CT scan of the anterior abdominal wall or an abdominal radiograph. Muscle and fascia infection is more extensively involved as the underlying microangiopathy of diabetes leads to occlusive disease. Such infections may occur on the lower anterior abdominal wall, the perineum, and pelvic areas where anaerobic organisms are common. These infections may occur in the extremities where the blood supply is compromised or along the deep fascial planes of the neck from infected teeth. The mortality rate in Stone's series was 85% for diabetics and 44% for nondiabetics.[11] Surprisingly, in these syndromes gas formation is more common with aerobic infections.

In yet another study of diabetic patients with nonclostridial gas gangrene of the lower extremities, only 3 of 83 organisms cultured were anaerobic.[3] *Clostridium perfringens* is penicillin sensitive; however, anaerobes such as bacteroides require clindamycin and cefoxitin. Extensive, prompt, and radical surgical debridement is the *sine qua non* of treatment and should be performed early in the course of these infections. Similar infections of the hand require careful debridement to minimize tissue loss and the later need for amputation. The majority of these infections are synergistic and, when left untreated or inadequately treated, will progress to polymicrobial osteomyelitis.

Malignant Otitis Externa

Over 90% of the recorded cases of malignant otitis externa (MOE) have occurred in diabetics over 35 years of age. With a mortality over 50%, this disease has an appropriate name. *Pseudomonas aeruginosa* is usually the offending organism and rarely are other organisms involved. These organisms invade and produce an infectious vasculitis, which compounds the treatment difficulties. These patients present with a chronic ear infection, otalgia, and a purulent discharge from the external auditory canal. Granulation polyps that develop in the floor of the external canal strongly suggest this disease. MOE spreads along the ridge between cartilage and bone in the auditory canal and, if untreated, progresses to involve the soft tissues of the parotid gland, temporomandibular joint, mastoid, and the seventh cranial nerve (the earliest neurologic complication). Mortality is quite high. Parenteral antibiotics (usually carbenicillin or ticarcillin plus tobramycin or gentamicin) combined with surgical debridement are the appropriate methods of management.[3,5,9]

Mucormycosis

Mucormycosis (mycoses due to fungi of the order *Mucorales* including species of *Mucor, Absidia,* and especially *Rhizopus*), a highly virulent infection, occurs most commonly in diabetics. The organisms initially colonize in the nose and paranasal sinuses and spread by direct extension to the orbit and periorbital tissues. Infrequently, ischemic infarction of the eyelid and orbital contents will develop, causing blindness and loss of sensation in the distribution of the trigeminal nerve (ophthalmic division). Black necrotic tissue may be seen in the nose or hard palate. If the disease progresses, it will invade the internal jugular vein, and cavernous sinus thrombosis will develop. Early biopsy of the nasal turbinates or pharyngeal tissues for culture and sensitivity will assist the diagnosis and management. Extensive surgical debridement is necessary and predictably disfiguring. Amphotericin is the antimicrobial agent of choice.[3,5,9]

Urinary Tract Infections (UTI)

Data available today lead to different conclusions regarding the increased incidence of wound infections in the urinary tract in diabetics. Wheat observed a two- to fourfold higher incidence of bacteriuria in diabetic women, while Gocke concluded that in the well-controlled diabetic UTI are no more likely than in nondiabetics.[1,4,13]

Within populations in whom the prevalence of UTI is increased, the diabetic is even more likely than a nondiabetic to develop UTI. Time-honored reasons for this increase in the diabetic is their neurogenic bladder with accompanying urinary stasis and frequent catheterizations often associated with underlying renal disease, and an impaired host defense system. Any diabetic not responding to adequate antimicrobial therapy within 3 to 4 days should provoke suspicion of a UTI or a perinephric abscess (PNA). The organisms usually associated with PNA are *Staphylococcus aureus,* which cause cortical abscesses by the hematogenous route. A well described but infrequent complication of UTI in the diabetic is renal papillary necrosis. This condition is related to renal ischemia and is accompanied by a rapid deterioration of renal function, fever, flank pain, and a poor response to antibiotics. Abdominal radiograms will confirm the diagnosis with the presence of mottled lucencies within the kidney, ureter, or bladder.[3,6,13]

In one study, 7% of diabetic patients developed septic shock after surgery compared with 1% for nondiabetics; in 86% of these cases that developed gram-negative shock, an *E. coli* UTI was the source of the bacteremia.[3] Fungal infections of the urinary tract in diabetic patients are not uncommon and probably result from the use of prolonged antibiotics for bacterial infections and subsequent *Candida* species overgrowth. Infections with the fungus *Torulopsis glabrata* occur in the elderly and may also infect the diabetic bladder. Patients who have a *Candida* colony of greater than 10,000/ml from a clean-catch specimen should be followed by a culture of a catheterized specimen. If the *Candida* colony count is still greater than 10,000/ml, then the patient should be treated as an actual UTI and not just colonization.[3,4]

Emphysematous Cholecystitis

This severe, fulminating infection caused by gas-producing organisms occurs frequently in diabetics. Of 136 proven cases, diabetes mellitus was found in 38%.[3,5] This disease differs from emphysematous pyelonephritis in that *Clostridium perfringens* is isolated in one half the cases. Although emphysematous cholecystitis presents with the same signs and symptoms as cholecystitis, the morbidity and mortality are alarmingly high. Gallbladder perforation and gangrene are frequent. The mortality is three to ten times higher than in the sporadic variety of acute cholecystitis. The male-to-female ratio is 3 : 1, the reverse of that seen in the commonly occurring acute cholecystitis. Diabetic vascular disease has been implicated in the pathogenesis of this unusual syndrome as it has been with the other gas-forming infections. The diagnosis is made by radiographic evidence of gas in the gallbladder wall (Fig. 11-4). Inasmuch as the presence of gas may be seen in the first 48 hours of infection and

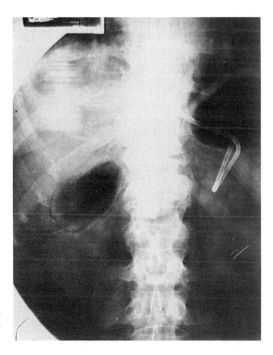

Figure 11-4.
Abdominal radiograph of a 72-year-old diabetic male with acute emphysematous cholecystitis.

spreads to surrounding tissues in the next 48 hours, abdominal flat films should be obtained every day for 4 days to track the emphysematous and perigallbladder involvement. The appropriate management of emphysematous cholecystitis is early surgical intervention. The antimicrobial coverage is penicillin, clindamycin, and an aminoglycoside. Closure of the abdominal incision by tertiary wound healing is preferred.[3,5,8,9]

SURGERY AND THE DIABETIC

Surgical conditions commonly associated with diabetes are occlusive vascular disease of the extremities, cholelithiasis, cataracts, and infections. During their lifetimes, 50% of the diabetic population will undergo one or more operations. Control of potential infections with antimicrobial agents in the diabetic whose resistance to bacterial invasion is reduced during hyperglycemia is important. Unsuspected infections in diabetics are common and may lead to sepsis in a patient whose resistance is lowered during stress-induced hyperglycemia. These patients benefit significantly from the appropriate management of fluids and electrolytes, nutritional replacement, and cardiopulmonary monitoring. A more aggressive management of diabetics with infections is both warranted and justified.

The preoperative recognition and evaluation of conditions known to be increased in diabetics (coronary, cerebral, and peripheral arterial disease) are essential to prevent complications during the perioperative period. Diabetic neuropathy may decrease vascular responses during periods of operative stress, provoke GI ileus and urinary retention. Alterations in renal function associated with diabetic neuropathy will cause disturbances in fluid and electrolyte balance. These recognizable risks in the surgical diabetic patient can be managed effectively if one obtains an adequate medical history with particular emphasis on the diabetic facts. Careful surveillance for conditions that may threaten overall surgical intervention is constantly needed.

Effects of Stress on Diabetes

Surgical stress will adversely affect the metabolic status of the diabetic patient through the influence of counterregulatory hormones, which increase the demand for insulin. In the type I diabetic patient, the catabolic effect of insulin deprivation results in (1) lipid mobilization and ketogenesis, (2) proteolysis with amino acid conversion through gluconeogenesis to increase the glucose pool and hyperglycemia, and (3) suppression of branch chain amino acid uptake by muscle. These changes are accelerated by the combined actions of catecholamines, cortisol, glucagon, and growth hormones. Such effects are related in magnitude to the severity of the stress and can be modified by matching insulin requirements with insulin administration.[5,6,8]

The type II patient experiencing operative stress will manifest similar alterations due to insulinopenia and resistance to insulin action is imposed by counter-insulin hormones. During major surgical procedures, insulin therapy is required for peripheral glucose utilization and prevention of increased gluconeogenesis. Inadequate treatment may lead to hyperosmolar nonketotic coma or, in severe cases, to ketoacidosis. Overly aggressive therapy will lead to hypoglycemia.[3,8]

Preoperatively, the medical and psychologic factors of diabetics warrant comparable attention. Analysis of their metabolic status including nutrition and blood glucose control is important to establish optimal conditions for surgical management. The surgeon must review the frequently occurring aspects of the diabetic syndrome (*i.e.,* neuropathic, retinal, renal, and vascular complications) as potential problems arising in the perioperative period. Between 20% and 25% of patients who have diabetes are initially discovered at the time of their hospital admission for an elective surgical procedure.[3] These patients should be managed with regular insulin given in divided doses, and the blood sugar should be lowered over a period of 24 to 48 hours. Emergency conditions, of course, would not permit such a gradual approach. In all cases, frequent intraoperative blood sugar determinations can be a useful monitor and guide to insulin and glucose therapy. The elective operation is best performed using regular insulin administered by the intravenous (IV) route. The insulin-dextrose infusion should be continued postoperatively until oral feedings are resumed. The diabetic state can then be stabilized during the convalescent period.

Preoperative medications are prescribed in lower doses than usual due to the increased depressing effects of these agents in diabetics and the elderly. The choice of anesthesia is based on the type of operation to be performed, the surgical risks, the medical status of the patient, and the skills of the anesthesiologist, without overriding concern for the diabetes. Spinal or intradural anesthesia will minimally affect blood glucose levels. Cardiopulmonary monitoring is now routine in all major surgical procedures.

Sustained hyperglycemia or hypoglycemia must be avoided during the operative procedure. Prolonged hyperglycemia induces urinary loss of water and electrolytes with a resulting hypovolemia and ketoacidosis. Hypoglycemia may result in serious central nervous system dysfunction. A blood glucose level between 100 and 200 mg/dl will provide protection against an unexpected drop or elevation in the blood glucose levels. Whether the diabetic patient should be scheduled in the early morning as opposed to the early evening is a moot question with regard to blood glucose control.

For elective surgery in type I diabetics, the use of regular insulin added to the IV glucose solution is preferred. Subcutaneous insulin is seldom used preoperatively. For type I diabetics using 40 units or less, 10 units of regular insulin added to the IV solution is adequate; 15 units should be added for those diabetics receiving 50 to 80 units of insulin per day; and 20 units should be added for those with a higher daily insulin dose.[8]

An alternate method would involve administering one third to one half of the total insulin dose subcutaneously the morning of the operation and replacing the morning feeding with a solution of 1000 ml of 5% dextrose. At the conclusion of the surgical procedure, a similar dose of insulin is administered in the recovery room. Blood glucose determinations are performed in the recovery room or in midafternoon (with both methods) as a guide to additional regular insulin doses. If the blood glucose is elevated to 250 mg/dl or above, an additional 6 units of regular insulin are given subcutaneously. If it is above 300 mg/dl, 8 to 10 units are given. During extended procedures, intraoperative blood glucose determinations will assist in recognizing and treating unexpected periods of hypoglycemia and hyperglycemia.[8, 13]

The type II diabetic patient is ketosis-resistant under normal conditions due to adequate endogenous insulin. Often the type II obese patient, with an insulin resistance and down-regulation of insulin receptors, will require additional insulin during stress.[8, 13] Blood glucose levels should be determined before and after the operation to recognize unsuspected hyperglycemia. Should the latter develop, exogenous insulin administration should be carried out as suggested for the type I diabetic.

For type II diabetics who demonstrate preoperatively a need for additional insulin support, the following regimen can be used: On the morning of the surgical procedure, 6 to 10 units of regular insulin are added to 1000 ml of 5% dextrose at a rate of 150 ml/hr. Blood sugar determinations are obtained in the recovery room and 8 hr postoperatively. Concentrations above 250 mg/dl will necessitate additional regular insulin, which may be administered subcutaneously.[3] Chemical hypoglycemia when encountered will necessitate lowering of the insulin content in the infused solution and, if symptomatic enough, a bolus of hypertonic glucose. Careful attention must be given to insulin administered by way of a 5% glucose solution due to the adherence of insulin to glassware and infusion equipment and its adsorption by the IV filter. This technique for monitoring and control of the diabetic undergoing major surgery using an insulin dextrose infusion is safe and effective.

Glucose-insulin fusions may be required for several days after the operation and will require blood sugar determinations at 8- to 12-hr intervals. Administration of insulin using the sliding scale based on urine glucose alone has not been satisfactory for determining insulin needs. Catheterization of the urinary bladder to obtain these results invariably leads to infection and should be avoided. Fluid and electrolyte replacement is continued until oral feedings are resumed. Additional fluids are required for elevated temperatures and extra renal losses (insensible and measured losses). The use of the insulin infusion pump, while having certain advantages, requires more frequent blood glucose determinations, and the possibility of pump failure always exists. The use of the artificial endocrine pancreas (Biostator) has created some intermittent interest. It is expensive and offers few advantages not already available.

The complications of diabetes mellitus are seldom totally prevented. Diabetics must be educated about diabetes if they are to lead a normal life. The diabetic can play a major role in reducing these risks to a bare minimum by not smoking; instituting regular eating habits; avoiding infection and trauma; protecting their feet by keeping them dry, warm, and clean; maintaining a normal weight; and routinely visiting their physicians. Attention to these details will minimize infection, increase limb survival, and prolong life.

REFERENCES

1. Bryan CS, Reynolds KL, Metzger WT. Bacteremia in diabetic patients: comparison of incidence and mortality with non-diabetic patients. Diabetes Care 1985;8(3):244.
2. Diabetes: facts you need to know. Alexandria, VA: The American Diabetes Association, 1985.

3. Ellenberg M, Refkin H. Diabetes mellitus, theory and practice. 3rd ed. New Hyde Park, NY: Medical Examination Publishing Co, 1972:667.

4. Gocke TM. Infections in the abnormal host. New York: Yorke Medical Books, 1980:585.

5. Larkin JG, Frier BM, Ireland JT. Diabetes mellitus and infection. Postgrad Med J 1985;6:233.

6. LeFrock JL, Joseph DPM. Lower extremity infections in diabetics. Infect Surg 1986;5(3):135.

7. Musher DM, McKenzie SO. Infections due to *Staphylococcus aureus*. Medicine 1977;56(5):383.

8. Rayfield EJ, Ault MJ, Keusch GT, et al. Infection and diabetes: the case for control. Am J Med 1982;72:439.

9. Sapico FC, Canwati HN, Witte JL. Quantitative aerobic and anaerobic bacteriology of the infected foot. J Clin Microbiol 1980;12:413.

10. Savin JA. Bacterial infections in diabetes mellitus. Br J Dermatol 1974;91:481.

11. Stone HH, Martin JD. Synergistic necrotizing cellulitis. Ann Surg 1972;175:702.

12. Warren S, LeCompte PM, Legg MA. Extremities, pathology of diabetes mellitus. 4th ed. Philadelphia: Lea & Febiger, 1966:284.

13. Wheat LJ. Infection and diabetes mellitus. Diabetes Care 1980;3(1):187.

12

○   ○   ○   ●   ●   ●

SURGICAL INFECTION IN NEUTROPENIC PATIENTS

Arthur E. Brown
Jerome J. DeCosse

In general, the principles of prevention and management of surgical infections in the neutropenic patient are similar to those principles already established for both the surgical patient and medical patient without neutropenia. Exceptions will be highlighted in this chapter. One must understand the problem and its magnitude, realize the likely causes of such infections, and know which therapeutic modalities are best applied.

We address the prevention and management of complications of neutropenia as seen by the surgeon. Serious "medical" complications of neutropenia, such as bacterial or fungal pneumonitis, are addressed peripherally. Detailed scrutiny of neutrophil physiology is provided in Chapter 23. General principles of management of surgical infections can be found in Chapter 7.

Magnitude of the Problem

Infection is a frequent cause of morbidity and the leading cause of death among patients with cancer.[3,7,9,10,38,51,52,58] Autopsy data from the National Cancer Institute and Memorial Sloan-Kettering Cancer Center (MSKCC)[34,42] from the mid-1950s through the earlier 1980s have demonstrated that infection is the leading cause of death among patients with leukemia[9] (Table 12-1). Both the increased risk of infection as well as its severity are related to profound suppression of host-defense mechanisms. Neutropenia is one of the most prominent examples of suppression of host-defense mechanisms. Neutropenia may be caused by hematologic neoplasms such as acute leukemia when there are very few functioning circulating granulocytic cells because the bone marrow has been replaced by blasts. Another major setting of neutropenia is the cancer patient who may have either a solid tumor or a hematologic malignancy and is receiving myelosuppressive chemotherapy, which leaves the bone marrow severely hypoplastic.

Although cancer chemotherapy, particularly in the leukemic patient, is by far the most common cause of neutropenia, neutropenia may also be seen in aplastic anemia, cyclic neutropenia, and after toxicity to certain drugs. Anemia and thrombocytopenia may also be associated with neutropenia.

Among experts in infectious diseases and oncology, it is agreed that the single most important factor determining the outcome of an infectious episode in the neutropenic patient is the absolute neutrophil count. Most conclude that the threshold for starting antibacterial therapy is an absolute neutrophil count of less than 1000/ mm^3. After initiation of therapy, the response of the absolute neutrophil count is a critical predictor of outcome. If the absolute neutrophil count falls below 100/mm^3 and remains at this low ebb for more than 10 to 14 days (*i.e.,* profound and prolonged neutropenia), the risk of a fatal infectious episode is magnified. Conversely, the rapid return of the absolute neutrophil count to more than 1000/mm^3 predicts a much more favorable outcome for the infectious episode.[3,7-10,38,51]

Table 12-1
Patterns of the Cause of Death in Autopsied Patients with Acute Leukemia

	NUMBER OF PATIENTS	HEMORRHAGE (%)	HEMORRHAGE AND INFECTION (%)	INFECTION (%)	OTHER (%)
1954–1959*	184	22	40	24	14
1960–1963*	182	14	23	44	19
1965–1971†	229	11	10	69	10
1976–1984‡	132	22	14	53	11

* *Data from Hersh EM, Bodey GP, Nies BA, et al. Causes of death in acute leukemia. JAMA 1965; 193:99.*
† *Data from Levine AS, Schimpff SC, Graw RG Jr, et al. Hematologic malignancies and other marrow failure states: progress in the management of complicating infections. Semin Hematol 1974; 11:141.*
‡*Pediatrics Department, Memorial Sloan-Kettering Cancer Center.*

Thus, because of the magnitude of this problem, empiric antibacterial therapy in the febrile, neutropenic patient with neoplastic disease has become standard care.

Organisms Causing Infections in the Neutropenic Patient

In order to understand the therapeutic choices that are to be applied in the febrile, neutropenic patient, the etiologic agents most likely responsible for infection in these patients must be understood. At initial presentation, bacterial organisms are of paramount concern. Patterns of infection in such patients are changing in the United States. Although gram-positive organisms[6,9,10,14,28,52,66] including *Staphylococcus epidermidis* are emerging as important pathogens in the setting of the febrile, neutropenic patient, the aerobic, gram-negative, enteric bacilli remain the principal bacterial pathogens against which antibacterial regimens must be directed.

Additional emphasis is given to this point when one considers the respective mortality in patients who are septicemic with organisms such as *Escherichia coli*, *Klebsiella* species, and *Pseudomonas aeruginosa* (Table 12-2). Startling mortality in excess of 50%[9,10,62] firmly supports the basis for beginning an empiric regimen that more than amply covers these pathogens. Initial empiric regimens must be directed against these organisms whenever there are no focal symptoms, signs, or laboratory evidence to suggest a specific microbiologic diagnosis, and thus more specific therapy.

Bacterial Infections

Initially, bacterial infections occur when febrile, neutropenic patients are first admitted to the hospital.[3,62] Both gram-positive cocci and enteric gram-negative bacilli are responsible for early infections in the febrile, neutropenic patient. After

Table 12–2
Etiology of Sepsis in Patients with Leukemia and Lymphoma

ORGANISM	PERCENTAGE OF TOTAL EPISODES (%)	PERCENTAGE MORTALITY (%)
Escherichia coli	23.6	25.4
Pseudomonas aeruginosa	14.9	54.3
Klebsiella species	10.8	66.0
Staphylococcus aureus	9.4	14.3
Candida species	4.7	71.5
Streptococcus pyogenes	3.4	20.0
Others	15.0	
Polymicrobic	16.9	56.0
Overall mortality		40.5

(Singer CF, Kaplan MH, Armstrong D. Bacteremia and fungemia complicating neoplastic disease: a study of 364 cases. Am J Med 1977; 62:731.)

prolonged hospitalization and treatment with various broad-spectrum, antimicrobial agents, infection may be caused by resistant nosocomial bacterial pathogens, either gram-positive or gram-negative, or infections may be caused by fungi.

Initial Gram-Positive Infections

Organisms that cause infections in normal hosts cause infections in the neutropenic host as well. The severity and duration of the infection is more marked in the neutropenic host compared to the normal host. Organisms to be anticipated are *Staphylococcus aureus, Streptococcus pyogenes*, and *Streptococcus pneumoniae* as etiologic agents of pneumonia and septicemia in the neutropenic host. Skin and supporting-structure infections may be due to *Staphylococcus aureus* and *Streptococcus pyogenes* either alone or in combination. Stomatitis may also result from *Staphylococcus aureus*.[3]

Later Gram-Positive Organisms

Septicemia due to *Staphylococcus epidermidis*,[28] viridans streptococci,[66] enterococci,[9,10] *Corynebacterium* species type CDC-JK,[6] and *Bacillus* species may be found in hospitalized patients who have received broad-spectrum antibiotic therapy for periods usually longer than 1 week and who develop a new fever. Often, *Staphylococcus epidermidis* infections are resistant to the semisynthetic penicillins (methicillin, oxacillin, nafcillin); they may require treatment with vancomycin. The isolation of viridans streptococci from blood should not be dismissed as a "contaminant," especially in a neutropenic patient who has a new temperature elevation and evidence of an oropharyngeal source of infection. More viridans streptococci resistant to penicillin are being reported, and vancomycin may need to be the treatment of choice until sensitivities are known.[10,66]

Superinfection with enterococci during hospitalization while a patient is neutropenic is a relatively new problem. At MSKCC,[9,10] we have seen enterococci emerge as a significant pathogen among patients treated with third-generation cephalosporins, particularly moxalactam. Although these organisms are susceptible to ampicillin, vancomycin is usually added when the microbiology laboratory reports that "gram-positive cocci" are seen on Gram's stain of a blood culture specimen. It is practical to change to ampicillin once the organism has been formally identified and the sensitivities are known. There have been both significant morbidity and mortality from such infections.

Corynebacterium species type CDC-JK is a gram-positive organism that may be mistaken for a contaminant. This organism is a variant of the common skin flora often referred to as "diphtheroids." Its special features make it recognizable to microbiologists and clinicians alike. Unlike the rod-shaped "diphtheroids," CDC-JK is more cocco-bacillary or even coccoid on Gram's stain. Most important, it is sensitive only to vancomycin. Skin colonization with CDC-JK may be the harbinger of sepsis due to this organism. Reduction of skin colonization with good personal hygiene techniques and use of a povidone–iodine-based soap has significantly reduced the frequency of CDC-JK bacteremia in our institution.[6]

A fifth gram-positive organism, which has more recently been found to be a problem in neutropenic, febrile patients who have been hospitalized for an extended period of time, is *Bacillus* species.[4,35,48] This organism has also been found among patients with indwelling intravascular lines, particularly Broviac and Hickman catheters. It has also been seen in intensive care unit settings where arterial lines have been used. Appropriate antimicrobial therapy and removal of the central line usually effect a cure of this infection.

Initial Gram-Negative Infections

Generally, patients who are febrile and neutropenic on admission to the hospital (not having been recently discharged from a hospital) are quite likely to be infected with *Enterobacteriaceae* (*Escherichia coli, Klebsiella* species, *Enterobacter* species, *Serratia* species, *Proteus* species) or *Pseudomonas aeruginosa*.[9,10,62] These organisms are among those most likely to cause the most serious and most life-threatening infections in the febrile, neutropenic patient. Therefore, the main thrust of initial empiric antibiotic therapy is aimed at these particular organisms. These organisms are responsible for the high mortality outlined at the opening of this chapter. Mortality ranging from 25% to 66% has been described.[9,10,62]

Furthermore, polymicrobial septicemia occurs frequently and is often fatal with mortality greater than 50%.[22,62] Traditionally, combinations of a beta-lactam antibiotic and an aminoglycoside have been used empirically to treat such presumed infections in febrile, neutropenic patients. These combinations may consist of two to three antibiotics, and the choice of combination may best be determined by the sensitivity patterns in a given hospital. Thus, the choice of which aminoglycoside (gentamicin, tobramycin, amikacin, or netilmicin) to use as the "first-line" drug may be different in New York than in Chicago, or different among different hospitals within the same city.

Later Gram-Negative Infections

Infection from highly resistant gram-negative bacilli pose difficult problems for the neutropenic patient who has become febrile again after an extended hospitalization. The choice of antimicrobial agent to add or substitute should be predicated by what is known about the microflora in a given hospital setting or even a given ward or given patient cohort. Second- and third-generation cephalosporins, extended-spectrum penicillins, combinations of beta-lactamase inhibitors with beta-lactam antibiotics, carbapenams, monobactams, and carboxyquinolones as well as tobramycin and amikacin all have a role here.

At the time of a new temperature elevation, it is essential that the patient be completely reevaluated and that all sites be recultured to allow a specific microbial diagnosis. On physical exam, there may be few clues as to the microbial cause of fever. These clues may be quite subtle, because the neutropenic patient may not have florid classic signs of inflammation—rubor, calor, tumor, and dolor. There will not be laudable pus. Instead, there may be only the slightest hint of erythema and tenderness.

Fungal Infections

Neutropenic patients who have been hospitalized for longer than a week, who have been treated with broad-spectrum antibacterial agents for presumed or proven sepsis, who have defervesced, and who have culture results that have been unrevealing with regard to a bacterial pathogen, particularly gram-positive cocci or bacilli, but who have a new temperature elevation, are the kind of patient in whom opportunistic fungal infections often are present. In this setting, invasive candidiasis, aspergillosis, and mucormycosis must all be considered. Environmental organisms such as *Trichosporon* species,[24,31,43,65] *Pseudallescheria boydii,* and *Fusarium* species[2,5,18,19,33,37,70] have also been reported to cause invasive disease in neutropenic patients.

Mortality ranging from 50% to 100% has been reported in cases of invasive fungal disease.[62] Amphotericin B remains the standard therapy against which all future antifungal agents must be judged regarding efficacy. Certain combinations of antifungal therapy, such as amphotericin B and 5-flucytosine, may be considered in the treatment of invasive candidiasis, but efficacy remains to be determined in prospective, randomized clinical trials. Whether new triazole antifungal agents will prove to be equal or better than amphotericin B also remains to be validated in clinical trials.

HOST-DEFENSE MECHANISMS IN NEUTROPENIA

Although neutropenia is defined here as an absolute neutrophil count below $1000/mm^3$, there are variations on this in terms of the degree of neutropenia and the duration of neutropenia. These variations have profound prognostic implications with regard to morbidity and mortality. Furthermore, additional factors, such as T-cell defects, B-cell defects, splenectomy, and interruption of mechanical barriers, which normally protect the host from invasive infectious disease, contribute to the outcome in hospitalized, neutropenic patients. Duration of hospitalization and the application of strict hospital infection-control techniques also influence the prognosis.

Duration of Neutropenia

Morbidity and mortality from infection are directly proportional to the length of time that a patient remains neutropenic and febrile. Prolonged neutropenia (longer than 10 days, as seen in leukemia during relapse–reinduction) is a risk factor for subsequent infection due to nosocomial bacteria and/or fungi. Conversely, patients with a solid tumor who receive myelosuppressive chemotherapy may be neutropenic for only 5 to 7 days and are less likely to have the same infectious sequelae as leukemic patients with prolonged neutropenia. Moreover, patients with a solid tumor have microbiologically documented infection less often, and fewer still have *Pseudomonas aeruginosa* septicemia and/or pneumonia.

The converse of the proposal (*i.e.*, that the rate of fall of the absolute neutrophil count is, in part, responsible for infectious mortality) also holds true for the rate of recovery of the absolute neutrophil count.[52] Because granulocyte precursors are suppressed for a more limited interval in an otherwise intact bone marrow, patients with a solid tumor who do not have bone marrow disease do better in terms of neutrophil recovery and, therefore, have less mortality from infection.[62] This may have a bearing on understanding of some clinical studies that employed monotherapy with success. Patients with short-term neutropenia will almost always get better so long as prompt and adequate empiric therapy is instituted.

Profound Neutropenia

Most oncologists and infectious-disease specialists agree with the definition of profound neutropenia as an absolute neutrophil count less than $100/mm^3$. Some believe that this is the true "benchmark" at which an infectious episode is most likely to begin.[9, 10, 51] After induction or reinduction chemotherapy, patients with leukemia almost invariably will have profound neutropenia, as will some patients with solid tumors. Depending on the chemotherapeutic regimen, profound neutropenia may persist for an interval varying from a few days to 6 weeks. Patients with profound and prolonged neutropenia are at the highest risk of dying from either an initial gram-negative bacillary sepsis, consequent nosocomial infection, or fungal infection.

Other Mechanisms

Because the complications of neutropenia occur particularly in the gastrointestinal tract of the cancer patient, other etiologic factors can be incriminated. Breaks in mucous membranes, either from chemotherapy or from trauma, permit bacterial colonization in these patients who are immunosuppressed. Administration of steroids, irradiation, and the presence of, or the consequences of, malnutrition surely contribute to these complications. Moreover, some chemotherapeutic agents, such as vincristine, by altering colonic motility and thereby modifying colonic microflora, may contribute to the necrotizing effects of profound neutropenia. Other chemotherapeutic agents can induce gastrointestinal ulcerations.

Other Immune Defects

Patients who are neutropenic may also have other immune defects (Table 12-3), such as decreased cell-mediated immunity (T-cell function) or diminished humoral immunity (B-cell function), or they may have undergone splenectomy or be physiologically asplenic, as after radiation to the spleen. Many of these defects may occur in combination.

Interruption of Mechanical Barriers (Table 12-4)

Breaks in the skin or mucous membranes of the gastrointestinal tract or respiratory tree allow microbial agents to become pathogens and lead to sepsis. Whether these are intentional breaks in the skin (*e.g.,* venipuncture or bone-marrow biopsy sites) or a chemotherapy-induced mucositis, the results are the same—infection may occur in a neutropenic patient.

Table 12–3
Immune Defects in Patients with Neoplastic Diseases

DEFECT	EXAMPLES
Neutropenia	Acute leukemia
	Chemotherapy
Impaired cell-mediated immunity (T-cell)	Hodgkin's disease
	Corticosteroids
	Chemotherapy
Abnormal immunoglobins (B-cell)	Multiple myeloma
	Chronic lymphocytic leukemia
	Corticosteroids
	Chemotherapy
Splenectomy	Staging laparotomy in Hodgkin's disease

(Brown AE. Neutropenia, fever, and infection. Am J Med 1984; 76:421.)

Length of Hospitalization

The longer a patient is hospitalized, the more likely is infection with a nosocomial organism, which may well be resistant to the administered antibiotic regimen.

Adherence to Hospital Infection-Control Practices

Simple measures among hospital staff, patients, and visitors, such as adherence to ordinary handwashing protocol, are essential preventive measures to keep neutropenic patients from becoming infected. Guidelines for vascular access and isolation must be followed scrupulously.

PREVENTION

There are many strategies to be considered for the prevention of sepsis in the neutropenic patient. Some take into consideration standard methods and techniques, whereas others are quite controversial. Most of these will be examined here, and an attempt will be made to put them in perspective.

Strategies for preventing infection in the neutropenic patient include: (1) protected environments, (2) gastrointestinal decontamination, (3) systemic prophylaxis, and (4) prevention of infection due to specific pathogens.

Protected Environments

The most rigorous hospital precaution, the laminar airflow unit, is appropriate in the bone-marrow transplant unit but is neither required nor fiscally feasible for routine care of the neutropenic patient.[2] Instead, good personal hygiene as well as

Table 12–4
Mechanical Defects and Organisms to be Anticipated in Patients with Neoplastic Diseases

DEFECTS	BACTERIA	FUNGI	VIRUSES	PARASITES
Interrupted integument				
Skin	*Staphylococcus aureus*	*Candida* species	Herpes simplex	
Venipuncture	*Staphylococcus epidermidis*		Varicella	
Finger stick	*Streptococcus pyogenes*			
Bone marrow biopsy	*Corynebacterium* CDC-JK			
Lumbar puncture	*Escherichia coli*			
Bladder catheter	*Klebsiella–Enterobacter–Serratia*			
Venous/arterial catheter	*Pseudomonas aeruginosa*			
	Other nosocomial antibiotic-resistant organisms			
Mucous membranes	*Staphylococcus aureus*	*Candida* species	Herpes simplex	
Cytotoxic chemo-therapy	*Staphylococcus epidermidis*			
Respiratory support	*Streptococcus pyogenes*			
Endoscopy	*Viridans streptococci*			
	Other streptococci			
	Corynebacterium CDC-JK			
	Escherichia coli			
	Klebsiella–Enterobacter–Serratia			
	Salmonella species			
	Pseudomonas aeruginosa			
	Bacteroides species			
	Other nosocomial antibiotic-resistant organisms			
Intravenous solutions and blood products	Enterobacteriaceae	*Candida* species	Cytomegalovirus	*Toxoplasma gondii*
			Epstein-Barr virus	*Plasmodium* species
			Hepatitis B	*Babesia* species
			Non-A/non-B hepatitis	*Trypanosoma Cruzi*
			HIV	
Surgical procedures	*Staphylococcus aureus*	*Candida* species	Herpes simplex	
	Streptococcus pyogenes			
	Enterobacteriaceae, *Salmonella* species			
	Pseudomonas aeruginosa			
	Bacteroides fragilis			
	Nosocomial bacteria			

(Brown AE. Neutropenia, fever, and infection. Am J Med 1984; 76:421.)

vigorous handwashing by patients, visitors, and staff with a povidone–iodine soap will provide much of the protection needed. Reverse isolation is not required of the staff and visitors outside of the laminar airflow unit.

Breaks in the skin or in mucous membranes of the gastrointestinal tract or respiratory tract permit access by microflora; therefore, a determined effort should be made to prevent or minimize these breaks. Dental prophylaxis before induction of chemotherapy will help prevent oral sepsis. Catheter lines need meticulous care. Tunneled catheters may be less likely to become infected; rigorous dressing changes are necessary.

In order to avoid anal sepsis, stool softeners should be administered to prevent constipation. Generally, neither rectal temperatures nor rectal suppositories are used. Rectal examinations are limited in frequency and are performed gently and with a well-lubricated examining finger.

Educational programs are important for both the patient and the hospital staff. For example, fresh fruit, vegetables, and salads are ill-advised in order to reduce enteric exposure to microorganisms. The patient with indwelling catheters should be advised not to swim.

Gastrointestinal Decontamination

Oral Nonabsorbable Antibiotics

Oral nonabsorbable antibiotics are not used routinely in the neutropenic patient at most U.S. cancer centers but are administered in Europe and South America. They are used here in bone-marrow transplant units where total decontamination and laminar flow are used in the cytoreduced patient about to undergo transplantation. Another difficulty with oral nonabsorbable antibiotics is the lack of patient compliance with the regimens devised; the taste is marginally acceptable. Other problems include emergence of organisms resistant to the oral agents.

Selective Decontamination

Partial decontamination with oral absorbable antibiotics such as sulfamethox-azole-trimethoprim, naladixic acid, norfloxacin, and ciprofloxacin lead to the attrac-tive concept of selective decontamination. Here, the concept of "colonization resist-ance factor" addresses a notion that one can obliterate the aerobic gut flora but leave intact the anaerobic gut flora, and that resistance will not emerge. It seems that this concept works only in highly selected patients who will be neutropenic for extended periods of time. There have been reports of resistant organisms developing while patients were receiving prophylaxis. With sulfamethoxazole-trimethoprim, there is a risk of more pronounced neutropenia from the sulfamethoxazole-trimethoprim itself.

Systemic Prophylaxis

The neutropenic patient can receive additional protection from a variety of oral and parenteral antimicrobial agents. These agents range in their activity from antibacterial, antifungal, antiprotozoan, and antihelmintic, to antiviral. Prevention of infection by specific pathogens is presented in terms of immunoprophylaxis by either active or passive immunization and by chemoprophylaxis.

Prevention of Infection-Specific Pathogens

Bacteria

Active immunization is feasible against *Streptococcus pneumoniae* by administering pneumococcal vaccine, preferably 7 to 10 days before splenectomy. Immunization with *Pseudomonas* vaccine is controversial. Passive immunization may be obtained by intravenous immune globulin, hyperimmune globulin, and emerging human and murine monoclonal antibodies. These are still investigational methods. Chemoprophylaxis against *Streptococcus pneumoniae* with penicillin is recommended for patients who have had splenectomy, in order to be protected from the overwhelming postsplenectomy sepsis syndrome due to pneumococcus. Even patients who have had pneumococcal vaccine before splenectomy should have penicillin prophylaxis.

Yeast

No current immunoprophylactic measures exist for preventing yeast infections in the neutropenic patient. Indeed, this is a fertile area for laboratory and clinical investigation. Chemoprophylaxis of yeast infection may be accomplished by one of several agents. Included among these are nystatin, ketoconazole, clotrimazole, amphotericin B, and miconazole. Triazole antifungal agents are currently in clinical trials to evaluate their prophylactic efficacy.

Parasites

The patient with acute lymphoblastic leukemia is at substantial risk to develop pneumonia with *Pneumocystis carinii*. This infection can be prevented by prophylaxis with sulfamethoxazole–trimethoprim and possibly aerosol pentamidine. *Strongyloides stercoralis* infestation can be inhibited by administering thiabendazole.

Viruses

Herpes simplex infection can be devastating in the neutropenic patient who has had a bone-marrow transplant. Risk can be reduced by chemoprophylaxis with acyclovir. Varicella can be prevented by active immunization with live, attenuated varicella vaccine or inhibited by passive immunization with zoster immune globulin. Cytomegalovirus (CMV) infection may also have its severity attenuated, or perhaps be prevented, by passive immunization with hyperimmune intravenous globulin preparations. Currently, murine and human monoclonal preparations are also being investigated for prevention and modification of CMV infection in bone-marrow transplant patients.

PRINCIPLES OF ANTIBIOTIC MANAGEMENT

The choice of antibiotic therapy among febrile, neutropenic patients with documented infection must be predicated on the organisms expected in such a setting. In many different clinical studies, various antibiotic combinations have been used with varying results. An overall efficacy rate of 75% to 85% should be anticipated from an antibiotic or combination of antibiotics before accepting its utility in the empiric treatment of febrile, neutropenic patients.

In the early 1960s, septicemia from *Pseudomonas aeruginosa* in a neutropenic patient meant almost certain death.[59] Until combination therapy with an amino-glycoside and a carboxypenicillin became available in the late 1960s, a mortality in excess of 90% was observed, one half of which occurred within the first 72 hours after the first drawing of blood for culture.[59] In contrast, patients with septicemia from *Pseudomonas aeruginosa* who were given gentamicin and carbenicillin had a mortality of 38.5%, a dramatic improvement. These experiences suggested that a combination of antibacterial agents, each bactericidal and acting at different sites, would produce what we now understand to be a synergistic combination superior to either drug alone.[60] This inference has been substantiated by studies that demonstrated that a significantly better outcome can be predicted when the pathogen is susceptible to more than one of the antibacterial agents used.[44]

Now, there are many more possible choices of antibiotics. Among these choices are: (1) combinations of an aminoglycoside and a beta-lactam antibiotic; (2) combinations of two beta-lactam antibiotics and an aminoglycoside; (3) double beta-lactam combinations; and (4) monotherapy. The first two choices employ the principle of synergy. Although the double beta-lactam combination would, at least theoretically, not lend itself to that concept, *in vitro* studies suggest that a double beta-lactam combination (moxalactam and piperacillin), although not synergistic, is not antagonistic and may indeed be additive.[47]

Aminoglycoside–Beta-Lactam Combinations

Various combinations of aminoglycosides and beta-lactams have been studied.[15,21,23,29,38,41,64,68] With one exception, no significant differences have been noted. In EORTC (the European Organization for Research on Treatment of Cancer) Trial III,[38] patients with microbiologically documented, gram-negative bacteremia treated with azlocillin–amikacin did significantly better than did patients given either ticarcillin or cefotaxime. However, the dose of cefotaxime administered in this study was only 100 mg/kg/day.

These comparisons of aminoglycoside–beta-lactam combinations demonstrated that nephrotoxicity, ototoxicity, and hypokalemia are all problems that must be considered. In EORTC Trial I,[23] patients given a combination of cephalothin–gentamicin experienced significantly more nephrotoxicity than did two groups given other drugs. However, in EORTC Trial II,[29] designed to compare two regimens with and without a cephalosporin (cefazolin), no significant difference in nephrotoxicity was found. The lack of nephrotoxicity was substantiated further in a four-way randomized study of a cephalosporin (cephalothin or cefamandole) in combination with an aminoglycoside (gentamicin or tobramycin) and carbenicillin in the empiric treatment of febrile, neutropenic patients with neoplastic disease.[11]

When the combination of moxalactam and amikacin was compared with ticarcillin and amikacin, de Jongh and co-workers found no differences in the incidence of nephrotoxicity and hypokalemia.[21] Winston and co-workers found that the combination of piperacillin–amikacin was associated with less hypokalemia but more nephrotoxicity than the combination of carbenicillin and amikacin.[68]

Although the MSKCC study did not demonstrate any significant differences among the three treatment regimens (ticarcillin–tobramycin, moxalactam–tobramycin, and piperacillin–tobramycin) with regard to hypokalemia or nephrotoxicity, subsequent infections occurred more frequently among the patients given piperacillin– tobramycin. Prolongation of the prothrombin time by more than 2 sec occurred more often in the moxalactam–tobramycin group. Moreover, among patients who received moxalactam–tobramycin and in whom the prothrombin time was prolonged by more than 2 sec, the incidence of clinical bleeding and the need for transfusion of both red blood cells and platelets was significantly higher.[15]

Double Beta-Lactam Combinations

The advent of more intensive chemotherapeutic regimens for the treatment of acute leukemia resulted in an increased incidence of initial and recurrent neutropenia. Moreover, these episodes were characteristically longer and the neutropenia more profound than had been seen previously. Consequently, there were more febrile episodes, and empiric antibacterial therapy was given more often and for longer periods of time. Because aminoglycosides were a traditional part of this empiric regimen, cumulatively more aminoglycosides were administered to more patients, thereby increasing the potential for nephrotoxicity and ototoxicity.

Concern about these side-effects and the coincident emergence of newer, extended-spectrum beta-lactam antibiotics led investigators to conduct clinical trials with combinations of two beta-lactam antibiotics,[20,26,27,36,67] after demonstrating in the laboratory that there was no antagonism between the agents proposed.[47] Not all penicillins and cephalosporins could be combined with ease because antagonism was demonstrated for some; mechanisms of induction of high-grade beta-lactamase were proposed.[39,55,56] However, a few combinations did emerge, and clinical trials were conducted. No significant differences in efficacy have been found in any study.

When the double beta-lactam combination was compared with a traditional aminoglycoside-containing combination, de Jongh and co-workers found significantly less ototoxicity and nephrotoxicity in the moxalactam–piperacillin group than in the moxalactam–amikacin group.[20] In the study at UCLA by Winston and co-workers, patients with *Pseudomonas aeruginosa* infections did significantly better if they received moxalactam–amikacin rather than moxalactam–piperacillin.[67] In that study, two episodes of relapsed *Pseudomonas aeruginosa* septicemia occurred with the development of beta-lactam resistance in patients receiving moxalactam-piperacillin. Emergence of resistance during therapy has been reported by others.[12,46,55]

In this same study, bacteremic enterococcal superinfections occurred significantly more often among patients receiving moxalactam–amikacin than in patients receiving moxalactam–piperacillin.[67] Enterococcal superinfection in conjunction with moxalactam use has also been observed by others.[9,10,71] The incidence of nephrotoxicity was not significantly different in the two treatment arms at UCLA.[42] All the patients in the UCLA study received prophylactic vitamin K, yet the incidence of prolongation of the prothrombin time by more than 2 sec was greater than 20%. Also, persistent, profound granulocytopenia (less than $100/mm^3$) occurred significantly more often in patients in the moxalactam–piperacillin group.[67]

Fainstein and co-workers did not find any differences in efficacy among two treatment arms studies: moxalactam–ticarcillin and moxalactam–tobramycin. Prolongation of the prothrombin time became apparent early in the study; thus, prophylactic vitamin K administration was incorporated into the protocol. No further significant elevations of the prothrombin time were mentioned, nor were any further episodes of clinical bleeding described.[26] The moxalactam–tobramycin group experienced more nephrotoxicity than did the moxalactam–ticarcillin group. Conversely, the moxalactam–ticarcillin group had more fungal superinfections than did the moxalactam–tobramycin group.

A study from the University of Maryland Cancer Center by Joshi and co-workers attempted to determine not only whether a double beta-lactam combination of antibiotics was less nephrotoxic and ototoxic, but also if such a combination would disrupt the "colonization resistance factor."[36] Initial results indicated that the ceftazidime–tobramycin group tended to have fewer subsequent infections than did the ceftazidime–piperacillin group; an anaerobe-preserving regimen may have been responsible for this finding. In a Canadian multicenter clinical trial comparing moxalactam–ticarcillin with tobramycin–ticarcillin, differences of nephrotoxicity were not observed, but the prothrombin time was prolonged more often in patients receiving moxalactam–ticarcillin.[27] Because of these results, that group recommended that all patients receiving moxalactam also be given prophylactic vitamin K.

Monotherapy

Some have approached the problem of avoiding various toxicities, such as the ototoxicity and nephrotoxicity of aminoglycosides and the hypokalemia associated with the antipseudomonal penicillin (particularly the disodium salt carboxypenicillins), by attempting to exploit the broad and extended spectrum of some of the "third-generation" cephalosporins and the carbapenems and monobactams, such as moxalactam, ceftazidime, cefoperazone, imipenem, and aztreonam, as monotherapy. Close observation is required when using single-agent therapy, because experience has shown that superinfections and the emergence of resistant organisms occur.[12,13,32,54,55] Certain investigators have compared these agents with conventional therapy, and the results were relatively consistent with those results of previously cited studies.[1, 49, 50, 53] However, one exception is the study by Pickard and co-workers[50] in which the results of the ticarcillin–tobramycin treatment arm seemed less than that observed in other studies using the same or very similar regimens. Although the study by Alanis and co-workers[1] indicated comparable results for both the moxalactam arm and the nafcillin–tobramycin arm, the latter treatment regimen would likely be inadequate if *Pseudomonas aeruginosa* and *Enterobacteriaceae* are the pathogens. In this study, the aminoglycoside provided only aerobic gram-negative rod coverage, and this has been found to be less than satisfactory. Pizzo and co-workers indicated that "this was not evidence of success, since neither of the comparative regimens was optimal."[52]

A study from the Institut Jules Bordet in Brussels found that cefoperazone alone was equivalent to the combination of cefoperazone–amikacin in the small group of neutropenic patients.[49] However, the authors caution that the study was conducted during a time when most of their clinical bacterial isolates were quite sensitive to cefoperazone and that this aspect could change.

The most definitive study regarding the treatment with monotherapy of the febrile, neutropenic patient comes from the National Cancer Institute.[53] Pizzo and co-workers found that ceftazidime alone as initial therapy of such patients was equivalent to that of the combination cephalothin–gentamicin–carbenicillin. As expected, toxicity was minimal in the monotherapy arm. The authors stressed that patients with documented infection or prolonged and profound neutropenia were likely to require additional or modified therapeutic regimens. Young[69] pointed out that "there is no substitute for knowledge of the local risks of nosocomial infection, the antimicrobial-susceptibility profiles of important pathogens, the clinical findings, and the patient's previous exposure to antimicrobial agents, before selection of empirical therapy."

Certain agents, such as the carbapenems (imipenem), which have significant postantibiotic effect,[17] may become useful for monotherapy in the febrile, neutropenic patient. Where carboxyquinolone compounds will fit into the antibacterial regimen for the neutropenic, febrile patient remains to be seen.

SURGICAL COMPLICATIONS
IN THE NEUTROPENIC PATIENT

General

Numerous inflammatory surgical emergencies are encountered in the neutropenic patient.[57] Two complications, necrotizing enterocolitis (typhlitis) and anorectal inflammation, stand out and are considered separately. Other septic complications include dental abscess, cholecystitis, often acalculous, and the range of common septic complications such as appendicitis and perforated viscus. Gastrointestinal hemorrhage may also occur.

Surgical complications arise most commonly from the gastrointestinal tract. The most frequently identified microbial causes of sepsis are *Escherichia coli* and *Pseu-*

domonas aeruginosa. About 11% of septic leukemic patients have blood cultures positive for *Klebsiella* species, and about 1 out of 6 patients has polymicrobial sepsis. Infection in the neutropenic patient is uncommonly from the genitourinary system.

The major factors in achieving patient survival are early physician recognition and timely operative intervention. The major difficulty in early recognition is the striking absence of the usual localizing signs of intra-abdominal sepsis. Reliance must be placed on suspicion and on integration of the patient's symptoms with basic clinical and laboratory determinants.

Neutropenic Enterocolitis

Neutropenic enterocolitis is a syndrome characterized by full-thickness ne-crosis of the intestine, particularly the cecum and ascending colon. Synonyms include neutropenic typhlitis and the ileocecal syndrome. Necrotizing colitis invariably occurs in association with neutropenia and immunosuppression and is most commonly seen in patients with acute myeloblastic leukemia.

Neutropenic enterocolitis was found in 46% of autopsied leukemic children.[45] This breakdown in the gastrointestinal barrier from chemotherapy and other causes probably provides a setting in which invasive infection occurs in a patient whose ability for repair is inhibited.

The presenting symptoms are those of vague abdominal pain, sometimes masked by steroids, vomiting, diarrhea which may be bloody, and fever. An elevated temperature in the range of 101°F to 104°F is usually seen. Exelby[25] found abdominal pain in 93% of patients with necrotizing colitis, vomiting in 81%, rebound tenderness in 69%, and abdominal distention in 62%. The typical peritoneal signs of an acute abdomen are ordinarily absent or blunted by steroids. Still, the abdominal pain ordinarily localizes in the right lower quadrant.

In this setting, the differential diagnosis includes appendicitis, intramesenteric hemorrhage, ischemic colitis, and pseudo-obstruction (Ogilvie's) syndrome. Other causes for diarrhea should be considered.[40] It is important to assay the stools for *Clostridium difficile* toxin.

An abdominal radiograph may be helpful. Enterocolitis may be associated with an ill-defined soft-tissue density on the right side of the abdomen, representing the dilated, fluid-filled, atonic cecum. The diagnosis of enterocolitis is unlikely if ordinary films of the abdomen show that the cecum retains its haustral markings and is distensible. Endoscopic examination of the colon may be helpful.

The patient who is neutropenic and develops abdominal pain and signs of sepsis without signs of peritonitis should be treated by nasogastric suction, intravenous hydration, and broad-spectrum antibiotic coverage. Antidiarrheal agents should be avoided. Appropriate adjustments in the chemotherapeutic treatment should be made. Peritoneal lavage may assist in establishing indications for operative interven-tion by detection of bacteria on Gram's stain.[30] Moreover, these patients must be investigated for pulmonary infiltrates and other possible causes for fever and sepsis.

The indications for operative intervention are difficult. Judgments tend to be conservative in these very sick patients. Nonetheless, clear-cut indications of peritonitis require exploration. If peritonitis is absent, symptoms will resolve with resolution of the neutropenia.

At exploration, it is not appropriate to remove only the appendix because extensive cecal necrosis is often associated. Mucosal ulcers are far more extensive than is apparent from a normal-appearing serosa. More appropriately, the patient should be treated by excision of the appendix and right colon, and construction of a temporary ileostomy and a mucous fistula of the right transverse colon. Gastrointestinal continuity can be restored subsequently when the patient is in remission.

Anorectal Complications

The neutropenic patient, particularly the patient with leukemia, is at great risk to develop life-threatening anorectal complications. Principles for management of the otherwise healthy patient with a fissure, fistula, or perirectal abscess are well-established and widely known. Management in the leukemic, neutropenic patient is, however, more complex.[61,63] In particular, a serious error in judgment can be made by failure to recognize anorectal sepsis or by inappropriate operative intervention. Incision into an indurated area may result in propagation of necrosis. Associated thrombocytopenia also adds to the risk of operative complications.

Any leukemic patient who complains of anal pain should be started on precautionary measures. Examination of the neutropenic patient who is complaining of anorectal pain may show minimal signs of sepsis. Induration without fluctuation results from the lack of suppuration due to absence of granulocytes. The induration may represent leukemic infiltration, and there may be extensive ulceration from leukemic cells. Crepitus may be associated with an invasive clostridial infection or a necrotizing infection from a mixed microflora.[16]

In the absence of clearly defined, drainable sepsis, patients with anorectal infection should be treated initially by conservative measures: warm compresses or sitz baths, stool softeners, analgesics, and broad-spectrum antibiotics. Operative drainage depends on the results of daily examinations. Local radiation therapy is indicated in leukemic patients who show indurated tender areas, which may be leukemic infiltrates. Therapy is limited to 300 to 400 rads daily over 1 to 3 days with a perineal port. After 3 to 5 days, the induration either subsides completely or drains spontaneously through necrotic tissue that forms over the indurated area. It may be helpful to pry open the necrotic tissue gently with a clamp to improve drainage. If a fistula occurs, it can be treated surgically when the patient is in remission. When the patient's white blood cells and platelet counts have returned to normal, standard surgical approaches, such as fistulotomy, sphincterotomy, or hemorrhoidectomy, may be performed.

REFERENCES

1. Alanis A, Graves S, Weinstein AJ. Moxalactam or nafcillin and tobramycin for empiric therapy of febrile granulocytopenic patients. Proceedings of the 22nd Interscience Conference on Antimicrobial Agents and Chemotherapy, Miami Beach, FL, October 4, 1982, Abstract 3.

2. Armstrong D. Protected environments are discomforting and expensive and do not offer meaningful protection. In: Brown AE, Armstrong D, eds. Infectious complications of neoplastic disease: controversies in management. New York:Yorke Medical Books, 1985:395.

3. Armstrong D. Infections in patients with neoplastic diseases. In: Verhoef J, Peterson PK, Quie PC, eds. Infections in the immunocompromised host: pathogenesis, prevention, and therapy. Amsterdam: Elsevier/North Holland Biomedical Press, 1980:129.

4. Banerjee C, Bustamante CI, Talley E, et al. *Bacillus* infections in patients with cancer. Proceedings of the 26th Interscience Conference on Antimicrobial Agents and Chemotherapy, New Orleans, September 29, 1986, Abstract 1051.

5. Blazar BR, Hurd DD, Snover DC, et al. Invasive *Fusarium* infections in bone marrow transplant recipients. Am J Med 1984;77:645.

6. Blevins A, Lange M, Sobeck K, et al. Prevention and control of *Corynebacterium* CDC JK bacteremia in cancer patients with prolonged neutropenia. Proceedings of the 85th Annual Meeting of the American Society for Microbiology, Las Vegas, March 3, 1985, Abstract L-57.

7. Bodey GP. Infection in cancer patients: a continuing association. Am J Med 1986;81(1A):11.

8. Bodey GP, Buckley M, Sathe YS, et al. Quantitative relationships between circulating leucocytes and infections in patients with acute leukemia. Ann Intern Med 1966;64:328.

9. Brown AE. Management in the febrile, neutropenic patient with cancer: therapeutic considerations. J Pediatr 1985;106:1035.

10. Brown AE. Neutropenia, fever, and infection. Am J Med 1984;76:421.

11. Brown AE, Quesada O, Armstrong D. Minimal nephrotoxicity with cephalosporin–aminoglycoside combinations in patients with neoplastic disease. Antimicrob Agents Chemother 1982;21:592.

12. Brown AE, Quesada O, Armstrong D. Moxalactam therapy of serious nosocomial *Serratia* infections in patients with neoplastic diseases. In: Periti P, Grassi GG, eds. Current chemotherapy and immunotherapy. Washington, DC: American Society for Microbiology, 1982:299.

13. Brown AE, Quesada O, Armstrong D. Empiric moxalactam therapy in febrile, neutropenic patients with cancer on nephrotoxic chemotherapy. Proceedings of the 21st Interscience Conference on Antimicrobial Agents and Chemotherapy, Chicago, November 4, 1981, Abstract 318.

14. Brown AE, Quesada O, Fiore A, et al. Changing patterns of enterococcal sepsis in patients with neoplastic disease. Proceedings of the 24th Interscience Conference on Antimicrobial Agents and Chemotherapy, Washington, DC, October 8, 1984, Abstract 374.

15. Brown AE, Quesada O, Murrer JA, et al. Empiric combination antibiotic therapy of febrile, neutropenic patients with neoplastic disease: results of a randomized study. Proceedings of the 13th International Congress of Chemotherapy, Vienna, Austria, September 2, 1983.

16. Bubrick MP, Hitchcock CR. Necrotizing anorectal and perineal infections. Surgery 1979;86:655.

17. Bustamante CI, Drusano GL, Tatem BA, et al. Postantibiotic effect of imipenem on *Pseudomonas aeruginosa.* Antimicrob Agents Chemother 1984;26:678.

18. Cho CT, Vats TS, Lowman JT, et al. *Fusarium solani* infection during treatment for acute leukemia. J Pediatr 1973;83:1028.

19. Collins MS, Rinaldi MG. Cutaneous infection in man caused by *Fusarium moniliforme.* Sabouraudia 1977;15:151.

20. De Jongh CA, Joshi JH, Thompson BW, et al. A double betalactam combination versus an aminoglycoside-containing regimen as empiric antibiotic therapy for febrile granulocytopenic cancer patients. Am J Med 1986;80:(5C)101.

21. De Jongh CA, Wade JD, Schimpff SC, et al. Empiric antibiotic therapy for suspected infection in granulocytopenic cancer patients. Am J Med 1982;73:89.

22. Elting LS, Bodey GP, Fainstein V. Polymicrobial septicemia in the cancer patient. Medicine 1986;65:218.

23. EORTC International Antimicrobial Therapy Project Group. Three antibiotic regimens in the treatment of infection in febrile granulocytopenic patients with cancer. J Infect Dis 1978;137:14.

24. Evans HL, Kletzer M, Lawson RD, et al. Systemic mycosis due to *Trichosporon cutaneum.* Cancer 1980;45:367.

25. Exelby PR, Ghandchi A, Lansigan, et al. Management of the acute abdomen in children with leukemia. Cancer 1975;35:826.

26. Fainstein V, Bodey GP, Bolivar R, et al. Moxalactam plus ticarcillin or tobramycin for treatment of febrile episodes in neutropenic cancer patients. Arch Intern Med 1984;144:1766.

27. Feld R, Louie TJ, Mandell L, et al. A multicentre comparative trial of tobramycin and ticarcillin versus moxalactam and ticarcillin in febrile neutropenic patients. Arch Intern Med 1985;145:1083.

28. Friedman LE, Brown AE, Miller DR, et al. *Staphylococcus epidermidis* septicemia in children with leukemia and lymphoma. Am J Dis Child 1984;138:715.

29. Gaya H. Rational basis for the choice of regimens for empiric therapy of sepsis in granulocytopenic patients. Schweiz Med Wochenschr 1983;113(suppl 14):49.

30. Geer DA, Lee YM, Barcia PJ. Peritoneal lavage as an aid in the surgical management of neutropenic colitis. J Surg Oncol 1986;31:222.

31. Gold JWM, Poston W, Mertelsmann R, et al. Systemic infection with *Trichosporon cutaneum* in a patient with acute leukemia. Cancer 1983;48:2163.

32. Gribble MJ, Chow AW, Naiman SC, et al. Prospective randomized trial of piperacillin versus carboxypenicillin–aminoglycoside combination regimens in the empirical treatment of serious bacterial infections. Antimicrob Agents Chemother 1983;24:388.

33. Gutmann L, Pore RS. Fusariosis, myasthenic syndrome, and aplastic anemia. Neurology 1975;25:922.

34. Hersh EM, Bodey GP, Nies BA, et al. Causes of death in acute leukemia. JAMA 1965;193:99.

35. Ihde DC, Armstrong D. Clinical spectrum of infection due to *Bacillus* species. Am J Med 1973;55:839.

36. Joshi J, Ruxer R, Newman K, et al. Double beta-lactam versus an aminoglycoside plus beta-lactam combination as empiric therapy for granulocytopenic cancer patients. Proceedings of the 24th Interscience Conference on Antimicrobial Agents and Chemotherapy, Washington, DC, October 8, 1984, Abstract 383.

37. Kiehn TE, Nelson PE, Bernard EM, et al. Catheter-associated fungemia caused by *Fusarium chlamydosporum* in a patient with lymphocytic lymphoma. J Clin Microbiol 1985;21:501.

38. Klastersky J. Prospective randomized comparison of three antibiotic regimens for empirical therapy of suspected bacteremic infection in febrile granulocytopenic patients. Antimicrob Agents Chemother 1986;29:263.

39. Kuch NA, Testa RT, Forbes M. *In vitro* and *in vivo* antibacterial effects of combinations of beta-lactam antibiotics. Antimicrob Agents Chemother 1981;19:634.

40. Kunkel JM, Rosenthal D. Management of the ileocecal syndrome. Dis Colon Rectum 1985;29:196.

41. Lau WK, Young LS, Black RE, et al. Comparative efficacy and toxicity of amikacin/carbenicillin versus gentamicin/carbenicillin in leukopenic patients. Am J Med 1977;62:959.

42. Levine AS, Schimpff SC, Graw RG Jr, et al. Hematologic malignancies and other marrow failure states: progress in the management of complicating infections. Semin Hematol 1974;11:141.

43. Libertin CR, Davies NJ, Halper J, et al. Invasive disease caused by *Trichosporon beigelii*. Mayo Clin Proc 1983;58:684.

44. Love LL, Schimpff SC, Schiffer CA, et al. Improved prognosis for granulocytopenic patients with gram-negative bacteremia. Am J Med 1980;68:643.

45. Moir DH, Bale PM. Necropsy findings in childhood leukemia, emphasizing neutropenic enterocolitis and cerebral calcification. Pathology 1976;8:247.

46. Mokhbat JE, Brown AE, Brooker DC, et al. Emergence of resistance of newer beta-lactams in *Pseudomonas aeruginosa* and *Serratia marcescens*. Proceedings of the 23rd Interscience Conference on Antimicrobial Agents and Chemotherapy, Las Vegas, October 25, 1983, Abstract 432.

47. Moody MR, Young VM, Schimpff SC. Synergistic activity of piperacillin-moxolactam-amikacin combinations. Proceedings of the 20th Interscience Conference on Antimicrobial Agents and Chemotherapy, New Orleans, LA, September 24, 1980, Abstract 752.

48. Pennington JE, Gibbons ND, Strobeck JE, et al. *Bacillus* species infection in patients with hematologic neoplasia. JAMA 1976;235:1473.

49. Piccart T, Klastersky J, Meunier F, et al. Single-drug versus combination empirical therapy for gram-negative bacillary infections in febrile cancer patients with and without granulocytopenia. Antimicrob Agents Chemother 1984;26:870.

50. Pickard W, Durack D, Gallis H. A randomized trial of moxalactam versus tobramycin plus ticarcillin in 50 febrile neutropenic patients. Proceedings of the 22nd Interscience Conference on Antimicrobial Agents and Chemotherapy, Miami Beach, FL, October 4, 1982, Abstract 5.

51. Pizzo PA. Empiric therapy and prevention of infection in the immunocompromised host. In: Mandell GL, Douglas RG Jr, Bennett JE, eds. Principles and practice of infectious diseases. 2nd ed. New York: John Wiley and Sons, 1984:1680.

52. Pizzo PA, Comers J, Cotton D, et al. Approaching the controversies in antibacterial management of cancer patients. Am J Med 1984;76:436.

53. Pizzo PA, Hathorn JW, Hiemenz J, et al. A randomized trial comparing ceftazidime alone with combination antibiotic therapy in cancer patients with fever and neutropenia. N Engl J Med 1986;315:552.

54. Quesada O, Brown AE, Won D, et al. Efficacy of ceftazidime in the treatment of selected cancer patient with serious infections. In: Ishigami J, ed. Recent advances in chemotherapy—antimicrobial section. Tokyo: University of Tokyo Press, 1985:974.

55. Sanders CC, Sander WE Jr. Emergence of resistance during therapy with the newer beta-lactam

antibiotics: role of inducible beta-lactamases and implications for the future. Rev Infect Dis 1983;5:639.

56. Sanders CC, Sanders WE Jr, Goering RV. *In vitro* antagonism of beta-lactam antibiotics by cefoxitin. Antimicrob Agents Chemother 1982;21:986.
57. Schaller RT, Schaller JE. The acute abdomen in the immunologically compromised child. J Pediatr Surg 1983;18:937.
58. Schimpff SC. Empiric antibiotic therapy for granulocytopenic patients. Am J Med 1986;80(5C):13.
59. Schimpff SC, Saterlee W, Young VM, et al. Empiric therapy with carbenicillin and gentamicin for febrile patients with cancer and granulocytopenia. N Engl J Med 1961;284:1061.
60. Sculier J, Klastersky J. Significance of serum bactericidal activity in gram-negative bacillary bacteremia in patients with and without granulocytopenia. Am J Med 1984;76:429.
61. Sehdeu MK, Dowling MD, Seal SH, et al. Perianal and anorectal complications of leukemia. Cancer 1973;31:149.
62. Singer CF, Kaplan MH, Armstrong D. Bacteremia and fungemia complicating neoplastic disease: a study of 364 cases. Am J Med 1977;62:731.
63. Vanheuverzwyn R, Delannoy A, Michaux JL. Anal lesions in hematologic diseases. Dis Colon Rectum 1980;28:310.
64. Wade JC, Schimpff SC, Newman KA, et al. Piperacillin or ticarcillin plus amikacin: a double-blind prospective comparison of empiric antibiotic therapy for febrile granulocytopenic cancer patients. Am J Med 1981;71:983.
65. Walsh TJ, Newman KR, Moody M, et al. Trichosporonosis in patients with neoplastic disease. Medicine 1986;65:268.
66. Weiner BC, Brown AE, Bell G, et al. Significant viridans streptococcal infections in children with cancer. Proceedings of the 21st Interscience Conference on Antimicrobial Agents and Chemotherapy, Chicago, November 4, 1981, Abstract 803.
67. Winston DJ, Barnes RC, Ho WG, et al. Moxalactam plus piperacillin versus moxalactam plus amikacin in febrile neutropenic patients. Am J Med 1984;77:442.
68. Winston DJ, Ho WG, Young LS, et al. Piperacillin plus amikacin therapy in febrile, granulocytopenic patients. Arch Intern Med 1982;142:1663.
69. Young LS. Empirical antimicrobial therapy in the neutropenic host. N Engl J Med 1986;315:580.
70. Young NA, Kwon-Chung KJ, Kubota TT, et al. Disseminated infection by *Fusarium moniliforme* during treatment for malignant lymphoma. J Clin Microbiol 1978;7:589.
71. Yu VK. Enterococcal superinfection and colonization after therapy with moxalactam. Ann Intern Med 1981;94:784.

13

○ ○ ○ ● ● ●

CAUSES AND RISKS OF WOUND INFECTION*

Albert T. McManus

Wounding disrupts a biologic barrier, and the resultant contamination increases the susceptibility to infection. The development of wound infections, however, requires a congruence of conditional, joint, and independent probabilities that relate to the size of the wound, the numbers and types of contaminating organisms, the saprophytic and pathogenic potentials of these organisms, and the ability of the host to resist microbial invasion. Most accidental wounds are contaminated immediately with organisms from the edges of the wound as well as from contact with the wounding environment. The observation that most small wounds that occur in the host's natural environment heal without difficulty speaks both for the lack of pathogenic mechanisms in the majority of microorganisms and for the presence of nonspecific and specific host defense mechanisms selected through evolution. Traumatic wounds or surgical wounds created in seriously ill patients in the hospital environment, however, may alter the conditions under which many of these evolutionary balances are effective.

---

* The opinions or assertions contained herein are the private views of the authors and are not to be construed as official or as reflecting the views of the Department of the Army or the Department of Defense.

The purpose of this chapter is to review the characteristics of organisms commonly causing infections in surgical patients as well as the host characteristics associated with increased risk of infections by specific organisms. It is hoped that this information will aid in improving the timely recognition of specific types of infection, and the choice and specificity of treatments.

ORGANISMS CAUSING WOUND INFECTIONS

Gram-positive cocci are the most common organisms causing wound infections requiring treatment. This appears to have been true before the development of antimicrobial therapy and before the knowledge that there was a microbial basis for infection. These organisms are from the genera *Staphylococcus* and *Streptococcus*.

Staphylococcus

These organisms are named for their distinctive morphology. The staphylococci are gram-positive cocci that have a peculiar postdivisional enzymatic process that translocates daughter cells to form characteristic irregular, grapelike clusters.[4] Staphylococci are moderately resistant to desiccation because their cell walls have the distinctive property of containing both teichoic acids and associated peptidoglycans. This combination gives the cells unusual mechanical strength, and their resistance to drying makes them more difficult to eliminate from the environment and allows for their ready distribution in the air or on fomites.

Staphylococci will grow readily on most meat infusion-based media. They have both respiratory and fermentative metabolic processes, and they produce catalase. Under anaerobic growth conditions, uracil and a fermentable carbon source are required. These organisms are relatively heat-resistant and will grow at 45°C; they are also salt-tolerant, and growth in 10% to 15% salt is not uncommon. This resistance to heat and salt makes these organisms and their extracellular toxins (see below) serious potential sources for food poisoning and a problem in canning and preserving.

The genus *Staphylococcus* contains at least 13 species, 6 of which have been associated with human disease.[3] The species causing human disease are *Staphylococcus aureus, Staphylococcus epidermidis, Staphylococcus saprophyticus, Staphylococcus simulans, Staphylococcus hominis,* and *Staphylococcus hemolyticus.* Historically, *Staphylococcus aureus* is by far the most common and serious pathogen.[8] Infection by *Staphylococcus epidermidis* appears to be rapidly increasing in incidence and is associated with the increased use of intraluminal catheters and other indwelling devices. *Staphylococcus aureus* can be isolated from 30% to 50% of normal humans and can readily be distinguished from the other members of the genus by its ability to clot plasma. This property is associated with both a bacterial cell-associated factor (clumping factor), which binds fibrinogen, and by extracellular enzymes (coagulases) that initiate thrombinlike activity. Another cell-associated property of *Staphylococcus aureus* is its production of protein A. This protein has the very unusual property of binding immunoglobulin G in the Fc region, which is thought to interfere with the activation of the alternate complement pathway by blocking normally activating peptidoglycans sites on the cell wall. This blockage inhibits immune recognition and phagocytosis. *Staphylococcus aureus* also has receptors that bind fibronectin, which may facilitate colonization of traumatized tissue.

Staphylococcus aureus produces a wide variety of potentially injurious extra-cellular products. The lethality for small animals of these substances present in growth media aroused early interest in this organism. Products such as collagenase, lipase, deoxyribonuclease, hyaluronidase, and fibrinolysin are commonly expressed. At least four (alpha, beta, gamma, and delta) red cell toxins have been described, as has a powerful white blood cell-disrupting toxin, Panton-Valentine (P-V) leukocidin. The food poisoning agents are called enterotoxins and exist as at least five distinct toxins. The syndrome associated with ingestion of these toxins is characterized by a delay of 2 to 3 hr, followed by acute gastrointestinal upset with vomiting, cramping, and diarrhea, which typically lasts more than 13 hr. The enterotoxins do not appear to be synthesized within the gut, and antimicrobial therapy is not useful.

There are several toxic conditions associated with *Staphylococcus aureus* tissue infections that, at least initially, must be diagnosed clinically. The oldest recognized condition is the staphylococcal scalded skin syndrome, which is most common in infants. The toxin is absorbed from a distant site of infection and produces a sunburnlike rash, which progresses to desquamation. The condition is commonly not fatal and responds when the primary infection is successfully addressed. The production of toxin is strain-specific and has been associated with nursery outbreaks. Definitive differentiation from more serious drug-induced allergic conditions, such as toxic epidermal necrolysis, depends on biopsy. A more recently recognized toxic condition is toxic shock syndrome. This condition is more serious than staphylococcal scalded skin syndrome and was originally associated with vaginal infections and tampon use, but the condition may also result from other localized infections, including wound infections. The production of the toxin, which has recently been shown to be identical to one of the staphylococcal enterotoxins noted above, is associated with lysogenic phages. The condition requires specific antistaphylococcal therapy as well as supportive care. The mortality associated with this toxemia is less than 10%.

Staphylococci have been continual targets for development of antibiotics. The initial success of native penicillin was short-lived. Modified penicillins that resist common staphylococcal beta-lactamases were released for clinical usage in the 1960s and were followed with the early generations of the cephalosporins. These developments have continually met with varying frequencies of clinically resistant strains. Currently, there appears to be a widening spread of so-called methicillin-resistant *Staphylococcus aureus* and *Staphylococcus epidermidis* strains in American hospitals. The mechanism of resistance of these strains is not that of antibiotic-inactivating enzymes such as beta-lactamase, but rather through alteration in penicillin-binding proteins in the cell membrane that are required for initiation of antimicrobial action. This alteration renders such strains resistant to all beta-lactam antibiotics. The rare incidence of toxicity and the current universal failure of the development of resistance to vancomycin have made it the drug of choice for such infections and for suspected staphylococcal infections in situations with significant epidemiologic risk of methicillin-resistant strains.

Streptococcus

This genus is also named for its morphology. Streptococcal cells divide by binary division in uniform planes, and daughter cells frequently remain attached. When growing cultures are examined, streptococci appear as winding chains of cells (Gr. *streptos,* winding). Streptococci can readily be distinguished from staphylococci on the basis of failure of streptococci to produce catalase. Streptococci are facultative anaerobes and have extensive growth requirements that include nucleic acid precursors, vitamins, and amino acids. However, most strains will grow on infusion-based media supplemented with blood. This requirement for blood agar was the basis for the earliest classification of streptococci. Colonies of these organisms, grown on infusion media containing 5% sheep red blood cells, produced characteristic hemolytic reactions. The most obvious reaction is clear hemolysis. Strains producing this see-through hemolysis are called beta-hemolytic. The second hemolytic type shows a zone of green discoloration surrounding colonies, and the third hemolytic type shows no hemolysis. The latter two types are called alpha and gamma hemolysis, respectively. The type of hemolysis caused by a strain is usually a stable property. Most strains of beta-hemolytic streptococci will form clear zones following surface growth. There are strains, however, that only produce clear hemolysis when the organisms grow below the surface of the agar. This fact can lead an inexperienced technician to miss an important organism in a specimen from an area normally containing high concentrations of nonpathogenic streptococci, such as the vagina or upper respiratory system. After inoculating a specimen from these areas, or with specimens suspected of containing streptococci, it is a common practice to stab the heavily streaked portions of the blood plate with the inoculating loop. This practice allows expression of the oxygen-suppressed streptolysin O, which is distinct from the surface-expressing, oxygen-stable streptolysin S.

Streptococci are normal flora at many sites in many species. Infections are most commonly associated with beta-hemolytic strains. The limited metabolic differences that exist among beta-hemolytic strains make metabolic subdivision of types impractical. The most widely used taxonomic scheme is based on the Lancefield system of immunotyping the carbohydrate antigens found in cell walls. There are, at present, 15 groups defined by the system, designated alphabetically from A to O. Most human disease is caused by group A beta-hemolytic strains. This antigen can be distinguished by most hospital laboratories and has been the target of recent rapid diagnostic techniques that allow identification of the designated single species of this group, *Streptococcus pyogenes.*

Streptococcus pyogenes is responsible for the majority of human infections and is capable of producing a wide variety of extracellular toxic products including hemolysin, deoxyribonuclease, hyaluronidase, streptolysin, and the plasminogen-activating enzyme, streptokinase.[1] Areas infected with *Streptococcus pyogenes* commonly contain other organisms, including both aerobes and anaerobes. This may become more obvious when a lesion containing a mixed flora, cellulitis, is treated with the universally active anti-*Streptococcus pyogenes* agent, penicillin. *Streptococcus pyogenes* may be quickly removed, but other antibiotics may be required to stop the infection. *Streptococcus pyogenes* is also associated with several systemic syndromes, including scarlet fever, acute rheumatic fever, and acute glomerulonephritis. These conditions do not commonly follow wound infections.

Most other streptococcal wound infections in humans are associated with two other Lancefield types, groups B and D. The name *Streptococcus agalactiae* is given to organisms of group B. This species is associated with neonatal sepsis and meningitis but may also cause wound infections. The Lancefield group D organisms are becoming more frequently recognized causes of human disease. In particular, the salt-tolerant (6.5%) strains common in the human gut are associated with infections in immunosuppressed patients in whom broad-acting antibiotics have been previously used. These salt-tolerant organisms, commonly called enterococci, can be divided into three species based on sugar fermentations, *Streptococcus* (enterococcus) *faecalis*, *Streptococcus* (enterococcus) *faecium*, and *Streptococcus* (enterococcus) *durans*. The enterococci are frequently nonhemolytic (gamma), but beta-hemolytic strains do occur. The enterococcus is commonly multiply-resistant to aminoglycosides and cephalosporin antibiotics.

Anaerobes

Anaerobic organisms are part of the microflora of most body surfaces. They are, by definition, sensitive to oxygen, but there is a variation in this sensitivity. Most anaerobic organisms recovered from infections are relatively aerotolerant and are rarely recovered as pure cultures. Sites of anaerobic wound infections generally have a predisposing pathologic condition limiting oxygen delivery or diffusion, such as traumatic tissue destruction, a foreign body, or a preexisting infection.[2] These defects must often be surgically addressed before antibiotics can be expected to be optimally effective.

The members of the genera *Bacteroides* and *Fusobacterium* are the most common gram-negative anaerobes found in infected wounds. Again, these organisms are rarely, if ever, found as pure cultures. The sources of both types of organisms are most likely endogenous, *Fusobacterium* from the upper respiratory tract and *Bacteroides* from the gastrointestinal tract. Although beta-lactamase activity against penicillin is becoming more common in *Bacteroides*, most strains are sensitive to ureidopenicillins.

Gram-positive anaerobes represent a much wider spectrum of organisms than the gram-negative anaerobes that cause wound infection. In the pre-penicillin era, anaerobic streptococcal genera that we now know as *Peptostreptococcus* and *Peptococcus* were serious and common causes for wound infections. Infections caused by these organisms, especially when mixed with *Streptococcus pyogenes* or *Staphylococcus aureus*, are devastating. Streptococcal gangrene has been recognized for more than 50 years but was probably the infectious gangrene known for much longer in hospitals and in stressful situations such as the prisoner-of-war camps during the

Civil War. The term streptococcal gangrene is rarely used today but is covered in this era by the term "necrotizing fasciitis." The name necrotizing fasciitis may also be given to mixed anaerobic infections such as nonclostridial anaerobic cellulitis, Fournier's gangrene, synergistic necrotizing cellulitis, and other necrotizing nonclostridial conditions that involve mixed aerobic and anaerobic flora. Again, the most effective and necessary treatment is surgery and coverage with penicillin. Other endogenous gram-positive organisms, the genera *Actinomyces* and *Propionibacterium* are rare causes of wound infections.

Organisms of the genus *Clostridium* are gram-positive spore-forming anaerobic rods commonly found in the soil and in the feces of many animals. The majority of the members of this genus are saprophytic, and relatively few species are associated with human disease. The species of concern to human health all produce toxins. Although very rare as a wound pathogen, *Clostridium botulinum* produces the most potent of all bacterial toxins.

Clostridium tetani, the cause of tetanus, produces two very potent toxins. The neurotoxin, tetanospasmin, and the lytic enzyme, tetanolysin, are normally produced within a local wound. The neurotoxin has a very strong affinity for neural tissue and has its main action on the anterior horn cells of the spinal cord. The spores of *Clostridium tetani* are very sensitive to oxygen and may remain dormant in viable tissue for extended periods before being activated by tissue necrosis. *Clostridium tetani* is not an invasive pathogen, and fatal toxemia can be produced by what appear to be relatively minor puncture wounds. Immunoprophylaxis with toxoid is the best protection against tetanus.

Two invasive and rapidly spreading clostridial conditions are myonecrosis (gas gangrene) and myositis. These conditions can be caused by several clostridial species, including *Clostridium histolyticum, Clostridium tetani, Clostridium septicum, Clostridium novyi, Clostridium oedematiens,* and *Clostridium bifermentans.* The conditions reflect both toxin and tissue-damaging enzymatic activities, with destruction of muscle and connective tissue. Collagenase, proteinase, hyaluronidase, lecithinase, and deoxyribonuclease are often produced by infecting strains. The best antimicrobial prophylaxis and treatment for all clostridial disease is the scalpel, with delayed closure accompanied by treatment with beta-lactam antibiotics and/or combinations with chloramphenicol and clindamycin.

Gram-Negative Bacteria

Nonfermentative Gram-Negatives

Pseudomonas aeruginosa is perhaps the best example of an opportunistic, nosocomial pathogen. Invasive wound infections with this organism are usually symptomatic of a serious underlying disease with an associated granulocyte or inflammatory defect. Patients with large burns or advanced lymphomas or other malignancies are susceptible to *Pseudomonas aeruginosa.* The presence of *Pseudomonas aeruginosa* in hospital wound infections can, in fact, be associated with improvements in the care of these diseases. In burns, for example, *Pseudomonas aeruginosa* only became a commonly reported burn pathogen after the development of fluid resuscitation. Prior to the development of effective resuscitation, patients with burns large enough to be susceptible to *Pseudomonas* usually died from shock or its complications in less time than that required for wound colonization and infection. The organism is characterized by oxidative metabolic activity that is distinct from the fermentative activity of the enteric gram-negative rods.

In susceptible hosts, *Pseudomonas aeruginosa* is an invasive organism.[7] A wide variety of virulence factors have been proposed. The organism frequently produces a variety of extracellular products, including collagenase and elastase, as well as two metabolic toxins. To date, the only factor that has been established as a requirement for invasion of intact burn wounds is the organism's active motility. Bacteremia may follow local invasion. Hematogenous spread with metastatic lesions in internal organs and unburned areas of skin (ecthyma gangrenosum) is common. Historically, *Pseudomonas aeruginosa* bacteremia has had a high associated mortality.[6] This may have been a reflection of the frequent antibiotic resistances associated with hospital strains. With improvements in antipseudomonal antibiotics, bacteremia-associated mortality may be decreasing.

Other less common wound pathogens with oxidative metabolism include the genera *Acinetobacter, Flavobacterium, Moraxella, Aeromonas, Achromobacter,* and marine *Vibrio.* Many of these organisms are found in the soil and water. *Acinetobacter* species, like *Pseudomonas aeruginosa,* are frequently resistant to disinfectants and have the ability to develop resistance, both by mutation and by plasmid acquisition, to toxic agents in the clinical environment. Because of their natural habitat, these organisms may also present in work-related trauma in farmers, fishermen, and others in contact with soil and water.

Enteric Gram-Negative Rods

The family Enterobacteriaceae includes 13 genera, most of which are included in the facultative flora of the human intestine. Three of the family (*Salmonella, Shigella,* and *Yersinia*) are considered pathogens, and their isolation from clinical materials is usually significant. The other members of the family are normally commensal with their host. However, in a compromised host or under conditions of excessive colonization of abnormal sites, these organisms are opportunistic. The genera *Escherichia, Proteus, Enterobacter, Serratia, Providencia,* and *Klebsiella* are the most common agents of this group causing human infections. The most obvious virulence factor for the group, and for that matter for most gram-negative organisms, is their characteristic lipopolysaccharide (endotoxin). This biologically active material is released during cell growth and may also accumulate in abscesses and wounds. Surgical manipulation of heavily contaminated tissue, as may occur during excision of burn wounds, can cause fever spikes and, on occasion, vascular collapse. Many members of this group also have capsular polysaccharides that, by virtue of antiphagocytic activity, are thought to increase virulence. The capsule may also protect the organism from the bactericidal activities of complement and antibodies. Such serum-resistant strains are thought to be more likely to cause infections.

The principal gram-negative organisms causing wound infections are often hospital-specific. That is, there is ample evidence that specific organisms can become endemic in clinical settings. Endemic organisms, by definition, can survive in the clinical situation where they are found. Resistance to cleaning agents and the cross-contamination from patient to patient by hand carriage is likely to result in strains also resistant to multiple antibiotics. Antibiotic resistance appears to be the common denominator for endemic enteric species.[9] Gentamicin resistance is commonly present as an antibiotic marker for endemic strains.

NOSOCOMIAL INFECTIONS: WHAT ORGANISM AND DOES IT MAKE A DIFFERENCE?

In the simplest terms, microbial pathogenicity is the relative ability of an organism to infect a host. In the laboratory, conditions can be established to relate dose of organisms in a challenge to outcome in controlled and susceptible animals. This methodology is the basis for comparing microbial species and is used to study virulence factors within a species. With few exceptions, much of what is written about nosocomial pathogens is based on epidemiologic observation and laboratory animal studies with infection-associated strains. A limitation of such data occurs when one tries to relate such pathogens to a human scale of host susceptibility.

Do identified nosocomial pathogens have different thresholds of patient resistance to overcome before they establish infection? Using the definition of pathogenicity as the ability to establish infection, would organisms with lower thresholds be more or less virulent? What relationship does infection with a particular type of organism that is treated under modern conditions have to mortality when compared to the patient's admission prognosis? The difficulty with these questions is, of course, to find large enough patient samples with documented infections that have a measurable underlying disease prognosis. Such a cohort may exist in burn patients. We have previously reported the association of bacteremia with burn mortality in a population of more than 5800 admissions to the U.S. Army Institute of Surgical Research—Burn Center.[5] Using multiple logistic techniques, the outcome of patients with bacteremia was related to that of patients with the same burn sizes and ages but without bacteremia. The results clearly showed that bacteremia with *Pseudomonas aeruginosa* or gram-negative enteric rods was associated with as much as a 50% increase in mortality when compared with the nonbacteremic group. Interestingly, in the same population, *Staphylococcus aureus* bacteremia was found to have no significant effect on mortality. These data, with the addition of three additional patient admission years, are summarized in Fig. 13-1. The left bar of each pair shows the observed mortality for each bacteremia group. The right bar of each group represents the expected mortality without bacteremia in the group and reflects the severity of injury associated with each group. When the three groups are compared, it is also seen that gram-negative bacteremia occurred in more severely injured patients. In that subset of burn patients, gram-negative organisms were more virulent than *Staphylococcus aureus* and once gram-negative bacteremia was established, gram-negative

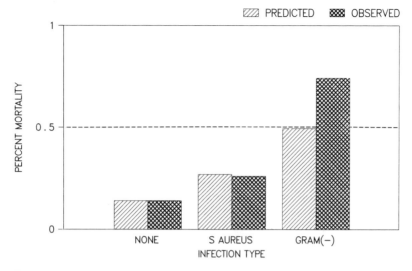

Figure 13–1.
Bacterimia-associated mortality in 6400 burned patients.

organisms were much more lethal. This observation documents a clear target for infection control efforts and predicts that elimination of gram-negative infections or prevention of antibiotic resistance in strains causing unavoidable infections will result in significant improvement in burned and, by inference, all infected patients.

REFERENCES

1. Bisno AL. Classification of streptococci and *Streptococcus pyogenes*. In: Mandell GL, Douglas RG Jr, Bennett JE, eds. Principles and practice of infectious diseases. 3d ed. New York: Churchill Livingstone, 1990:1518.
2. Finegold SM. Anaerobic bacteria in human disease. New York: Academic Press, 1977.
3. Kloos WE. Natural populations of the genus *Staphylococcus*. Annu Rev Microbiol 1980;34:559.
4. Koyama T, Yamada M, Matsuhashi M. Formation of regular packets of *Staphylococcus aureus* cells. J Bacteriol 1977;129:1518.
5. Mason AD Jr, McManus AT, Pruitt BA Jr. Association of burn mortality and bacteremia: a 25-year review. Arch Surg 1986;121:1027.
6. McManus AT, Mason AD Jr, McManus WF, et al. Twenty-five year review of *Pseudomonas aeruginosa* bacteremia in a burn center. Eur J Clin Microbiol 1985;4:219.
7. Pruitt BA Jr, McManus AT. Opportunistic infections in severely burned patients. Am J Med 1984;76(3A):146.
8. Sheagren JN. *Staphylococcus aureus*—the persistent pathogen. N Engl J Med 1964;310:1368.
9. Weinstein L. Gram-negative bacterial infections: a look at the past, a view of the present, and a glance at the future. Rev Infect Dis 1985;7(4):S538.

14

INFECTION IN OPEN-HEART SURGERY

Jeffrey P. Gold
O. Wayne Isom

    Infectious complications following surgical procedures that involve extracorporeal circulation remain a small but definite source of mortality and major morbidity. It is estimated that either superficial or deep-seated infections will occur in anywhere from 1% to 5% of all patients undergoing mediastinotomy and open cardiac surgery. Because of the significant mortality and morbidity associated with these infections, it is of paramount importance for physicians dealing with this subset of patients to understand the pathogenesis of these infections and, using this information, to attempt to prevent them or treat them when they occur. As a direct result of the study of the microbiology and pathophysiology of these disease processes over the last 10 years, the overall mortality has been significantly reduced.

PROPHYLAXIS: MICROBIOLOGY

As depicted in Table 14-1, most superficial and deep-seated wound infections occurring in patients undergoing cardiopulmonary bypass surgical procedures are caused by organisms carried by the patient. Stapholococcal species as well as streptococci and certain gram-negative organisms, therefore, remain the most common organisms encountered. Because surgical procedures that involve cardiopulmonary bypass tend to be somewhat more lengthy than other types of general surgical and subspecialty procedures, the incidence of wound colonization, which varies as a function of time, tends to be somewhat higher. In one study where the operative field as well as the blood bags, pump reservoirs, tubing, and so forth, were cultured, 71% of patients had a positive culture. It is of interest that all of these patients underwent a prosthetic valve implantation at the same time and none of them subsequently developed postoperative endocarditis. As with most other surgical procedures, multiple factors are in play here, most of which are related to the host situation surrounding the colonization at the time of surgery.

It is important for each institution doing a significant volume of open-heart surgery to become very familiar with their own hospital microbiologic flora. Certain patterns of resistance, as well as the relative incidence of polymicrobial or synergistic infections, are distinct to various institutions and services and, therefore, cannot be generalized. It is quite important, however, for the institution to be aware of these patterns so that empiric therapy and prophylaxis can be specifically aimed in the

Table 14–1
Microbiology of Postoperative Sternal
Wound Infections

Gram-Positive Organisms	
Staphylococcus aureus	30%
Staphylococcus epidermidis	26%
Streptococcus faecalis	4%
Other gram-positives	1%
Gram-Negative Organisms	
Klebsiella species	11%
Pseudomonas aeruginosa	10%
Escherichia coli	5%
Proteus species	5%
Serratia species	3%
Enterobacter species	3%
Other gram-negatives	4%
Fungi	
Candida albicans	4%
Multiple Isolates	16%

appropriate direction. Well-kept records of operating room as well as cardiopulmonary bypass equipment cultures, which can be compared to patient cultures when and if significant wound infections develop, can provide the basis for this detailed statistical analysis. As is mentioned above, it is presently theorized that all such deep-seated sternal wound infections are the result of contamination in the operating room or immediately following the surgical procedure and develop based on multiple ambient host-related factors. The remainder of this section will discuss these factors.

PROPHYLAXIS: THE PATIENT

In many instances, the nature and timing of the specific cardiac surgical procedures are not optional in that the patient in question needs to undergo the surgical procedure immediately and time does not permit better preparation to lower the risk for infection. Patients with ongoing infections such as acute or subacute bacterial endocarditis who become hemodynamically impaired fall into this group. Although the subsequent prosthetic valve endocarditis rate and wound infection rate are significantly above average in this group, these risks need to be accepted under appropriate antibiotic coverage because the hemodynamic lesion if left untreated would remain life-threatening. Table 14-2 lists some of the general and specific risk factors known to be associated with poor wound healing and subsequent mediastinal infection.

Table 14–2
General and Specific Risk Factors for Impaired Wound Healing and Mediastinal Infection

Nutritional (deficiency or excess)
Hypoxemia
Malignancy
Systemic infection or distant localized infection
Diabetes mellitus
Renal or hepatic insufficiency
Immunoincompetence (iatrogenic or other)
Arteritis (radiation or other)
Low cardiac output or IABP requirement
Leukocyte abnormalities
Prolonged surgical procedure or prior sternotomy
Bilateral internal mammary grafts
Foreign bodies
Osteopenic sternum
Sternal fractures of malalignment
Reexploration for postop bleeding or 2.5-liter transfusion
Tracheostomy or prolonged ventilation
Emergency postop sternotomy or cardiac massage

Other concomitant infections such as those involving the urinary tract, skin, mucous membranes, lungs, and so forth, should be dealt with as best as is possible prior to the initiation of the surgical procedure. Ongoing serious dental infection is another major source of secondary intracardiac infection. Therefore, these lesions should be evaluated and fully dealt with under antibiotic coverage prior to initiation of any cardiac surgical procedure, particularly valve replacement. Intervals of at least 24 to 48 hr between dental extractions and anticipated valve replacement should be allowed to clear any bacteremia. A longer interval, if possible, would be desirable.

Ongoing serious metabolic abnormalities, which include severe malnutrition, electrolyte imbalances, and hyperglycemia, that are not under control can, with the appropriate inoculum, produce an excellent host for the initiation of a deep-seated sternal wound infection. The assessment of peripheral arterial blood flow and venous return in patients who are to undergo coronary artery revascularization is also of critical importance. Patients who have problems with distal arterial or venous blood flow should, if possible, have vein conduit harvested from the upper legs when necessary. Patients with prior surgery or intertriginous skinfold infection should attempt to have this treated preoperatively and then undergo harvesting of lower leg saphenous vein as necessary. Ongoing or recent infection in the line of either the sternal or leg incision is also a relatively strong contraindication to proceeding and should be either drained or treated with appropriate antimicrobial medication for an adequate time prior to the contemplated cardiac surgical procedure.

PROPHYLAXIS: TECHNICAL ASPECTS

Most surgeons believe that the major steps to prevent infectious complications of cardiac surgical procedures occur in the operating room. Meticulous attention to detail as well as curtailing the time of the surgical procedure is paramount in this regard. This care begins with the skin shave and prep, which should be no more than 12 hr prior to the initiation of the procedure but should not occur in the operating theater itself because the hair removed tends to form foreign bodies, which can easily fly into the wound site during the prepping and draping procedures. The need for multiple central venous and arterial access lines in these patients provides yet another avenue for organisms and subsequent infection. These lines must be handled meticulously during their placement and management and must be removed early in the postoperative period.

Although many acceptable skin preparation procedures exist, most centers have presently gone to one in which a povidone–iodine compound is used with or without a subsequent alcohol wash. The use of a plastic barrier drape and circumferential drapes around the legs in coronary bypass patients has seemed to decrease further wound infection rates.

From a technical point of view, old scars, if possible, should be excised rather than reincised because of the possibility of unrecognized indolent infection trapped within the scar tissue itself. Hemostasis should be meticulous, and any devitalized tissue should be removed. It is of paramount importance to preserve the midline sternal incision so that the blood supply of the sternum and the stability of the sternum remain uncompromised during the postoperative period. Because of the recent emphasis on the use of single or double internal mammary arteries for coronary revascularization, the resulting devascularization of the sternum makes the midline secure closure even more important. The use of bilateral internal mammary grafts or the use of a unilateral internal mammary graft in an obese, female, and diabetic patient raises the risk of sternal wound dehiscence and/or infection and must be considered when this particular type of conduit is selected. Irrigation of the pericardial space prior to the initiation of cardiopulmonary bypass not only removes particulate debris but dilutes any organisms and removes them prior to their being fed directly into the bypass circuit. Minimal use of cardiotomy suction thereafter will reduce trauma of the formed blood elements and also decrease the incidence of entrained organisms. The minimization of foreign material, such as bone wax, pledgets, and suture material, will further decrease infection. If electrocautery is used, it should be used sparingly.

With the increasing use of pericardial substitutes, either glutaraldehyde-preserved bovine pericardium or polytetrafluroethylene (PTFE) pericardial substitute, a foreign body is placed in the anterior mediastinal space between the heart and the sternum. Although initial data do not suggest an increased wound infection rate, the long-term follow-up is lacking. The minimal amount of this material necessary to serve its purpose should be used, with adequate drainage on either side.

As noted, meticulous attention to sternal closure is paramount in the reduction of wound infection rates. Many authors agree that instability of the sternum with secondary dehiscence predisposes to the development of deep-seated wound infections. After adequate mediastinal hemostasis has been obtained and drains have been placed, the sternum should be reapproximated. Any bleeding points on the periosteal surface should be individually dealt with, but a major attempt should be made to not devitalize the anterior and posterior periosteal tables. Small amounts of bleeding from the marrow cavity may be accepted because it will tend to be self-tamponaded on closure. Excessive amounts of bone wax, another foreign material, must be avoided. Multiple types of sternal closures have been employed successfully. Combinations of mattress as well as simple heavy stainless steel sutures have been successful in that they produce both lateral and vertical stabilization of the resutured sternal tables. Any sternal bone fragment that has been fractured and is considered significantly devitalized should be removed because this can serve as a nidus for sternal osteomyelitis at a later time. Following apposition of the sternum, the musculofascial elements of the chest wall should then be anatomically approximated. Most centers now employ running absorbable sutures rather than interrupted braided permanent sutures. Clearly, multiple techniques for dealing with the skin closure are acceptable. This should also be done in a very meticulous fashion because skin edge overriding and uneven apposition may result in a site for bacterial spread beneath the surface.

Occlusive postoperative dressing should be used around the wound, pacing wires, and chest tube sites, and should be painted on a daily basis with a povidone–iodine compound. All indwelling transthoracic devices, which include chest tubes, pacing wires, thermistors, and plastic monitoring lines, should be removed at the earliest possible opportunity when they are no longer necessary, because they can all serve as a tract for later colonization and infection.

Major morbidity resulting from leg wound infections can, in most instances, be prevented at the time of saphenous vein harvesting. An inexperienced surgeon, making multiple attempts to locate the course of the greater saphenous vein, may create a tissue flap of varying size. This flap, with the attendant devitalized fatty tissue in the obese patient, will serve as a nidus for later infection. Direct incision over the saphenous vein wherever possible and the absence of a skin and soft tissue flap will help to guard against these related problems. Irrigation of the wound with either saline or other antimicrobial solutions to dislodge and remove any devitalized fatty tissue or foreign body is also helpful. Absolute hemostasis is important as well. Drainage, although used in some institutions, has not been a major contribution to the prevention of subsequent seromas or deep-seated leg wound infections. The use of running absorbable suture with meticulous skin closure has been important. Many centers have attempted to keep these incisions from entering the inguinal crease, bridging the knee joint, and extending below the ankle, all of which should prevent subsequent abrasion and breakage in the skin closure, which may result in infection. A sterile absorbent postoperative leg wound dressing followed by a compressive elastic dressing to aid with hemostasis has also contributed to the resolution and prevention of some hematomas, seromas, and infectious complications. Postoperative edema is one of the most important factors contributing to dehiscence and subsequent infection of a lower extremity wound. Elevation and diuretic management in patients with postoperative leg edema is key to both the prevention and treatment of dehiscences and infection. Avoidance of compressive elastic dressings, tight closures, and "tension-reducing" retention sutures will all contribute to minimizing lower leg infections.

PROPHYLAXIS: ANTIBIOTICS

There is no subject in cardiac surgery more controversial than prophylactic antibiotics. It appears that most centers have developed their own regimen for the selection and administration of prophylactic antibiotics and are willing to defend their regimen against all others. From the myriad of publications and discussions surrounding this subject, certain facts appear to have emerged.

As seen in Table 14-1 on the microbiology of deep sternal wound infections, it appears that antistaphylococcal and antistreptococcal agents would be the optimal drugs for surgical prophylaxis. As we are excluding from this subject general thoracic procedures in which infected lung or bronchii are transsected, we are relegating our discussion only to "clean" open-heart operations. Therefore, with the exception of those patients with ongoing intracardiac infections, namely endocarditis, all of these antibiotics are employed in a truly prophylactic fashion.

With the need for ongoing cost containment in the health-care industry, it should be recognized that antimicrobial drugs account for approximately 35% of the total pharmacy cost in many large hospitals. Prophylactic antibiotics are responsible for between 10% and 15% of this total. Clearly, the cost of these drugs to the health-care industry is immense, and, if safely possible, their use should be minimized.

The noneconomic morbidity of prophylactic antibiotics extends in many directions. This includes those patients who have allergic reactions to the antibiotics in all of their forms and those patients who develop either ototoxicity or nephrotoxicity as a direct result of antibiotics. The incidence of oral and esophogeal candidiasis is increasing following antibiotic prophylaxis and appears to be related to the duration of the antimicrobial therapy employed. Hemodynamic aberrations, intestinal mucosal changes, and so forth, are all too common. An additional and perhaps most serious complication is that of the development of multiply resistant organisms in patients who are susceptible hosts. This not only puts the individual patient at risk for a difficult-to-treat deep sternal wound infection, but puts the entire unit and perhaps hospital at risk in that these multiply resistant organisms can be spread from unit to unit and be extremely difficult to treat with conventional antimicrobial therapy. A delicate balance needs to be struck for each of these indications and agents when used in a prophylactic fashion.

Multiple studies have been undertaken looking at the duration of preoperative treatment necessary to reduce the incidence of subsequent wound infections. Most authors now agree that a single high dose of drug given prior to the onset of skin incision, preferably 30 to 60 min before the surgical procedure begins, will result in adequate levels of antibiotic in the serum pericardial fluid and cardiac tissue. In particular, levels of antibiotics present in sternal cortical bone, marrow, and atrial appendage have demonstrated this fact as well. The dilution effects of the cardio-pulmonary bypass reservoir appear to decrease the circulating levels of antibiotics, and, therefore, put the patient at a somewhat increased risk for infection. This can be managed either by adding antibiotics to the bypass circuit or by supplementing the antibiotic dosage following the discontinuation of cardiopulmonary bypass. The renal clearance of most drugs is altered transiently as a direct result of cardiopulmonary bypass. Clearance of most such drugs decreases following the bypass run and lasts for approximately 24 hr following the procedure. Dosing, particularly with nephrotoxic antibiotics, needs to be adjusted for this specific requirement.

Introduction of antimicrobial drugs into the pericardial cavity, into the subcutaneous tissues, as well as rarely into the heart itself, has met with variable success. Again, it appears to be the irrigation and dilution of the microbial innoculum rather than the antimicrobial effect of the drug that have the major effect here. Meticulous surgical technique seems to be more important than the irrigation with specific antimicrobial agents.

A plethora of studies have been undertaken to look at the duration of antibiotic treatment required postoperatively to reduce the incidence of wound infections. Treatment courses, particularly in valve replacement patients, have ranged from 7 days postoperatively down to 24 hr. Most authors now agree that 48 hr should serve as an outside limit for any prophylactic regimen. Trials in which even a single postoperative dosage of antibiotics, when compared to longer duration of therapy, seem to show no advantage for either of these courses. Due to the multiple negative aspects of prolonged antibiotic treatment, most studies now favor a limited dosage regimen. Cultures and antibiotic levels from chest tube effluent demonstrate that adequate levels of antibiotics can be reached in the thoracic drainage material. Most authors would, therefore, continue their antibiotic coverage until intramediastinal foreign objects such as chest tubes and monitoring lines have been removed. The infectious complications surrounding transthoracic intracardiac monitoring lines, which include left atrial, right atrial, and pulmonary artery lines, are rare and perhaps need not be covered with prophylactic antibiotics for the duration of their existence.

Multiple studies have been undertaken in comparing many agents with anti-staphylococcal activity in an attempt to determine the optimal drug for prophylaxing patients undergoing open-heart surgery. Although the dosages of these drugs, as well as the resultant drug levels present in serum, urine, cardiac tissue, sternum, and chest tube drainage, appear to be tremendously variable, the resultant incidence of significant wound infection apparently is independent of all of these factors. There appears to be little rationale other than economic and practical, in terms of dosing intervals and so forth, to guide the selection of one drug over another. Cephalosporins have enjoyed the major popularity in this area. Cephalothin has been used in many centers for long periods of time with good results. Because of somewhat better serum and tissue levels, a recent change to cefazolin from cephalothin has occurred. As a result of the emergence of a broader spectrum of organisms in some institutions, a switch to a third-generation drug, such as cefamandole or cefoxitin, has occurred. Longer acting cephalosporins, such as cefonicid, have gained popularity in other institutions because of the simple dosing procedures. It is imperative that each cardiac surgical program identify the organisms unique to their institution and select an appropriate prophylactic agent. The cephalosporin agents that have been studied are listed in Table 14-3. Figure 14-1 depicts the serum levels for three widely used cephalosporin agents given at a time prior to skin incision. This demonstrates that cefamandole has extremely high levels, which can correlate well with good soft tissue and bone penetration as well. Other agents, such as amoxicillin and oxacillin, have enjoyed popularity in other centers as well but are not in as widespread use as the second- and third-generation cephalosporin agents.

Topical agents, such as povidone–iodine solution, available as both irrigation and topical sprays have been widely used in many centers prior to wound closure. Recent data on inhibition of wound healing might theoretically discourage the use of these agents, but the practical experience has been quite favorable. Randomized prospective studies looking at the efficacy of antibiotic versus plain saline irrigation of the mediastinum and presternal space demonstrate no additional benefit from the

Table 14–3
Antibiotic Prophylaxis for Postoperative
Sternal Wound Infections: Cephalosporin
Agents

Cephalothin
Cefazolin
Cefamandole
Cefonicid
Ceforanide
Ceftriaxone
Moxalactam

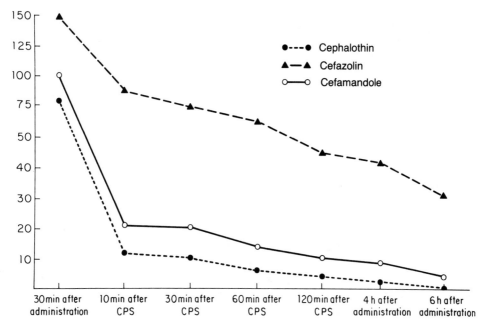

Figure 14–1.
Mean concentrations of cephalothin, cefazolin, cefamandole in serum during and after cardiopulmonary bypass procedures. (Eigel P, et al. Infection 1978; 6(1):23)

addition of antimicrobial solution and indeed, the group treated with dilute antimicrobial irrigation had a slightly higher, although not statistically significant, incidence of wound infection.

The use of a single high-dose short-duration agent should accompany any long-term antimicrobial treatment that a given patient is undergoing. For instance, if such a patient is admitted to the surgical service following his 6-week course of penicillin and gentamicin for streptococcal encocarditis, these two specific agents should be continued through the perioperative period pending microbiologic and histologic evaluation of any excised valvular tissue. A single preincision dose of any third-generation cephalosporin combined with 24 hr of postoperative coverage protecting the patient against the skin and soft tissue flora would be of additional benefit in this setting.

Much of the literature concerning the indication for prophylactic antimicrobial therapy in open-heart surgery results from the early years of cardiac valvular implantation. There are really equal amounts of literature on both sides of the issue for patients undergoing coronary revascularization in which an intravascular foreign body is not routinely used. In these patients, the indications for antibiotic prophylaxis for what is otherwise a clean operation are more questionable. It is, however, clear that if one is to use prophylactic antibiotics in this patient setting, and most centers do, they should be high-dose, short-duration, broad-spectrum drugs, with coverage of staphylococcal organisms.

Patients with a demonstrated history of serious reactions to cephalosporin form a special subgroup deserving comment. Included in this group are those patients with historically demonstrated serious penicillin reactions as well. Because of the 10% to 15% cross-reactivity of these two groups of antibiotic moieties, these patients should be considered together. Agents such as clindamycin and vancomycin have enjoyed widespread use for these allergic patients. Caution concerning the administration of these two drugs should be mentioned because neither of these agents is as innocuous as the cephalosporins previously discussed.

MANAGEMENT: CLASSIFICATION

Most of the serious infections associated with open-heart surgery are those involving the sternotomy incision site. These infections can range from the mildest forms of cutaneous and subcutaneous cellulitis to those that involve all of the subcutaneous tissues with fat necrosis extending deeper to involve the bone with frank osteomyelitis and costochondritis. The most serious form of these infections involves all of the above combined with mediastinitis in which purulent debris is present within the pericardial cavity as well as involving all of the bone and soft tissue. A classification of these infections is found in Table 14-4.

Infections involving the lower extremities following saphenous vein harvesting are an all too common problem complicating aortocoronary bypass procedures. Again, technical care involved in harvesting the vein and managing the wound post-operatively can avoid most of these deep-seated infections. When they are manifest clinically, confirmation by multiple techniques, including ultrasonography (US), computerized tomography (CT), and magnetic resonance imaging (MRI), can be useful. The assessment of their extent can, from time to time, be problematic. Usually, prompt incision and drainage and appropriately prescribed antibiotic coverage will produce satisfactory resolution in the overwhelming majority of cases. Attempts at secondary closure of these wounds are usually unsuccessful, and they should, therefore, be allowed to granulate until a clean, healthy bed of tissue exists. Secondary skin grafting procedures may be necessary but usually are not. These can frequently be managed in an outpatient setting with frequent follow-up visits complemented by topical lavage, debridement, and antibiotics, if necessary.

Table 14–4
**Classification of Postoperative Sternal
Wound Infection by Depth of Involvement**

Skin
Subcutaneous tissue
Fascia and muscle
Bone and periosteum
Mediastinal contents

Those leg infections that result from arterial or venous insufficiency in the extremity or ongoing secondary infection, such as untreated osteomyelitis, are much more difficult to eradicate, and attention should be directed at the primary course rather than the local wound caused by the saphenous vein harvesting.

Infections of intracardiac prosthesis, such as artificial heart valves, septal patches, and so forth, are extremely difficult to manage and shall not be the topic of this section. Suffice it to say that long-term, high-dose, antibiotic therapy, coupled with aggressive surgical debridement and a series of ingenious extra-anatomic bypass techniques have somewhat improved the survival in this extremely high-risk group. These infections can frequently be anticipated in that they tend to occur in patients with ongoing active infections at other sites. Once established, these are difficult to eradicate, carrying a high morbidity and mortality rate.

MANAGEMENT: DIAGNOSIS

The diagnosis of sternal infections remains a clinical one. The patients frequently complain of pain in their sternal area, which may or may not be combined with infra- and intrascapular back pain. This pain frequently radiates to the shoulders and the neck. The pain may be at first related to motion but later is present at all times. Spiking fevers and chills are frequent accompaniments of this syndrome.

Physical examination usually reveals an extremely ill-appearing patient with erythema surrounding their sternal wound. Exceptions to this may occur, with patients demonstrating few if any physical findings. Examination usually further reveals tenderness along the lines of the sternal wound and, more often than not, the sternal tables are somewhat unstable. It is extremely important to differentiate between a sternal sterile dehiscence, which may occur postoperatively, and deep-seated sternal wound infections. The former condition, which results merely from the separation of the sternal tables, is usually a self-limited process, which usually resolves with fibrous union without any significant morbidity. The latter infectious condition requires aggressive treatment, usually surgical, and carries with it a relatively high morbidity and mortality.

If deep sternal wound infection is clinically suspected, aggressive management should be undertaken. Broad-spectrum antibiotics aimed at organisms specific to the hospital environment should be initiated by parenteral route. This is by no means a substitute for aggressive surgical debridement but can limit the bacteremia while any other diagnostic or preliminary measures are undertaken. Plain chest roentgenography with lateral views may sometimes demonstrate air in the retrosternal space. Although not diagnostic, this finding is highly suggestive. US and CT, when combined with MRI, can sometimes further assist in the diagnosis of purulent mediastenitis and sternal osteomyelitis. Changes that occur in the bone can be diagnostic at times but, more frequently, are very difficult to separate from the usual changes that occur in the sternum following a sternotomy and normal subsequent healing. Bone scanning is almost uniformly positive in all patients following sternotomy and, unless the infection is quite late in the patient's course, is not a useful modality. Frequently, CT or MRI scanning of the chest will reveal "dirty fat" in the retrosternal space, which can be a marker for significant sternal wound infection but more frequently accompanies routine uncomplicated sternotomy incisions. Pericardial fluid, as demonstrated on two-dimensional echocardiography, can also be consistent with the diagnosis of deep-seated sternal wound infection but again, more often than not, is present following routine uncomplicated sternotomy, particularly if any degree of postcardiography syndrome is present. Indium-labeled white cell scans are also used in some institutions for difficult diagnostic problems but, again, produce an indeterminate diagnosis in most instances.

All of the above mentioned diagnostic tests (Table 14-5) have been used with some degree of success in the assessment of patients suspected of having deep sternal wound infections. These laboratory findings can be helpful; however, the majority of the time, mediastinitis remains a clinical diagnosis. In many respects, the diagnosis is based more on the clinician's level of suspicion than any of the diagnostic tests available. The aspiration of the midline wound, a bedside test, using a medium-gauge sterile needle inserted between the tables of the sternum, can frequently be helpful. Frequently patients with well-established mediastinal wound infection will drain spontaneously between their skin sutures, making the diagnosis all too obvious to even the least experienced member of the surgical team. The true challenge in these patients, aside from the prevention of this serious complication, is the early recognition, which, when combined with aggressive management, will reduce significantly the morbidity and mortality. Culture and Gram's stain of any material aspirated from the wound is key to identify any unusual organisms that might be present and to be sure that the systemic antibiotic coverage employed is appropriate.

MANAGEMENT: SURGICAL THERAPY

Only patients with mild peri-incisional cellulitis may be treated successfully with only parenteral antiobiotics. These should be continued until well after the tenderness and erythema dissipate, and the patient should be observed to be sure that a recurrence of the infection does not occur.

Table 14—5
Diagnostic Examinations Available for
Postoperative Sternal Wound Infections

Aspiration of wound
PA and lateral chest x-ray
Computerized tomography
Technetium bone scan
Gallium scan
Ultrasound scan
Magnetic resonance scan
Labeled white cell scan
Sinogram

Patients with simple subcutaneous fat necrosis complicated by secondary soft tissue infection may be managed by opening of the skin incision and with debridement and drainage of the subcutaneous space. These wounds should be left open, copiously irrigated, and well drained. Careful daily inspection of these wounds will quickly tell the clinician whether there is adequate improvement. When deeper seated infection is not present, these wounds should heal quickly. Almost any regimen of topical therapy, including saline, dilute betadine, dilute sodium hypochloride, and so forth, can be successful in eradicating these infections. If at the time of debridement there are exposed sternal wires or bone, suspicion of a deeper infection should occur, and the patient should be managed more aggressively. Any foreign material identified in these wounds, which is the usual inciting cause, such as suture, devitalized fat, or necrotic subcutaneous fascia, should be debrided at the time of the initial procedure.

When evidence of deeper seated infections occurs, these patients need to be managed more aggressively. Under general anesthesia with adequate invasive intra-cardiac monitoring, these patients should all undergo repeat sternotomy. Frequently, the sternum has been rendered unstable, and it is a simple matter to remove any of the remaining indwelling sternal wires and separate the halves of a sternum. On careful inspection, it will be noticed frequently that the sternum has multiple transverse fractures where the wires have cut through and that the fragments are relatively free floating. This will be discussed subsequently in the section on reclosure. After the sternal edges are separated, the mediastinum can be exposed and assessed. If there is frankly purulent material in the mediastinum, there is usually a moderate amount of necrotic debris as well. This should all be removed using a combination of blunt and sharp dissection techniques. These should all be debrided down to healthy tissue. The sternum should likewise be debrided, frequently with a laminectomy-type angulated bone cutting rongeur to healthy bleeding sternal bone and periosteum. Electrocautery and suture material should be minimized because these techniques both serve as foreign bodies for subsequent reinfection. The full extent of the pericardial cavity should be explored, including the diaphragmatic and lateral surfaces of the heart, to evacuate and drain any loculated purulent collections that may be present there. The great vessels and other sites of suture or anastomosis should be inspected carefully and gently debrided. Infections of this nature tend to erode through vessels, particularly along suture lines. In patients having undergone aortic valve replacement, this can be a life-threatening problem. Any unnecessary foreign material, such as bone wax and free bits of suture and pledget material, should be removed at this time. The pericardial space should be irrigated copiously with large amounts of warm saline solution or dilute antimicrobial solution until all of the obvious fibrinous debris has been removed. The subcutaneous tissues and skin edges may require debridement as well.

At this stage, an assessment needs to be made of the feasibility of reclosing the patient's sternum. Although modern techniques of ventilatory support and wound care have minimized the long-term morbidity of not closing the sternum, this still remains a major source of difficulty in these patients. If possible, the sternum and remaining wound should be reapproximated. Patients who are seriously immunocompromised, patients with extensive infections that can be debrided only partially, patients with severely fractured and fragmented sternums, and patients with aggressive gram-negative or polymicrobial infections are frequently not good candidates for primary sternal reclosure. Other patients, presenting with gram-positive organisms and only minimal amounts of tissue necrosis, can be successfully reclosed after adequate debridment and drainage.

Figure 14-2 depicts the irrigation drainage system used in numerous centers quite successfully. It involves one or two irrigation catheters placed laterally with multiple side ports for the infusion of an antimicrobial solution. A single midline chest tube is placed in a dependent stab wound and sutured into the skin. All previously present chest tubes, chest tube sutures, pacing wires, and so forth, are removed because they serve as a nidus for ongoing infection. After placement of the drains and irrigating catheters, the irrigation and drainage with 50 ml/hr of sterile saline solution divided between the two catheters is begun. Hemostasis should be established carefully, and any debridable infected or nonviable material should be removed. If the decision has been made to reclose the sternum, then the sternal edges need to be assessed carefully. The sternal fractures, if present, should be noted, as well as the relative symmetry of the previously made sternal incision. Many centers have adopted the approach of a woven or a mattress sternal closure, taking special care to fix the fracture fragments of the edges of the sternum. In our center we have tended to avoid woven sternal closures unless absolutely necessary, because they jeopardize sternal blood supply and may jeopardize healing. An alternating simple and mattress wire

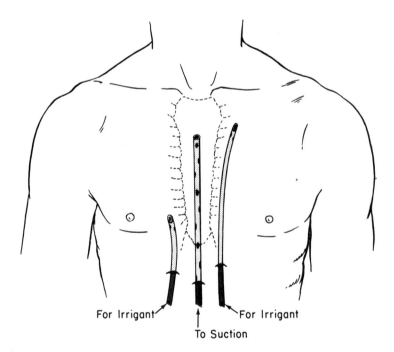

For Irrigant   For Irrigant

To Suction

Figure 14–2.
Arrangement of drainage and irrigation catheters used with closed management of postoperative mediastinitis.

closure has been very successful (Fig. 14-3). This is particularly true in patients who have undergone unilateral or bilateral internal mammary artery harvesting and are completely dependent on their intercostal collaterals for revascularization of the sternal bone and cartilage. Regardless of the technique of sternal closure employed, the important outcome of this is a stable osseus closure. This will allow adequate union of the sternum and prevention of subsequent dehiscence and infection. Following this, the subcutaneous tissue should be irrigated copiously, and all infected and necrotic debris should be removed. If it is possible, this should be closed in an anatomical fashion using interrupted absorbable sutures. If necessary, a deeply placed drain can be inserted and set to suction for the initial postoperative days. The skin, if possible, should be approximated loosely using multiple broad-based nonabsorbable nylon retention sutures. Bolsters made of latex rubber are frequently helpful in this setting because they prevent suture knots from eroding into the patient's skin.

Cultures and histologic specimens of mediastinal fat, anterior and posterior sternal tables, and any obvious loculated collections, should be dispatched immediately. Although these will not aid in the initial assessment and management, these will help aid in the decision concerning duration of therapy and overall prognosis.

In patients where the judgment has been made that the sternal wound cannot be primarily closed but the debridement is adequate, muscle interposition or omental pull up with secondary closure can be safely done. The viability of the muscle flap is contingent to some extent on whether the internal mammary artery has been utilized. Input from our plastic surgery colleagues is invaluable. The use of irrigation systems beneath muscle or omental flaps has been tried in a number of institutions; however,

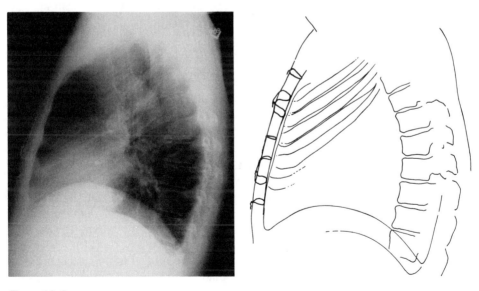

Figure 14–3.
Alternating simple and mattress sternal wire closure technique used with closed management of postoperative mediastinitis.

most applications of this technique are successful without the need for continuous substernal lavage. Unless great care is exercised it is possible that the placement of such catheter irrigation systems could interfere with the blood supply of the flap.

In patients where the assessment is made that the sternal wound cannot be primarily closed, it has not been our preference to place irrigating catheters. We have used large-bore sump drains in the open mediastinal wound to collect any effluent. The wounds then are packed with a lint-free roll gauze material, which can be changed in the postoperative setting. It is quite important to be sure that the packing extends into all of the loculations of the retrosternal space. Bridges of rigid material, such as short interconnecting pieces of rubber or plastic, can be used to support the edges of the sternum to protect them from collapsing and loculating the retrosternal space. These can be removed subsequently in the postoperative period without the need for general anesthesia. Because many patients will require later plastic surgical flap reconstruction, we have elected to involve the plastic surgical team as early as possible and find it useful to have them in the operating theater at the time of the initial debridement. This provides our colleagues with an excellent perspective in the assessment and timing of the patients for secondary closure.

MANAGEMENT: POSTOPERATIVE THERAPY

Most patients undergoing adequate surgical debridement with concomitant appropriate antimicrobial systemic therapy will have a prompt and sustained resolution in the systemic symptoms associated with their infection. Rapid improvement in mental status associated with near complete afebrility and slow normalization of the white blood cell count are the rule rather than the exception. Management regimens for patients with open and closed drainage procedures are outlined in Fig. 14-4.

Patients having been treated with closed drainage and catheter irrigation should be managed by continuous irrigation for 7 to 10 days postoperatively. The irrigation with solutions such as dilute povidone–iodine or specific antimicrobial therapy should be complemented with long-term parenteral antimicrobial therapy. Although early experience with dilute povidone-iodine irrigation was relatively successful, most centers presently employ a specific dilute antimicrobial therapy aimed at the offending organism or organisms cultured from the patient's wound. Until specific culture identification is made, dilute povidone-iodine, broad spectrum antimicrobial solutions, or normal saline can be successfully employed.

With deep-seated sternal wound infections, it is unlikely that the histologic evaluation of the edges of the sternum will reveal anything other than evidence of osteomyelitis, and, therefore, long-term antimicrobial therapy is indicated. In most cases, it is possible to discontinue the irrigation and drainage system after the patient has demonstrated an adequate clinical response. Careful and frequent inspection of the wound and catheter sites needs to be made to detect recurrent or persistent infection in these critical areas. Systemic antibiotics need to be continued for a long period of time, as discussed below.

In patients in whom closed treatment is not possible, the wound that has been

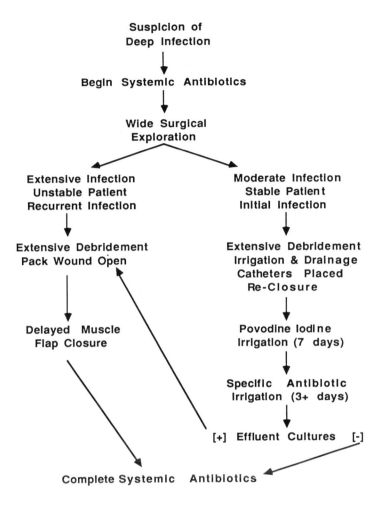

Figure 14–4.
Management scheme for deep postoperative sternal and mediastinal wound infections.

packed with antibiotic- or saline-soaked lint-free gauze should be inspected by the physician on at least a daily basis, with the dressings being changed twice or three times daily. It is important to use aseptic technique because these cardiac and other mediastinal structures are readily visible beneath the gaping edges of the sternal wound. These wounds tend to granulate quickly and become relatively fixed and stable, permitting rapid weaning and discontinuation of mechanical ventilation. Daily sharp debridement of any visible necrotic material should be conducted and combined with return trips to the operating theater when necessary to debride completely any and all nonviable tissue.

It is possible to return these patients to the operating room after adequate control of their infection and healthy granulation tissue has formed for closure of this sternum and closure of the skin and soft tissues superficial to the sternum. As a practical matter, it is frequently more expeditious to allow for a fibrous union of the sternum to occur and either perform merely a skin and soft tissue closure with localized flap advancement or to perform a rotation myocutaneous skin flap closure of the presternal deficit. Assistance in planning from plastic surgical colleagues is very helpful at these stages.

MANAGEMENT: ANTIMICROBIAL THERAPY

Concomitant with the surgical debridement and subsequent open or closed treatment, it is important to begin and maintain the patient on appropriate antimicrobial therapy. At the earliest suggestion of a significant sternal wound infection, broad-spectrum antimicrobial therapy should be initiated because these patients are usually quite ill and are not stable enough to allow enough time for careful microbiologic laboratory determinations by culture and sensitivity methods. Once the causative organism has been identified and the most appropriate antibiotic has been selected, this should be maintained during the entire treatment. It is frequently helpful to enlist the assistance of the infectious diseases specialist to follow these patients as well to be sure that the peak and trough antibiotic levels are therapeutic and not toxic and that the minimum inhibitory concentrations of the drugs relative to the patient's own organism does not change, ensuring that the entire course of treatment is optimally therapeutic. Duration of treatment is extremely variable depending on the organism and the extent of infection. Superficial cellullitic or subcutaneous infections require 10 to 14 days parenteral or oral antimicrobial therapy. Infections involving the bone or deeper tissues will usually require 4 to 6 weeks of parenteral antimicrobial therapy dated from the initiation of antibiotic therapy and drainage of the wound. As with any long-standing course of antimicrobial therapy, a careful surveillance must be made for the insidious toxic effects, namely deafness and renal insufficiency. Bone marrow abnormalities, as well as multiple other less common changes, can occur in these patients, and they need to be watched for carefully. Intestinal and other mucosal flora changes can produce annoying symptoms, which can be usually managed by either minor alterations in the antibiotic or by oral antimicrobial or supressant administration. Rarely, secondary complications, such as acquired drug allergy, drug fever, stomatitis, dermatitis, and so forth, can be so severe that they require the change of the antimicrobial therapy. The total course of therapy, however, unless very extenuating circumstances are present, should remain unchanged from the initial plan.

Following discharge, many centers have used an additional 2- to 4-week course of appropriately selected oral antimicrobial therapy in patients with extensive mediastinal or sternal involvement. It is felt that the additional benefit of this without the morbidity of additional hospitalization has some merit. This remains unproven but is associated with little subsequent morbidity and is the subject of ongoing research trials.

The selection of agents for irrigation of the mediastinum is also the subject of a great deal of debate. It is thought that the physical irrigation and dilution of the mediastinal space organisms with washout of the bacteria and debris are perhaps the most important aspects. For this reason, the total irrigation should equal 100 ml/hr with half being instilled through each catheter. It is extremely important for the bedside nurse and the physician managing the patient to be quite cognizant of the hourly output and input to be sure that mediastinal tamponade does not occur from obstruction of the effluent catheter or uncontrolled inflow. For this reason, calibrated pleurovac drainage or some suction drainage is used frequently for the effluent, and a mechanical pump is used for the inflow measurement. Dilute povidone–iodine solution is used frequently initially until definitive microbiology is available. In many centers, the povidone–iodine solution is used for irrigation for the first 5 to 7 days, and the terminal 5 to 7 days of irrigation are done with a dilute solution of the appropriate specific antimicrobial therapy. This is not a mandatory requirement because there still remain many centers that use normal saline or other combinations of nonspecific antimicrobials for mediastinal wound irrigation.

MANAGEMENT: GENERAL CONSIDERATIONS

After the appropriate surgical drainage and selection and administration of the antibiotics have been undertaken, many other considerations need to be made in these critically ill patients. They are usually initially managed in an intensive care unit setting and weaned from ventilatory support as rapidly as possible. Ongoing hemodynamic compromise secondary to infection or initially depressed cardiovascular function can complicate their recovery and frequently make weaning from the ventilator or inotropic support more difficult. Nutritional support is critical in these patients, and, if they cannot be fed by oral or enteral route, they should receive their nutritional support from a parenteral route. These patients frequently require 25 to 35 kcal/kg in the initial postoperative period because of their extreme catabolic state and have requirements for fatty acids as well. When possible, this should be switched to the enteral route because this is easier to manage and, in many respects, is safer, particularly as related to the removal of any indwelling intravascular access lines. This will also provide the theoretic advantages of nonspecific gut-related immunocompetence. The changing of all access lines should be accomplished at least every 3 days or more frequently if persistent infection occurs.

Attention to the other metabolic requirements of the patient is also quite important, and, because many of the antimicrobial agents employed can produce metabolic alteration, their careful monitoring is essential. If the patient cannot be weaned successfully from the ventilator in a reasonable period of time, temporary tracheostomy should be considered. Because of the communication of most tracheostomy stomas with the mediastinal wound, a desirable period, 14 to 21 days, should be allowed to elapse before tracheostomy is undertaken. This should be done as high as possible with a transverse skin incision in an attempt to keep the two incisions separate. This is particularly difficult with open mediastinal wounds, but every attempt should be made to separate these wounds and delay tracheostomy. The use of low pressure, controlled, soft-cuffed endotracheal tubes has markedly minimized the incidence of long-term tracheal complications and allowed for safer and longer endotracheal intubation periods. Many centers have recently employed a temporary crycothyroidotomy rather than a classical tracheostomy in patients with open or infected mediastinal wounds. Their experiences have indicated that the morbidity of this type of respiratory access in this particular setting is acceptable.

Chest and general physical therapy are an important part of the remainder of these patients' hospitalization. Because they tend to be in the hospital for long periods of time, they may become sedentary and depressed. This can result in poor nutrition, skin pressure and stasis problems, deep venous thrombosis, pulmonary embolization, and a generally negative mental attitude. Adequate ambulation and physical therapy can help to prevent this. Support from the well-counseled family and primary physician are also helpful in this area. Formal psychiatric intervention may become necessary under unusual circumstances.

MANAGEMENT: TREATMENT FAILURES

Patients who have been treated by either the open or closed technique have a small but definite incidence of treatment failure. The incidence of early failure is higher in patients who are treated with the closed technique. Any patients who remain systemically ill after a reasonable period of time or who redevelop sternal wound drainage with instability of the closure should be considered a treatment failure and should be re-explored aggressively. It is important to have close and careful surveillance of these patients to be sure that they are not relocating a collection in the mediastinal wound and developing recurrent sepsis. Should any suspicion of this occur, it is critical to return these patients as early as possible to the operating room where they are reopened and redebrided. At this juncture, in spite of how well they can be debrided and how much of the necrotic debris can be evacuated successfully, the temptation to reclose them should be resisted. Because they have already failed closed treatment once, the chance of their having a successful result the second time is small. Patients who have failed a closed irrigation technique may benefit from a subsequent debridement with either open packing or muscle/omental flap interposition if the clinical condition dictates. Frequently these patients are quite ill and operative intervention should be limited at this stage. The open technique is rapid, safe, and highly effective. Patients who are treated initially with open drainage may also require multiple return trips to the operating room for debridement and to break up and drain posterior or lateral intrapericardial loculations, which cannot be reached without undue hemodynamic lability and discomfort at the bedside. Late treatment failures may result from unrelated sources of infection, namely colonization of central venous access lines, bladder, lung, and so forth, but until proven otherwise, all "septic" appearing episodes should be considered to represent recurrent mediastinal wound infection and should be be evaluated aggressively.

MANAGEMENT: PEDIATRIC PATIENTS

The management of significant sternal wound infections in the pediatric age group, and in particular, in the infant age group, is significantly different from that employed in most adults. Although the microbiology of the infection is usually the same, these infections rarely involve the deepest mediastinal structures and can usually be managed by local wound treatment and systemic antibiotics. Because of the small amount of tissue involved and the extremely dense blood supply, it is usually possible to manage even deep sternal wound infections without debridement, lavage, irrigation, or drainage. Clearly, subcutaneous and subxyphoid loculations of purulent material should be locally drained and adequate microbiologic evaluation obtained. Broad spectrum, parenteral antimicrobial therapy should be carried out for a significant course depending upon the organism and the extent of infection.

With meticulous control of therapeutic blood levels, rapid diverescence and clinical resolution is the rule. A prolonged septic course manifested by fever, irritability, or other laboratory evidence after a reasonable course of therapy should be considered as a treatment failure, and the patient offered an open debridement technique. Open debridement has been successful in limited number of these patients. It should be pointed out, however, that even exposed bone or deeper structures are not necessarily an indication for further surgical debridement. Rapid granulation with control of the infection by antimicrobial means frequently occurs, making flap closure unnecessary.

When surgical debridement is necessary because of the small size of sternum present, near total sternectomies are frequently required. Debridements of costal-chondral junctions and costal arch material are often necessary as well. These major osseous deficits can be quite devastating both from a functional and later cosmetic perspective. The reconstruction can be very challenging.

Although sternal wound infections are rare in children following cardiac surgery, when they occur they will involve the same prolonged hospitalization and attendant morbidity as associated with adult infections. Outcome of treatment is frequently more dependent upon the underlying metabolic, nutritional, and structural cardiac defect than it is on the success of the local debridement and antimicrobial approach.

MANAGEMENT: RESULTS

The long-term outcome of patients treated for deep-seated sternal wound infections has improved over the last 10 years. These improvements most likely represent more attention to metabolic and nutritional details, with better selection of antibiotics, and more aggressive surgical drainage. Indeed, better understanding of the pathophysiology of these infections has allowed the mortality to be reduced from

80% to approximately 12%. The results of many studies have demonstrated that patients with gram-negative infections still have a poorer prognosis than those with gram-positive infections and that those patients who have failed closed drainage at one time have a poorer prognosis than those that can be treated with a single closed drainage procedure. The mortality for irrigation and drainage with sternal reclosure runs between 5% and 10%, with the corresponding mortality for debridement and open drainage between 25% and 50%. Series reviewing debridment and closure alone uniformly report mortalities in excess of 50%.

The cosmetic results of all of these closures are obviously not as ideal as the usual fine-healed sternotomy wound, but they are not terribly deforming either. Even the fibrous union of the sternum, which could theoretically pose significant problems, is tolerated extremely well by most patients. Figure 14-5 shows a representative technique frequently used for closure of a wound treated with open drainage. Latissimus dorsi flaps, pectoralis flaps, and advancement flaps can be used successfully to close these wounds and markedly shorten the duration of the patient's hospitalization.

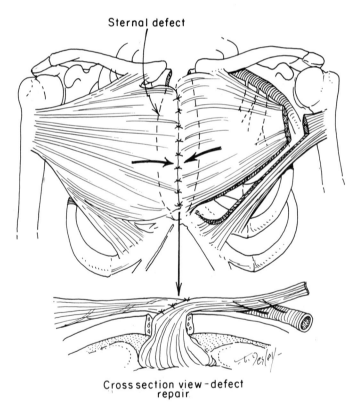

Sternal defect

Cross section view – defect
repair

Figure 14–5.
Pectoralis muscle flap advancement to close a large defect following open management of postoperative mediastinitis. (Pairolero PC, Arnold PG. JTCVS 1984; 88:357)

The key to all of these closures is, of course, that a new and stable blood supply is brought to the wound edges with the flap, which further adds to controlling infection and closure of the defect. Although the absolute survival and the degree of morbidity suffered by patients sustaining deep-seated sternal wound infections has improved over the last number of years, and the secondary osseus and cosmetic defects have become less and less prominent, these infections do require a minimum of 4 to 6 weeks of hospitalization and frequently a number of staged surgical procedures. Prevention, if possible, would be the ideal solution to this problem. The combination of careful attention to the points stressed above and early recognition of established infections should minimize resultant morbidity and mortality. Study of the needs of each cardiac surgical center, regional microbiologic flora, and surgical techniques will serve to produce the best combination of prophylaxis and treatment.

BIBLIOGRAPHY

Amoury RA. Infection following cardiopulmonary bypass. In: Norman JC, ed. Cardiac Surgery. 2nd ed. New York: Appleton-Century-Crofts, 1972:555.

Arnold PG. Reconstruction of the chest wall. In Mathes SJ, Nahai F, eds. Clinical applications for muscle and musculocutaneous flaps. St. Louis: CV Mosby, 1982:236.

Ashleigh EA (ed). Pathophysiology and techniques of cardiopulmonary bypass. Vol 1. Baltimore: Williams & Wilkins, 1982:132.

Austin TW, Coles JC, Finley R, et al. Prophylactic antibiotic therapy and heart valve replacement. Can J Surg 1976;19:349.

Baffes TG, Blazek WV, Fridman JL. Postoperative infections in 1,136 consecutive cardiac operations. Surgery 1970;68:791.

Barois A, Grosbius S, Simon N, et al. Treatment of mediastinitis in children after cardiac surgery. Intensive Care Med 1978;4:35.

Benner EG. Metabolism of antibiotics during cardiopulmonary bypass for open-heart surgery. Antimicrob Agents Chemother 1968;8:373.

Breyer RH, Mills SA, Hudspeth AS, et al. A prospective study of sternal wound complications. Ann Thorac Surg 1984;37:412.

Brook I. Microbiology of postthoractomy sternal wound infection. J Clin Microbiol 1989;27(5):806.

Brown AH, Braimbridge MV, Panagopoulos P, et al. The complications of median sternotomy. J Thorac Cardiovasc Surg 1969;58:189.

Burnakis TG. Surgical antimicrobial prophylaxis: principles and guidelines. Pharmacotherapy 1984;4(5):248.

Coleman JJ 3d, Bostwick J. Rectus abdominis muscle-musculocutaneous flap in chest-wall reconstruction. Surg Clin North Am. 1989;69(5):1007.

Conte JE, Cohen SN, Roe BB, et al. Antibiotic prophylaxis and cardiac surgery. Ann Intern Med 1972;76:943.

Cruse PJE, Foord R. A five-year prospective study of 23,649 surgical wounds. Arch Surg 1973;107:206.

Culliford AT, Cunningham, JN, Zeff RH, et al. Sternal and costochondral infections following open-heart surgery. J Thorac Cardiovasc Surg 1976;72:714.

Donaldson RM, Ross DN. Homograft aortic root replacement for complicated prosthetic endocarditis. Circulation 1984;70:178.

Eigel P, Tschirkov A, Satter P, et al. Assays of cephalosporin antibiotics administered prophylactically in open-heart surgery. Infection 1978;6(1):23.

Engelman RM, Williams CD, Gouge TH, et al. Mediastinitis following open-heart surgery. Arch Surg 1973;107:772.

Fanning WJ, Vasko JS, Kilman JW. Delayed sternal closure after cardiac surgery. Ann Thorac Surg. 1987;44(2):1969.

Fernando B, Muszynski C, Mustoe T. Closure of a sternal defect with the rectus abdominis muscle after sacrifice of both internal mammary arteries. Ann Plast Surg. 1989;21(5):468.

Firmin RK, Wood A. Postoperative sternal wound infections. Infections in Surgery, 1987.

346

Fong IW, Baker CB, McKee DC. The value of prophylactic antibiotics in aorta-coronary bypass operations. J Thorac Cardiovasc Surg 1979;78:908.

Gilbert DN, Tice AD, Marsh PK, Craven PC, Preheim LC. Oral ciprofloxcin therapy for chronic contiguous osteomyelitis caused by aerobic gram-negative bacilli. Am J Med 1987;82(4A):254.

Grmoljez PF, Barner HH, Willman VL, et al. Major complications of median sternotomy. Am J Surg 1975;679.

Grossi EA, Culliford AT, Krieger KH, et al. A survey of 77 major infectious complications of median sternotomy: a review of 7,949 consecutive operative procedures. Ann Thorac Surg 1985;40(3):214.

Heath BJ, Bagnato VJ. Poststernotomy mediastinitis treated by omental transfer without postoperative irrigation or drainage. J Thorac Cardiovasc Surg 1987;94(3):355.

Hehrlein FW, Herrman H, Kraus J. Complications of median sternotomy in cardiovascular surgery. J Cardiovasc Surg 1972;13:390.

Iacobucci JJ, Stevenson TR, Hall JD, Deeb GM. Sternal osteomyelitis: treatment with rectus abdominis muscle. Br J Plast Surg 1989;42(4):452.

Johnson JA, Gall WE, Gundersen AE, Cogbill TH. Delayed primary closure after sternal wound infection. Ann Thorac Surg 1989;47(2):270.

Jurkiewicz MJ, Arnold PG. The omentum. An account of its use in the reconstruction of the chest wall. Ann Surg 1977;185:548.

Jurkiewicz MJ, Bostwick J, Hester TR, et al. Infected median sternotomy wound: successful treatment of muscle flaps. Ann Surg 1980;191:738.

Kluge RM, Calia FM, McLaughlin JS, et al. Sources of contamination in open-heart surgery. JAMA 1974;230:1415.

Kluge RM, Calia FM, McLaughlin JS, et al. Serum antibiotic concentration pre- and post cardiopulmonary bypass. Antimicrob Agents Chemother 1973;4:270.

Martin RD. The management of infected median sternotomy wounds. Ann Plast Surg 1989;22(3):243.

Miller JI, Nahai F. Repair of the dehisced median sternotomy incision. Surg Clin North Am 1989;69(5):1091.

McKenna RJ Jr, Mountain CF, McMurtrey MJ, Larson D, Stiles QR. Current techniques for chest wall reconstruction: expanded possibilities for treatment. Ann Thorac Surg 1988;46(5):508.

Myerowitz PD, Caswell K, Lindsay WG, et al. Antibiotic prophylaxis for open-heart surgery. J Thorac Cardiovasc Surg 1977;73:625.

Nahai F, Morales L Jr, Bone DK, et al. Pectoralis major muscle turnover flaps for closure of the infected sternotomy wound with preservation of form and function. Plast Reconstr Surg 1982;70:471.

Nahai F, Rand RP, Hester TR, Bostwick J 3d, Jurkiewicz MJ. Primary treatment of the infected sternotomy wound with muscle flaps: a review of 211 consecutive cases. Plast Reconstr Surg 1989;84(3):434.

Nuutinen L, Hollmen A. Cardiopulmonary bypass time and renal function. Ann Chir Gynaecol 1976;65:191.

Ottino G, DePaulis R, Pansini S, et al. Major sternal wound infection after open-heart surgery: a multivariate analysis of risk factors in 2,579 consecutive operative procedures. Ann Thorac Surg 1987;44(2):173.

Pairolero PC, Arnold PG. Intrathoracic transfer of flaps for fistulas, exposed prosthetic devices, and reinforcement of suture lines. Surg Clin North Am 1989;69(5):1047.

Pairolero PC, Arnold PG. Management of recalcitrant median sternotomy wounds. J Thorac Cardiovasc Surg 1984;88:357.

Pairolero PC, Arnold PG, Piehler JM, et al. Intrathoracic transposition of extrathoracic skeletal muscle. J Thorac Cardiovasc Surg 1983;86:809.

Penketh ARL, Wansborough-Jones MH, Wright E, et al. Antibiotic prophylaxis for coronary artery bypass graft surgery. Lancet 1985;1:1500.

Peterson CD, Lake KD. Reducing prophylactic antibiotic costs in cardiovascular surgery: the role of the clinical pharmacist. Drug Intell Clin Pharm 1986;20(2):134.

Porter GA, Kloster FE, Herr RJ, et al. Relationship between alterations in renal hemodynamics during cardiopulmonary bypass and postoperative renal function. Circulation 1966;34:1005.

Rapp RP, Blue D. The role of the extended half-life second-generation cephalosporins in surgical prophylaxis. Drug Intell Clin Pharm 1985;19(3):214.

Rooney R, Neligan MC, Hone R, et al. Cephradine and cefamandole in coronary artery bypass surgery. Int Congr Symp Ser R Soc Med 1985;85:93.

Sanfelippo PM, Danielson GK. Complications associated with median sternotomy. J Thorac Cardiovasc Surg 1972;63:419.

Sarr MG, Gott VL, Townsend TR. Mediastinal infection after cardiac surgery. Ann Thorac Surg 38:415.

Scully HE, Leclerc Y, Martin RD, et al. Comparison between antibiotic irrigation and mobilization of pectoral muscle flaps in treatment of deep sternal infections. J Thorac Cardiovasc Surg 1985;90:523.

Sebening F, Meisner H, Kloevekorn WF. Six years experience with Betadine solution in heart surgery. In: Proceedings of the 2nd World Congress on Antisepsis. City TK, Perdu Frederick, 1980:151

Serry C, Bleck PC, Javid H, et al. Sternal wound complications: management and results. J Thorac Cardiovasc Surg 1980;80:861.

Seyfe AE, Shriver CD, Miller TR, et al. Sternal blood flow after median sternotomy and mobilization of the internal mammary arteries. Surgery 1988;104(5):899.

Shafir R, Weiss J, Herman O, et al. Faulty sternotomy and complications after median sternotomy. J Thorac Cardiovasc Surg 1988;96(2):310.

Shamberber RC, Welch KJ. Surgical repair of pectus excavatum. J Pediatr Surg 1988;23(7):615.

Shumacker HB Jr, Mandelbaum I. Continuous antibiotic irrigation in the treatment of infection. Arch Surg 1963;86:384.

Simpson LC, Peters GE. Poststernotomy infections presenting as deep neck abscess. Arch Otolaryngol Head Neck Surg 1988;114(8):909.

Slama TG, Sklar SJ, Misinski J, et al. Randomized comparison of cefamandole, cefazolin, and cefuroxime prophylaxis in open-heart surgery. Antimicrob Agents Chemother 1986;29(5):744.

Snow N, Gerding R, Horrigan TP, et al. Coverage of the open sternotomy wound with biobrane dressing. J Thorac Cardiovasc Surg 1987;94(6):914.

Stahl RS, Kopf GS. Reconstruction of infant thoracic wounds. Plast Reconstr Surg 1988;82(6):1000.

Sutherland RD, Martinez HE, Guynes WA, et al. Postoperative chest wound infections in patients requiring coronary bypass: a controlled study evaluating prophylactic antibiotics. J Thorac Cardiovasc Surg 1977;73:944.

Tector AJ, Davis L, Gabriel R, et al. Experience with internal mammary artery grafts in 298 patients. Ann Thorac Surg 1976;22:515.

Teranova W, Crawford FA Jr. Treatment of median sternotomy wound infection and sternal necrosis in an infant. Ann Thorac Surg 1989;48(1):122.

Thurer RJ, Bognolo D, Vargas A, et al. The management of mediastinal infection following cardiac surgery. An experience utilizing continuous irrigation with povidone–iodine. J Thorac Cardiovasc Surg 1974;68:962.

Tobin GR. Pectoralis major muscle-musculocutaneous flap for chest wall reconstruction. Surg Clin North Am 1989;69(5):991.

Vasu MA, Icenogle TB, Williams RJ, et al. Management of difficult sternal closure after sternal infection. Ann Thorac Surg 1989;48(2):315.

Walesby RK, Goode AW, Spinks TJ, et al. Nutritional status of patients requiring cardiac surgery. J Thorac Cardiovasc Surg 1979;77:570.

Wallace RJ Jr, Musser JM, Hull SI, et al. Diversity and sources of rapidly growing mycobacteria associated with infections following cardiac surgery. J Infect Dis 1989;159(4):708.

Williams CD, Cunningham JN, Falk EA, et al. Chronic infection of costal cartilages after thoracic surgical procedures. J Thorac Cardiovasc Surg 1973;66:592.

Williams DJ, Steele TW. Cephalothin prophylaxis assay during cardiopulmonary bypass. J Thorac Cardiovasc Surg 1976;71:207.

Yew WW, Kwan SY, Ma WK, et al. Combination of ofloxacin and amikacin in the treatment of sternotomy wound infection. Chest 1989;95(5):1051.

15

INFECTION IN ORTHOPEDIC SURGERY

Paul M. Pellicci
Eduardo A. Salvati
Philip D. Wilson, Jr.

Editorial constraints render impossible an all-encompassing treatise on orthopedic infections. Rather, in this chapter, we will discuss concepts of prevention and management of surgical infection as applied to the most commonly performed orthopedic procedures at The Hospital for Special Surgery and The New York Hospital. Management of infections following specific procedures not covered in this chapter may be found in texts dealing with those particular operations.

We begin this chapter with a brief general discussion of osteomyelitis. The reader should understand that not all postoperative surgical infections result in clinical osteomyelitis. For instance, infection following knee ligament repair may only involve the joint or the extra-articular soft tissues. Infections following joint replacement surgery early on may only involve the soft tissues surrounding the implant or the bone–cement interface at the edges of the implant. Conversely, infections following open reduction and internal fixation of fractures may more likely result in osteomyelitis and have important implications for fracture healing.

These issues will be dealt with in later sections of this chapter.

OSTEOMYELITIS

Osteomyelitis can be subdivided into three types: hematogenous osteomyelitis, osteomyelitis associated with vascular insufficiency, and osteomyelitis secondary to a contiguous focus of infection. This last type is most commonly the result of infection developing in an operative site or an open fracture.

Osteomyelitis secondary to a contiguous focus of infection differs from the other two types with regard to pathogenesis, the bones involved, the microorganisms responsible, and therapy. Staphylococci are the most frequent pathogens, but infection with gram-negative organisms is not uncommon.

The antimicrobial therapy of osteomyelitis secondary to a contiguous focus of infection must be based on the results of cultures obtained from the infected bone. *Escherichia coli, Proteus mirabilis,* and the majority of isolates of *Klebsiella pneumoniae* are susceptible to cephalosporin antibiotics. When these species have been isolated from the bone of a patient with osteomyelitis secondary to a contiguous focus of infection, a cephalosporin antibiotic may effectively be employed. However, if other aerobic gram-negative bacilli have been isolated, alternative antimicrobial therapy must be administered.

Although *Enterobacter* species and indole-positive *Proteus* species (*Proteus morgani, Proteus rettgeri, and Proteus vulgaris*) are not susceptible to first-generation cephalosporins (cephalothin, cephaloridine, cefazolin, cephradine, and cephapirin), these organisms are susceptible, in varying degrees, to the second-generation cephalosporins, cefamandole and cefoxitin. The majority of isolates of *Enterobacter aerogenes, Enterobacter cloacae,* and indole-positive *Proteus* species are susceptible to cefamandole, and this antibiotic may be safely and effectively used in the therapy of osteomyelitis due to these organisms. Cefoxitin is effective against some indole-positive *Proteus* species and may be administered when the infection is produced by *Proteus vulgaris.*

The antimicrobial agents most active against aerobic gram-negative bacteria are the aminoglycoside antibiotics. The aminoglycosides most frequently used in the modern antibiotic era are gentamicin, tobramycin, and amikacin. The compounds are active against *Escherichia coli, Proteus mirabilis,* indole-positive *Proteus* species, *Enterobacter* species, *Klebsiella pneumoniae, Pseudomonas aeruginosa,* and *Serratia marcescens.* A comparative microbiologic assessment of the aminoglycoside antibiotics suggests that tobramycin is most active against *Pseudomonas aeruginosa* and that gentamicin is most active against *Serratia marcescens.*[49] There is very little difference in the ability of the three compounds to inhibit other aerobic gram-negative microorganisms.[49]

In addition to their broad spectrum of aerobic gram-negative activity, the aminoglycoside antibiotics are characterized by their potential for the production of toxic effects. All of the aminoglycoside antibiotics may produce ototoxicity, nephrotoxicity, and, rarely, neuromuscular blockade. Nonoliguric acute renal failure is the most common renal toxic effect of the aminoglycosides; following discontinuance of the antibiotic the renal failure is reversible in virtually all patients. Either vestibular or auditory dysfunction may result from the administration of these compounds. Associated with the potential for the wide variety of untoward effects involving the blood-forming elements, caution must be exercised when the drug is administered.

Sulfonamide antibiotics and tetracyclines also are active against some aerobic gram-negative organisms. However, because these agents are bacteriostatic, their role in the treatment of osteomyelitis must be severely limited.

Although the parenteral administration of a bactericidal antibiotic for 6 weeks provides the greatest likelihood of successful therapy of hematogenous osteomyelitis, this is not the case when osteomyelitis has developed as the result of spread from a contiguous focus of infection. The treatment of this form of osteomyelitis must include not only the administration of antimicrobial agents, but also debridement of infected bone. The combination of effective surgical debridement of devitalized bone with appropriate antibiotic administration will afford the patient the greatest chance for successful eradication of this form of osteomyelitis.[48]

INFECTED FRACTURES

Successful management of infected fractures depends on early diagnosis and institution of prompt treatment to prevent spread of infection from soft tissue to bone.

Open fractures are classified into three categories. Type I open fractures include open fractures with clean wounds less than 1 cm long. Usually a spike of bone pierces outward.

Type II open fractures consist of open fractures with a laceration more than 1 cm long, without extensive soft-tissue damage, flaps, or avulsion, and no crushing component.

Type III open fractures indicate high severity of muscle, periosteal, and bone damage with increased potential bacterial contamination, providing an avascular environment conducive to bacterial growth.

The incidence of wound infection in open fractures varies according to the magnitude of trauma, ranging from less than 2% for type I and II fractures to 10% for type III fractures.[20]

Type III open fractures comprise the following: (1) extensive lacerations, flaps, severe crushing injury to the soft tissue; (2) segmental fracture of long bones, irrespective of the size of the wound; (3) farm injuries (potential soil contamination), irrespective of the size of the wound; gas gangrene should always be borne in mind as a potential complication of farm injuries; (4) vascular injuries; (5) gunshot injuries; (6) traumatic amputation; and (7) open fractures over 8 hr old.

Management of type III open fractures should commence within 8 hr of injury to prevent a contaminated wound from becoming an infected wound. Debridement and irrigation of the wound should be carried out in the operating room. Clear recognition of muscle viability comes with experience. However, reliable criteria, as described by Scully[46] and co-workers, must be used: (1) consistency, (2) ability to bleed, (3) contractility, and (4) color. Consistency and contractility are best determined by response to forceps pinch or stimulation under low-power coagulation. Viable muscles obviously will bleed when cut. This bleeding must be differentiated from arterial bleeding when cutting into small blood vessels. Color appears to be the least reliable indicator of muscle viability, particularly when there is improper lighting in the operating room. Debridement of skin should be conservative, particularly in the lower extremities where closure is essential. The fracture site must be exposed with an elliptical or longitudinal incision that could be converted into extensile exposure if internal fixation becomes necessary. Bone ends should be exposed and any foreign material, such as dirt or clothing, must be meticulously removed. Pieces of free bone fragments must be removed, unless they provide stability, in which case they should be retained. The wound should be irrigated at frequent intervals with normal saline solution or 0.1% bacitracin–polymixin solution using jet lavage. One should try to accomplish adequate debridement and irrigation at first surgery in a systematic manner, as efficiently and completely as possible.

Routinely, all type III open fractures must be brought back to the operating room for repeat inspection, debridement, and irrigation of the wound under general anesthesia within 24 hr. The wound should be left open and packed with Betadine gauze or Kerlix soaked with bacitracin–polymyxin solution (0.1%).

Administration of appropriate and adequate antibiotics for a short period of time should be considered therapeutic, and not prophylactic, in the management of type III open fractures. Preoperative antibiotics reduce the infection rate in open fractures.[19] A cephalosporin is the antibiotic of choice, based on culture and sensitivity studies of bacteria isolated in open fractures on admission. Antibiotics should be changed if necessary according to results of culture of the wound during various stages of its care.

The wound should be left open in all type III open fractures, even with the use of internal fixation and in open joint injuries. Delayed primary closure should be accomplished in 5 to 7 days by direct skin suture, or in the presence of tension or inadequate coverage, by split-thickness skin grafts or muscle pedicle flaps. The concept that the wound cannot be left open just because metal or articular cartilage is exposed has been proven wrong. The presence of metal per se does not promote bacterial growth *in vitro*. Indeed, recent clinical studies by Chapman and Mahoney[10] and Rittman and co-workers,[39] using early internal fixation of open fractures while leaving the wound open with an exposed joint and/or metal, revealed 10.6% and 7% infection rates, respectively, comparable to conservatively treated series of type III open fractures.

When the wound in an open fracture is left open for several days, because of the large soft-tissue defects, and healing by either granulation tissue and subsequent split-thickness skin graft or by secondary intention, prolonged antibiotic therapy is not recommended. It would be difficult to keep such a large open wound sterile for long periods of time, even with antibiotic therapy. Resistant-strain organisms can select out and develop an infection, which becomes a more difficult problem.

Fracture stability must be achieved to allow easier soft tissue management and to preserve soft tissue integrity. Primary internal fixation of type III open fractures should be considered in the following situations:

1. In multiple-trauma patients, primary internal fixation of open fractures allows for early mobilization, ease of transfer and care of patients requiring frequent diagnostic and therapeutic procedures, and better nursing care. Primary internal fixation also prevents shock lung.
2. In massive and mutilating soft-tissue injury requiring repeated surgical procedures. In limb salvage, stable internal fixation is an important factor in the care of soft-tissue injuries.
3. In floating extremity (ipsilateral fracture of femur and tibia) including ligamentous knee instability, occasionally associated with displaced acetabular fractures.
4. In arterial injury requiring repair. If it is an isolated arterial injury, traction may be used instead of primary internal fixation for a period of 4 to 6 weeks. Then one decides whether to continue traction and spica cast treatment, cast bracing, or delayed open reduction and internal fixation.
5. Intra-articular fractures. Joint congruency must be restored by internal fixation followed by early motion. Joints should be left open and then closed in 4 to 5 days.

Primary intramedullary nailing is contraindicated in type III open fractures. The periosteal circulation, as well as the extraperiosteal circulation provided by the surrounding muscles, is interrupted. When intramedullary nailing of type III open fractures is used, one completes the devascularization process of the fractured bone, particularly at the fracture site, by destroying the remaining endosteal circulation. Studies by Hansen,[21] as well as Rittman and co-workers,[39] have shown increased incidence of infection and difficult ostitis of the entire femur or tibia in early nailing of type III open fractures. Studies by Rhinelander[38] have shown the importance of intact muscular, periosteal, and endosteal circulation in fracture healing, even with stable fixation. External fixation, such as the Hoffman device or plating, would be the preferred method of achieving early stability if indicated. Plating is particulary indicated when the fracture is already largely exposed by extensive lacerations or wound flaps, thus additional surgical exposure for plating is not needed or is minimal.

The wound should be inspected daily, the examiner being alert for potential complications, particularly infection, including gas gangrene. Because of the long period that such wounds are open, superinfection, usually with gram-negative organisms, may be a problem. Because these organisms are usually difficult to control by antibiotics alone, prolonged aminoglycoside therapy, particularly for *Pseudomonas,* is dangerous and of questionable value. Daily soaking of the open wound with hydrogen peroxide, acetic acid, or plain normal saline solution or 0.1% bacitracin–polymixin solution helps to control infection and enhance the formation of granulation tissue.

Even if all the above principles are followed, the wound may still become infected. Proper management begins with surgical debridement. The wound should be opened widely. All nonabsorbable suture material should be removed, and all devitalized tissue should be debrided. Irrigation with antibiotic solution (bacitracin–polymixin) using jet lavage is recommended. The wound should be left open initially. Delayed primary closure may be performed in 4 to 5 days. A closed suction irrigation system may be used for 3 to 5 days thereafter.

If internal fixation has been used initially, it should be left in place if it still provides stability. If not, it should be removed, and traction or an external fixation device should be used for 4 to 5 days. At the time of delayed primary closure, a new internal fixation device may be used.

If there is inadequate soft tissue coverage, various techniques for wound closure may be employed, depending on the state of the bone and the presence or absence of exposed metal. If there is no bone loss with intact periosteum, granulations will form and the wound can be managed by split thickness skin grafting. Granulations will also form if cortical bone is removed to bleeding cancellous bone. If there is bone loss, primary cancellous bone grafting should be carried out over which granulations can be allowed to form. When hardware is exposed, muscle pedicle flaps or free vascularized tissue transfers should be considered.

Antibiotic therapy is not started until appropriate wound cultures are taken from the deeper part of the wound. Wound cultures taken superficially or inside the sinus tract can be misleading as to the real infecting organism inside the deep part of the wound. In the treatment of infected open fractures or infected wounds following open reduction and internal fixation of closed fractures, antibiotic therapy cannot be the only treatment of the problem.

After appropriate cultures have been taken, a cephalosporin should be started. Once the bacteria has been identified and sensitivity studies have been done, appropriate intravenous antibiotic therapy is selected for a minimum of 3 weeks, followed by oral antibiotics for another 3 weeks. This is adequate for an acute wound infection with relatively good prognosis compared to chronic wound infection with bony involvement. When an infection that has not been recognized in the first 3 to 6 weeks following an open fracture or open reduction and internal fixation of a closed fracture occurs, bone involvement should be suspected.

Intravenous antibiotics should be given for at least 4 to 6 weeks intravenously, followed by oral antibotics for 3 to 6 months. Whether prolonged, massive antibiotic therapy will prevent osteomyelitis or recurrent osteomyelitis in the future has not been supported or contradicted by any good, controlled studies.

INFECTIONS ASSOCIATED WITH PROSTHETIC IMPLANTS

In 1985 approximately 100,000 total hip and 40,000 total knee replacements were performed in the United States. This widespread use of total joint replacements fixed by acrylic bone cement has brought the problem of complicating sepsis to the fore for two important reasons. The first and more important is that, in contrast to the usual dramatically successful outcome of such surgery when uncomplicated, the development of deep infection almost invariably leads to painful loosening of the prosthetic components. This requires their eventual removal and leaves in their place large skeletal defects, important extremity shortening, and disastrous physical impairment. The second is the increased cost of hospital care, which, based on past experience, averages about $40,000 (four times more than the cost for the original prosthetic joint replacement). Approximately 1% to 2% is a reasonably conservative estimate of the current incidence of early and late deep infection associated with prosthetic joint surgery. Therefore, roughly 1400 to 2800 infections will occur in 1 year from hip and knee replacement surgery alone, at an approximate hospitalization cost of $56 to $112 million.

Prevention

The origin of deep postoperative periprosthetic infection is multifactorial. Contamination appears to come from both the patient and surgical team. The prime considerations in prevention are surgical asepsis, reduction of traffic and number of people in the operating room, the use of gowns impervious to contamination, double gloves, meticulous surgical technique, hemostasis, and gentle handling of tissues.

Patients should be selected carefully, and potential sources of infection should be recognized and eradicated prior to surgery, especially urinary tract infections. Obese patients should be required to lose weight, and they usually need help doing this. A low-calorie diet, a weight chart, a reasonable weight goal, and the incentive that surgery will be denied until they have met their goals are helpful techniques.

Patients with chronic debilitating diseases such as rheumatoid arthritis deserve special care and attention. The increased susceptibility to infection of rheumatoid patients is well recognized, particularly while on steroid therapy. The infection rate after joint replacement is higher in rheumatoid arthritis than in osteoarthritis.

Any patient who has had previous surgery should be evaluated carefully for possible infection, especially if an implant is still present. In such cases, preoperative aspiration of the joint under x-ray control is advisable to rule out occult infection.

The incidence of infection may be reduced remarkably by special precautionary prophylactic measures. Charnley,[11,13] a pioneer in the development of total joint replacement and in the use of methylmethacrylate bone cement, has championed the cause of reduction of exogenous operative wound contamination by the use of an enclosure, unidirectionial vertical airflow, ultrafiltered air, rapid air changes, ultrafine fabrics for clothing and draping, and air exhaust systems for the operative team.[12]

Clean Air

The effect of clean air has been studied at The Hospital for Special Surgery in New York.[1] The air flowing over the wounds of patients operated on in an enclosure with horizontal unidirectional filtered airflow contained fivefold less microorganisms than air near the wound in an enclosure without laminar airflow. Within the enclosure, wound cultures before surgical closure showed significantly less contamination when horizontal unidirectional filtered airflow was used. The organisms most frequently recovered in these studies from incisions, surgical field, and air flowing over the wound were coagulase-negative staphylococci.

Recently, a definitive study was published on the efficacy of ultraclean air. In a multicenter study of sepsis after 8000 total hip or knee replacements, Lidwell and co-workers[26] concluded that the infection rate was about one half when operations were performed with ultraclean air systems, compared with operations in conventional surgical suites. Furthermore, when whole body exhaust-ventilated suits were worn in a theater ventilated by an ultraclean air system, the incidence of sepsis was about one quarter of that found in conventional operating rooms.

A significant reduction of infections was also observed in those patients who received prophylactic antibiotics.

However, a recent study performed at The Hospital for Special Surgery[42] demonstrated that horizontal laminar airflow may produce adverse as well as beneficial effects, depending on whether the technique is properly performed. A significant reduction of infections in total hip replacement was shown, but, in total knee replacement, the infection rate was actually increased, probably because during the surgery members of the surgical team must stand between the source of the horizontal laminar airflow and the open wound. Because the surgeons did not use whole body exhaust-ventilated suits, they were probably shedding their own bacteria onto the open wound during total knee replacement.

Others have championed the use of ultraviolet (UV) light in surgery, but, despite reported successes, it is probably fair to state that the most widely used means of prophylaxis in current use is preoperative, intraoperative, and early postoperative antibiotics.

Operative wound infections come from endogenous sources as well as from exogenous contamination of the open wound. An additional factor in the immediate postoperative period is contamination from percutaneous sutures, suction drains, intravenous lines, indwelling catheters, and so forth. When one considers the multiple sources of contamination, both exogenous and endogenous, prophylactic antibiotics provide a more prolonged protection of the operative wound than do measures that affect only wound contamination at the time of surgery.

Prophylactic Antibiotics in Clean Surgery

The experience of the authors, and of others, has demonstrated that prophylactic antibiotics are highly efficacious. At The Hospital for Special Surgery, a program of prophylactic antibiotic treatment was instituted in December 1969 after an early experience with total joint replacement had shown a very high incidence of infection, particularly of the latent deep type. Because most of these infections were due to gram-positive organisms, particularly to coagulase-negative staphylococci (*Staphylococcus epidermidis;* Tables 15-1 through 15-4), a semisynthetic penicillin (oxacillin) was selected so as to have antimicrobial activity against penicillinase-producing organisms. In patients allergic to penicillin (nonimmediate type reactions), intra-

Table 15–1
Infected Arthroplasty by Diagnosis

Osteoarthritis	28
Rheumatoid arthritis	8
Failed prosthesis	16 (6*)
History of sepsis	7 (6*)
Osteonecrosis	2
Radiation for cancer	2
Systemic lupus erythematosus	1
Fusion	1
	59

* Same hips.

Table 15–2
**Gram-Positive Isolates from 59 Infected Total Hip Prostheses
(42 Gram-Positive [71%])**

Staphylococcus epidermidis	16
Staphylococcus aureus	11
Streptococci	7
Micrococci	2
Diphtheroids	3
Listeria monocytogenes	1
Staphylococcus epidermidis plus microaerophilic streptococci	1
Other gram-positive cocci	1

Table 15–3
**Gram-Negative Isolates from 59 Total Hip Prostheses
(13 Gram-Negative [22%])**

Escherichia coli	6
Proteus species	3
Klebsiella species	2
Pseudomonas species	2
Hemophilus influenzae plus *Staphylococcus epidermidis*	1
Culture negative*	3 (5%)

* Despite the negative cultures, the laboratory, radiologic, pathologic, and clinical findings were consistent with infection.

Table 15–4
Final Outcome of 59 Infected Hip Arthroplasties

Removal	23
Prosthesis in place and "healed"	18
Still infected	12 (2 died)
On antibiotics	4
Awaiting surgery	2

venous cephalothin was administered. (Thus far, significant allergic reactions from cross-sensitivity have not been encountered.)

There is considerable experimental and clinical evidence to show that the use of short duration, bactericidal prophylactic antibiotics in clean surgery is beneficial in lowering the infection rate. Sandusky[43] reviewed over 30 studies in the surgical literature that demonstrated a reduction in the infection rate when prophylactic antibiotics were used. He recommended that their use be routine when implants were to be used.

The risk of osteomyelitis and its sequelae with grave implications for patients makes it prudent to employ prophylactic antibiotics routinely, even in clean cases. Pollard and co-workers[34] and Hill and co-workers[22] were able to reduce their infection rates with the use of prophylactic antibiotics.

The use of perioperative antibiotics may even decrease the incidence of late infections.[9,18] Using an experimental skin model, Burke[7] was able to document the optimum time to administer prophylactic antibiotics. He showed that for antibiotics to be effective, they must be present in the tissues at adequate levels before bacterial inoculation. This presumably prevents the rapid exponential growth of the bacteria and allows the host to eradicate the infection.[5,28,29]

The pharmacokinetics of beta-lactam antibiotics require that they be given no more than 1 hr preoperatively.[33,44,51] They should be discontinued within 24 to 48 hr[50] when the drainage tubes and intravenous lines are discontinued.

Bone Penetration by Antibiotics

It is apparent from many studies that all classes of bactericidal antibacterial agents that produce significant serum levels also penetrate into bone. Many penicillins (penicillin G, ampicillin, oxacillin, nafcillin, methicillin, carbenicillin, ticarcillin), cephalosporins (cefazolin, cephalothin, cefamandole), cefoxitin, tobramycin, amikacin, vancomycin, clindamycin, lincomycin, and metronidazole have been evaluated by quantitative analysis of human bone biopsies, by study in experimental rabbit bone infection, and by observation of clinical effectiveness in human osteomyelitis.[15]

Methodologic considerations limit the accuracy of all results from antibiotic levels in osseous tissue. Because bone samples are perfused by blood *in vivo*, the blood-associated antibiotic content must be distinguished from the osseous tissue to determine the true bone level. Present quantitative elution techniques do not permit adequate removal of this blood "contamination" from bone without the risk of an artifactual reduction in bone antibiotic content. Furthermore, most studies are performed on normal, uninfected bone, which may not accurately reflect the penetration of antimicrobial agents into infected bone, which has an enriched vascular supply. However, on the basis of presently available data, the bone level of most antibiotics approximates 10% to 30% of the serum level. The degree to which variations in the protein-binding of an antimicrobial agent influences osseous penetration remains controversial.[16,47]

With the knowledge that bone antibiotic levels are substantially less than serum levels, antimicrobial regimens are usually designed to produce serum bactericidal activity (serum bactericidal titer) several times higher than the quantitative susceptibility of the pathogen to the therapeutic agent (minimum bactericidal concentration). It has been an often quoted clinical axiom that a serum bactericidal titer of 1 : 8 constitutes effective antimicrobial therapy for osteomyelitis although no data have been collected to substantiate this assertion.[14,25]

Joint and Synovium Penetration by Antibiotics

Most antimicrobial agents diffuse easily from the blood into infected joint spaces. Synovial fluid bactericidal activity bears a linear relationship to the serum bactericidal activity for penicillins, cephalosporins, clindamycin, and the tetracyclines.[30] Adequate joint penetration by all antibacterial agents that attain significant serum levels is likely. Occasionally, when the clinical effectiveness of a particular agent or therapeutic regimen is questioned, synovial fluid bactericidal activity can be assayed using available *in vitro* tests (tube-dilution technique). Protein binding does not appear to alter significantly the effectiveness of antibiotics in treating septic arthritis.[30] Synovial fluid antibiotic levels are substantially higher in infected joints than in noninfected joints.[30]

Penetration of Hematomas by Antibiotics

Antimicrobials administered intravenously have been shown to penetrate collections of human blood (hematomas) up to 4 days after their formation.[52] Penetration may depend on the size of the collection, because larger hematomas may not have demonstrable antibiotic content. Penicillins, cephalosporins, and aminoglycosides have been measured within hematomas.[3] In an experimental model devised to study the penetration of antibiotics into hematomas *in vivo*, fibrin clots were inserted subcutaneously into rabbits.[4] An inverse correlation was found between the penetration of antibiotics (penicillins) and the extent to which these agents were protein-bound by serum. Penetration into hematomas by these antibiotics was closely related to the level of "free" (unbound) drug in the blood. The maximal concentration found in fibrin clots was 19% to 25% of the peak level of free antibiotic in serum after single bolus injections. Repeated bolus injections or continuous infusions of antibiotics produced a two- to threefold increase in hematoma penetration.[2]

Local Antibiotics

Because most, if not all, antibacterial agents diffuse readily into infected joints from the blood, it is not necessary to employ intra-articular therapy in the standard treatment of septic arthritis. Occasionally, it may be necessary to confirm that adequate synovial fluid bactericidal activity has been achieved when a relatively new antibiotic agent is in use, or when clinical effectiveness is uncertain. If *in vitro* testing (tube dilution assay) does not confirm an adequate therapeutic level, then an alternative intravenous antimicrobial agent should be selected rather than supplementation by the intra-articular route. Intra-articular antibiotics can be irritants to the synovium inducing a severe chemical synovitis. In addition, intra-articular antibiotics are readily absorbed systemically, which can result in toxic serum levels. Moreover, intra-articular administration may predispose to contamination and superinfection of the involved joint. These principles also apply to the use of antibiotics in irrigation tubes in postoperative orthopedic patients.

The rapid penetration of bacteria deep into wound tissues appears to defeat the purpose of surface therapy. Recent studies have shown that antibiotic solutions failed to eradicate bacteria from wounds even when irrigation was commenced 1 min after contamination.[31]

Hematogenous Infection of Joints with Prostheses

With the increased numbers of total hip and knee arthroplasties being performed, there is an increased population of patients at risk for metastatic hematogenous spread of infections. Secondary prophylaxis against these infections must be instituted prior to any procedure that might produce transient bacteremia. Metastatic hematogenous spread of infection has been reported from various sites, including dermal abscesses, genitourinary tract, gastrointestinal tract, oropharyngeal, and respiratory sources. The following protocols are in effect at The Hospital for Special Surgery for secondary prophylaxis against metastatic hematogenous infections (Table 15-5).

All drugs are given parenterally 30 to 60 min prior to the procedure. This obviates the need for patient compliance or variations in intestinal absorption. The protocol should be effective in preventing the secondary spread of infections to orthopedic prosthetic devices.

Pathogenesis of Infection

The proliferation of a significant number of pathogenic microorganisms in viable tissue produces local edema, necrosis, and inflammation, which in turn impair local tissue circulation with consequent reduction of the local levels of antibodies, leuko-

Table 15–5
Protocol for Prophylactic Antibiotics to Prevent Metastatic Hematogenous
Infection of Total Joint Prostheses

A. Oropharyneal procedures
Procaine penicillin G (1.2 million units, IM) 30–60 min before the procedure
followed by penicillin V (500 mg, PO) every 6 h for eight doses.
For patients allergic to penicillin:
Clindamycin (600 mg, IM/IV) 60 min before the procedure followed by clinda-
mycin (300 mg, PO) every 6 hr for eight doses or
Cefazolin (1 g, IM/IV) 30–60 min before the procedure followed by cephradine
(500 mg, PO) every 6 hr for eight doses
B. Genitourinary or gastrointestinal procedures
Procaine penicillin G (2.4 million units, IM) 30–60 min before the procedure
and every 8 hr for three doses, or
Ampicillin (1 g, IM/IV) 30–60 min before the procedure and every 8 hr for
three doses, plus
Gentamicin (1 mg/kg, IM/IV) (not to exceed 80 mg) 30–60 min before the pro-
cedure and every 8 hr for three doses
For patients allergic to penicillin:
Vancomycin (1 g, IV) 30–60 min before the procedure and every 12 hr for two
doses, plus
Gentamicin (1 mg/kg, IM/IV) (not to exceed 80 mg) 30–60 min before the pro-
cedure and every 8 hr for three doses
C. Tissues infected/colonized with *Staphylococcus aureus*
Nafcillin (2 g, IM/IV) 30–60 min before the procedure followed by dicloxacillin
(500 mg, PO) every 6 hr for eight doses, or
Cefazolin (1 g, IM/IV) 30–60 min before the procedure followed by cephradine
(500 mg, PO) every 6 hr for eight doses, or
Clindamycin (1.2 g, IM/IV) 30–60 min before the procedure followed by (300
mg, PO) every 6 hr for eight doses

---

cytes, oxygen, and tissue nutrients. Waste products and bacterial toxins accumulate
and the acidity increases. The phagocytes, unable to function in this environment,
eventually die, releasing cytolytic enzymes that increase the suppuration and tissue
destruction. The bacteria persist at a phase of stationary growth. Incision, drainage,
and debridement permit a fresh serous exudate to reach the lesion, starting a new
cellular and humoral immunologic process.

Deep periprosthetic infections depend, as any other infection in general, on the
interplay between the microorganism and the resistance of the host. Factors such as
type, number, and virulence of infecting bacteria; localization; cellular and humoral
immune mechanisms play an essential role. However, the presence of a foreign body
enhances the risks of infection by interfering with the host defense mechanisms,
mainly at the foreign body–tissue interface. Neither the cellular defense (phagocytic
cells, neutrophils, macrophages, reticuloendothelial system) nor the humoral defense
factors (lymphocyte mediators, transfer factor, opsonins) can act adequately in the
presence of a foreign body. The fibrinogenesis and tissue reaction cannot localize the
infection nor the inflammatory process, which spreads along the surface of the foreign
body.

In 1957, Elek and Conen demonstrated the increased incidence of infection when a foreign body was introduced.[17] The subcutaneous injection of up to 1 million *Staphylococcus aureus* organisms did not produce infection in human volunteers. The immunity of the host was sufficient to control this amount of inoculation. The injection of 2 to 8 million *Staphylococcus aureus* organisms was enough to produce local infection. However, if a foreign body was present, the injection of only 100 *Staphylococcus aureus* organisms would produce an infection. Charnley,[12] in view of his experience with clean-air operating rooms, has suggested that the number of bacteria causing infection in total hip replacement must be less than previously considered.

There is *in vitro* evidence that methylmethacrylate, at very low concentrations, significantly decreased the efficiency of leukocytes for phagocytosis and killing of bacteria, due to a direct toxic effect.[32] Furthermore, insoluble wear products around implanted prosthesis could facilitate late infections by impairing local reactions to bacteria.[36]

Early deep infections tend to be more virulent, with local signs of inflammation as well as systemic symptoms. Late, latent, or delayed infections usually follow a more silent course, persistent hip pain being the main indication of its presence.[55] In spite of their late onset, metastatic or hematogenous infections produce a more acute and severe symptomatology, resembling early deep infections in their manifestations.[40]

DEPTH AND VARIETY OF INFECTIONS: GENERAL CONSIDERATIONS OF DIFFERENTIAL DIAGNOSIS

There are three general types of surgical hip wound infections: acute suprafascial or subcutaneous infections, acute subfascial or deep infections, and latent deep wound infections. Although it is not always easy, it is important to distinguish one from the other because the management and prognosis are quite different for each group.

Acute suprafascial infection manifests itself clinically by incisional pain, inflammation, and/or drainage, associated (but not invariably so) with fever and leukocytosis. It usually becomes manifest early (within 2 weeks of operation) and is particularly prone to occur in patients with thick subcutaneous tissues. It therefore should be watched for in overweight patients. It almost invariably runs a short course and, with proper treatment, carries a good prognosis.

Acute, deep, or subfascial hip wound infections vary in their mode of presentation depending on the virulence of the organism involved and individual resistance. The mode of presentation may be modified further by treatment measures such as the use of antibiotics, the development of spontaneous drainage, or incision and drainage. The variation runs from an acute prostrating and potentially fatal illness of very early potoperative onset to a low-grade indolent infection manifested by pain and little else. In The Hospital for Special Surgery's experience, the former have almost invariably been associated with beta-hemolytic streptococcal infections, and fortunately they have been rare. They were manifested by high fever, usually developing the night of surgery with septic shock, and required massive intravenous antibiotics and fluid replacement, and wide-open wound drainage for control. Once controlled, secondary closure or closure by skin-grafting has been possible and successful without sacrificing the prosthesis.

The more common deep-wound infections due to staphylococci have been less fulminating. In such infections, the hip and thigh are swollen. Often there is little if any superficial incisional inflammation or tenderness. The patients, however, complain of more than the usual degree of postoperative pain or their pain fails to lessen with time and is aggravated by activity. There is often deep hip joint tenderness unrelated to the incision. There may or may not be associated fever, and, when it is present, it tends to be quite low grade. This is also true of leukocytosis, but there is usually a left shift of polymorphonucleocytes. Diagnosis depends on recovery of organisms. The results of blood cultures are disappointing because there is rarely, if ever, a bacteremia or septicemia. The diagnosis is usually made by aspiration of the hip joint or, alternatively, by incision and drainage or wound biopsy.

In prosthetic arthroplasty of the hip, deep wound infections of this kind may be overlooked because the major clinical indication is pain and the pain may be assumed to be due to other causes. The persistence or recurrence of joint pain is almost always a cause for alarm. However, a safe rule to follow is that the persistence of troublesome pain after the early postoperative period should always raise the question of deep wound infection in the surgeon's mind.

Latent infections present a different problem and by definition are not manifest before discharge from the hospital and usually not until after 3 months or more have passed and the incision appears to have healed uneventfully. Many of the patients who develop such infections give no early indications of trouble, while others if questioned closely will admit that they have had pain in the hip ever since the primary procedure. The leading indication of such a complication is pain, a pain bothersome enough so that the hip is not really used for weight bearing. Examination of the hip usually gives no indication of an inflammatory process. There is often a very good range of passive movement, although movement is painful in the extreme range. Pain can also prevent or impede active hip movements. There is usually no fever and no leukocytosis, but often the sedimentation rate is elevated. Radiographs frequently show a gradual loss of bone density and varying degrees of prosthetic loosening, depending on the length of time from operation and the degree to which the patient is able to use the limb. Although some periostitis may become manifest around the femoral shaft, this finding has been rare in our experience. Again, diagnosis depends on obtaining positive cultures of organisms from hip aspiration, or pseudocapsular biopsy.

Diagnosis

Bone imaging by nuclear scanning can give valuable information.[37] Technetium 99 polyphosphate, gallium, and other radioactive agents have been used with variable success. Recently, the use of indium 111-labeled autologus polymorphonuclear leukocytes has been shown to be more specific and reliable in the diagnosis of infection.[35] However, the only definite and conclusive diagnostic tool remains the isolation and identification of the infecting organism. Thus, to establish the diagnosis the procedure of choice is a hip aspiration, preferably performed under the image intensifier with strict antiseptic precautions and local anesthesia. The fluid aspirated is sent immediately to the bacteriology laboratory for direct-smear (Gram's stain), aerobic, anaerobic, mycobacterial, and fungal cultures and sensitivities. The infecting organism can be a susceptible fragile bacteria. To increase the chances of growth, the aspirate should be inoculated as soon as possible into the appropriate medium. The use of a transport system with a culture medium to support the bacteria during the time of transport can also be helpful. The phenomenon of "sterile" infections may well be due to the difficulty of recovering and growing this fragile type of bacteria.

Immediately after hip aspiration, an arthrogram should be performed.[41] It will give valuable information as to the extent of the septic process, presence of abscesses, and loosening of the components. However, in certain cases, the injected contrast agent can fail to demonstrate loosening because it will tend to accumulate in the sites of least resistance, that is, where the abscesses are. It may also fail to dissect into the bone–cement interface when it is filled with granulation tissue. Although a larger volume of contrast agent could be injected to overcome this problem, it should be avoided because it entails a risk of producing septicemia or a distant seeding of the infection. Thus, in the presence of infection, the possibility of having a false-negative arthrogram should be kept in mind.

A complete cell count and differential count of the hip aspirate also may give valuable information. If the complete count shows more than 20,000 white blood cells/ml and the differential count more than 75% of polymorphonuclear leukocytes, infection should be suspected. Obviously, the higher these numbers, the greater the possibility of infection. If enough fluid is obtained, glucose and protein levels could also be helpful in making the diagnosis. In infection, the synovial glucose level will be less than half the blood glucose value because there is a decreased entrance and an increased utilization of glucose by the inflamed synovial tissue and the higher number of cells and bacteria present in the synovial fluid. On the other hand, the protein levels will be elevated; normal synovial fluid contains only one third as much protein as the serum and none of the recognized factors in the blood clotting system. But, in infection, there is an augmented passage of plasma proteins into the joint, including clotting factors.

When the hip is "dry," the injection of a small amount of sterile saline (without antiseptic preservative as in solutions for intravenous use) for irrigation of the joint with subsequent reaspiration may yield positive cultures. An arthrogram can also be helpful if there is any question as to whether the pseudocapsule has been actually entered. A negative culture from aspirate or from irrigation should not be accepted as conclusive if the other findings strongly suggest infection. In such cases, a biopsy of the pseudocapsular tissue or other suspicious tissues might be indicated. The specimen obtained should be smeared for Gram's stain and subjected to frozen section. If the Gram's stains are negative for bacteria, the presence of acute inflammatory cells in frozen section should caution the surgeon, and the wound should be closed to await the final results of cultures. Not infrequently, a reasonable judgment of the degree of inflammation may be made from gross findings only, but the fact that prior antibiotic treatment may modify the tissue response must always be borne in mind.

Sinograms can also provide useful information as to the depth and extent of the infectious process. Several organisms can be recovered from the sinus tract that do not necessarily correspond to the ones causing the deep periprosthetic infection.

Antibiotic Therapy

The effectiveness of antibiotic therapy is closely related to the intensity of the bacterial metabolism. Wood and Smith[56] demonstrated in 1956 that bacteria were killed promptly when penicillin was added early, during the logarithmic phase of bacterial growth, but failed to occur if the addition of antibiotics was delayed until the stationary growth phase. In thick purulent exudates, penicillin exerted only a slow bactericidal effect. The bacteria tended to persist at a stationary growth phase.

In infections complicating total hip replacements, antibiotic therapy might suppress the symptoms of infection and may be indicated as a temporizing measure if surgery is contraindicated due to medical reasons or if the patient does not accept it. However, it is unlikely to cure the infectious process. Successful suppression occurs in about 50% of patients. Its use can also complicate the problem by selecting genetically or phenotypically resistant strains or by inducing spontaneous mutation to resistant strains, while still not resolving the underlying infection.

If an infection involving an implant is diagnosed, the ideal treatment is early, adequate, and prolonged bactericidal antibiotic therapy combined with incision, drainage, thorough debridement of the involved tissues, and removal of the foreign body.

Depending on the sensitivity of the infecting organism, bactericidal drugs of first choice should be given in high doses intravenously for at least 6 weeks, followed by oral antibiotics for 3 to 6 months or even longer in some instances, particularly if the prosthesis is retained. While, ideally speaking, selecting the drug of choice from the large number of antibiotics available should not be difficult, several factors limit the selection of the antibiotic, such as the drug resistance of the organism and the general health and tolerance of the patient.

All these factors should be thoroughly assessed prior to deciding what antibiotic regimen is to be used, and not infrequently we may have to resort to antibiotics of second choice. If they produce adverse effects, we are forced then to switch to a drug of third choice, narrowing the alternatives even further. The need for careful monitoring of patients on antibiotics should be kept in mind, considering the high doses and prolonged time necessary for adequate treatment.

A combination of three antibiotics, acting at different sites on the bacterial metabolism, has been recommended. Because of the significant toxic potential, we have used this combination only in selected cases, working in close relation with the infectious disease specialist.

Surgical Considerations

The treatment of suprafascial subcutaneous wound infections follows the principles of treatment of all surgical wounds. Recovery of the organisms and the establishment of effective antibiotic treatment is of primary importance. Adequate drainage to evacuate loculated hematomata or abscesses is also important. How extensive the drainage will have to be varies, but it should be adequate to evacuate thoroughly the area involved so as to permit its rapid cleansing by frequent changes of dressing. Depending on the size, early closure, delayed primary closure, or coverage by split-thickness skin grafts should be considered in order to reduce the chance of secondary contamination. Secondary closure might be indicated in selected cases.

For the surgical treatment of deep periprosthetic infections, the patient should be typed and cross-matched for at least 6 to 8 units of blood. When the acute inflammation is severe, profuse bleeding can be expected, particularly if radical excision and debridement of the inflamed tissues are carried out. Spinal anesthesia proves advantageous for this type of surgery. The amounts of total blood loss and corresponding blood replacement during total hip replacement operations are less with spinal than with general anesthesia.[45]

Removal of the prosthetic components and acrylic cement can prove to be a difficult task, particularly if the septic process is of recent onset. The prosthetic components may not yet be loose, and removal of the tight interdigitation between bone and cement demands a laborious, patient, and meticulous technique if unnecessary loss of bone stock is to be avoided. In infections of longer duration, the septic process dissects along the bone–cement interface and loosens the components and acrylic cement by bone destruction, facilitating their removal.

The previously osteotomized greater trochanter is advanced and sutured to the proximal and lateral part of the femur. The proximal femoral shaft can be left outside the acetabulum, resembling a Girdlestone procedure (resection arthroplasty), or introduced into the acetabulum as in the Colonna or Whitman reconstruction (trochanteric arthroplasty). Advantages of the resection arthroplasty usually include less pain and freer range of passive motion. Increased shortening, telescoping, hip instability, and poor muscle control are the main disadvantages. In the trochanteric arthroplasty the opposite is true; usually it is a more stable joint, although it can be painful due to bony contact. The shortening and telescoping are not as severe, but the hip is more prone to stiffness. Considerations such as age, sex, and occupation might influence the choice of procedure. At The Hospital for Special Surgery we feel that resection of the superolateral acetabular margin is contraindicated, because it compromises a later prosthetic reconstruction and its value in improving the results of simple removal of the prosthetic component remains to be proved.

Following incision, debridement, and removal of the foreign body, including all acrylic cement, if the acute inflammation of the tissues is severe, the wound should be packed open for 3 to 4 days. A delayed primary closure can then be performed. This approach is safer than a primary closure over closed suction-irrigation. Qualitative and quantitative determination of the number of bacteria present in the wound tissue prior to closure has been suggested as a means of determining the best time for closure. Whenever the number of bacteria exceeds the critical level of 10^5/ml of tissue, secondary closure is preferred. However, we have not tested the practicality of this principle in our cases.

If primary wound closure is considered safe, a closed suction-irrigation system should be used. A meticulous complete closure of the fascia is mandatory to avoid leakage. Multiperforated polyethylene tubes are used, two for irrigation and two for suction. Two tubes are placed within the femoral shaft (one inflow, one outflow) and two within the femoral shaft (one inflow, one outflow) and two within the acetabulum. Large tubes are preferable. They clog less and allow an easier flow in and out of the wound. We have not followed the practice of using detergents, surfactants, antibiotics, or antiseptics in the irrigation fluid. Two Emerson suction systems should be used, maintaining a constant vacuum of about 100 to 200 mmHg. The outflow empties into a sterile bottle.

To reduce the chances of clogging, the suction-irrigation should be started promptly, as soon as the fascia is adequately sutured. Profuse irrigation in the amount of 6 to 10 liters is advisable for the first day. As soon as the system functions properly, with the outflow matching the inflow, the amount of irrigation can be reduced progressively and kept at about 4 liters/day. Close surveillance of the patient's medical conditon, electrolyte balance, fluid balance, and hematologic parameters is essential.

Cultures of the outflow are recommended. Gram-negative enteric bacteria are occasionally recovered and are usually considered contaminants unless the same single organism is repeatedly isolated. The cultures are likely to be negative if antibiotics are added to the inflow.

If wound healing progresses satisfactorily, the irrigation is discontinued after 2 or 3 days and all four tubes are converted to suction. Twenty-four hours later or when the outflow ceases, the tubes are removed, first the two inflow tubes and 8 to 12 hr later both outflow tubes.

When the closed system is maintained for longer periods of time, exogenous superinfections with hydrophilic opportunistic invaders can occur. Thus, particular care to avoid contamination is essential when changing bottles and so forth. The site of entrance of the tubes into the skin should be inspected daily. Preferably they should be placed anterolaterally, at least 5 cm away from the wound, to reduce the chances of sinus tract formation following removal of the tubes.

The lower extremity is kept in balanced suspension with tibial skeletal traction for 4 to 5 weeks. During this period, active muscle setting, limited range of motion, and deep breathing exercises are performed under the supervision of a physical therapist. Occupational therapy helps in keeping these patients interested and motivated. It is advisable to discontinue isolation as soon as the wound is healed to reduce the possibilities of emotional depression.

Prophylactic anticoagulation is advisable to reduce the danger of thromboembolism in view of the long period of recumbency. We prefer to start anticoagulation after the closed suction-irrigation system has been discontinued to decrease the risk of wound bleeding.

Four to 5 weeks after surgery, once acceptable scarring and stability of the hip are obtained, the skeletal traction is removed and the patient is started on gentle, progressive, active range-of-motion exercises. This is followed by dangling, standing, and partial weight-bearing ambulation with a walker, attended by a physical therapist. Pool therapy can be of particular help. Patients are progressed in their rehabilitation program as tolerated.

Reinsertion of a Total Hip Prosthesis

Treatment of subacute or recently arrested sepsis of the hip by total joint replacement and antibiotics is a relatively recent method of therapy in the United States. As already mentioned, past practice in such cases has been that of thorough debridement, removal of all foreign material, antibiotics with possible ingress and egress tubes, and resection or trochanteric arthroplasty.[24,27] Recently, because of the superiority of total hip replacement over these procedures, attempts have been made either to debride the hip in one stage, removing all foreign material and reconstructing the joint with a total hip prosthesis, or to delay this reconstruction to a second operative session. In either case, massive antibiotic therapy is administered.[6,8,53]

We have reimplanted total hip prostheses in cases of subacute, latent, or recently arrested hip sepsis, provided the wound was closed and the infecting organism was preferably gram-positive.[23,54] Frozen tissue sections at the time of surgery and the macroscopic appearance of the wound should show only mild to moderate inflammation. The Gram's stain should be negative. All scarred and devitalized tissues should be excised, leaving viable, well-irrigated, healthy tissues.

Adequate preoperative planning is essential to have available appropriate prosthetic components to facilitate a satisfactory biomechanical reconstruction when there is a bone stock deficit.

We have carefully selected the patients with latent deep infections in which we have used this procedure. Open wound drainage, pus, gram-negative or mixed flora, acute inflammation, and granulation tissue all constitute contraindications to one-stage debridement and reconstruction. The presence of a draining wound suggests a severe infection with marked exudate that had to decompress itself spontaneously through drainage. Infections caused by gram-negative or mixed flora are difficult to control, requiring intensive antibacterial therapy, close to toxic levels. Active pus formation implies a continuous process of leukocyte necrosis because of the virulence of the microorganisms. Acute inflammation or the presence of granulation tissue also demonstrates the severity of the infection. The reinsertion of a foreign body would further compromise the situation in these instances. Once clean, dry wound healing has been achieved, a second-stage reconstruction may be considered if other factors are favorable, and provided the cellular and humoral immune mechanism is normal.

REFERENCES

1. Aglietti P, Salvati EA, Wilson PD Jr, et al. Effect of a surgical horizontal unidirectional filtered air flow unit on wound bacterial contamination and wound healing. Clin Orthop 1974;101:99.
2. Barza M, Brusch J, Bergeron MG, et al. Penetration of antibiotics into fibrin loci *in vivo*. III. Intermittent versus continuous infusion and the effect of probenecid. J Infect Dis 1974;129:73.
3. Barza M, Samuelson T, Weinstein L. Penetration of antibiotics into fibrin loci *in vivo*. II. Comparison of nine antibiotics: effect of dose and degree of protein binding. J Infect Dis 1974;129:66.
4. Barza M, Weinstein L. Penetration of antibiotics into fibrin loci *in vivo*. I. Comparison of penetration of ampicillin into fibrin clots, abscesses and "interstitial fluid." J Infect Dis 1974;129:59.
5. Bowers WH. A rational plan for the use of preventive antibiotics in orthopaedic surgery. In: AAOS Instructional Course Lectures. Vol 26. St Louis: CV Mosby, 1977:30.

6. Buchholz HW, Englebrecht H, Rottger J, et al. Erkenntnisse nach Wechsel von uber 400 infizierten Huftendoprosthesen. Orthop Prox 1977;12:1117.
7. Burke J. The effective period of preventative antibiotic action in experimental incisions and dermal lesions. Surgery 1961;161.
8. Carlson AS, Josefsson G, Lindberg L. Revision with gentamicin-impregnated cement for deep infection in total hip arthroplasties. J Bone Joint Surg 1978;60A:1059.
9. Carlson VS, Lidgren L, Lindberg L. Prophylactic antibiotics against early and late hip infection after total hip replacements. Acta Orthop Scand 1973;48:405.
10. Chapman MW, Hahoney M. The role of early internal fixation in the management of open fractures. Clin Orthop 1979;138:132.
11. Charnley J. Low friction arthroplasty of the hip: theory and practice. Springer-Verlag, 1979.
12. Charnley J. Postoperative infection after total hip replacement with special reference to air contamination in the operating room. Clin Orthop 1972;87:167.
13. Charnley J. Acrylic cement in orthopaedic surgery. Baltimore: Williams & Wilkins, 1970.
14. Coleman DL, Horwitz RI, Andriole VT. Association between serum inhibitory and bactericidal concentration and therapeutic outcome in bacterial endocarditis. Am J Med 1982;73:260.
15. Cunha BA, Grossling HR, Pasternak HS, et al. The penetration characteristics of cefazolin, cephalothin and cephradine into bone in patients undergoing total hip replacement. J Bone Joint Surg 1977;59A:856.
16. Dombusch K, Carlstom A, Hugo H, et al. Antibacterial activity of clindamycin and lincomycin in human bone. J Antimicrob Chemother 1977;3:153.
17. Elek SD, Conen PE. The virulence of *Staph. pyogenes* for man: a study of problems of wound infection. Br J Exp Pathol 1957;38:573.
18. Ericson C, Ledgren L, Cindler L. Cloxacillin prophylaxis of postoperative infections of the hip. J Bone Joint Surg 1973;55A:80.
19. Gustilo RB. Use of antimicrobials in the management of open fractures. Arch Surg 1979;114:805.
20. Gustilo RB, Anderson JT. Prevention of infection in the treatment of one thousand and twenty five open fractures of long bones. J Bone Joint Surg 1976;58A:453.
21. Hansen ST, Winguist RA. Closed intramedullary nailing of the femur: Kuntscher technique with reaming. Clin Orthop 1979;138:56.
22. Hill C, Mazas F, Flamant R, et al. Prophylactic cefazolin versus placebo in total hip replacement. Lancet 1981;8224:795.
23. Hughes PW, Salvati EA, Wilson PD Jr. Treatment of subacute sepsis of the hip by antibiotics and joint replacement: criteria for diagnosis with evaluation of twenty-six cases. Clin Orthop 1979;141:143.
24. Hunter G, Dandy D. The natural history of the patient with an infected total hip replacement. J Bone Joint Surg 1977;59B:293.
25. Jordan GW, Kawachi MM. Analysis of serum bactericidal activity in endocarditis, osteomyelitis and other bacterial infections. Medicine 1981;60:49.
26. Lidwell OM, Lowbury EJJ, Whyte W, et al. Effect of ultraclean air in operating rooms on deep sepsis in the joint after total hip or knee replacement. A randomized study. Br J Med 1982;1(14):253.
27. Nelson JP. Deep infection following total hip arthroplasty. J Bone Joint Surg 1977;59A:1042.
28. Nelson CL, Bergfeld JA, Schwartz J, et al. Antibiotics in human hematoma and wound fluid. Clin Orthop 1979;108:138.
29. Nelson C, Schurman DJ. Preventative antibiotics. In: AAOS Instructional Course Lectures. Vol 31. St Louis: CV Mosby, 1982.
30. Parker RH, Schmid FR. Antibacterial activity of synovial fluid during therapy for septic arthritis. Arthritis Rheum 1971;14:96.
31. Petty W. Quantitative determination of the effect of antimicrobial irrigating solutions on bacterial contamination of experimental wound. 25th Annu. Orthop Res Soc 1979;9.
32. Petty W. The effect of methylmethacrylate on chemotaxis of polymorphonuclear leukocytes. J Bone Joint Surg 1978;60A:492.
33. Polk HC, Trachtenberg L, Finn MP. Antibiotic activity in surgical incisions. JAMA 1980;244(12):1353.
34. Pollard JP, Hughes SPF, Scott JE, et al. Antibiotic prophylaxis in total hip replacement. Br J Med 1979;6165:707.
35. Propst SL, Dillingham MF, Stanford JP, et al. Use of indium-111 labeled leukocyte scanning in orthopaedics. AAOS 47th Annual Meeting, February, 1980.
36. Rae T. A study on the effects of particulate metals of orthopaedic interest on murine macrophages *in vitro.* J Bone Joint Surg 1975;57B:444.
37. Reinig CM, Richin PF, Kenmore PI. Differential bone scanning in the evaluation of a painful total joint replacement. J Bone Joint Surg 1979;61A:933.

38. Rhinelander PW. Fractures of the tibial shaft. Clin Orthop 1974;105:34.
39. Rittman WW, Schibli M, Matter P, et al. Open fractures: long term results in 200 consecutive cases. Clin Orthop 1979;138:132.
40. Rubin R, Salvati EA, Lewis R. Infected total hip replacement after dental procedures. Oral Surg 1976;41:18.
41. Salvati EA, Freiberger RH, Wilson PD Jr. Arthrography for complications of total hip replacement: a review of thirty-one arthrograms. J Bone Joint Surg 1971;53A:701.
42. Salvati EA, Robinson RP, Zeno SM, et al. Infection rates after 3175 total hip and total knee replacements performed with and without a horizontal unidirectional filtered air-flow system. J Bone Joint Surg 1982;64A:525.
43. Sandusky WR. Use of prophylactic antibiotics in surgical patients. Surg Clin North Am 1980;60(1):83.
44. Schurman DJ, Hirshman HP, Burton DS. Cephalothin and cefamandole penetration into bone, synovial fluid and wound drainage fluid. J Bone Joint Surg 1980;62A:981.
45. Sculco TP, Ranawat C. The use of spinal anesthesia for total hip replacement arthroplasty. J Bone Joint Surg 1975;57A:173.
46. Scully RE, Artz C, Sako Y. An evaluation of the surgeons' criteria for determining viability of muscle debridement. Arch Surg 1956;73:1031.
47. Tetzlaff TR, Howard JB, McCracken GH Jr, et al. Antibiotic concentrations in pus and bone of children with osteomyelitis. J Pediatr 1978;92:135.
48. Waldvogel FA, Medoff G, Schwart MN. Osteomyelitis: a review of clinical features, therapeutic considerations and unusual aspects. N Engl J Med 1970;282:198.
49. Watanakmakorn C, Kaufman CA. *In vitro* susceptibility of gentamicin and/or tobramycin resistant gram-negative bacilli to serum aminoglycosides. Infection 1978;6:111.
50. Wicks MH, Rich GE, Rattliff RM, et al. The importance of cephradine in hip surgery. J Bone Joint Surg 1981;63B:413.
51. Wiggins CE, Nelson CL, Clarke R, et al. Concentration of antibiotics in normal bone after intravenous injection. J Bone Joint Surg 1978;60A:93.
52. Wilson FC, Worchester NN, Coleman PD, et al. Antibiotic penetration of experimental bone hematomas. J Bone Joint Surg 1971;53A:1622.
53. Wilson MR, Fitgerald RH Jr, Coventry MB. Reconstruction (delayed) by total hip arthroplasty after resection arthroplasty for infection. In: Nelson CL, ed. The hip: proceedings of the Sixth Open Scientific Meeting. St Louis: CV Mosby, 1978.
54. Wilson PD Jr, Aglietti P, Salvati EA. Subacute sepsis of the hip treated by antibiotics and cemented prosthesis. J Bone Joint Surg 1974;56A:879.
55. Wilson PD Jr, Salvati EA, Aglietti P, et al. The problem of infection in endoprosthetic surgery of the hip joint. Clin Orthop 1973;96:213.
56. Wood WB Jr, Smith MR. An experimental analysis of the curvature action of penicillin in acute bacterial infections. I. The relationship of the antimicrobial effect of penicillin. II. The role of phagocytic cells upon the antibacterial action of the drug. J Exp Med 1956;103:487.

16

○　　○　　○　　●　　●　　●

INFECTION IN VASCULAR SURGERY

Malcolm O. Perry

INTRODUCTION

In 1851, Koch described the treatment of a 22-year-old patient with rheumatic fever who died as a result of rupture of an aneurysm of the superior mesenteric artery.[13] Thirty-four years later, Sir William Osler coined the term "mycotic aneurysm" when he observed a patient with multiple aneurysms of the thoracic aorta, which Osler thought had the appearance of fungus vegetations.[21] He subsequently described the pathophysiologic mechanism—bacterial endocarditis with embolization of the arterial wall. Primary vascular infections are serious, especially when the infecting organism is *Salmonella,* or a resistent hospital-based organism such as *Staphylococcus aureus.*[11,18] With appropriate therapy directed toward the prevention and treatment of rheumatic fever and valvular disease, primary infections have been reduced in number. Because of the tremendous increase in direct vascular reconstructions, particularly those employing prosthetic grafts, secondary vascular infections have become more frequent.[32] Most vascular infections, whether primary or secondary, eventually require resection of the infected artery or removal of the infected graft, although in some cases intensive antibiotic therapy has been successful in either eradicating the infection or holding it in check.[31]

The incidence of vascular infections following reconstructive procedures varies between 0.25% and 6%, although most reports suggest there is an infection rate of approximately 2%; over three fourths of these involve the femoral arteries in the groin.[3,31,32] Untreated, such infections of vascular grafts almost invariably lead to suture line disruption or arterial rupture, bleeding, thrombosis, and generalized sepsis, threatening the limb and life of the patient.

ETIOLOGY

Primary vascular infections may be caused by many different types of bacteria, including various staphylococci, *Diploccocus pneumonia, Hemophilus influenzae,* streptococci, *Escherichia coli,* and even unusual organisms such as *Candida.*[4,9,10] *Salmonella* and *Campylobacter* seem to have a predilection for vascular endothelium, more so when the artery has atherosclerosis.[17,18] *Salmonella* causes a particularly virulent and dangerous vascular infection, especially when it involves the aorta.

The most common bacterial flora cultured from infected vascular repairs includes *Staphylococcus* and some gram-negative and anaerobic bacteria.[8] These organisms may be hospital-based and can be relatively resistant to the usual antibiotic programs.

PATHOPHYSIOLOGY

Although in the past hematogenous spread from endocarditic lesions was thought to be the most common cause of primary arterial infections, treatment of these diseases and the availability of antibiotics have reduced this problem. More often, direct inoculation may occur as a result of contamination during an operation, or perhaps as a result of bacteremia from concomitant illnesses at the time of implantation of a graft.[8,10] On rare occasions there is extension of an infectious process from a surrounding area (the inoculation of a graft placed near an abscess). In other cases, lymphatic-borne organisms from infections in the foot or leg infect a graft to the femoral artery.[1,20] The tendency for vascular infections to arise primarily in groin wounds is not unexpected because such wounds are in proximity to the perineum and are surrounded by lymph nodes that not only drain the extremity but may drain areas around the anus. Bacteremia, as a result of a remote infection in some other organ system (gallbladder, colon, urinary tract), can be a source of graft infection, but this is apparently a less frequent problem.[20]

Direct seeding of the wound or the graft during the operative procedure is always a risk.[8] If the graft is permitted to come in contact with the skin edges or with other organs, or if there is inadvertent bowel or urinary tract injury during a vascular procedure, contamination and subsequent infection are serious threats. Because a significant number of arterial graft infections are caused by hospital-based resistant organisms, it appears that direct contamination in the perioperative period is a recurring problem.

PREVENTION OF INFECTION

In emergency operations such as the treatment of an acute ischemic limb, or an operation on a patient for a ruptured aneurysm, prophylactic antibiotics may be administered before the operation, but it may not be possible in all instances to eradicate concomitant problems. In elective surgery, however, every effort should be made to ensure that the risk of infection is reduced to the absolute minimum. If such patients have a urinary tract infection or an upper respiratory infection, the operation should be deferred until these are identified and completely eradicated. Similarly, if a patient is being operated on for limb salvage and has an infected lesion on the foot or the leg, all dead and devitalized tissue should be removed and all pus should be drained prior to surgery.[10] Associated diseases such as cholecystitis or diverticulitis may require surgical correction prior to the elective vascular reconstruction.[9,31]

Although most vascular surgeons employ a mechanical preparation of the large bowel prior to operation, antibiotic regimens such as are used to prepare patients for bowel surgery are not routinely chosen. In unusual circumstances when the vascular repair cannot be deferred, and the patient has intercurrent colon problems, a more extensive bowel preparation is recommended, similar to that which might be used if the patient were to undergo bowel surgery.

Prophylactic Antibiotics

Most vascular surgeons employ some form of antibiotic prophylaxis, although the practice is not supported by conclusive data. Prospective studies in patients undergoing general surgery strongly suggest that the preoperative administration of antibiotics significantly reduces the incidence of postoperative wound infections.[29] Studies by Pitt and associates and Kaiser and co-workers show a significant reduction in graft infections if a prophylactic antibiotic regimen is employed.[12,24] In the past, penicillin and streptomycin and subsequently cephalosporins were chosen; more recently cephamandole and cefoxitin have been used. Changing bacterial flora encountered in a hospital setting mandate the use of a more potent antibiotic.

If prophylactic antibiotics are to be given, they should be begun prior to the operation; it is a common practice to administer the antibiotics beginning the evening before or the morning of operation. The aim is to obtain adequate tissue levels prior to the incisions. During the vascular procedure, it is also common practice to administer a second bolus of the antibiotic timed to increase the level in the blood during the interval in which the graft is being inserted into the arterial system. Although formerly the antibiotics were continued for 3 to 5 days postoperatively, now many vascular surgeons continue the drugs only for 48 hr after the operations. There are data suggesting that this confers adequate protection without encouraging the overgrowth of opportunistic bacteria, which might produce infections in other areas.[24,29] In some hospitals, the antibiotics are continued as long as the patient has a central line or a urinary catheter in place. There are no data supporting one practice over the other, and the decision to continue antibiotics further into the postoperative period is basedlargely on individual experience and judgment. Wherever possible, specific antibiotic therapy is employed, but in those patients in whom the offending organism cannot be easily identified, broad-spectrum antibiotics are administered if serious soft tissue infections appear postoperatively.

Skin Preparation

Although it is recognized that no method of skin preparation is perfect, and it is agreed that the effects of cleansing the skin are transient at best, various iodine solutions have been used successfully.[33] The addition of cleansing also with alcohol has merit, and some studies suggest that this may be the most desirable method of skin preparation. It is clear, however, that shaving prior to surgery is associated with an increased incidence of wound infection, particularly if the patient is shaved a day or two prior to the operative procedure. This permits the skin nicks and scrapes to become infected, usually with the *Staphylococcus* so often present on the skin. Inspection of the skin of a patient who has been shaved the day before almost invariably reveals scattered areas of folliculitis and tiny pustules where the razor has injured the skin. Shaving or removal of hair is generally not necessary unless the hair is so long as to pose a mechanical problem in the area of the surgical incision. In those cases, simple clipping of the hair just prior to the operation is recommended.

It has been suggested that transfemoral percutaneous catheter arteriography by the Seldinger method is likely to produce local infection along the punctured tract.[15] If the operation is performed prior to healing of the tract, the possibility of a groin wound infection may be enhanced. Although the data supporting this assumption have not been confirmed, some studies suggest that this is a real danger. Positive cultures can be obtained from these arteriographic puncture sites within a few days following the arteriogram. If, for example, an aortofemoral graft is to be inserted, it would be desirable to defer the procedure until the groin wound is entirely healed, but if that is not possible because of the necessity of treating an ischemic extremity, it is best to perform the operation the day following the arteriogram, covering the patient with specific antibiotics. At the time of operation, culture of the groin wounds is recommended on a routine basis in order to identify organisms that might later be responsible for an infection of the femoral artery.

After surgery, wounds closed with percutaneous sutures should be protected. This especially pertains to groin wounds (a urinary catheter should not be allowed to lay across a fresh suture line). Experimental studies suggest that percutaneous sutures permit the migration of bacteria from the skin surface into the depths of the wound; it is prudent to protect such wounds from gross contamination, although the incision itself may be well sealed within 24 hr.[28] As described above, it is common practice to use a program of prophylactic antibiotic administration for patients undergoing vascular reconstructive procedures, especially if prosthetic graft material is to be used.

Some studies suggest that the local irrigation of the wounds at the time of the vascular operation offers as much protection as the administration of systemic antibiotics, but there is no unanimity of opinion in this matter. Many surgeons choose to do both: give prophylactic antibiotics systemically and also irrigate the wounds and the prosthetic material with a topical solution of antibiotics at the time of operation.[32]

Several experimental studies are exploring the possibility of direct incorporation of antibiotics into the plastic grafts.[1] The incorporation of antibiotic or chemotherapeutic agents (silver-containing compounds) into the graft is being investigated. At present, no decision can be made as to whether this practice will be successful. Perhaps it will expose the patient to allergic reactions against the substances placed in the grafts. Because bacteremic contamination of a graft that is not thoroughly incorporated by fibrous tissue is always a threat, such methods clearly should be explored. The final decision as to the usefulness of such techniques has not yet been reached.

Wound Closure and Care

The closure of the wound in the neck, upper extremities, or the abdomen is straightforward and requires only that the tissue be brought into apposition without residual accumulations of blood, serum, or devitalized structures. Most surgical wounds are closed by sutures placed in the fascia and the skin—only rarely is it necessary to use subcutaneous tissue to obliterate dead space.

The groin incision is the one most often infected. The femoral sheath should be closed, then the fascia and skin are closed separately with interrupted monofilament sutures. These closures should be tight and meticulously placed.[1] It is also important that all lymphatics be ligated or excised because there are data suggesting that open lymphatics can contribute to bacterial contamination.[25] Postoperatively, if there is a superficial wound infection or the accumulation of a seroma that requires drainage, removal of sutures and opening the skin do not expose the graft because it is protected by two other layers.

Delayed Infection

If the graft is thoroughly incorporated by an external capsule and a thinner internal fibrous capsule, there is less tendency for bacteremic inoculation at a later date.[20] Unfortunately, most arterial prostheses do not heal entirely on their inner surface, nor do they remain healed. Thus, the grafts have exposed areas from time to time, and bacterial invasion is possible in a patient with bacteremia. Dental operations and urinary tract procedures can cause such bacteremia. It is prudent in these people to administer prophylactic broad-spectrum antibiotics prior to the procedure in order to reduce the chance of direct graft inoculation. This practice should be continued for the remainder of the patient's life.

Concomitant Operations

During the course of intra-abdominal vascular operations, the usual surgical principles should be observed. As described above, all intercurrent infections should be identified and eradicated prior to an elective vascular procedure, but in some patients vascular repair may be necessary despite the presence of other intra-abdominal pathology, such as symptomatic cholelithiasis. In such situations, because postoperative cholecystitis is one of the most common of the intra-abdominal complications occurring after surgery, following completion of the aortic operation and after closure of the retroperitoneal space, removal of the gallbladder is indicated.[30] In such patients, this is preferable to leaving a diseased organ in place to cause other postoperative complications. Incidental operations, such as removal of an asymptomatic appendix, are contraindicated.

If disease of the colon is encountered at the time of the elective vascular procedure, the unexpected abdominal pathology should be treated initially and the patient should return at a future date for the vascular repair. In other situations, for example, an operation being performed for a very large but asymptomatic abdominal aortic aneurysm, treatment of a nonobstructing colon lesion might be deferred for a later date and the life-threatening aneurysm can treated as planned. These are individual decisions the vascular surgeon must make according to the nature of the pathology. The danger of subsequent infection will depend on the extent and nature of the problems.

It has been shown that the subsequent development of aortic-enteric fistulae is probably related to erosion of the bowel by the relatively rigid prosthetic graft.[5, 22] Proper interposition of tissue between the graft and the intestine will eliminate this danger in most cases. In aneurysm operations, the aneurysm wall can be used to place a barrier between the graft and the small intestine, but in instances where the sac is too small or the retroperitoneal tissue is too scanty to permit this maneuver, a pedicle of omentum can be brought through the transverse colon to cover the graft and thus protect the small bowel. With this method of protection, the dreaded complication of aortoenteric fistula can be almost completely eliminated.

GRAFT INFECTION

Clinical Features

Infections of aortofemoral or femoral-popliteal grafts most commonly present as groin infections. There may be a mass, perhaps fluctuant, or development of a draining sinus. Occasionally the wound may dehisce, especially if the infection occurs early postoperatively.[8, 31, 32] If the suture line, or neointima is infected, local bleeding, thrombosis, or distal septic embolization can occur. If the suture line disruption is limited, a false aneurysm may appear. Any or all of these findings can be accompanied by generalized sepsis.

Upper gastrointestinal bleeding is the most common presentation of aortic graft infections, although some patients will have only sepsis.[32] Others may have only mild symptoms suggesting infection, usually recurrent fever and malaise. The aortic or iliac suture line is susceptible to disruption and bleeding or aneurysm formation, as well.

The infection may manifest itself within the first few days following the vascular operation, but there may be a delay of several years before there is evidence of infection. In some patients the only signs of graft infection are intermittent episodes of a low-grade fever, gastrointestinal discomfort, or recurrent episodes of diarrhea.[31]

Diagnostic Tests

Vascular infections occurring in grafts placed in the extremities are usually easily diagnosed on the basis of the clinical features and local findings, but infections of grafts in the aortoiliac position are more difficult to detect.[1] Any patient with a prosthetic graft and signs of sepsis or unusual clinical symptoms should be considered to have a graft infection. Venous and arterial blood cultures may be needed to identify the organism. A positive blood culture in any patient with a prosthetic graft is an alarming finding that mandates an extensive and thorough evaluation. In some cases, venous blood cultures may not be positive, and downstream arterial blood cultures taken distal to the location of a prosthetic graft may grow the offending organism. Because many of the patients may have had prophylactic antibiotics and at the time of evaluation may be on other antibiotics, careful culture techniques often are required to isolate and identify the organism. In some patients, there may be distal septic emboli in the lower extremity, for example, as a result of infection of an aortoiliac graft. In such cases, downstream cultures may be positive, or perhaps a local punch biopsy of one of the septic emboli may be diagnostic.

Standard x-ray examinations are usually of little value except for detecting the presence of a mass or displacement of other organs. In rare instances the presence of gas in an abscess may be seen.

When a sinus tract exists, sinography may be helpful in delineating the extent of the graft infection, and perhaps in some instances the graft itself may be visualized as the contrast material layers along its outer surface. A negative sinogram does not rule out a graft infection, of course, because a remote focus of infection may exist even in the presence of a normal study. In addition, intraluminal or neointimal graft infection, or suture line infection may be present yet not be in continuity with a sinus tract.

Ultrasonography, particularly B-mode gray-scale scanning, may be helpful in patients in whom the suspected area of infection is deep and inaccessible to clinical evaluation. The sonogram is not specific for graft infection, but it may detect a mass and determine if the mass is solid or cystic.[1,32] In other cases false aneurysms of anastomotic aneurysms may be examined by sonography. Such masses can be aspirated carefully under sonographic control, and the aspirated fluid can be examined with appropriate stains and cultures to determine if the fluid is infected or not.

Perhaps of more value is a careful computerized tomography (CT) scan, which may reveal the graft and the normal or infected artery proximal and distal to the graft. In addition, a careful CT scan may also show disruption of the suture line and in some cases show a perigraft hematoma or abscess. Dynamic contrast studies are particularly helpful in these situations. A surrounding hematoma may show delayed enhancement with the contrast medium.

Arteriography may be useful in some graft infections, but as with sonography it is not diagnostic unless there is extravasation of the contrast material into a false aneurysm, or through a disrupted suture line.[22] The arteriogram may be entirely normal. Radioisotope techniques, which include gallium- and indium-tagged white blood cells apparently, are especially useful in the detection of aortic prosthetic graft infection. Autologous white blood cells can be tagged with ^{111}indium or ^{99}technetium, reinfused, and serial scans can be performed.[19,26] Although such studies are not necessarily specific, they do have a high degree of correlation with vascular graft infections and are recommended in those situations in which graft infections are suspected but not confirmed by more standard techniques.

Antibiotics

The discovery of a prosthetic graft infection is a clear indication for intensive antibiotic therapy. If the offending organism can be identified by arterial or venous blood cultures or by direct aspiration, then specific antibiotics can be begun. Although the response in patients who have primary arterial infections is more likely to be satisfactory than those with secondary graft infections, there are reported instances in which such patients have been treated satisfactorily with intensive antibiotic therapy. In most patients who have an arterial prosthesis in place, removal of the graft and repair by some other method will be required.

Operative Management

It has been helpful in planning the management of infected grafts to divide the procedures according to the type of graft and the extent of involvement.[8] There are suggestive, although not conclusive, data that indicate that grafts made of polytetrafluroethylene (PTFE) are more resistent to bacterial infection than fabric grafts made of Dacron.[1] When they are infected, on occasion, they can be treated by drainage, topical antibiotic irrigation, systemic antibiotic administration, and local debridement.

A patient who has a paraprosthetic graft infection that involves only the body of the graft may respond to intensive antibiotic therapy, local drainage, and irrigation. If the shaft of the graft at the time of surgical exploration is the only portion involved, an attempt to eradicate the infection with continuous recirculation of triple antibiotic solution (neomycin, bacitracin, polymixin) or intermittent irrigation with a one to ten dilution of povidone–iodine solution may successfully clear the infection without removal of the graft. Connolly and co-workers have reported successful treatment of graft infections by continuous irrigation techniques.[14]

In contrast, experience from the Ford Hospital suggests that in certain situations graft removal is mandatory.[8] These include an aortoenteric fistula with erosion into the duodenum. Moreover, if the suture line is involved, graft removal will be required. If there is infection of the neointima, as manifested by continuing sepsis or distal septic embolization, it will be necessary to remove the graft. If other complications, such as bleeding, thrombosis, or embolization, occur, graft removal will also be required. It is clear, therefore, that only in a small and select group of patients will it be possible to treat the patient without removal of the prosthesis.

When it is necessary to remove the graft for the aforementioned indications, management of the residual infected arterial stumps continues to pose serious problems. It is desirable at the time of graft removal to debride the arterial bed extensively and to remove all dead, devitalized, and infected tissue. This may require repeated examination of sections of arterial wall prepared with Gram's stains, and perhaps frozen sections to determine if there are residual bacteria or inflammatory cells in the tissue to be left behind. This is particularly a difficult problem in the management of the proximal aortic stump after removal of an aortic graft. If the patient was treated for aneurysmal disease, the suture line will be just below the origin of the renal arteries, and it may be difficult to debride the aortic stump adequately to reach uninfected aortic tissue and ensure a safe closure.

Several investigators have suggested that this closure be performed in two layers with monofilament sutures (and/or staples) and that the suture line be buttressed by bringing a pedicle of omentum through the transverse mesocolon to cover the closed aortic stump.[1,8] Other surgeons have suggested that the anterior longitudinal ligament be transected distally, brought over the aortic stump, and sutured to further buttress the closures. None of these methods has been shown to be universally successful although they may be helpful in selected instances. Leather and Karmody have suggested an alternative method. These surgeons prepare a Roux-en-Y segment of jejunum by removing mucosa and using the small segment of vascularized bowel as a patch over the closed proximal aortic stump.[2]

Restoration of Blood Flow

In cases where it is necessary to remove an aortic graft, there are several methods for revascularization of the lower extremity. These basically center on the insertion of a remote subcutaneous graft, usually from the second portion of the axillary artery to the femoral artery (to the common femoral if it is not involved, or to the superficial femoral or profunda artery if the common femoral artery is involved in the infection). If it is known prior to operation that removal of the aortic graft is contemplated, most surgeons recommend placing the axillary-femoral and its adjunctive femoral-femoral bypass through clean tissue planes under the protection of systemic antibiotics prior to removal of the aortoiliac graft. In patients who had an aortic graft inserted for aneurysmal disease with an end-to-end anastomosis at the renal arteries, it will be necessary to remove the aortic graft and to use some type of remote bypass graft. If the patient had an aortic tube graft, an axillary-femoral graft may be put in place, and then it may be possible to restore vascular continuity to the contralateral extremity by either sewing the common iliac arteries together end-to-end or anastomosing one iliac artery end-to-side to the opposite iliac artery. This would complete a crossover revascularization with autogenous tissue performed in the retroperitoneal space. If such a repair is not possible, a standard femoral-femoral graft can be inserted. Once these grafts are in place and the wound is closed, then the infected aortic graft may be removed.

If the initial operation was for obstructive arterial disease and the native aorta remains in place, an autogenous reconstruction as advocated by Ehrenfeld and his associates can be accomplished.[7] In these situations, an aortoiliac endarterectomy can be performed after removal of the infected prosthetic graft. Vascular reconstruction of the lower extremity is therefore accomplished by using only autogenous tissues.

In some patients it has been recommended that lifetime antibiotic suppression be employed. Broad-spectrum antibiotics, penicillin, or, in some instances, trimethoprim–sulfamethoxazole have been used.

Aortoenteric Fistulae

Patients who have aortoenteric fistulae must be treated aggressively.[5,6] Usually the proximal aortic graft and the fourth portion of the duodenum are involved. Any patient who has an aortic prosthesis in place and experiences gastrointestinal hemorrhage must be assumed to have such a complication. Although careful upper and lower bowel endoscopy may, on occasion, confirm the presence of an aortoenteric fistula, negative endoscopic examinations, negative x-ray contrast studies, and negative arteriograms do not rule out the possibility of such a fistula. Even in the absence of positive studies, a patient with sepsis and gastrointestinal bleeding requires surgical exploration. It is prudent in these patients to obtain proximal control above the celiac artery prior to exploration of the aortic graft. Exposure of an aortoenteric fistula is usually accompanied by profuse hemorrhage.

In an emergency operation for aortoenteric fistula, early construction of remote subcutaneous bypass grafts is usually not feasible. Bleeding is controlled by temporarily occluding the supraceliac aorta, and then, when distal aortic exposure is completed, vascular clamps can be shifted to below the renal arteries.[22] The infected graft must be removed, and usually the sites of aortic and iliac anastomoses are closed with monofilament sutures, perhaps with reinforcement as described above.

Most patients will require some type of bypass grafting to restore blood flow to the lower extremities. The patient is given systemic heparin, and the abdomen is closed after debridement and drainage procedures are completed. In a few cases Doppler and physical examination may reveal that the legs are viable without further surgery, although this is rare in the author's experience.[16] More often, it is appropriate to return the patient to the operating room under clean conditions and to place remote subcutaneous grafts. Usually, left-sided axillary-femoral and femoral-femoral connections are preferred to restore blood flow. Under intravenous antibiotic coverage these can be performed with a low risk of infection of the new grafts.

Femoral-Popliteal Graft Infection

Although less likely to cause immediate death, infections in these areas are equally dangerous overall. The limb is often immediately in jeopardy if bleeding, thrombosis, or embolism occurs, and generalized sepsis is always a threat.

Some patients who were treated for calf claudication can tolerate removal of a femoral-popliteal prosthetic graft without severe limb ischemia. The sites of graft anastomosis to the arteries can be closed with autogenous tissue patches (superficial femoral artery segments or portions of saphenous vein). With antibiotic protection and careful coverage of the repaired artery by normal tissue, such repairs are often successful.[27]

If the leg cannot survive without the bypass graft, an alternative must be sought. Remote subcutaneous grafts using autogenous veins or perhaps PTFE are usually favored.[23] Iliopopliteal, femoral-popliteal, or femoral-tibial grafts may be placed laterally or anteriorily in the leg through uninfected tissue planes prior to removal of the infected graft. Although it is feasible at a later date, when all the wounds are healed, to return the graft to a more normal position, this has not been necessary in most cases.

Follow-up

Delayed suture line disruption with fatal hemorrhage can occur at any time, even after many symptom-free years. The aortic stump just beyond the renal arteries is particularly a danger, despite innovative methods of closure. These patients should be followed carefully for the remainder of their lives.[32]

Follow-up should include daily monitoring of temperature and intermittent evaluation of the erythrocyte sedimentation rate. If these are elevated, another check of the white blood cell count should also be obtained. Any evidence of infection suggests the need for ultrasound or CT scans of the suspected areas, usually the aortic and iliac site of the previous infection. Repeat blood cultures and perhaps repeat scanning using indium- or technetium-labeled white blood cells may be needed to find the infection. If these studies are positive, then surgical exploration will almost certainly be required to accomplish satisfactory drainage of abscesses and removal of infected tissue. An aggressive program of follow-up and early surgical intervention is essential if these delayed complications are to be adequately managed.

REFERENCES

1. Bernhard VM, Towne JB: Complications in vascular surgery. In: Moore WS, ed. Vascular surgery—a comprehensive review. New York: Grune & Stratton, 1984:737.
2. Buchbinder D, Leather R, Shah D, et al: Pathologic interactions between prosthetic aortic grafts and the gastrointestinal tract. Am J Surg 1980;140:192.
3. Casali RE: Infected prosthetic grafts. Arch Surg 1980;115:577.
4. Collins GJ, Rich NM, Hobson RW, et al: Multiple mycotic aneurysms due to *Candida* endocarditis. Ann Surg 1977;186:136.
5. Connolly JE, Kwaan JHN, McCart M, et al: Aortoenteric fistula. Ann Surg 1981;194:402.
6. Daugherty M, Shearer GR, Ernst CB: Primary aortoduodenal fistula: extra anatomic vascular reconstruction not required for successful management. Surgery 1979;86:399.
7. Ehrenfeld WK, Wilbur BC, Olcott CN, et al: Autogenous tissue reconstruction in the management of infected prosthetic grafts. Surgery 1979;84:82.
8. Elliot JP, Smith RF, Szilaygi DE: Aortoenteric and para prosthetic-enteric fistulas: problems of diagnosis and management. Arch Surg 1974;479.
9. Fry WJ, Lindenauer SM: Infection complicating the use of plastic arterial implants. Arch Surg 1967;94:600.
10. Goldstone J, Moore WS: Infection in vascular prostheses. Am J Surg 1974;128:222.

11. Johanson K, Devin J: Mycotic aortic aneurysm. Arch Surg 1983;118:583.
12. Kaiser AB, Clayson KR, Mulherin JL, et al: Antibiotic prophylaxis in vascular surgery. Ann Surg 1978;188:283.
13. Koch L: Ueber aneurysma der arterial mesenterichae superioris, in Inaug Dural-A Bhandlung. Erlangen JJ Barfus' schen Universitats—Buchdovckerd 1851:5.
14. Kwaan JHM, Connolly JE: Successful management of prosthetic graft infection with continuous povidone–iodine irrigation. Arch Surg 1981;116L:716.
15. Landrencan MD, Raji S: Infections after elective bypass surgery for lower limb ischemia: the influence of preoperative transcutaneous arteriography. Surgery 1981;90:956.
16. Ledgewood HM, Lucas CE: Biological dressings for exposed vascular grafts: a reasonable alternative. J Trauma 1975;15:567.
17. Martz AT, Webb TA, Stubbs K, et al: Inflammatory abdominal aortic aneurysm infected by *Campylobacter* fetus. JAMA 1983;249:1190.
18. Mendelowitz DS, Ramstedt R, Yao JST, et al: Abdominal aortic salmonellosis. Surgery 1979;85:514.
19. Miller DC: White cell scanning pinpoints infection. JAMA 1982;247:737.
20. Moore WS, Rosson CT, Hall AD, et al: Transient bacteremia: a cause of infection in prosthetic vascular grafts. Am J Surg 1969;117:342.
21. Osler W: The Gulstonian lectures on malignant endocarditis. Br Med J 1855;1:467.
22. Perdue GD, Smith RB, Ansley JD, et al: Impending aortoenteric hemorrhage. Ann Surg 1980;192:237.
23. Perry MO: Remote bypass grafts for managing infected popliteal artery lesions. Arch Surg 1979;114:605.
24. Pitt HA, Postier RG, MacGowan WAL, et al: Prophylactic antibiotics in vascular surgery. Ann Surg 1980;192:356.
25. Rubin JR, Malone JM, Goldstone J: The role of the lymphatic system in acute arterial prosthetic graft infections. J Vasc Surg 1985;2:92.
26. Serota AI, Williams RA, Rose JG, et al: Uptake of radiolabeled leukocytes in prosthetic graft infection. Surgery 1981;90:35.
27. Shah PM, Ito K, Clauss RH, et al: Expanded microporous polytetrafluroethylene (PTFE) grafts in contaminated wounds: experimental and clinical study. J Trauma 1983;23:1030.
28. Stillman RM, Bella FJ, Seligman SJ: Skin wound closure. Arch Surg 1980;115:674.
29. Stone HH, Honey BB, Kobb LD, et al: Prophylactic and preventative antibiotic therapy. Ann Surg 1979;189:691.
30. String ST: Cholelithiasis and aortic reconstruction. J Vasc Surg 1984;1:664.
31. Szilagyi DE, Smith RF, Elliot JP, et al: Infection in arterial reconstruction with synthetic grafts. Ann Surg 1972;176:221.
32. Talkington CM, Thompson JE: Prevention and management of infected prostheses. Surg Clin North Am 1982;62:515.
33. Wlrich JA, Beck WC: Surgical skin prep regimens: comparison of antimicrobial efficacy. Inf in Surg 1984;Aug:569.

17

○   ○   ○   ●   ●   ●

PEDIATRIC SURGERY INFECTIONS

S. Frank Redo

Surgical infection in the pediatric age group is not significantly different from that in the adult patient. It may be localized to the incision at the operative site, "wound or incisional infection," or may be deep to the incision site as an abscess and in the body cavity in which the operation was performed.

The incidence of postoperative infection in the general surgical patient has been reported to be 7.5% overall, rising to 30% or more following certain types of operations.[1] Surgical procedures have been divided into four categories of risk for development of postoperative infection: clean, clean–contaminated, contaminated, and dirty or infected[4,12] (Table 17-1). The incidence of wound infection increases markedly as the surgery progresses from clean to dirty or infected cases.[4] The incidence of surgical infection in the pediatric patient is not readily available. The overall infection rate for 3264 general surgical operations in pediatric patients at the New York Hospital–Cornell Medical Center for the period 1980 to 1985 was 2.2%. The incidence was only 0.6% for clean cases but rose to 25% for dirty or infected cases (Table 17-2).

Table 17–1
Classification of Surgical Procedures by Degree of Contamination

Clean	Elective, primarily closed, no drains
	Nontraumatic, not infected or inflamed
	No break in sterile technique
	No entry into respiratory, GU, GI, oropharyngeal tracts
Clean–contaminated	Minor break in sterile technique
	Appendectomy
	GI, GU, respiratory tracts entered under controlled conditions and without unusual contamination
	Oropharynx, vagina entered
	GU tract entered in absence of culture-positive urine
	Biliary tract entered in absence of infected bile
	Mechanical drainage
Contaminated	Major break in sterile technique
	Open, fresh traumatic wounds
	Gross spillage from GI tract
	Entry into GU or biliary tracts in presence of infected urine or bile
	Incisions encountering acute, nonpurulent inflammation
Dirty and infected	Wounds with retained devitalized tissue, foreign bodies, fecal contamination, delayed treatment or from dirty source
	Perforated viscus
	Acute bacterial infection with pus encountered

(Adapted from Altemeier WA, Burke JF, Pruitt BA, et al, eds. Manual on control of infection in surgical patients. Philadelphia: JB Lippincott, 1984:10 [Table 2-2] and Mollitt DL. Pediatric surgical infection and antibiotic usage. Pediatr Infect Dis 1985;4:326.)

Table 17–2
Incidence of Surgical Infection as Related to Wound Classification

YEAR	TYPE OF CASE			
	Clean	Clean–Contaminated	Contaminated	Dirty
1981	520	118	15	16
1982	534	107	18	13
1983	529	76	34	24
1984	408	130	36	25
1985	539	80	24	18
Total	2530	511	127	96
Number of infections	15	22	12	24
Percent incidence	0.6%	4.3%	9.4%	25%

Total operations: 3264
Total infections: 73
Overall infection incidence: 2.2%

Specific types of postoperative infections and their seriousness are related to the age of the patient (*i.e.,* premature, newborn, toddler, or older child) as well as to the problem for which the surgery was performed.

Length of anesthesia and the operation, lack of immunologic response by the patient, and quality of surgical technique contribute to the development of infection following surgery. The nutritional and metabolic status of the patient related to prematurity, inanition, and underlying pathologic condition also are important factors. Obviously the possibility for postoperative infection increases as the category of surgery progresses from clean to dirty.

Nosocomial infections not related to surgery are not infrequent in the pediatric patient. These include such diseases as chickenpox, measles, group A streptococcal pharyngitis, viral gastroenteritides, and bacterial diarrhea.

PROPHYLACTIC MEASURES

Steps to minimize the development of infections in surgery begin with a careful assessment of the patient preoperatively. This includes history of exposure to communicable diseases, recent upper respiratory infection, current illnesses in siblings or family as well as a thorough physical examination, complete blood count, and urinalysis. Elective procedures should be postponed if the white blood cell count is elevated or if there is any evidence of otitis media, pharyngitis, superficial skin infections or prodromal signs of a viral or communicable disease.

In the operating room, careful and thorough preparation of the operative area should be done. This consists of scrubbing and painting the proposed surgical field with betadine solution followed by the application of sterile towels and drape.

An important source of incisional, superficial wound infections is the operating team itself. Thus, proper scrubbing techniques, appropriate operating room attire, and prevention of individuals with dermatitis, furuncles, paronychia or other draining lesions from participating in the surgery are of great importance in decreasing the number of such infections. Whistling and excessive or boisterous talking should be avoided in order to minimize contamination of the field with pharyngeal organisms.

The efficacy of the use of antibiotics for prophylaxis or prevention of surgical infections has been demonstrated by several studies in adults and has been applied to pediatric surgical patients. In many instances, antibiotics were used inappropriately.[10]

Antibiotic prophylaxis is considered appropriate if the drug is given parenterally within 4 hours before surgery, every 3 hours during surgery or within 1 hour of completion of surgery.[5, 17] Antibiotic prophylaxis in the postoperative period is considered appropriate if the drug is discontinued within 72 hours following surgery.[7,8]

Antibiotics for prevention or prophylaxis of surgical infection are used to minimize the danger of lodgement and to prevent colonization of bacteria in tissues. There is no need for prophylactic antibiotics in clean cases, except in the setting of hernia repair in patients with ventriculoperitoneal shunts, where an antistaphylococcal agent should be given a few hours preoperatively and for 48 hr after surgery. Antibiotics are not needed for hernia repair in patients with cardiovascular lesions.

In clean–contaminated cases, prophylactic antibiotics are indicated. The choice of antibiotic is based on the bacteria most likely to be encountered. Contaminated and dirty cases require antibiotic coverage that may be considered therapeutic rather than prophylactic.

Basically, the most commonly encountered clean–contaminated cases in pediatric surgery include appendectomy for uncomplicated appendicitis, repair of intestinal atresia, colostomy, gastrostomy in the aseptic newborn, and Meckel's diverticulectomy. Contaminated and dirty cases include those in which there has been gross spillage of contents of the gastrointestinal tract and contamination of the abdominal cavity such as with perforation of viscera due to necrotizing enterocolitis, meconium ileus, distally obstructed bowel, volvulus, trauma, perforated or gangrenous appendix, as well as definite intra-abdominal or intrapelvic abscesses.

Antibiotic Prophylaxis for Appendicitis

There has been a great deal of controversy regarding the use of antibiotic prophylaxis for appendicitis. It is generally agreed that antibiotics are not needed for a patient suspected of having acute appendicitis without evidence of peritonitis to suggest abscess or perforation. In patients with appendicitis complicated by perforation or gangrene, antibiotics are indicated. Altemeier observed that appendicitis–peritonitis was a polymicrobial infection due to aerobic and anaerobic organisms.[2,3] Thus, the choice of antibiotics must be such that aerobic and anaerobic, gram-negative and gram-positive organisms will be controlled. King and co-workers[11] compared the effectiveness of the use of ampicillin and gentamycin to the use of ampicillin, gentamycin, and clindamycin and recommended the routine use of these three drugs for all children with complicated appendicitis. David and co-workers[9] reviewed 300 cases of acute gangrenous and perforated appendicitis in pediatric patients and reported markedly fewer wound infections and abscesses in children treated with ampicillin, gentamycin, and clindamycin. Antibiotics were administered for 5 to 7 days and longer if there was ongoing sepsis. Other investigators think that one of the new tertiary cephalosporins (*e.g.,* moxolactam), which has broad-spectrum coverage, might be as effective and require only one drug. The pediatric infectious disease division at the New York Hospital recommends cefoxitan (150 mg/kg/day in four divided doses) for its effect on gram-negative and anaerobic organisms and ampicillin to cover gram-positive organisms such as enterococci.

In those patients who require antibiotic prophylaxis for appendicitis–peritonitis, antibiotics are given within 4 hr of surgery (usually 1 hr before). If there is no evidence of perforation or gangrene of the appendix at surgery, antibiotics are stopped after the one dose by many physicians. Some continue them for 24 to 48 hr. If the appendix is found to be gangrenous but not perforated, antibiotics are used for 48 to 72 hr. When the appendix is noted to be perforated, antibiotics are continued for 5 to 7 days. If there is generalized peritonitis or localized peritonitis without an established abscess, a drain is not used. In cases where there is an abscess, transperitoneal drains are employed and brought out through a separate stab wound, not the incision site. Usually three drains are placed, one up to the subhepatic region, a second into the pelvis, and the third down to the right gutter near the base of the cecum. The drains are left in place for 7 days after which they are twisted and gradually removed over the next 2 to 3 days, by which time a definite tract should have developed. Once the drains are out, the tract should be kept open by means of an indwelling "pin" tube (a short segment of rubber tubing through which a safety pin is inserted to prevent migration of the tube). The tract should be allowed to close in from the deep to the superficial portion. The skin edges must not be allowed to seal over until the tract has closed.

Antibiotic prophylaxis for contaminated and dirty cases arising from gross contamination of the abdomen as a result of perforation of a segment of the gastrointestinal tract, especially when this is in terminal small bowel or colon, is based on the usual microflora associated with this type of leakage. The organisms involved are the Enterobacteriaceae, including *Escherichia coli, Klebsiella, Enterobacter, Serratia,* and *Proteus,* the Streptococcaceae and Micrococcaceae as well as *Clostridium,* Bacteroidaceae, and Pseudomonadaceae.[6, 15] Thus, appropriate antibiotic prophylaxis requires an agent or agents effective against gram-negative, gram-positive, aerobic and anaerobic organisms. A proven combination has been ampicillin, gentamycin, and clindamycin. These are begun within 4 hr of surgery and continued for 7 to 10 days postoperatively. As in the case of perforated appendicitis with perforation, cefoxitan and ampicillin may be as effective as triple drug therapy. Specimens for anaerobic and aerobic cultures are obtained at the time of surgery and changes are made in the antibiotics being used as may be indicated by the culture and sensitivity reports.

Pediatric patients who are to undergo surgery of the stomach, duodenum, or biliary system will not require antibiotic prophylaxis. In those patients for whom elective distal small bowel or colon surgery is planned, preoperative bowel preparation is indicated. This should include both mechanical and antibiotic measures. Mechanical cleansing of the bowel consists of a clear fluid diet for 48 hr and saline enemas. Oral neomycin (100 mg/kg in four doses) and erythromycin are given for 24 hr prior to surgery. In addition, cefoxitan and ampicillin are given 1 to 2 hr before surgery and continued for about 72 hr postoperatively, depending on whether there is any spillage of ileal or colon contents. When a colostomy is done in an unprepared bowel, antibiotics should be continued for 3 to 5 days.

Careful attention to technical details in performing surgery is important in preventing surgical infection. This technical prophylaxis includes minimizing bacterial contamination by suitable preparation of the patient and wound site and proper attire and conduct of the operating team. Delicate handling of tissues, discriminate employment of cautery, avoidance of clamping and ligation of large masses of tissue, removal of any devitalized tissue or foreign body, prevention of collection of serum or blood by careful hemostasis, obliteration of dead space, judicious use of drains, quick but fastidious and thorough surgery, attention to closure of the wound, or leaving wound open for delayed closure in cases where subcutaneous tissue is potentially contaminated are all of extreme importance in minimizing possible postoperative infection.

SURGICAL INFECTION

The type of postoperative infection that may develop depends on the bacteria involved. The pathogens cultured from infections in the New York Hospital series and those reported from the National Nosocomial Infection Study are listed in Table 17-3. In the New York Hospital group, *Staphylococcus aureus* and *epidermidis* were the organisms most commonly recovered from clean cases. Group A streptococcus and beta-hemolytic streptococcus were found in four infections. No gram-negative bacteria were cultured from wounds in clean cases. In clean–contaminated, contaminated, and dirty cases wound infections cultured chiefly *Klebsiella, Escherichia coli, Enterobacter,* and *Streptococcus faecalis.* In 12 patients the wounds also grew out *Staphylococcus epidermidis.*

WOUND INFECTION

This may occur at any time from the first to fourteenth postoperative day. Infections caused by group A streptococcus usually are evident within 24 hr and are associated with fever, cellulitis, spreading erythema, and minimal, serous type of drainage. Treatment consists of systemic penicillin and application of continuous warm soaks to the area. It is not necessary to open or drain the wound. Resolution of the process is usually prompt.

Wound infections due to staphylococci become apparent most often from the third to fifth postoperative day. There is usually tenderness, swelling, induration,

Table 17–3
Postoperative Wound Pathogens of Pediatric Surgical Infections

	NYH-CMC		NNIS*	
	Number	%	Number	%
Staphylococcus aureus	23	27	133	30
Escherichia coli	15	18	77	17
Klebsiella pneumoniae	12	14	—	—
Streptococcus fecalis	10	12	—	—
Staphylococcus epidermidis	8	10	—	—
Enterobacter cloacae	3	4	—	—
Pseudomonas aeruginosa	2	2	50	11
Beta-hemolytic streptococcus	2	2	7	2
Group A streptococcus	2	2	8	2
Other or no culture	7	8	167	38
Total	84	99	442	100

* *Pediatric and newborn combined. From Hospital Infections. National Nosocomial Infection Study. Washington, DC, US Public Health Service, January 1970 through August 1973, Table 16–5.*

erythema, and purulent discharge. Therapy includes incision and drainage and loose packing of the wound as well as antistaphylococcal antibiotics that should be given intravenously. Infections due to enteric organisms usually occur 7 to 14 days post-operative and may be delayed even longer if the patient has been on antibiotics. There is usually induration, limited erythema, slight purulent or seropurulent discharge, and fever. Severe toxic signs may be manifested if gram-negative sepsis ensues. Treatment consists of drainage of purulent collections, debridement of necrotic tissue, local wound care, and antibiotics to combat bacterial dissemination and prevent systemic toxicity.

INTRACAVITARY INFECTIONS

The most common intracavitary infections encountered in general pediatric surgery are intraperitoneal. These usually are related to surgery for appendicitis, visceral perforation, bowel resection, or splenectomy. Abscesses may develop, which may be subphrenic, subhepatic, midabdominal, or pelvic. One or all of these may arise as the result of contamination during surgery, and the location of the abscess may not be related to the operative site per se. The abscess may be symptomatic as early as 5 to 7 days postoperatively or may not be evident until later if the patient has been on antibiotics. Persistent fever, ileus, intestinal obstruction, pain and tenderness, diarrhea, pleural effusion, and a mass are suggestive of an intraperitoneal abscess.

In addition to physical examination, diagnosis and location of the abscess can be established usually with the use of appropriate abdominal radiographs, sonography, and computerized tomography (CT) scans. Treatment consists of drainage of the abscess and culture and sensitivity studies of the contents. Until culture and sensitivity results are available, an antibiotic to cover the anticipated bacterial contaminant should be used intravenously. In the past, adequate drainage could be done only by surgical means. However, currently, many intra-abdominal abscesses and fluid collections can be drained by percutaneous techniques. Successful drainage without operation was achieved in 83.6% of 250 percutaneous procedures with only 8.4% failures and 8% recurrences.[13,16] The success rate is related to the experience of the interventional radiologist, appropriate drainage catheter size, and proper catheter management. A large-bore double lumen sump (12F to 14F) is preferred for drainage of frank pus, while medium or small-bore non-sump catheters can be used for drainage of nonviscid fluids. Catheter irrigation initially, and subsequently for patency, is usually done with saline. Although the initial irrigation may require several hundred milliliters of saline, delayed or subsequent irrigation using 10 to 25 ml is a simple bedside procedure that should be done several times daily at the outset and gradually decreased to once a day.

Withdrawal of the catheter depends on marked diminution or cessation of drainage and development of a well matured drain-tract. Ultrasound (US), CT, or fluoroscopic abscessograms can be employed to obtain information regarding the status of the abscess (Figs. 17-1, 17-2, and 17-3). The patient's physical signs are also of help in evaluating the efficacy of the drainage.

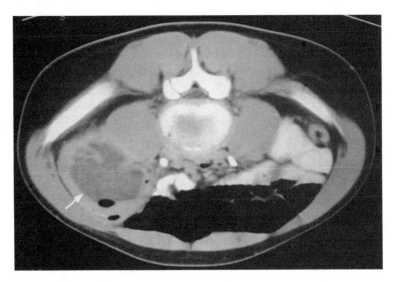

Figure 17–1.
CT scan of abdomen of 13-year-old boy transferred to New York Hospital 10 days following appendectomy because of fever and suspected intraperitoneal abscess. There is a right lower quadrant mass (*arrow*) inseparable from terminal ileum, cecum, and proximal ascending colon. The mass measures 7 cm in width and 5 cm in anteroposterior diameter. It contains fluid and gas with an air fluid level and a thick, somewhat nodular wall. There is soft tissue infiltration of the adjacent fat at the base of the small bowel mesentery, consistent with lymphadenopathy and post-operative change.

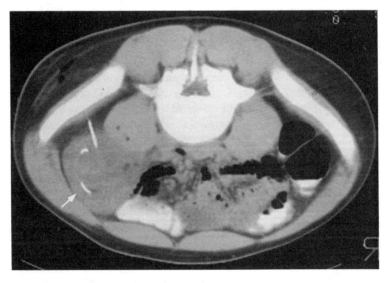

Figure 17–2.
CT scan after percutaneous CT-guided placement of catheter in the abscess cavity (*arrow*) in right lower quadrant.

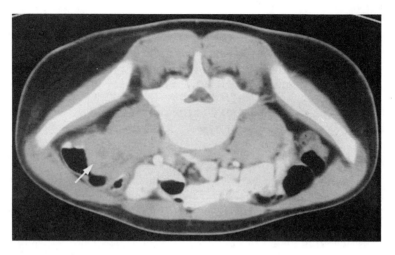

Figure 17–3.
CT scan after removal of catheter following 6 days of drainage. There is only small amount of residual thickening of tissues at abscess site (*arrow*). The patient was afebrile with normal CBC. He was discharged and had no further abdominal complaints.

If the percutaneous drainage cannot be done successfully or if the abscess is not able to be drained by way of the catheter that has been inserted, open surgical drainage should be done.

INFECTIONS OTHER THAN WOUND INFECTIONS IN THE POSTOPERATIVE PERIOD

Less prevalent in children than in adults but still potentially hazardous are infections related to the overall operative procedure rather than the wound per se. These include pulmonary and urinary tract infections and those related to indwelling venous or arterial catheters. Not uncommonly these infections are manifested by fever in the early postoperative period, when there is no evidence of inflammation of the wound. Pulmonary atelectasis and progression to pneumonia are not as common in pediatric surgical patients as in older patients but may occur secondary to poor or traumatic placement of endotracheal tubes, aspiration of gastric contents, tenacious tracheal or bronchial secretions, ineffective cough, or oversedation. The diagnosis should be suspected by findings on physical examination and confirmed by roentgenograms of the chest. Treatment is usually supportive and includes chest physiotherapy, incentive spirometory, and antibiotics.

Urinary tract infections in the postoperative period are not common in children largely because indwelling urethral catheters are not used as often or for as long as in adult patients. Fever is the usual manifestation of such infection. Diagnosis is suspected by microscopic examination of a urine specimen that reveals pyuria or bacilluria, and is confirmed by urine culture with colony count greater than 10^5/ml of urine. Treatment includes hydration and antibiotics, usually Bactrim, until sensitivity results are available, after which the most appropriate antibiotic should be employed.

INFECTIONS ASSOCIATED WITH VENOUS AND ARTERIAL CATHETERS

In many pediatric patients and especially newborn infants, venous or arterial access, or both, may be necessary for blood sampling or pressure measurements, chemotherapy or antibiotic instillation, or hyperalimentation. Lines may be inserted percutaneously or by cut-down on the vessel. In either event, the catheter should be placed with sterile technique. The exit site of the catheter from the skin should be as distant as possible from the entry site into the vessel. The exit site should be cleaned, antibiotic ointment should be placed over it, and the area should be redressed every other day. If erythema, swelling, tenderness, or discharge develop at the exit site or along the course of the catheter, the catheter should be removed, and the infected area should be treated appropriately with hot soaks, antibiotics, or incision and drainage as may be warranted. If signs of sepsis develop and blood cultures are positive, the catheter should be removed and the tip should be cultured. If venous access is still required, a new catheter should be inserted through a different site, once repeat blood cultures are negative.

If there is infection of a segment of vein with obvious suppuration, the affected portion of vein should be excised, and a sample of it should be cultured. Appropriate antibiotics should be administered to the patient. A common cause of nosocomial bacteremia is the indwelling venous catheter, including the infusion solution and connecting tubings. The incidence of bacterial colonization has been estimated to be approximately equal to the square of the number of days the line has been in place (*e.g.*, 4% at 2 days, 9% at 3 days).[14] This predicted incidence of infection is not applicable to central venous lines placed under strict aseptic (sterile) conditions in the operating room. Such catheters may remain in place for periods of several years, if properly managed postoperatively.

REFERENCES

1. Ad Hoc Committee of the Committee on Trauma, Division of Medical Sciences, National Academy of Sciences—National Research Council. Postoperative wound infections: the influence of ultraviolet irradiation of the operating room and various other factors. Ann Surg 1964;160(Suppl):1.
2. Altemeier WA. The pathogenecity of the bacteria of appendicitis peritonitis. Ann Surg 1941;114:158.
3. Altemeier WA. The bacterial flora of acute perforated appendicitis with peritonitis. A bacteriologic study based upon one hundred cases. Ann Surg 1938;107:517.
4. Altemeier WA, Burke JF, Pruitt BA, et al, eds. Manual on control of infection in surgical patients. Philadelphia: JB Lippincott, 1984:10 (Table 2-2).
5. Burke JF. Preventing bacterial infection by coordinating antibiotic and host activity: a time-dependent relationship, South Med J 1977;70:24.

6. Chang JHT. The use of antibiotics in pediatric abdominal surgery. Pediatr Infect Dis 1984;3:195.
7. Chodak GW, Plaut ME. Use of systemic antibiotics for prophylaxis in surgery. Arch Surg 1977;112:326.
8. Crossley K, Gardner LC. Antimicrobial prophylaxis in surgical patients. JAMA 1981;245:722.
9. David IB, Buck JR, Filler RM. Rational use of antibiotics for perforated appendicitis in childhood. J Pediatr Surg 1982;17:494.
10. Kesler RW, Guhlow LJ, Saulberry FT. Prophylactic antibiotics in pediatric surgery. Pediatrics 1982;69:1.
11. King DR, Browne AF, Birken GA, et al. Antibiotic management of complicated appendicitis. J Pediatr Surg 1983;18:945.
12. Mollitt DL. Pediatric surgical infection and antibiotic usage. Pediatr Infect Dis 1985;4:326.
13. Mueller PR, Van Sonnenberg E, Ferrucci JT Jr. Percutaneous drainage of 250 abdominal abscesses and fluid collections. Part II. Radiology 1984;151:343.
14. Stone HH. Surgical infections and antibiotics. In: Welch KJ, ed. Complications of pediatric surgery. Philadelphia: WB Saunders, 1982:78.
15. Stone HH, Kolb LD, Geheber CE. Bacteriologic considerations in perforated necrotizing enterocolitis. South Med J 1979;72:1540.
16. Van Sonnenberg E, Mueller PR, Ferruci JT Jr. Percutaneous drainage of 250 abdominal abscesses and fluid collections. Part I. Radiology 1984;151:337.
17. Veterans Administration Ad Hoc Interdisciplinary Advisory Committee on Antimicrobial Drug Usage. Prophylaxis in surgery. JAMA 1977;237:1003.

18

BILIARY SEPSIS

Leon D. Goldman
William A. Silen
Michael L. Steer

Biliary tract sepsis is a major problem that affects thousands of people each year. It is estimated that gallstones, the major marker for biliary disease, affect about 10% of the American population,[116] but exact figures as to the true incidence are not available. About 400,000 cholecystectomies are performed each year in the United States. Without antibiotic prophylaxis the incidence of wound infections for elective biliary tract operations is about 11% to 20% overall.[147] The incidence of septicemia (as defined by positive blood cultures) can be as high as 0.8% of patients undergoing biliary operations.[111] Septic complications of nonoperative biliary tract interventions, such as percutaneous transhepatic cholangiography, endoscopic retrograde cholangiography, or endoscopic papillotomy, have been reported to be around 0.8%.[6] It is clear from these data that tens of thousands of individuals each year are affected by biliary tract infections or their sequelae. The prevention and treatment of this problem thus assume major social and financial importance.

Effective treatment of biliary sepsis requires an understanding of the normal anatomy of the biliary tree, its microbiology, and a knowledge of how these factors affect clinical disease. Therapy is aimed at removing or altering those conditions that promote bacterial growth and/or invasion, and at maximizing those factors that either eliminate bacteria or foster a more benign relationship between the organisms and their host. With this in mind, the goals of this chapter are (1) to present an overview of how normal anatomy relates to protection against infection, (2) to examine the means by which bacteria gain access to the biliary tree, and the consequences of bacterial invasion, (3) to present current concepts of prophylactic and therapeutic use of antibiotics, and (4) to review specific conditions that affect the biliary tree.

ANATOMY

Standard texts on biliary surgery usually concentrate on the extrahepatic biliary tree and its anatomical variations[8, 88] with little if any attention to the intrahepatic bile ducts and canaliculi, important routes of entry of bacteria in certain situations. From the hepatocytes distally, the biliary tree is made up of the biliary canaliculi, ductules of Hering, bile ductules, bile ducts, extrahepatic bile ducts, gallbladder and cystic duct, and the ampulla of Vater with its sphincteric system.

The canaliculi are formed by spaces between adjacent hepatocytes[114] (Fig. 18-1). Disse's space, the space between the hepatocyte and the sinusoid, is separated

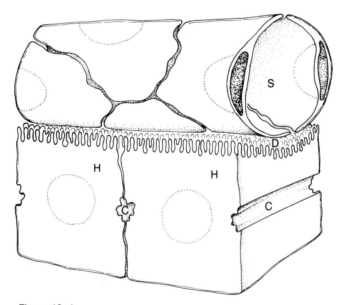

Figure 18–1.
Schematic representation of hepatocytes and relation of space of Disse (*D*) to hepatocytes (*H*) and canaliculi (*C*). *S* = sinusoidal lumen.

from the canaliculi by the tight junctions of the hepatocytes. To date, no connections between the canaliculi and Disse's space have been demonstrated in the normal animal. This suggests that the reticuloendothelial system, consisting mainly of Kupffer's cells, and the various constituents of the portal venous blood do not have direct access to the biliary system except through the hepatocyte, and vice-versa.

Bile flows from canaliculi to the ductules of Hering, which are simply spaces between the canaliculi and the bile ductules. The ductules of Hering are lined by both hepatocytes and biliary epithelium.[114] From these, bile enters the bile ductules and then proceeds to the larger bile ducts in the portal tracts, where the ducts are completely lined by biliary epithelium. Bile then flows to larger ducts, enters the extrahepatic bile ducts, and finally empties into the duodenum by way of the ampulla of Vater (Fig. 18-2).

Bile flow into the duodenum is thought to be a passive event mostly under the control of the sphincter of Oddi.[88] The bile ducts contain virtually no smooth muscle,[68] and coordinated peristalsis of the bile duct is not believed to occur in humans. What few smooth muscle fibers are present are thought to cause shortening of the ducts, which may affect bile flow by changing the length/volume relationship of the duct.[88]

The ampulla of Vater with its sphincteric system is a complex and intriguing structure whose function is, even now, poorly understood. One of the earliest descriptions of this area was by Ruggero Oddi in 1887.[68] In 1898, Hendrickson gave a detailed description of the comparative anatomy of the ampullary area,[68] and, more recently, Boyden[10] again described the anatomy of the choledochoduodenal junction. He showed this area to be a complex of interlacing muscle bundles divided into three parts—a superior and an inferior choledochal sphincter, and a papillary sphincter. Boyden believed that these parts could act independently. Until recently, the choledochoduodenal junction was viewed as a simple valve system relaxing or opening in response to food or enteric hormones (*e.g.,* cholecystokinin). This relaxation along with the contraction of the gallbladder results in the discharge of bile into the duodenum.[88] Recently reported manometric studies, however, have shown that phasic pressure changes are present in the sphincter.[52, 163] Hauge and Mark[66] have shown pressure activity within the sphincter that they believe represents a rhythmic ampullary emptying and filling. These pressure changes in the sphincteric area can be observed without change in the pressure of the proximal bile duct. Tansy has postulated that the epithelium of the distal bile duct and its vasculature is actively involved in the control of sphincter function.[157] Thus, the choledochoduodenal sphincter is more than a simple valve that is either open or closed. It is a complex structure whose function is just beginning to be elucidated.

ETIOLOGY OF BILIARY INFECTIONS

The development of clinical infection depends both on the presence of sufficient numbers of bacteria and on the breakdown of normal defense mechanisms. A knowledge of the anatomy as described above is important because part of the defense of

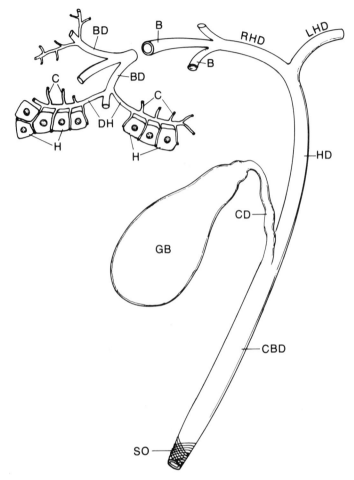

Figure 18–2.
Schematic representation of biliary system. Canaliculi (*C*) collect bile from hepatocytes (*H*) and carry it by way of ductules of Hering (*DH*) to bile ductules (*BD*). The bile ductules merge into bile ducts (*B*) and eventually form the right (*RHD*) and left (*LHD*) hepatic ducts. Other structures shown are the main hepatic duct (*HD*), cystic duct (*CD*), gallbladder (*GB*), common bile duct (*CBD*), and sphincter of Oddi (*SO*).

the biliary tree against bacteria is found in its anatomy, especially an intact sphincter of Oddi.

The normal biliary tract does not harbor bacteria.[97,141] How the biliary tract maintains this sterile state is not entirely clear. Bacteria have three potential routes of access to the biliary tree. The first is the lymphatics, a route that was presumed for many years to be the primary and most important route. Bacteria theoretically could gain access to the biliary tree by way of the lymphatics in the region of the pancreas and the duodenum. However, some studies suggest that the flow of lymph in this area is away from the hilum of the liver and the gallbladder.[37] Furthermore, Kune and co-workers[87] showed that bacteria could not be recovered from the bile after the injection of bacteria into the intestinal wall. If a lymphatic source were most important, then the gallbladder wall should be colonized first and the luminal bile subsequently, with the gallbladder wall containing more bacteria than the bile. But, the gallbladder wall has been shown not to have more bacteria than the bile,[97,118] and the majority of evidence indicates that the lymphatics are not a major route of access of bacteria into the biliary tree.

A second possible route of biliary invasion by bacteria is the portal vein. Dineen[37] in a series of experiments on guinea pigs showed that the portal vein was the most significant route of delivery of bacteria to the biliary tree. Ong,[125] while studying the pathogenesis of oriental cholangiohepatitis, was able to produce biliary inflammation and stones in rabbits by the injection of organisms into the portal vein. Ong felt that the streaming of portal venous blood[27] could explain the left-sided predilection for the infections seen in oriental cholangiohepatitis.[125] It is not at all clear, however, that portal bacteremias occur normally in humans. Orloff and co-workers[126] found that portal venous blood taken at operation in patients with a variety of conditions was sterile. Schatten and co-workers[139] in a similar study found positive portal venous blood cultures in 32% of patients studied and proposed that portal bacteremias do indeed occur in humans. Nolan pointed out that the development of spontaneous *Escherichia coli* bacteremias in cirrhotics are believed to be of intestinal origin. He concluded that portal bacteremias do occur in humans.[120] Whether or not portal bacteremias occur, the intact biliary tree is an effective barrier to intravenous bacteria, as evidenced by the inability to produce high bacteria counts in bile in normal animals after either the systemic or portal intravenous (IV) injection of bacteria.[37,118]

Ascent of bacteria through the ampulla of Vater is a third potential route of biliary infection. Early arguments favoring this route were based on the fact that the concentration of bacteria is greater in the gallbladder bile than in its wall.[43] More recently, studies in animals[135] and in humans[62] have shown that ablation of the sphincter results in colonization of the biliary tree with enteric organisms within a few weeks to months. Arguments against the importance of this route are based on the fact that in the normal, fasting, nonchlorhydric individual the proximal small intestine is essentially sterile.[38,158] Some foods have been shown to contain high concentrations of coliform organisms,[131] and after eating there is transiently a rise in the numbers of luminal bacteria, including Enterobacteriaceae, in the proximal small bowel and in the periampullary region of normal individuals.[40] An ascending route of infection is more clear in the case of stone disease associated with juxtapapillary duodenal diverticula. In patients with duodenal diverticula, the incidence of stone disease rises as the location of the diverticulum becomes closer to the papilla.[91] The incidence of bactobilia associated with cholelithiasis is higher in patients with duodenal diverticula compared to patients without diverticula.[44,97,100] Also, there is evidence for dysfunction of the choledochal sphincter in patients with juxtapapillary duodenal diverticula.[101] All of these findings suggest that the bacteria gain access and ascend the common duct through an abnormal sphincter. Further, stones found in patients with juxtapapillary diverticula tend to be pigment stones associated with β-glucuronidase-producing bacteria.[98, 99] The bulk of evidence strongly suggests that the most important route by which bacteria gain access to the biliary tree is ascent through the papilla of Vater.

DEFENSE MECHANISMS

An understanding of the defense mechanisms that keep the biliary tree free of organisms is a requisite to the proper treatment of biliary infections, because the normal biliary tree is sterile.[88] Clearly, organisms cannot become established unless normal defense systems break down.

The normal biliary tree is for all intents and purposes a closed system. Tight junctions separate the canaliculi from the sinusoids at the hepatic end,[133, 134] and the choledochoduodenal sphincteric system protects the distal portion of the system. Within the bile ducts there are no circulating macrophages to combat bacteria. In addition, there is no muscular contraction to empty the common bile duct, although contraction of the gallbladder, when present, may, in part, play a role in ridding the bile of bacteria. Once the barriers at either end are breached, the bile duct becomes colonized and may not be able to cleanse itself.[48, 49, 62, 135, 160]

At the hepatic end, the canaliculi do not normally connect to the sinusoids or to Disse's space. Bacteria arriving at the liver are, therefore, normally efficiently removed before reaching the bile ducts,[76, 118] but when cholestasis is present, the clearance of bacteria is impaired. Dineen[37] showed that, in animals with bile duct obstruction, biliary infections are easily produced by injecting bacteria into the portal vein. Cardoso[14] has also shown impaired clearance of bacteria in the presence of cholestasis, and Tanaka[156] demonstrated increased mortality in animals challenged with intravenous bacteria when bile duct obstruction was present as compared with nonobstructed animals. Just how cholestasis impairs the clearance mechanism has yet to be elucidated.

The barrier to bacteria at the hepatic end of the system (probably the Kupffer's cells and the tight junctions) fails in the face of bile duct obstruction, but the reasons for this failure are not clear. Impaired Kupffer's cell activity has been observed during cholestasis,[41] and it has been postulated that reflux of bile acids and bilirubin into Disse's space is responsible for breakdown of the canaliculosinusoidal barrier.[41] While this may explain the impaired hepatic clearance of bacteria during cholestasis, it does not readily explain why bacteria do not appear in the biliary tree unless biliary obstruction causes a mechanical break in the canaliculosinusoidal barrier. Discontinuities in the junctional network providing a direct pathway between the canalicular lumen and the intercellular space have been shown by some investigators who performed freeze-fracture ultrastructural studies of the livers of patients with extrahepatic cholestasis.[113, 133, 134] However, Carpino[16] could not demonstrate such disruptions and postulated an endocytic transfer of molecules across the hepatocyte to account for the increased permeability of the canaliculosinusoidal barrier found with bile duct obstruction. In our opinion available evidence favors a mechanical breakdown of the barrier.

That the choledochoduodenal sphincter is a barrier to bacteria has not been proven beyond doubt, although there is a reasonable body of circumstantial evidence to support this proposal. Ablation or bypass of the sphincter almost invariably leads to bactobilia. Also, conditions in which there is sphincteric dysfunction are also associated with bactobilia.[44, 49, 62, 96, 98, 99, 100, 102, 135] The close association of sphincteric dysfunction and bactobilia strongly suggests that the normal sphincter system is an effective barrier to bacteria.

In summary, the normal biliary tree is protected from bacterial invasion by barriers at both ends. Various disease states alter these protective mechanisms, and, once these mechanisms are altered, bacteria gain access to the system. Bacteria can remain within the biliary system for long periods without causing symptoms.[49, 165] The damage, if any, that bacteria cause by their mere presence is not known. However, given the proper conditions, they can invade their host and cause a multitude of clinical problems (to be discussed below).

ANTIBIOTICS

Biliary tract infections develop when bacterial invasion occurs, an event thought to happen only with elevated intraductal pressure or with injury to the biliary epithelium. Acute cholecystitis does not develop merely as a result of the presence of bacteria in the gallbladder. Rather, obstruction of the gallbladder and/or injury to its epithelium is also necessary.[2, 25, 51, 60, 146, 159] Huang[72] demonstrated that elevated intraductal pressures were needed for bacteremia to develop as a result of organisms present within the bile duct. In cases where cholangitis develops in the absence of ductal obstruction (*e.g.*, the "sump syndrome" following choledochoduodenostomy), the degree of bacterial contamination is thought to be important.[58] However, in the majority of cases, ductal obstruction and biliary epithelial injury in the presence of bacteria are the commonest causes of invasive biliary infection. Relief of obstruction and mitigation of injury to the biliary epithelium remain the primary modes of treatment of established biliary infection. Antibiotic treatment affects the systemic symptoms of infection but does not affect the icterus or pain in patients with common duct obstruction,[140, 173] nor does antibiotic treatment affect the incidence of empyema of the gallbladder in patients with acute cholecystitis.[173] Antibiotic therapy alone will not resolve biliary infections, and, for that reason, antibiotics must be regarded as an adjunctive form of therapy.

The choice of antibiotic is determined by the susceptibility of the organism to be treated and the ability of the drug to penetrate the tissues in sufficient quantities. It is illogical to treat biliary infections with drugs that will neither successfully eradicate the invasive organisms nor reach susceptible organisms. In the case of an infection by known organisms with known drug sensitivities, the choice of an antibiotic is relatively simple.

However, culture results are not immediately available in most patients with acute biliary infections. Usually, the initial choice of antibiotic is based on an understanding of the organisms most likely to cause the infection. In the case of the biliary tree, there is a large body of knowledge concerning the organisms present in various disease states.[49,62,65,81-83,100,108,153,156] Of the aerobes, the commonest organisms are *Escherichia coli, Klebsiella* species, *Proteus* species, and enterococci. *Bacteroides* species, and *Clostridia* species are the predominating anaerobes. Aerobic infections are far more common than anaerobic ones, and the antibiotic chosen should, at a minimum, be effective against these aerobic organisms. Whether it is necessary to treat the anaerobes is not clear. The incidence of recovery of anaerobes from cultures of the biliary tree varies from 1% to 40%.[39,103] This variability is not solely due to culture technique because studies using very careful anaerobic methods have not produced a very high incidence of positive cultures.[35,103] For these reasons, some authors feel that aerobic coverage is sufficient,[103] while others advocate the use of antibiotics directed against both aerobic and anaerobic organisms.[39] Because established anaerobic infections in other areas result in considerable morbidity,[59] it seems reasonable to us to include anaerobic coverage for most established biliary infections and also for prophylaxis, provided the risks of the drug chosen are not out of proportion to the gain expected from their use.

Other factors also enter into considerations regarding the choice of antibiotics. Host factors including drug allergies and associated illnesses clearly affect these decisions. The ability of the antibiotic to penetrate the biliary tree must also be evaluated, although it is not clear how much weight should be given to this factor. A drug with good serum levels is more protective against septic complications of biliary surgery than is one with high levels in the bile.[83] In addition, abnormal liver function or bile duct obstruction result in poor excretion of all antibiotics in the bile, regardless of levels obtained in the absence of bile duct obstruction. Thus, the potency and serum levels of antibiotics are far more important than the level obtained in the bile during the treatment of biliary infection, especially in the presence of biliary obstruction.

While antibiotics are an adjunctive treatment for acute biliary infections, they are of prime importance in prophylaxis against wound infections and abscesses. The incidence of infectious complications of biliary surgery is high when bacteria are present in the bile[20,82] and can be decreased considerably by the use of prophylactic antibiotics,[82,152] although antibiotics are not completely without hazard. In view of this, efforts have been made to identify patients at high risk of having bacteria in their biliary tree. The factors that have been identified are: (1) emergency operation, (2) common duct stones (with and without jaundice), (3) age over 70 years, and (4) previous biliary operation. To be effective prophylactically the drug must be started preoperatively. There is some evidence that a single dose of the appropriate drug is an effective form of prophylaxis,[94] although most authorities recommend a total of three doses.

In choosing an antibiotic for the treatment of biliary infections, one desires a safe drug that is effective against the common pathogens. The cephalosporins are, for many, the first line drug,[150] although they are without activity against enterococci. The newer penicillins such as piperacillin and mezlocillin, on the other hand, do have activity against these organisms. For this reason, the latter two drugs may be a better choice in patients who are not allergic to penicillin. Costs and local custom may dictate the final decision. For the patient who is allergic to penicillin, an aminoglycoside might be required. It is probably not necessary to cover the anaerobes when treating prophylactically, although if it is possible to do so with little added risk to the patient, it seems a reasonable thing to do. The second- and third-generation cephalosporins and newer penicillins provide this coverage (Table 18-1). With these factors in mind, a reasonable choice for prophylaxis might be cephazolin 1 g, IV, or mezlocillinn 3 g IV, (single dose).[39] For established infection, one might use mezlocillin 4 g IV every 6 hr, or cefoxatime 1 g every 6 hr, plus gentamycin 80 mg, IV, every 8 hr, and metronidazole 500 mg, IV, every 8 hr. Other regimens could be used keeping the above guidelines in mind.

ACUTE CHOLECYSTITIS

Etiology

Acute cholecystitis is an acute inflammatory process that affects approximately 25% of patients with gallstones.[149] While about 70% of patients with acute cholecystitis will have positive biliary cultures, bacteria alone are probably not primarily responsible for the development of acute cholecystitis.[2, 43, 51, 60, 159] One possible exception to this general rule is the variant of cholecystitis known as emphysematous cholecystitis. In these cases, bacterial infection with gas-forming organisms may precipitate acute cholecystitis.[112] However, in the more common nonemphysematous cholecystitis, obstruction of the cystic duct would appear to be the most important etiologic factor because most cases of acute cholecystitis occur in patients with

Table 18–1
Relative Susceptibility of Biliary Tree Pathogens to Commonly Used Antibiotics

	Ampicillin	Cephalothin	Cefamandole	Cefoxitin	Cefotaxime	Gentamicin	Mezlocillin	Moxalactam	Piperacillin
Enterococcus	+ +	−	−	−	−	−	+ +	−	+ +
Staphylococcus aureus	−	+ +	+	+	+	−	−	±	−
Streptococcus species	+ +	+ +	+ +	+	+ +	−	+ +	±	+ +
Enterobacter species	−	−	+	±	+ +	+ +	+	+ +	+
Escherichia coli	+	+	+	+	+ +	+ +	+	+ +	+
Indole & *Proteus*	−	−	±	±	+ +	+ +	+	+ +	+
Klebsiella	−	±	+	+	+ +	+ +	+	+ +	+
Proteus mirabilis	+	+	+	+	+ +	+ +	+ +	+ +	+ +
Pseudomonas aeruginosa	−	−	−	−	±	+	+	±	+
Bacteroides fragilis	−	−	−	+ +	±	−	+ +	+ +	+ +
Other anaerobes	±	±	±	+ +	±	−	+ +	+ +	+ +

occlusion of the cystic duct by gallstones. Acute cholecystitis may develop, however, in the absence of cystic duct obstruction (*e.g.,* in acalculous cholecystitis), suggesting that factors other than obstruction must be involved. Many believe that toxic agents within the bile are responsible.[51,60,149,159] Lysolecithin is one such substance that has been studied extensively.[60,149] Whatever the exact etiology, bacterial invasion seems to be a secondary event.

Clinical Syndrome and Diagnosis

As with any disease, the mainstay of diagnosis is a careful history and physical examination. Most often patients have upper abdominal pain, usually in the right upper quadrant and/or in the epigastrum. Nausea and vomiting are also common. Fever and chills may be present.[50,54-56] Jaundice is present in about 20% of patients, but this abnormality does not necessarily indicate that common duct stones are present.[21,42,50] On physical examination, there usually is right upper quadrant abdominal tenderness, which may be associated with guarding and signs of parietal peritoneal inflammation. A mass can be felt in approximately 50% of patients with acute cholecystitis.

No single laboratory test is diagnostic of acute cholecystitis. Blood studies, including liver function tests, are nonspecific and cannot be relied on to make the diagnosis. Radiologic studies may provide important information. A plain film of the abdomen can be diagnostic of emphysematous cholecystitis if gas is seen within the gallbladder lumen, gallbladder wall, or bile ducts.[112] Ultrasound (US) is extremely useful for determining the presence or absence of gallstones but is not reliable for making the specific diagnosis of acute cholecystitis.[26] Some authors feel it is helpful in diagnosing acute cholecystitis if one carefully assesses the thickness of the gallbladder wall.[32] Given a patient in whom the diagnosis of acute cholecystitis is suspected on the basis of the history and physical examination, a radionuclide cholescintigram can be diagnostic[170,174] if the radionuclide is detected within the common bile duct and small intestine but not the gallbladder. Viewed in this context, US is a means of detecting gallstones, and the radionuclide scan is a method of diagnosing acute cholecystitis.

Treatment

Initially, a patient suspected of having acute cholecystitis should have nothing by mouth and should be started on IV fluids while studies are undertaken to establish the diagnosis. The use of nasogastric suction should be determined by the patient's symptoms. There is nothing specific about nasogastric suction that directly treats acute cholecystits. Its value lies in keeping the stomach empty in patients who are vomiting, thus decreasing the risk of aspiration.

The use of antibiotics can be debated because bacterial infection of the gallbladder is a secondary event in acute cholecystitis. Antibiotics do not treat the underlying process and do not decrease the risk of empyema or perforation, but they do decrease the risk of septicemia and associated symptoms[173] and clearly have a role perioperatively in preventing postoperative infectious complications.[81,82] In our opinion, the use of antibiotics is recommended in patients with acute cholecystitis, initially to protect against the systemic effects of bacterial infection and perioperatively to decrease the incidence of postoperative septic complications.

Cholecystectomy is the treatment of choice for acute cholecystitis.[50–52,54–56] Cholecystostomy is reserved for those patients in whom cholecystectomy cannot be performed safely and for the few patients who are so seriously ill that the procedure must be brief or must be done under local anesthesia. There is debate over the timing of cholecystectomy for acute cholecystitis. The proponents of early nonoperative treatment of acute cholecystitis[30] point out that approximately 90% of patients initially treated nonoperatively will improve sufficiently to allow subsequent elective cholecystectomy at a later time, usually at 6 to 8 weeks.[30] Early operation, however, is not accompanied by a higher complication rate.[89,96] In addition, it eliminates the need for the patient to return to the hospital at a later date. Further, early operation obviates the possibility of an undesirable acute exacerbation during the waiting period. Controlled trials have shown that early cholecystectomy can be performed as safely as an elective operation, and that early operation reduces total hospital stay.[79] Delay in operation is unwise in patients over the age of 60 because nonoperative treatment usually fails in this group.[115] Glenn[54] points out that in the elderly an aggressive approach to the diagnosis and treatment of acute cholecystitis is the safest course. In emphysematous cholecystitis, delay in operation is clearly contraindicated.[112] In our opinion, early cholecystectomy is the treatment of choice for acute cholecystitis. Operation should be delayed only long enough to establish the diagnosis. A trial of nonoperative therapy is not justified as a routine except under unusual circumstances such as during an acute myocardial infarction, or in the face of hemodynamic instability. If, in the judgment of the surgeon, cholecystectomy is too risky, a cholecystostomy can safely solve the immediate problem.

ACUTE CHOLANGITIS

Definition

Acute cholangitis spans a broad spectrum of disease from brief, self-limited episodes to progressive, unrelenting, and ultimately fatal sepsis in the absence of decompressive intervention. While there has been exceptional emphasis on the latter fulminating form, which has been referred to as "acute suppurative cholangitis,"[57] this group comprises only about 15% of all cases of acute cholangitis.[9] Furthermore, it has become clear that not all cases that require urgent operation because of clinical deterioration actually have pus in the common duct and conversely there are many patients who are ultimately found to have purulent material in the common duct, but who have promptly responded to nonoperative treatment.[9,122] Because there is relatively little correlation between the clinical picture and the pathologic findings,[123] it has been suggested that the term suppurative cholangitis be discarded.[9] The severity of acute cholangitis should be judged more on clinical than on pathologic criteria, and perhaps the term refractory cholangitis would be more appropriate for those cases that require urgent operation.

Clinical Syndrome and Diagnosis

The classical triad of jaundice, abdominal pain, and chills and fever so characteristic of cholangitis was described in 1877 by Charcot.[18] A pentad was created when Reynolds and Dargon[132] added to these findings the presence of shock and obtundation of the central nervous system. This pentad has been observed in only about 5% of cases, however, whereas Charcot's triad is present in over 90%.[9] Physical findings consist usually of mild tenderness in the right upper quadrant and, occasionally, hepatomegaly. The relative paucity of findings is helpful in differentiating these cases from those patients who have acute cholecystitis in which much more tenderness is usually present. Elevations of the white blood count, serum bilirubin, and serum transaminases are common, but total white blood counts of less than 10,000/ml and a serum bilirubin of 2 mg% or less have been observed in as many as 15% to 20% of cases.[9, 137]

The diagnosis can usually be established on clinical grounds alone, and percutaneous transhepatic cholangiography (PTC) or endoscopic retrograde cannulation of the papilla (ERCP) are usually reserved for difficult cases, for those in which simultaneous therapeutic maneuvers may be indicated (see below), or for accurate anatomical delineation of the abnormalities of the biliary system immediately preoperatively. PTC and ERCP by themselves occasionally produce or accentuate the clinical syndrome of cholangitis.[6, 24] Ultrasonography is a simple, noninvasive method of demonstrating dilated intrahepatic ducts and may be useful for this purpose, although cholangitis can occur in patients with ducts of relatively normal size.

Etiology

Role of Bacteria and Obstruction. There is general agreement that large, sudden increases in intrabiliary ductal pressure in the presence of bacterial organisms are frequently associated with the development of acute cholangitis.[76, 80, 105, 119, 137] Jacobson and co-workers,[78] using radiolabeled bacteria, demonstrated reflux of these organisms from the biliary tree into portal veins and estimated a 90% filtration rate by the liver. In addition, many substances as large as 300 A injected into obstructed ducts at a pressure just greater than secretory pressure have been recovered in systemic blood.[73] Clinically, the incidence of acute cholangitis is far greater when dyes are injected under pressure than when gravity, alone, is applied.[34] That obstruction is not mandatory for the development of cholangitis, however, is clear because instances of cholangitis have been documented in the absence of obstruction, especially under circumstances in which bacterial overgrowth is abundant, such as in cases of achlorhydria or where juxtapapillary duodenal diverticula are present.[58] It is possible in these cases that only the slightest physiologic increases in pressure, which in instances of only mild bacterial contamination are innocuous, can cause cholangitis when the bacterial population is abundant. Huang and co-workers[72] have shown that elevated intraductal pressures are required for the development of bacteremia from infected bile.

The importance of the role of bacteria in the development of cholangitis is underscored by the fact that cholangitis is relatively rare in patients with malignant obstruction of the extrahepatic biliary tract unless operative or radiologic intervention has occurred, primarily because the bile is initially sterile in at least 90% of the cases.[49,139,142] The major controversy surrounding bacterial contamination of the biliary tree in previously unoperated cases is whether the bacteria derive from an ascending route by way of the duodenum or whether they enter by way of the bloodstream. While experimentally the portal venous route has been suggested as being the most important,[37] portal venous blood has been shown to be sterile in almost all humans undergoing laparotomy for a variety of reasons.[126] One would expect a high incidence of biliary infection in patients with complete malignant obstruction if the bloodstream was an important route of entry of bacteria, but, as mentioned above, such is not the case.

The higher incidence of biliary infection in association with calculi has been generally attributed to partial obstruction of the bile duct.[142] Indirect evidence for the importance of the papilla of Vater in preventing ascending infection is derived from the observation that infection is absent in children with biliary atresia when the gallbladder can be anastomosed to the porta (remainder of extrahepatic ducts are intact as is the papilla), whereas infection is the rule when a Roux-en-Y is anastomed to the porta.[95] The high incidence of biliary infection in association with juxtapapillary duodenal diverticula[58,102] also suggests that the ascending route is of primary importance. The role of the lymphatics is unclear, although some have suggested that lymphatic obstruction enhances the development of infection.[37,69]

The role of foreign bodies and a connection with the external environment by means of surgically placed tubes in the pathogenesis of serious biliary infection should not be underestimated.[58,148] It is clear that the longer a tube is in place in the biliary tract, the more likely it is that bacterial contamination might occur, so that by 14 days bactobilia is invariably present.[148] Such infections can never be eradicated so long as the tube or other foreign body, such as a nonabsorbable suture, is present.

A rare but important type of acute cholangitis has been described in patients with the toxic shock syndrome[75] in which jaundice is present in about 50% of cases. The extrahepatic biliary tree is normal, and it has been suggested that the severe microscopic intrahepatic cholangitis is caused by a circulating toxin rather than by bacterial infection.

Organisms Associated with Cholangitis. These are predominantly the aerobic enteric organisms *Escherichia coli, Klebsiella, Streptococcus faecalis,* and *Proteus vulgaris. Pseudomonas* species is uncommon except following surgical or radiologic intervention. Anaerobes, especially *Bacteroides* and *Clostridium,* can be isolated from approximately 40% of infected bile samples and are found more frequently in patients who have had multiple biliary operations or biliary-intestinal anastomoses. Pure cultures of anaerobes are very unusual, and mixtures of multiple aerobic organisms is common. Some evidence has been accrued that aerobic and

408

anaerobic organisms are synergistic in producing intrahepatic abscesses and death.[80,119]

Associated Clinical Conditions. Approximately 50% to 60% of cases of cholangitis are associated with iatrogenic strictures and calculi, about equally divided between these two conditions.[9,161] Malignancy accounts for an additional 10%, and recently PTC and especially ERCP have become an increasingly frequent source of patients with cholangitis. Postoperative T-tube cholangiograms, sump syndrome after choledochoduodenostomy, sclerosing cholangitis, and foreign bodies (sutures) comprise the remainder of causative factors in most series.

Treatment

Initial Nonoperative Treatment. Virtually all authorities agree that the initial therapy for patients with acute cholangitis should be nonoperative.[9,122,161] Bismuth and co-workers,[7] even in the presence of acute renal failure, prefer to provide an initial period of nonoperative treatment. There is absolutely no diagnostic test that will determine whether a given patient with cholangitis will respond to nonoperative therapy except a trial of such treatment. It has been shown that such a trial may enhance the final outcome rather than being detrimental, even in patients who ultimately require urgent operation.[7] Because about 85% of patients with acute cholangitis will respond to nonoperative treatment and will *not* require emergency operation, all patients with acute cholangitis should receive such treatment initially. At least 6 to 8 hr will be required to ascertain whether the patient is responding favorably. If so, nonoperative treatment is continued until the episode is concluded, but if improvement is not clear by 8 hr, emergency operation will be required. Persistent hypotension and fever and a serum bilirubin of greater than 4 mg% should alert the surgeon to the need for an emergent procedure.[9]

The mainstays of nonoperative treatment consist of adequate hydration achieved with suitable monitoring, and antibiotics. In aged patients with cardiovascular disease, a Swan-Ganz catheter may be necessary. The choice of antibiotics is extremely important. Although the complications of biliary infection may be prevented by therapeutic levels of an appropriate antibiotic in the serum, the importance of antibiotic excretion in the bile is not as clear.[39,83] It would be reasonable, however, to choose an antibiotic that is excreted in the bile, with all other things being equal in patients with acute cholangitis. The factors that influence the biliary excretion include molecular weight, polarity, and hepatic metabolism, but the relative importance of each is not known. Table 18-2 shows the biliary excretion of various antibiotics into human bile. The effectiveness of a given agent is not solely dependent on the concentration in the bile because of differing potencies of antibiotics. Because initial treatment of acute cholangitis is begun before the responsible organisms are known, broad-spectrum coverage is appropriate until the results of cultures become available. A combination of an ureidopenicillin, such as mezlocillin, or a cephalosporin, such as cefoxatime, with an aminoglycoside is probably the most suitable combination.[39] Great care should be exercised in the use of aminoglycosides in the patient with

Table 18–2
Biliary Excretion of Antibiotics Into Common Bile Duct in Humans in the
Absence of Biliary Obstruction or Abnormal Liver Function Tests

POOR (Bile/Serum Ratio <1)	MODERATE (Bile/Serum Ratio 1–4)	GOOD (Bile/Serum Ratio >4)
Ticarcillin	Ampicillin	Mecillinam
	Carbenicillin	Mezlocillin
Cephazolin		Piperacillin
Cefotaxime		
Ceftazidime		Cefamandole
Cefuroxime		Cefoperazone
Sulphamethoxazole	Trimethoprim	
		Rifampicin
Amikacin	Metronidazole	Erythromycin
Gentamicin	Clindamycin	Tetracyclines

incipient renal failure, however. Metronidizole is probably preferable to clindamycin for treatment of anaerobes because of the enhanced possibility of development of pseudomembranous enterocolitis with the latter. An example of a reasonable regimen has been given above. It is possible that such new broad-spectrum agents such as imipenem might be considered as a single drug, but further studies are necessary before that can be recommended. There are no strict rules and no data to determine how long treatment should be continued, especially in patients who respond to the treatment. It is unlikely that more than 7 days is advantageous, and longer than that is probably deleterious.

Nonsurgical Interventions. While many gastroenterologists, internists, and radiologists are intrigued with the new techniques of ERCP[74,85] and percutaneous transhepatic drainage[31] of the biliary system as possible means to avoid operation, it should be emphasized that these procedures should not even be considered for patients with acute cholangitis until the initial nonoperative therapy has been instituted, and possibly even only after it has failed. These methods are to be regarded in the same light as emergent open operations and are thus applicable only for no more than 15% of cases.[9] Because there are no controlled trials to compare these techniques with open operations, we believe that they are best reserved for aged, debilitated, and otherwise severely ill patients, and should be used only when an expert radiologist or endoscopist is available. In addition, the underlying condition may influence the choice in favor of one of these techniques. For example, transhepatic drainage is probably preferred for the patient with an iatrogenic stricture or carcinoma who fails to respond to the initial nonoperative treatment because even simple drainage by open operation is likely to be difficult. On the other hand, ERCP would be most useful for calculus disease but is contraindicated in most cases of iatrogenic stricture. Unless all or most calculi can be removed from the common duct through an endoscopic papillotomy, or an iatrogenic stricture can be dilated successfully trans-hepatically, it is likely that such techniques will fail to provide the urgently required biliary drainage. Therefore, we should not impose procedures such as PTC or ERCP unless there is a high likelihood of success of relief of biliary obstruction in these seriously ill individuals.

Surgical Drainage. The term surgical drainage rather than surgical treatment is used because, in most instances, only simple drainage of the biliary tree, usually by means of a T-tube, is the treatment of choice. These seriously ill patients should not be subjected to a definitive procedure in most instances. Fortunately, most patients who have strictures or tumors that may be hazardous to repair or remove under emergent circumstances will respond to nonoperative treatment. The various definitive procedures used for the elective operations in these patients are not within the purview of this chapter and will not be discussed here. While some authors have claimed that internal drainage in the form of choledochoduodenostomy is preferable to simple external drainage for patients with suppurative cholangitis,[104] it is clear that many, if not most, of the patients in that report,were operated on semielectively 48 hr after admission and when their condition had stabilized. For most patients with calculi of the common duct, simple drainage of the duct itself is preferred, whereas cholecystostomy is to be avoided unless the cystic duct has been shown to be widely patent by operative cholangiography.[138]

Complications

The most frequent complications of cholangitis are the formation of calculi and the development of hepatic abscesses (discussed below). Pigment calculi often develop in the presence of bacteria in the bile, even when acute cholangitis or overt infection has not been present. Maki[107] and others[98,154] have shown that certain bacteria, especially *Escherichia coli* and *Klebsiella*, produce β-glucuronidases that cause the breakdown of conjugated bilirubin to unconjugated bilirubin. The latter, in contrast to the former, avidly binds the calcium present in bile to precipitate as calcium bilirubinate, the classical black pigmented stone associated with infection. These calculi are often tiny (less than 1 mm in size) and are frequently present by the thousands. These calculi will continue to form *even in the absence of biliary obstruction* unless the infection is eradicated.

Mortality

It is extremely difficult, if not impossible, to characterize mortality and morbidity in these cases of acute cholangitis because of the unfortunate use in the literature of the term suppurative cholangitis without specific definition of the kinds of cases that have been treated. Because recent series have been enlightened and have adopted the policy of initial nonoperative treatment, a reasonable approximation of overall mortality and morbidity can be reached. In three such series,[7,9,137] the mortality has been from 15% to 20%. It is clear that the mortality will approach 100% if cases that do not respond to initial nonoperative treatment are not drained.[122] In addition, overly aggressive early operation without an initial period of intensive treatment is similarly likely to result in mortalities approaching 100%.[7]

ORIENTAL CHOLANGIOHEPATITIS

Definition

Oriental cholangiohepatitis, also called recurrent pyogenic cholangitis, is endemic in southeast Asia and is especially common among the Chinese population of Hong Kong and Singapore. The disease is characterized by recurrent attacks of fever associated with chronic, often suppurative inflammation of the bile ducts and portal tracts. Enteric organisms, mainly *Escherichia coli*, can generally be cultured from the bile. Multiple hepatic abscesses are common, and the gallbladder is often normal with no or few stones. Recurrent pyogenic cholangitis is distinct from the Western cholangitis, which complicates cholesterol cholelithiasis. The disease is not restricted to the Chinese in the Orient but occurs also in Chinese migrants in North America and Australia.[15, 23]

Etiology

The pathogenesis of recurrent pyogenic cholangitis is not well understood. Although infestation with parasites, particularly *Clonorchis sinensis*, has been implicated, this organism is found in only approximately 20% of cases.[23, 171] *Ascaris lumbricoides* has been found in from 5% to 15% of cases and, therefore, also cannot be regarded as the primary causative factor. Bacteria, especially *Escherichia coli* have been isolated from the liver, bile, and wall of the gallbladder in from 60% to 95% of cases,[23, 171] but the route of entry of these organisms has been debated. A variety of other aerobic bacteria including *Proteus, Pseudomonas,* and *Klebsiella,* as well as some anaerobic organisms have also been isolated from these cases. Gallstones, usually of the earthy brown or black pigment type and composed mainly of calcium bilirubinate, have been found in 60% of the cases.[162] The disease is most prevalent among poor socioeconomic classes.

Most authorities believe that biliary sludge is the factor that produces stasis and converts otherwise innocuous transient bacteria into pathogens.[23] This view is supported by the ERCP findings, which demonstrate that early cholangitic changes are detectable only in those ducts that already harbor stones. The prevalence of the calcium bilirubinate stone is said to be related to a deficiency of glucaro—1:4—lactone in the bile, presumably caused by a low-protein diet. Glucaro—1:4—lactone normally inhibits glucuronidase so that its absence or deficiency allows the glucuronidase to hydrolyze conjugated bilirubin into free bilirubin, which can form a complex with calcium and, hence, calcium bilirubinate stones. It is interesting that the incidence of pigment stones in Japanese people has decreased markedly since World

War II, presumably due to an increased consumption of protein. Portal bacteremia is thought to be an important source of the organisms in the bile of patients with oriental cholangiohepatitis because the early pathologic lesion is thought to be thrombophlebitis and pericholangitis in the portal tracts.[23] Once infection is established, the concentration of glucuronidase in bile increases as a result of its production by bacteria. More stones are thus formed with consequent stasis, and ultimately a vicious cycle ensues.

Clinical Manifestations

The most common symptoms are pain, chills, fever, and jaundice. Repeated attacks are almost invariable. Ultimately, if untreated, biliary cirrhosis with splenomegaly, portal hypertension, and esophageal varices ensues. Pancreatitis is sometimes associated with recurrent pyogenic cholangitis, possibly as a result of pigment stones incarcerated transiently at the papilla of Vater. The natural course of both treated and untreated oriental cholangiohepatitis is not readily discerned from the literature on this subject.

Treatment

The treatment of acute attacks should be identical to that for Western forms of acute cholangitis described above. The preferred elective treatment has been placement of a Roux-en-Y of jejunum to the transected common hepatic duct,[22, 127, 143, 164] but long-term results of this treatment are not available in the literature. During all operations for this disease, careful assessment of the intrahepatic biliary tree must be made by appropriate cholangiographic studies for the presence of strictures of the intrahepatic ducts. Occasionally, resection of infected and obstructed segments of the liver, especially the left lobe, are required in association with hepaticojejunostomy. Surgeons have generally eschewed the use of operative sphincteroplasty because it is impossible to drain exceptionally large ducts by this means. However, recently, endoscopic papillotomy has yielded excellent results approaching those of operation.[90] The mortality of endoscopic papillotomy was 1.5% compared with an operative mortality of 7%.[90]

PYOGENIC ABSCESS

Etiology

Many processes can lead to the development of pyogenic liver abscesses. The large number and variety of events that can result in liver abscesses reflect the fact that bacteria can reach the liver by many routes (Table 18-3). Before the advent of antibiotics, most patients with pyogenic liver abscesses were young and developed this lesion as a consequence of portal bacteremia during acute appendicitis.[121] Pyogenic liver abscesses can also occur after portal bacteremia caused by other

Table 18–3
Route of Entry for 398 Cases of Pyogenic Liver Abscess[4, 33, 62, 93, 129, 136]

	NUMBER OF PATIENTS	(%)
Biliary tract	173	43
Portal vein	67	17
Hepatic artery	32	8
Penetrating trauma	23	6
Direct extension	28	7
Cryptogenic	75	19

processes such as diverticulitis, umbilical cord infection, and inflammatory bowel disease. Liver abscess may also develop in immunocompromised patients whose gastrointestinal barrier to bacterial invasion has been lost. Currently, most patients with hepatic abscess develop this lesion as a consequence of biliary tract disease and cholangitis.[4, 11, 33, 61, 70, 93, 110, 129, 136, 145] Pyogenic liver abscess can also develop as a result of direct extension into the liver of a perihepatic pyogenic process such as acute cholecystitis or subphrenic abscess. Hepatic arterial bacteremia during subacute bacterial endocarditis can also lead to the development of pyogenic liver abscess. Secondary bacterial infection of metastatic malignant lesions in the liver or of intra-hepatic hematomas are relatively uncommon causes of liver abscess. Penetrating liver injuries may become infected as a result of organisms carried inward to the liver at the time of the trauma. Finally, pyogenic liver abscess may develop in the absence of an identifiable cause, and, in most series reported to date, these cryptogenic liver abscesses account for 20% to 25% of the patients.[4, 11, 33, 61, 70, 93, 110, 129, 136, 145]

Pathology

Pyogenic liver abscesses may be single or multiple, superficial or deep, large or small. They are found most often in the right lobe of the liver.[12, 36, 70, 145] When only deep-seated or small abscesses are present, the hepatic surface may be normal to inspection and palpation. When superficial abscesses are present, however, thickening of the capsule, a fibrinous exudate, and a fluctuant mass can often be detected.

Clinical Presentation

The clinical presentation of patients with hepatic abscesses can be quite variable.[4, 11, 61, 70, 110, 121, 136, 145] The most common symptom is fever, frequently associated with rigors, sweats, malaise, anorexia, and weakness. Weight loss is a frequent symptom. Patients with large abscesses, especially those whose abscess is superficial, may complain of epigastric or right upper abdominal quadrant pain. Those whose abscess is immediately below the diaphragm may note pleuritic chest pain, cough, and shortness of breath.

Surprisingly, in spite of large abscesses, the physical examination may be unremarkable. On the other hand, hepatomegaly, liver tenderness, a tender upper abdominal mass, pleural rubs, rales, and a pleural effusion may be noted. Jaundice is present in 25% to 50% of patients with hepatic abscess,[4, 11, 33, 61, 70, 93, 110, 129, 136, 145] and laboratory tests may, in addition to hyperbilirubinemia, detect anemia, leukocytosis, hypoalbuminemia, elevated transaminase levels, and an elevation of the prothrombin time.

Diagnosis

The diagnosis of pyogenic liver abscess may be difficult and elusive. A high index of suspicion is of paramount importance. A number of relatively recently developed noninvasive tests may be of benefit in the detection of this lesion. Hepatic scans, using compounds such as ^{99m}Tc–sulfur colloid, can usually identify lesions larger than 2 cm, although they cannot discriminate between solid and fluid-filled lesions.[4, 11, 61, 70, 110, 136, 145] Agents such as ^{67}Ga, which are likely to be localized to pyogenic collections, have also been used as imaging agents for the detection of liver abscesses, but the results have been varied. US may be a particularly sensitive method of detecting liver abscesses and of determining whether a lesion seen on liver scan is solid or cystic.[86] Computerized tomography (CT), however, is the most sensitive method of detecting liver abscess, and, when contrast enhancement is used, CT scans can reliably detect abscesses 1 cm in diameter.[11, 33, 61, 63, 70, 93, 110, 129, 136, 145]

Treatment

Antibiotic therapy is the mainstay of treatment when multiple or small abscesses are present. A variety of organisms may be present in these abscesses. Those most frequently encountered include *Escherichia coli, Bacteroides fragilis, Clostridium, Pseudomonas,* and *Staphlococcus.*[4, 11, 33, 61, 70, 93, 110, 129, 136, 145] Thus, until definitive identification of the offending organism(s) is obtained, antibiotic therapy should be broad-spectrum and directed against both aerobes and anaerobes. The combination of chloramphenicol with ampicillin, ampicillin with gentamycin and clindamycin, or ampicillin with gentamycin and metronidazole or either mezlocillin, or cefotaxime with gentamycin and metronidazole would be appropriate.[4, 19, 32] The appropriate duration of antibiotic therapy has not been determined, and recommendations have varied between 10 days and 6 months.

In addition to parenteral antibiotic therapy, large liver abscesses should be treated by drainage. This can be accomplished by an open surgical procedure performed by way of a transperitoneal approach and, if possible, designed to result in dependent drainage of the abscess cavity.[1, 121] Alternatives to this approach include percutaneous needle aspiration with instillation of antibiotics into the abscess and percutaneous catheter drainage with subsequent periodic transcatheter irrigation of the cavity.[53, 86] Both of these procedures can be performed using US or CT scan to localize the abscess and monitor the drainage procedure. These percutaneous nonoperative approaches should be considered as the treatment of choice when the necessary radiologic expertise is available and a large or solitary abscess is present. Using these techniques, a successful outcome can be anticipated for most patients.

Prognosis

Untreated pyogenic abscess is associated with a mortality rate of 80% to 100%.[1,4,61,129] A number of complications can occur, including rupture into the peritoneal cavity with the subsequent development of peritonitis. The pleura may be involved in 15% to 20% of patients, and empyema can result if the abscess ruptures above the diaphragm. With contained rupture below the diaphragm, subphrenic abscess can develop.

AMOEBIC ABSCESS

Etiology[12,71,84]

Amoebic abscesses occur in 5% to 10% of patients with intestinal amoebiasis caused by *Entamoeba histolytica*. Infection with this organism is usually mediated by way of the fecal–oral route. The trophozoites present in the feces are in a cyst stage, which is resistant to drying and to acid *p*H. Thus, they can traverse the acidity of the stomach without being damaged and subsequently rupture in the intestine, releasing metacystic trophozoites. The latter elaborate enzymes, such as proteases, hyaluronidases, and mucopolysaccharidases, which can injure tissue and which enable the organism to penetrate the wall of the colon. The disease may remain confined to the colonic mucosa for many years, and invasion may never occur. On the other hand, invasion may occur, with resulting hematogenous spread of organisms by way of the portal venous system to the liver. The factors that regulate invasiveness have not, unfortunately, been defined.

Pathology

Hepatic amoebic abscesses may vary in size from a few millimeters to several centimeters in diameter. They may be single or multiple, with single cysts occuring in 90% of patients. Amoebic abscesses typically contain a creamy or reddish "anchovy sauce" material, which is sterile when cultured for bacteria. These abscesses occur more often in men than in women and are more common in the right than in the left lobe. Amoebic abscesses of the liver may appear after overt evidence of active intestinal disease has disappeared, and they can enlarge relatively rapidly over a period of weeks.[12,71,84]

Amoebic abscesses typically are composed of several different zones of activity.[12,84] At the periphery, there is a layer of hepatic cells involved in an inflammatory process in which parasites cannot be identified. The active trophozoites can frequently be found, however, on the inner edge of this zone. Further inward, the abscess contains liquefied tissue debris, which has been degraded by the digestive enzymes elaborated by the amoeba, and between these layers is a zone containing hepatocytes in various stages of degradation. When appropriately treated with amoebicidal agents, the trophozoites are destroyed and the lesion regresses. A fibrotic scar may persist, or the lesion may resolve completely. Calcification of the lesion can occur, but this is rare.

Clinical Presentation

Amoebic abscesses of the liver can occur in patients of any age. They are, obviously, most common in areas that are endemic for amoebiasis, but they are not rare in the United States or Western Europe. Usually there is the insidious onset of right upper abdominal quadrant pain, fever, malaise, and weight loss.[12,71,84] On the other hand, the presenting complaint may be the acute onset of hepatic pain and rigors. Chest symptoms are common, usually consisting of right lower chest pain, pleuritic pain, and/or cough. Diarrhea is noted by less than one fourth of the patients, and jaundice is unusual. Over 90% of the patients have tender hepatomegaly or a tender right upper abdominal mass.

Diagnosis

Laboratory tests usually show a normochromic normocytic anemia, leukocytosis, elevated eythrocyte sedimentation rate, and hypoalbuminemia. An elevated alkaline phosphatase and transaminases are frequently found. Abdominal radiographs are usually normal, but chest x-rays may show an elevated right hemidiaphragm, atelectasis, and/or a pleural effusion. A number of serologic tests have been developed to identify patients with invasive amoebiasis, and a positive serology can be expected in 90% of patients with hepatic amoebic abscesses.[12,71,84] Other tests for this disease include radionuclide liver scans, US, and CT. The radionuclide scan is of greatest value is demonstrating the site and number of lesions,[29] but it cannot distinguish amoebic abscess from other hepatic lesions such as metastatic malignant tumors. US, by demonstrating fluid within the mass, is ideal for identifying the cystic nature of the lesion.[109,130] Diagnostic needle aspiration, guided by physical findings, US, or CT may allow the clinician to distinguish between amoebic and pyogenic liver abscess.

Amoebic abscesses must be distinguished from other parasitic liver lesions such as hydatid disease of the liver. The latter lesion, caused by *Echinococcus,* occurs almost exclusively in areas endemic for that parasite, because specific snails act as obligate intermediate hosts for the *Echinococcus.* Hydatid cysts are frequently calcified and multiple, and are almost always associated with a positive Casoni skin test.[144] Percutaneous, or even open operative drainage of hydatid cysts is contraindicated because inadvertent spill of the cyst contents into the peritoneal cavity can trigger an anaphylactic reaction.

Treatment

Amebic liver abscesses can be effectively treated with a 7- to 10-day course of metronidazole. In the past, a number of amoebicidal drugs were used, but, currently, metronidazole is the drug of choice, and successful treatment can be expected in over 90% of patients. Surgical drainage may be considered as a method to establish the diagnosis if the latter is in doubt and if hydatid disease is unlikely. Surgical drainage may also be of value if multiple amoebic abscesses are present, particularly if they are large and if the response to medical management has been poor. Surgical drainage is mandatory if there is impending rupture, if rupture has already occurred, or if secondary bacterial infection has developed.[12,71,84]

Prognosis

The prognosis for treated amoebic abscess is very good.[12,71,84] Major complications usually result from rupture of the abscess in untreated patients. In this regard, rupture into the pleural space, lung, or pericardium is associated with high mortality.

SCLEROSING CHOLANGITIS

Etiology

Sclerosing cholangitis is a poorly understood inflammatory disease of the bile ducts of uncertain etiology.[92,168] It has been arbitrarily divided into two types—primary and secondary. Previous reviewers have not always used the same criteria to distinguish between these two types. Some have defined primary sclerosing cholangitis as that which occurs without the presence of one of the various underlying disease processes known to be associated with sclerosing cholangitis[5,155] (see below). More often, primary sclerosing cholangitis has been defined as that type which occurs in the absence of underlying bile duct disease (*i.e.*, stricture, prior surgical manipulation, cancer). If this latter convention is adopted, sclerosing cholangitis can be said to be a lesion that, in 70% to 80% of patients, occurs in association with some other disease process. Ulcerative colitis, the most common of these associated disease processes, has been noted in 40% to 70% of patients with sclerosing cholangitis.[5,92,155,166,168,169] On the other hand, less than 1% of patients with ulcerative colitis develop sclerosing cholangitis. The severity of the sclerosing cholangitis need not parallel that of the colonic disease, and, in fact, the onset of sclerosing cholangitis may precede identifiable colonic disease or, alternatively, follow panproctocolectomy for ulcerative colitis. Other diseases associated with sclerosing cholangitis include retroperitoneal fibrosis, sclerosing mediastinitis, pancreatitis, Riedel's struma, immunodeficiency states, and Crohn's disease.[5,92,155,166,168,169] Association with some of these disease processes has suggested that sclerosing cholangitis may involve a form of autoimmune reaction.[5,92,155,166,168,169] On the other hand, the observation that sclerosing cholangitis can complicate inflammatory bowel disease has suggested to some that it results from bacterial injury to the liver and periductal structures as a result of portal bacteremia. Bactobilia and signs of infection are not consistent features of the disease, however, especially if the biliary tree has not been instrumented or intubated.

Pathology

The distinction between sclerosing cholangitis and pericholangitis may be difficult. Some believe that the latter is an early stage of sclerosing cholangitis.[92,168] In its fully manifest form, sclerosing cholangitis is characterized by a dense, fibrous, inflammatory reaction around and involving the bile duct wall but, for the most part, sparing the epithelial lining.[5, 92, 155, 166, 168, 169] The large ducts are usually the most severely involved, but almost any pattern of distribution can be encountered, including pure involvement of extrahepatic ducts, intrahepatic ducts, both intra- and extrahepatic ducts, or only segmental ducts. There are usually scattered areas of narrowing with intervening non-narrowed areas giving rise to a beaded appearance. As a result of biliary stasis in these segments, stones may develop, but their presence usually does not precede significant ductal changes. More often than not, the inflammatory process does not involve the gallbladder. The distinction between sclerosing cholangitis and a sclerosing cholangiocarcinoma may be extremely difficult or even impossible on pathologic grounds, particularly when only localized disease is present. The coexistence of ulcerative colitis does not aid in this distinction because the incidence of both sclerosing cholangitis and cholangiocarcinoma are increased in ulcerative colitis. In addition, sclerosing cholangitis may predispose to the development of cholangiocarcinoma.[169]

Clinical Presentation

The disease is most often first manifest in the fourth and fifth decades. The major clinical features result from biliary obstruction.[5, 92, 155, 166, 168, 169] Thus, jaundice, acholic stools, pruritus, and abnormal liver function tests are commonly present. In addition, vague upper abdominal pain, malaise, anorexia, and weight loss are usually noted. Chills, fever, and other manifestations of sepsis are relatively uncommon because the bile is usually sterile prior to operative intervention.

Diagnosis

The diagnosis should be suspected in patients with diseases known to be associated with sclerosing cholangitis (*e.g.,* ulcerative colitis) who develop signs and symptoms of biliary tract obstruction. The absence of ductal dilation and of stones on US examination in this setting should further arouse suspicion.[17] Endoscopic retrograde cholangiography can be diagnostic if the "pruned tree" appearance of ducts is noted or, alternatively, if diffusely scattered areas of narrowing and beading of the ducts are demonstrated.[45, 106, 168] Ultimately, exploratory laparotomy and biopsy of thickened ducts may be required to distinguish this lesion from a sclerosing cholangiocarcinoma, and, occasionally, even that procedure may fail and the diagnosis may only be made at the time of autopsy.

Treatment

Treatment of sclerosing cholangitis is difficult and usually unrewarding. The value of proctocolectomy for patients who have ulcerative colitis and who have sclerosing cholangitis has been controversial. There are some reports of success,[124] but more frequently colon resection does not alter the course of the liver disease.[169] When sclerosing cholangitis is limited to the extrahepatic ducts, biliary obstruction can be alleviated by a variety of bypass procedures. With intrahepatic lesions, treatment usually involves splinting of narrowed segments with indwelling tubes (T-tubes, percutaneous transhepatic tubes, Y-tubes, and so forth).[13, 128, 172] Corticosteroids and long-term broad-spectrum antibiotics have been advocated, but the results obtained are usually poor.[169] Liver transplantation should be considered in selected patients with sclerosing cholangitis.[169]

Prognosis

The course of sclerosing cholangitis is usually characterized by progressive evidence of biliary cirrhosis, liver failure, and portal hypertension. Life expectancy after diagnosis is usually 4 to 6 years, and most of the patients die of either progressive hepatic failure or variceal hemorrhage.[5, 92, 155, 166, 168, 169]

REFERENCES

1. Altemeier WA, Schowengerdt CG, Whiteley DH. Abscesses of the liver: surgical considerations. Arch Surg 1970;101:258.
2. Aronsohn HG. and Andrews E. Experimental cholecystitis. Surg Gynecol Obstet 1938;66:748.
3. Babb RR. The use of antibiotics in biliary tract disease. Am J Gastroenterol 1975;63:37.
4. Balasegaram M. Management of hepatic abscess. Curr Probl Surg 1981;18:285.
5. Benjamin IS, Blumgart LH. Biliary bypass and reconstructive surgery. In: Weight R, Alberti KGMM, Karran S, et al, eds. Liver and Biliary Disease. London: WB Saunders, 1979:1124.
6. Bilbao MK, Dotter CT, Lee TG, et al. Complications of endoscopic retrograde cholangiopancreatography (ERCP): a study of 10,000 cases. Gastroenterology 1976;70:314.
7. Bismuth H, Kuntziger H, Corlette MB. Cholangitis with acute renal failure: priorities in therapeutics. Ann Surg 1975;181:881.
8. Blumgart LH. The biliary tract. London: Churchill Livingstone, 1982.
9. Boey JH, Way LW. Acute cholangitis. Ann Surg 1980;191:264.
10. Boyden EA. The anatomy of the choledochoduodenal junction in man. Surg Gynecol Obstet 1957;104:641.
11. Brandborg LL. Bacterial and miscellaneous infections of the liver. In: Zakim D, Boyer TD, eds. Hepatology. Philadelphia: WB Saunders, 1982:1036.
12. Brandborg LC. Parasitic diseases of the liver. In: Sakim D, Boyer TD, eds. Hepatology. Philadelphia: WB Saunders, 1982:1010.
13. Cameron JL, et al. Sclerosing cholangitis: Biliary reconstruction with Silastic transhepatic stents. Surgery 1983;94:324.
14. Cardoso V, et al. The effect of cholestasis of the hepatic clearance of bacteria. World J Surg 1982;6:330.
15. Carmona RH, Crass RA, Lim RC Jr, et al. Oriental cholangitis. Am J Surg 1984;148:117.
16. Carpino F, et al. A scanning and transmission electron microscopic study of experimental extrahepatic cholestasis in the rat. J Submicrosc Cytol 1981;3:581.
17. Carroll BA, Oppenheimer DA. Sclerosing cholangitis: sonographic demonstration of bile duct wall thickening. AJR 1982;139:1016.
18. Charcot JM. Lecons ser les maladies du foie des voices biliares et des reins Paris: Faculte de Medecinde de Paris Recueilles et pibliees par Bourneville et Sevestre, 1877.
19. Chattopadhyay B. Pyogenic liver abscess. J Infect 1983;6:5.
20. Chetlin SH, Elliott DW. Biliary bacteremia. Arch Surg 1971;102:303.
21. Cheung LY, Maxwell JG. Jaundice in patients with acute cholecystitis. Am J Surg 1975;130:746.
22. Choi TK, Wong J, Ong GB. Choledochojejunostomy in the treatment of primary cholangitis. Surg Gynecol Obstet 1982;155:43.
23. Chou S-T, Chan CW. Recurrent pyogenic cholangitis: a necropsy study. Pathology 1980;12:415.
24. Clouse ME, Evans D, Costello P, et al. Percutaneous transhepatic biliary drainage: complications due to multiple duct obstructions. Ann Surg 1983;198:25.

25. Cole WH, Novak MV, Hughes EO. Experimental production of chronic cholecystitis by obstructive lesions of the cystic duct. Ann Surg 1941;114:682.

26. Cooperberg PL, Burhenne HJ. Realtime ultrasonography. N Engl J Med 1980;302:1277.

27. Copher GH, Dick BM. "Stream line" phenomena in the portal vein and selective distribution of portal blood in the liver. Arch Surg 1928;17:408.

28. Csendes A, et al. Pressure measurements in the biliary and the pancreatic duct systems in controls and in patients with gallstones, previous cholecystectomy, or common bile duct stones. Gastroenterology 1979;77:1203.

29. Cuaron A, Gordon F. Liver scanning analysis of 2500 cases of amebic hepatic abscesses. J Nucl Med 1970;11:435.

30. Dawson JL. Cholecystitis and cholecystectomy. Clin Gastroenterol 1973;2:85.

31. Dawson SL. Nonoperative management of biliary obstruction. Annu Rev Med 1985;36:1.

32. Deitch EA, Engel JM. Acute acalculous cholecystitis, ultrasonic diagnosis. Am J Surg 1981;142:290.

33. de la Maza LM, Naeim F, Berman L. The changing etiology of liver abscess. JAMA 1974;227:161.

34. Dellinger EP, Kirshenbaum G, Weinstein M, et al. Determinants of adverse reaction following postoperative T-tube cholangiogram. Ann Surg 1980;191:397.

35. Dey M, MacDonald A, Smith G. The bacterial flora of the biliary tract and liver in man. Br J Surg 1978;65:285.

36. Dietrick RB. Experience with liver abscess. Am J Surg 1984;147:288.

37. Dineen P. The importance of the route of infection in experimental biliary obstruction. Surg Gynecol Obstet 1964;119:1001.

38. Donaldson RM. Normal bacterial populations of the intestine and their relation to intestinal function. N Engl J Med 1964;270:938.

39. Dooley, Hamilton-Miller, Brumfitt, Sherlock. Antibiotics in the treatment of biliary infection. Gut 1984;25:988.

40. Drasar BS, Shiner M, McLeod GM. Studies on the intestinal flora. I. The bacterial flora of the gastrointestinal tract in healthy and achlorhydric persons. Gastroenterology 1969;56:71.

41. Drivas G, James O, Wardle N. Study of the reticuloendothelial phagocytic capacity in patients with cholestasis. Br Med J 1976;1:1586.

42. Dumont AE. Significance of hyperbilirubinemia in acute cholecystitis. Surg Gynecol Obstet 1976;142:855.

43. Edlund YA, Mollstedt BO, Ouchterlony P. Bacteriological investigation of the biliary system and the liver in biliary tract disease correlated to clinical data and microstructure of the gallbladder and liver. Acta Chir Scand 1958/1959;116:461.

44. Eggert A, Teichmann W, Wittmann DH. The pathologic implication of duodenal diverticula. Surg Gynecol Obstet 1982;154:62.

45. Elias E, Summerfield JA, Dick R, et al. Endoscopic retrograde cholangiography in the diagnosis of jaundice associated with ulcerative colitis. Gastroenterology 1974;67:907.

46. Engstrom J, Hellstrom K. The duodenal microflora in relation to various symptoms and manifestations in patients with extrahepatic biliary disease. Acta Med Scand 1973;193:267.

47. Engstrom J, Hellstrom K. The duodenal microflora and the incidence of malabsorption in non-icteric patients with extrahepatic biliary disease. Acta Med Scand 1973;193:273.

48. Feretis CB, et al. Long term consequences of bacterial colonization of the biliary tract after choledochostomy. Surg Gynecol Obstet 1984;159:363.

49. Flemma RJ, Flint LM, Osterhaut S, et al. Bacteriologic studies of biliary tract infection. Ann Surg 1967;166:563.

50. Gagic N, Frey CF, Gaines R. Acute cholecystitis. Surg Gynecol Obstet 1975;140:868.

51. Gatch WD, Battersby JS, Wakim KG. The nature and treatment of cholecystitis. JAMA 1946;132:119.

52. Geenen JE, et al. Intraluminal pressure recording from the human sphincter of Oddi. Gastroenterology 1980;78:317.

53. Gerzof SG, Johnson WC, Robbins AH, et al. Intrahepatic pyogenic abscesses: treatment by percutaneous drainage. Am J Surg 1985;149:487.

54. Glenn F. Surgical management of acute cholecystitis in patients 65 years of age and older. Ann Surg 1981;193:56.

55. Glenn F. Acute acalculous cholecystitis. Ann Surg 1979;189:458.

56. Glenn F. Acute cholecystitis. Surg Gynecol Obstet 1976;143:56.

57. Glenn F, Moody FG. Acute obstructive suppurative cholangitis. Surg Gynecol Obstet 1961;113:265.

58. Goldman LD, Steer ML, Silen W. Recurrent cholangitis after biliary surgery. Am J Surg 1983;145:450.

59. Gorbach SL, Bartlett JG. Anaerobic infections. N Engl J Med 1974;290:1177.

60. Gottfries A. Lysolecithin: a factor in the pathogenesis of acute cholecystitis. Acta Chir Scand 1969;135:213.

61. Greenstein AJ, et al. Continuing changing patterns of disease in pyogenic liver abscess: a study of 38 patients. Am J Gastroenterol 1984;79:216.

62. Gregg JA, De Girolami P, Carr-Locke, DL. Effects of sphincteroplasty and endoscopic sphincterotomy on the bacteriologic characteristics of the common bile duct. Am J Surg 1985;149:668.

63. Halvorsen EA, et al. The variable CT appearance of hepatic abscesses. Am J Res 1984;142:941.

64. Hancke E, Marklein G, Helpap B. Route of infection of the biliary tree: experimental evidence for an enterohepaticobiliary cycle. Langenbecks Arch Chir 1980;353:121.

65. Hatfield ARW, et al. The microbiology of direct bile sampling at the time of endoscopic retrograde cholangiography. J Infect 1982;4:119.

66. Hauge CW, Mark JBD. Common bile duct motility and sphincter mechanism. Ann Surg 1965;162:1028.

67. Helm EB, et al. Elimination of bacteria in biliary tract infections during cefitizomine therapy. Infection 1982;10:67.

68. Hendrickson WF. A study of the musculature of the entire extra-hepatic biliary system, including that of the duodenal portion of the common bile-duct and of the sphincter. Johns Hopkins Hosp Bull 1898;90–91:221.

69. Hirsig J, Kara O, Rickham PP. Experimental investigations into the etiology of cholangitis following operation for biliary atresia. J Pediatr Surg 1978;13:55.

70. Holdstock G, et al. The liver in infection. In: Wright R, et al, eds. Liver and Biliary Disease. London: WB Saunders, 1979:1155.

71. Holdstock G, et al. The liver in infection. In: Wright R, et al, eds. Liver and Biliary Disease. London: WB Saunders, 1979:1163.

72. Huang T, Bass JA, Williams RD. The significance of biliary pressure in cholangitis. Arch Surg 1969;98:629.

73. Huitborn A, Jacobson B, Rosengren B. Cholangiovenous reflux during cholangiography. Acta Chir Scand 1962;123:111.

74. Ikeda S, et al. Emergency decompression of bile duct in acute obstructive suppurative cholangitis by duodenoscopic cannulation: a lifesaving procedure. World J Surg 1981;5:587.

75. Ishak KG, Rogers WA. Cryptogenic acute cholangitis—association with toxic shock syndrome. Am J Clin Pathol 1981;76:619.

76. Jackman FR, et al. Experimental bacterial infection of the biliary tract. Br J Exp Pathol 1980;61:369.

77. Jackman FR, Hillson GRF, Lord Smith of Marlow. Bile bacteria in patients with benign duct stricture. Br J Surg 1980;67:329.

78. Jacobson B, Kjellander J, Rosengren B. Cholangiovenous reflux. Acta Chir Scand 1962;123:316.

79. Jarvinen HJ, Hastbucka J. Early cholecystectomy for acute cholecystitis. Ann Surg 1980;191:501.

80. Justesen T, Nielsen ML. Anaerobic infection of the liver and biliary tract in experimental common duct occlusion. Scand J Infect Dis [Suppl] 1979;19:35.

81. Keighley MRB Jr, Flinn R, Alexander-Williams J. A multivariate analysis of clinical and operative findings associated with biliary sepsis. Br J Surg 1976;63:528.

82. Keighley MRB, et al. Infections and the biliary tree. In: Blumgart LH, ed. The biliary tract. London: Churchill Livingstone, 1982:219.

83. Keighley MRB, et al. Antibiotics in biliary disease: the relative importance of antibiotic concentrations in the bile and serum. Gut 1976;17:495.

84. Knight R. Hepatic amebiasis. Semin Liver Dis 1984;4:277.

85. Kozarek RA. Transnasal pancreatiobiliary drains. Am J Surg 1983;146:25.

86. Kuligowska E, Connors SK, Shapiro JH. Liver abscess: sonography in diagnosis and treatment. Am J Roentgenol 1982;138:253.

87. Kune GA, Hibbard J, Morahan R. The development of biliary infection. Med J Aust 1974;1:301.

88. Kune GA, Sali A. The practice of biliary surgery. Oxford:Blackwell Scientific Publications, 1980.

89. Lahtinen J, Alhava EM, Aukee S. Acute cholecystitis treated by early and delayed surgery. A controlled clinical trial. Scand J Gastroenterol 1978;13:673.

90. Lam SK. A study of endoscopic sphincterotomy in recurrent pyogenic cholangitis. Br J Surg 1984;71:262.

91. Landor JH, Fulkerson CC. Duodenal diverticula. Arch Surg 1966;93:182.

92. LaRusso NF, et al. Primary sclerosing cholangitis. N Engl J Med 1984;310:899.

93. Lazarchick J, Nichols DR, Washington JA. Pyogenic liver abscess. Mayo Clin Proc 1973;48:349.

94. Lewis RT, et al. A single preoperative dose of cefazolin prevents postoperative sepsis in high-risk biliary surgery. Can J Surg 1984;27:44.

95. Lilly JR, Hitch DC. Postoperative ascending cholangitis following porteonterostomy for biliary atresia: measures for control. World J Surg 1978;2:581.

96. Lindahl F, Cedeqvist CS. The treatment of acute cholecystitis. Acta Chir Scand [Suppl] 1969;396:9.

97. Lotveit T. Bacterial infections of the liver and biliary tract. Scand J Gastroenterol [Suppl] 1983;85:33.

98. Lotveit T. The composition of biliary calculi in patients with juxtapapillary duodenal diverticula. Scand J Gastroenterol 1982;17:653.

99. Lotveit T, Foss OP, Osnes MC. Biliary pigment and cholesterol calculi in patients with and without juxtapapillary duodenal diverticula. Scand J Gastroenterol 1981;16:241.

100. Lotveit T, Isnes M, Aune S. Bacteriological studies of common duct bile in patients with gallstone disease and juxtapapillary duodenal diverticula. Scand J Gastroenterol 1978;13:93.

101. Lotveit T, et al. Studies of the choledocho-duodenal sphincter in patients with and without juxtapapillary duodenal diverticula. Scand J Gastroenterol 1980;15:875.

102. Lotveit R, Isnes M, Larsen S. Recurrent biliary calculi. Duodenal diverticula as a predisposing factor. Ann Surg 1982;196(1):30.

103. Lou MA, et al. Bacteriology of the human biliary tract and the duodenum. Arch Surg 1977;112:965.

104. Lygidakis NJ. Acute suppurative cholangitis: comparison of internal and external biliary drainage. Am J Surg 1982;143:304.

105. Lygidakis NJ, Brummelkamp WH. The significance of intrabiliary pressure in acute cholangitis. Surg Gynecol Obstet 1985;161:465.

106. MacCarty RL, et al. Cholangiographic and pancreatographic features of primary sclerosing cholangitis. Radiology 1983;149:39.

107. Maki T. Pathogenesis of calcium bilirubinate gallstone: role of *E. coli*, glucuronidase and coagulation by inorganic ions, polyelectrolytes and agitation. Ann Surg 1966;164:90.

108. Mason GR. Bacteriology and antibiotic selection in biliary tract surgery. Arch Surg 1968;97:533.

109. Matthews AW, et al. The use of combined ultrasonic and isotope scanning in the diagnosis of amoebic liver abscess. Gut 1973;14:50.

110. McDonald MI, et al. Single and multiple pyogenic liver abscesses. Natural history, diagnosis and treatment, with emphasis of percutaneous drainage. Medicine (Baltimore) 1984;63:291.

111. McLeish AR, et al. Selecting patients requiring antibiotics in biliary surgery by immediate Gram stains of bile at operation. Surgery 1977;81:473.

112. Mentzer RM, Jr, et al. A comparative appraisal of emphysematous cholecystitis. Am J Surg 1975;129:10.

113. Metz J, et al. Morphologic alterations and functional changes of interhepatocellular junctions induced by bile ducts ligation. Cell Tissue Res 1977;182:299.

114. Millward-Sadler GH, Jezequel AM. Normal histology and ultrastructure in the liver. In: Wright R, et al, eds. Liver and Biliary Disease. London: WB Saunders, 1979:34.

115. Morrow DJ, Thompson J, Wilson SE. Acute cholecystitis in the elderly. Arch Surg 1978;113:1149.

116. Motson RW, Way LW. Cholecystitis. In: Blumgart LH, ed. The Biliary Tract. London: Churchill Livingstone, 1982:121.

117. Nagar H, Berger SA. The excretion of antibiotics by the biliary tract. Surg Gynecol Obstet 1984;158:601.

118. Nielsen ML. Route of infection in extrahepatic biliary tract disease. Scand J Gastroenterol [Suppl] 1976;37:11.

119. Nielsen ML, Asnaes S, Justesen T. Susceptibility of the liver and biliary tract to anaerobic infection in extrahepatic biliary tract obstruction. Scand J Gastroenterol 1976;11:263.

120. Nolan JP. Bacteria and the liver. N Engl J Med 1978;299:1069.

121. Ochsner A, DeBakey M, Murray S. Pyogenic abscess of the liver: an analysis of forty-seven cases with review of the literature. Am J Surg 1938;40:292.

122. O'Connor MJ, et al. Acute bacterial cholangitis: an analysis of clinical manifestation. Arch Surg 1982;117:437.

123. O'Connor MJ, Hatton WS, Schwartz ML. The clinical and pathologic correlations in mechanical biliary obstruction and acute cholangitis. Ann Surg 1982;195(4):419.

124. Olsson R, Hulten L. Concurrence of ulcerative colitis and chronic active hepatitis: clinical courses and results of colectomy. Scand J Gastroenterol 1975;10:331.

125. Ong GB. A study of recurrent pyogenic cholangitis. Arch Surg 1962;84:199.

126. Orloff MJ, Peskin GW, Ellis HL. A bacteriologic study of human portal blood. Ann Surg 1956;148:738.

127. Peng SY, et al. Aspects of treatment at the Zhejiang Medical College, China. Ann Royal College of Surg Engl 1983;65.

128. Pitt HA, et al. Primary sclerosing cholangitis: results of an aggressive surgical approach. Ann Surg 1982;196:259.

129. Pitt HA, Zuidema GD. Factors influencing mortality in the treatment of pyogenic hepatic abscess. Surg Gynecol Obstet 1975;140:228.

130. Ralls PW, et al. Gray-scale ultrasonography of hepatic amoebic abscesses. Radiology 1979;132:125.

131. Remington JS, Schimpf SC. Please don't eat the salads. N Engl J Med 1981;302:433.

132. Reynolds BM, Dargan RL. Acute obstructive cholangitis. Ann Surg 1959;150:299.

133. Robenek J, Herwig J, Themann H. The morphologic characteristics of intercellular junctions between normal human liver cells and cells from patients with extrahepatic cholestasis. Am J Pathol 1980;100:93.

134. Robenek J, Rassat J, Themann H. A quantitative freeze-fracture analysis of gap and tight junctions in the normal and cholestatic human liver. Virchows Arch (Cell Pathol) 1981;38:39.

135. Rosseland AR, Midtvedt T, Aasen AO. Gallbladder and duodenal bacterial flora after papillotomy in rabbits. Scand J Gastroenterol 1982;17:785.

136. Rubin RH, Swartz MN, Malt R. Hepatic abscess: changes in clinical, bacteriologic and therapeutic aspects. Am J Med 1974;57:601.

137. Saharia PC, Cameron JL. Clinical management of acute cholangitis. Surg Gynecol Obstet 1976;142:369.

138. Saik RP, Greenburg AG, Peskin GW. Cholecystectomy hazard in acute cholangitis. JAMA 1976;235:2412.

139. Schatten WE, Desprez JD, Holden WD. A bacteriologic study of portal-vein blood in man. Arch Surg 1955;71:404.

140. Schoenfield LJ. Biliary excretion of antibiotics. N Engl J Med 1971;284:1213.

141. Scott AJ. Bacteria and disease of the biliary tract. Gut 1971;12:487.

142. Scott AJ, Khan GA. Origin of bacteria in bile duct bile. Lancet 1967;2:790.

143. Seel DJ, Park YK. Oriental infestational cholangitis. Am J Surg 1983;146:366.

144. Shearman DJC, Finlayson NDC. Diseases of the gastrointestinal tract. Edinborough: Churchill Livingstone, 1982:419.

145. Shearman DJC, Finlayson NDC. Diseases of the gastrointestinal tract. Edinborough: Churchill Livingstone, 1982:510.

146. Shimada K, et al. Biliary tract infection with anaerobes and the presence of free bile acids in the bile. Rev Infect Dis 1984;6(Suppl 1):s147.

147. Shorey BA. Systemic antibiotic prophylaxis in gastrointestinal surgery. In: Strachan CJL, Wise R, eds. Surgical Sepsis. New York: Grune & Stratton, 1979.

148. Silen W, Wetheimer M, Kirshenbaum G. Bacterial contamination of the biliary tree after choledochotomy. Am J Surg (Festschrift Ed) 1978;135:325.

149. Sjodahl R, Tagesson C, Wetterfors J. On the pathogenesis of acute cholecystitis. Surg Gynecol Obstet 1978;199.

150. Smith BR, LeFrock, J. Biliary tree penetration of parenteral antibiotics. Infect in Surg 1983;110.

151. Sobel JD, Kaye D. Host factors in the pathogenesis of urinary tract infections. Am J Med 76(5A):122.

152. Strachan CJL, et al. Prophylactic use of cephazolin against wound sepsis after cholecystectomy. Br Med J 1977;1:1254.

153. Suzuki Y, et al. Bacteriological study of transhepatically aspirated bile. Dig Dis Sci 1984;29:109.

154. Tabata M, Nakayama F. Bacteria and gallstones. Etiological significance. Dig Dis Sci 1981;26:218.

155. Tan EGC, Warren KW. Diseases of the gallbladder and bile ducts. In: Schiff L, Schiff ER, eds. Diseases of the Liver. Philadelphia: JB Lippincott, 1982:1532.

156. Tanaka N. Biliary sepsis. Bulletin No. 52, Dept of Surg, University of Lund, Sweden, 1985.

157. Tansy MF, et al. The mucosal lining of the intramural common bile duct as a determinant of ductal pressure. Am J Dig Dis 1975;20:613.

158. Thadepalli H, et al. Microflora of the human small intestine. Am J Surg 1979;138:845.

159. Thomas CG, Womack NA. Acute cholecystitis, its pathogenesis and repair. Arch Surg 1952;64:590.

160. Thomas E, et al. Bacterial flora in the duodenum of patients after biliary fenestration. Br J Surg 1973;60:107.

161. Thompson JE, Tompkins RK, Longmire WP. Factors in management of acute cholangitis. Ann Surg 1982;195:137.

162. Ti TK, Yuen R. Chemical composition of biliary calculi in relation to the pattern of biliary disease in Singapore. Br J Surg 1985;72:556.

163. Toouli J, et al. Sphincter of Oddi motor activity: a comparison between patients with common bile duct stones and controls. Gastroenterology 1982;82:111.

164. Turner WW Jr, Cramer CR. Recurrent oriental cholangiohepatitis. Surgery 1983;93:397.

165. Twiss JR, Carter RF, Fishman BS. Infection in chronic cholecysitits. JAMA 1951;147:1266.

424

166. Vierling JM. Hepatobiliary complications of ulcerative colitis and Crohn's disease. In: Zakim D, Boyer TD, eds. Hepatology. Philadelphia: WB Saunders, 1982:818.

167. Wacha H, Helm EB. Efficacy of antibiotics in bactobilia. J Antimicrob Chemother 1982; 9(Suppl)A:131.

168. Wiesner RH, LaRusso NF. Clinicopathologic features of the syndrome of primary sclerosing cholangitis. Gastroenterology 1980;79:200.

169. Wiesner RH, et al. Diagnosis and treatment of primary sclerosing cholangitis. Semin Liver Dis 1985;5:241.

170. Weissmann HS, et al. Rapid and accurate diagnosis of acute cholecystitis with ^{99m}Tc-HIDA cholescintigraphy. AJR 1979;132:523.

171. Wong WT, Teoh-Chan CH, Huang CT. The bacteriology of recurrent pyogenic cholangitis and associated diseases. J Hyg (Lond) 1981;87:407.

172. Wood RAB, Cuschieri A. Is sclerosing cholangitis complicating ulcerative colitis a reversible condition? Lancet 1980;2:716.

173. Zaslow J. Antibiotics in diseases of the biliary tree. JAMA 1953;152:1683.

174. Zeman RK, et al. Diagnostic utility of cholescintigraphy and ultrasonography in acute cholecystitis. Am J Surg 1981;141:446.

19

○ ○ ○ ● ● ●

INFECTIOUS COMPLICATIONS IN TRANSPLANT SURGERY

David L. Dunn
John S. Najarian

Infection in the normal mammalian host involves a complex interaction between invading microbes and host defenses, which include specific defense mechanisms such as the activation of humoral and cellular immunity, as well as more general systems such as phagocytosis and microbial killing by leukocytes and complement. In the transplant recipient maintenance of allograft function requires suppression of the host immune system, which concomitantly diminishes the capacity of host defenses to cope with microbial invasion. The immunosuppressed allograft recipient is therefore predisposed to infection from a wide and varied number of agents of disease. In fact, many series report that over 30% of patients develop some type of significant infection after transplantation. Thus, while the overall rates of infection and mortality have declined progressively, infectious disease processes still represent a significant problem following transplantation.[40,44,66,76,78,86,87,102,126,149,198,214,217,220,256,266,337]

A number of factors have been shown to predispose patients to infection after transplantation. These include diabetes mellitus, hepatitis, leukopenia, splenectomy, persistent uremia with renal allograft dysfunction, receiving a cadaveric allograft, and repeated treatment of persistent or recurrent rejection leading to host overimmunosuppression. The latter two factors are probably related, due to the fact that recipients of cadaveric allografts typically require more immunosuppression than well-matched living related allograft recipients, and have a higher incidence of allograft dysfunction. It is well known that the patient who is repeatedly subjected to antirejection therapy (corticosteroids, antilymphocyte globulin, or both) is at higher risk for infectious complications.[44,52,76,86,126,200,209,256,266,271,308]

In the immediate postoperative period, transplanted patients are exposed to infection at the allograft site. A complex interaction probably occurs in which the allografted tissues as well as the host tissues react to the trauma of the operative procedure. In addition, the response of the host immune system may be immediate and vigorous or prolonged and minimal, each leading to changes in the local and systemic host defense milieu. Thus, renal transplant patients most typically develop urinary tract infections, hepatic transplant patients develop intra-abdominal sepsis, and heart and heart–lung recipients contract infections of the lung and pleural cavity. Subsequently, the often global depression of immune defenses subjects the transplant patient to a higher incidence of infection at distant sites as well.

The immunosuppressed transplant patient is predisposed to both common and unusual infections. Microbial agents that are nonpathogenic in the immunologically intact host may cause a severe infection in the transplant patient, and those that normally cause a serious infection may be lethal. Although the various immunosuppressive agents currently used in transplantation (corticosteroids, azathioprine, cyclophosphamide, cyclosporine, antilymphocyte globulin, OKT3 murine monoclonal antibody) provide excellent immunosuppression by a variety of mechanisms, they do not provide selective immunosuppression and prevention of rejection without simultaneously depressing antimicrobial host defenses. It may be possible to develop more selective immunosuppressants, or use those currently available in more suitably balanced combinations, in order to maintain allograft function without a high infection rate. Our experience is that this is indeed the case.[47,226,290,313]

In this immunosuppressed patient population, the symptoms and signs of even common disease processes may be masked, and the clinical picture can be extremely confusing to the clinician. In many cases this leads to a delayed or an incorrect diagnosis. The usual paradigms the clinician uses to evaluate a patient must often be modified when attempting to establish a diagnosis in the transplant patient. In particular, when infection occurs in the transplant patient, the usual signs and symptoms (fever, chills, elevated white count) may be minimal or absent. The presence of any of these signs or symptoms mandates a thorough clinical evaluation (Fig. 19-1). In many cases thought must be given to instituting empiric antimicrobial treatment prior to establishing the diagnosis, as well as tapering immunosuppression

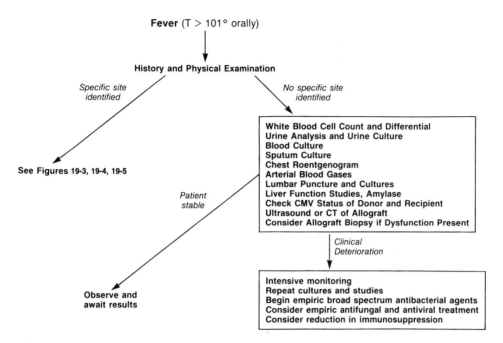

Fever (T > 101° orally)

History and Physical Examination

Specific site identified

No specific site identified

White Blood Cell Count and Differential
Urine Analysis and Urine Culture
Blood Culture
Sputum Culture
Chest Roentgenogram
Arterial Blood Gases
Lumbar Puncture and Cultures
Liver Function Studies, Amylase
Check CMV Status of Donor and Recipient
Ultrasound or CT of Allograft
Consider Allograft Biopsy if Dysfunction Present

See Figures 19-3, 19-4, 19-5

Patient stable

Clinical Deterioration

Intensive monitoring
Repeat cultures and studies
Begin empiric broad spectrum antibacterial agents
Consider empiric antifungal and antiviral treatment
Consider reduction in immunosuppression

Observe and await results

Figure 19-1.
Algorithm for the diagnostic evaluation of fever occurring in a patient after organ transplantation.

should clinical deterioration occur. Reevaluation of a specific diagnosis must then take place frequently based on the patient's response to initial therapy. In the following sections, the viral, bacterial, fungal, protozoan, and parasitic infections that patients develop after solid organ transplantation and the means by which they may be diagnosed and treated will be reviewed.

VIRAL INFECTIONS

Viral infections are probably the most frequent form of infection to which the transplant patient is subjected.[253,256,289,291,292] They assume a wide variety of forms, which range from asymptomatic infection diagnosed solely on the basis of a progressive increase in antibody titer to fulminant disease, which may cause rapid host demise. Viral infections may be caused by latent host viruses, or by way of exposure of the immunosuppressed host to viral agents within the environment.

Herpes Viruses

Infection with various herpes group viruses is known to occur with increased frequency after organ transplantation. Infection due to cytomegalovirus (CMV) has protean manifestations, occurring primarily in neonates, after transfusion of blood products to immunocompetent as well as immunodeficient patients, and after organ transplantation and other forms of immunosuppression. CMV disease has been extensively studied in relation to its impact on patient survival after transplantation and can present as fever and leukopenia, cecal ulceration with gastrointestinal hemorrhage, pancreatitis, retinitis, hepatitis, or interstitial pneumonia.[29,30,97,103,179,221,227,243,246,254,262,277,291,297,311] Both primary and reactivation CMV disease can occur, and naive recipients who receive an organ from a donor in which a CMV titer is present (in most cases indicative of latent donor CMV infection) are at highest risk for development of disease. CMV thus represents perhaps the foremost example of transmission of disease from a donor organ to the host.

The reported incidence of CMV infection after renal transplantation is 25% to 96%.[19,53,98,175,179,193,254,291,292] The majority of these infections are made on the basis of either cultural evidence or a greater than fourfold rise in the antibody titer. Peterson and co-workers[254] demonstrated in a prospective study that CMV infections occur primarily within the first several months after renal transplantation and exert a significant detrimental effect on both patient and allograft survival. Cheeseman and co-workers[53] noted that beginning several months after transplantation there is a subgroup of patients who continue to excrete CMV for many years. The spectrum of syndromes that CMV can cause vary from mild fever and leukopenia to a lethal syndrome consisting of hypoxemia, weakness, hypotension, gastrointestinal hemorrhage, bacterial and fungal superinfection, and death. It is not clear, however, why certain patients develop more severe forms of the disease, although overimmunosuppressed CMV naive patients are clearly at higher risk for lethal sequelae.[98,254,291,292]

Herpes simplex virus (HSV) typically presents as oropharyngeal or vesicular skin lesions that are painful and crust over within several days. Isolated cases of disseminated HSV epidermal infection, diffuse gastrointestinal tract involvement, fulminant hepatitis, pneumonia and encephalitis have also been reported (Fig. 19-2).[10,12,13,74,88,173,213,227,245,309] Most cases, however, do not produce lethality, and a detrimental effect of HSV alone on either patient or allograft survival has not been documented. On the basis of cultural evidence, Lopez and co-workers were able to demonstrate that approximately 21% of patients developed HSV infection in the immediate post-transplantation period.[175] Other investigators have reported HSV infection to occur in 14% to 70% of patients after renal transplantation.[12,227,243,245]

Naraqi and co-workers found in a prospective study that 73% of renal allograft recipients had evidence for HSV infection after renal transplantation, the majority within the first 6 months.[227] Armstrong and co-workers determined by serologic testing that HSV infection occurred in 38% of renal transplant patients.[12] This figure rose to 48% when both serologic and cultural evidence was used. Pass and co-workers found that the most commonly involved anatomical site was the oropharynx and reported an HSV infection rates of 70% after transplantation.[243,245] Shedding of HSV was found to peak within the first month after renal transplantation. These investigators also examined serum antibody titers to HSV in patients prior and subsequent to renal transplantation. No patients were found to shed HSV prior to transplantation, and those patients identified as having a prior significant antibody titer were found to be at high risk for the development of HSV after renal transplantation. Current therapy for HSV disease consists of acyclovir, which appears to shorten the duration of

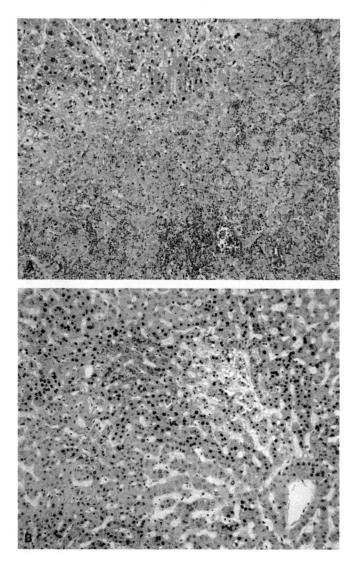

Figure 19-2.
Fulminant herpes simplex virus (HSV) type I hepatitis occurring after pancreas transplantation. Note the extensive parenchymal damage and hemorrhagic necrosis (*A*, 120× hematoxalin and eosin), and the large areas staining specifically for HSV (*B*, 120× immunoperoxidase).

infection. Many centers are examining the effect of prophylactic acyclovir therapy in the immediate post-transplant period.

Both HSV and CMV infections may occur concurrently with other severe infections. The occurrence of disease generally coincides with the immediate post-transplantation period of maximal immunosuppression. Some authors have noted that treatment with antilymphocyte globulin appears to predispose patients to CMV infection.[52,254,271,291,292] Both CMV and HSV become latent after the initial infection and thus are difficult to combat by vaccination. Lopez and co-workers noted that 14% of patients had combined HSV and CMV infection after renal transplantation.[175] Similarly, Naraqi and co-workers reported a 20% incidence of this combined disease.[227] Balfour and co-workers noted that 25% of patients had simultaneous HSV and CMV infection after renal transplantation, and considered that the clinical course of these patients was more severe than that of patients with single viral infections.[19]

Dunn and co-workers demonstrated that while HSV spillage alone produced no significant detrimental effect on mortality and allograft loss, spillage of CMV led to diminished patient and allograft survival after renal transplantation.[83] Although the presence of HSV alone appeared to have no detrimental effect, concurrent HSV and CMV infections were associated with increased allograft loss and patient mortality over and above the effect of CMV alone. Nearly 40% of the patients within this group underwent a concurrently treated rejection episode, but the onset of rejection treatment did not correlate with viral spillage. Marker and co-workers, in a similar examination of patients with CMV infection, found that 51% of patients with CMV experienced a treated rejection episode, but the timing of treatment bore no relation to the viral infection.[193]

In an attempt to reduce both the incidence and lethality of CMV disease after transplantation, an attenuated CMV virus (Towne strain) has been developed for use as a vaccine. In healthy persons, this vaccine induces a suitable antibody response, but immunosuppressed patients have a poorer response in many cases.[194,264,275,305] In addition, this vaccine has not yet unequivocally been shown to be efficacious in this setting, although several reports have provided evidence that a reduction in morbidity due to CMV disease may occur in renal allograft recipients who are vaccinated.[18,258,259] Several vaccines are being developed to prevent and treat HSV infection and are currently being tested clinically.[131,203,296]

Several studies have demonstrated the efficacy of anti-CMV immunoglobulin pooled from human sources to reduce CMV-associated lethality when administered prophylactically to bone marrow allograft recipients.[60,206] Although anecdotal evidence exists regarding the ability of anti-CMV immunoglobulin to prevent mortality due to CMV disease in solid organ transplant recipients, this has not yet been completely substantiated.[41] Therapy with agents such as acyclovir has not been uniformly successful, although newer agents with better activity against CMV (ganciclovir, foscarnet) are available and are undergoing clinical testing.

Other herpes viruses also cause infection and morbidity, but generally after the immediate post-transplant period. Epstein-Barr virus (EBV) has been shown to cause post-transplantation B-cell lymphoma, as well as an occasional case of fatal mononucleosis.[37,117,192] Varicella-zoster virus (VZV) typically causes the manifestations of shingles causing pain along a certain dermatome with or without skin eruptions, but may also cause severe disseminated infection, particularly in pediatric patients never previously exposed to chickenpox.[141,180,207] Zoster immune globulin may be preventive when administered soon after exposure but is not generally thought to be helpful in the treatment of severe disease. Mild VZV infection typically responds rapidly to acyclovir therapy, but more severe forms of infection that are disseminated with pneumonitis or encephalitis may be lethal. In mild cases, however, a complete response may be achieved without a reduction in immunosuppression.

Viral Hepatitis

Both the surgical patient and the surgeon are exposed to hepatitis B virus frequently through contact with blood products. The infection is diagnosed clinically by the identification of alterations in liver enzymes, the presence of surface antigen in the bloodstream, and the development of an antibody response to surface antigen as well as the core and other viral antigens. Exposure to hepatitis B virus carries the risk of mild to fulminant hepatitis with hepatic coma and death, as well as the potential sequelae of chronic hepatitis with eventual hepatic failure and the risk of hepatic carcinoma.

Chronic hepatitis occurs in 6% to 40% of patients after renal transplantation.[28,51,68,85,133,272] Both non-A, non-B hepatitis and hepatitis B infection are most probably the causative agents, and both may be acquired while on hemodialysis or by way of transfusion of blood products while awaiting transplantation. Progressive liver dysfunction can occur in patients with chronic antigenemia after transplantation, and this is associated with an increased incidence of fatal infections at other sites due to other microbial pathogens.[133,257,322] HSV, CMV, EBV, VZV, and adenovirus have also been implicated in the etiology of progressive liver disease after transplantation, but the evidence that these agents commonly cause chronic progressive hepatitis is lacking. HSV hepatitis is rare but can present as a fulminant form of hepatitis. Azathioprine has been implicated in the etiology of liver dysfunction after transplantation, but in many cases the liver function abnormalities do not resolve when the drug is discontinued.[10]

Limiting the exposure of patients to blood products prior to transplantation is often difficult, but both blood products and potential organ donors should be evaluated for the presence of hepatitis B in order to avoid transmission of this agent. Hepatitis B immune globulin is available (pooled from human sources) for use in conjunction with hepatitis B vaccine and should be administered to nonimmunized patients as soon as possible after exposure. It is not clear at present whether this form of passive immunotherapy invariably prevents the disease, reduces the severity of disease, or merely prolongs the incubation period.[263]

A hepatitis B vaccine has been tested in a number of trials and demonstrated to be efficacious in reducing the incidence of infection due to this agent by 80% to 95% when vaccinees receive all three recommended immunizations.[71,128,314] Persons at high risk for hepatitis B exposure (surgeons, operating room staff, dentists, oral hygienists and oral surgeons, hemodialysis patients and personnel, homosexuals, drug addicts) should receive the vaccine.[268] Concern over the transmission of human T-cell lymphotropic virus (HTLV-III) by the vaccine has not been borne out.[70] Lack of response in certain normal persons as well as immunosuppressed and hemodialysis patients has been noted and may be eventually overcome by additional doses, higher dose vaccination, or vaccination with immunoenhancing agents being concomitantly administered.[307] It is not clear whether patients will require booster injections at various intervals to maintain protective antibody titers.

Other Viruses

Papilloma viruses cause verrucae, which occur much more frequently in immunosuppressed transplant patients, but are rarely responsible for serious disease. Human polyoma viruses are excreted with increased frequency after transplantation and have been implicated in the development of malignancy, multifocal leukoencephalopathy, ureteral stricture, renal allograft dysfunction, and pancreatitis.[100,136] Adenoviruses typically cause respiratory tract infection, conjunctivitis, and hemorrhagic cystitis in the normal population. These viruses can cause similar, but much more severe disease in immunosuppressed patients, such as diffuse interstitial pneumonia, which may be lethal.[119,225]

Probable transmission of human immunodeficiency virus (HIV), the causative agent of acquired immunodeficiency syndrome, by way of an organ from donors with HIV-positive serology has recently been reported. Several recipients developed an acute viral syndrome with splenomegaly and leukopenia. Patients with positive HIV serology have undergone renal transplantation and may have a higher rate of infectious complications after transplantation.[164,235,288]

BACTERIAL INFECTIONS

Bacterial infection continues to be a major problem in clinical transplantation leading to substantial morbidity and mortality. One of the major means by which bacterial infection may be avoided after transplantation is by careful screening of patients prior to the procedure and judicious treatment of existing infectious problems (Table 19-1). Each patient should first have a thorough history obtained and should undergo a complete physical examination. A complete dental examination is mandatory to identify the presence of oropharyngeal infection, such as an abscessed tooth, which must be removed prior to transplantation.[107] Access sites used for hemodialysis or peritoneal dialysis must be examined. Extremity ulcers may not heal prior to transplantation, but it is often possible to place the allograft in the iliac fossa opposite the extremity with ulceration, to avoid either further limb ischemia or the transection of contaminated lymphatics draining that region. Urine cultures are obtained, and any infection is treated prior to transplantation. Occasionally, a patient requires chronic antimicrobial therapy prior to transplantation, but in this setting a thorough investigation of the urogenital system is mandatory. An intravenous pyelogram (IVP) may reveal significant ureteral reflux, calyceal and cortical changes indicative of pyelonephritis, or even a perinephric abscess. In the presence of persistently positive urine cultures and IVP abnormalities, an elective bilateral nephrectomy (and ureterectomy if significant reflux is present) is performed in preparation for transplantation. A routine chest roentgenogram should be obtained to determine whether any form of pulmonary disease is present.

At the time of transplantation, irrigation of the bladder and wound takes place with topical antimicrobial agents, and systemic antimicrobial agents are also administered. A second-generation cephalosporin, such as cefamandole, may be used in renal transplant recipients because this agent is efficacious against both gram-positive and gram-negative organisms. Broader spectrum coverage with several agents in combination or an extended spectrum cephalosporin or penicillin agent may be administered for prophylaxis in either hepatic and pancreatic transplant recipients in which enteric contamination may occur. Subsequently, trimethoprim–sulfamethoxazole may be administered once a day for long-term prophylaxis against urinary tract infection and has the added benefit of preventing pneumocystis, nocardial, and listerial infections (see below). Penicillin or erythromycin may be administered to patients with a history of significant allergic reactions to sulfonamide drugs.

Urinary Tract Infection

Urinary tract infection is the most common form of bacterial infection to which the renal transplant patient is exposed. The reported incidence of bacteriuria after renal transplantation has been between 8% and 83%.[109, 116, 139, 145, 156, 157, 189, 250, 261, 266, 267, 270, 272, 315, 321, 333] The majority of these infections occur in the early post-transplant period, during maximal immunosuppression. During this time, these infections can be associated with systemic sepsis or wound sepsis and, therefore, are extremely important in terms of morbidity and mortality. If infection occurs early after transplantation, aggressive therapy (systemic followed by oral antimicrobial agents) should be instituted. Prevention of urinary tract infections in the immediate period after transplantation can be accomplished by a combined approach in which the bladder is irrigated with topical antimicrobial agents, prophylactic systemic antibiotics are administered prior to cystotomy, meticulous surgical technique is used, and early catheter removal takes place.

Urinary tract infections occurring 6 months or longer after transplantation are less frequently associated with systemic sepsis and mortality and generally may be treated with a 10- to 14-day course of an oral antimicrobial agent.[65, 109] While several studies have demonstrated that these late infections do not adversely affect either graft or recipient survival in renal transplant patients, many centers employ the use of prophylactic oral antimicrobial agents to prevent both early and late urinary tract infections, which can produce lethality. Since 1975, we have administered either sulfasoxazole or trimethoprim–sulfamethoxazole in combination to our patients on a long-term basis with a low incidence of urinary tract infections.[250] Presumably as a direct consequence, few of our patients who adhere to this regimen have contracted infection due to *Pneumocystis carinii, Nocardia* species, *Listeria monocytogenes,* or *Toxoplasmosis gondii.* Tolkoff-Rubin and co-workers reported a controlled trial in which trimethoprim–sulfamethoxazole significantly reduced the incidence of urinary tract infections in the immediate post-transplant period.[321] A simultaneous reduction in systemic bacterial sepsis was also noted.

We therefore recommend long-term prophylaxis with trimethoprim–sulfamethoxazole for all transplant patients. Prophylaxis against urinary tract infections occurring late after transplantation is controversial, but the added benefit of prevention of several types of superinfections would seem to outweigh any detrimental effects. Overgrowth of *Candida* species may occur in these patients, and oral antifun-

Table 19–1
Preoperative Preparation of the Potential Transplant Recipient

POTENTIAL INFECTION SITE	EVALUATION	TREATMENT
Oropharynx, esophagus		
Dental abscess	Dental exam	Dental extraction
Oropharyngeal candida	Oral exam	Oral nystatin
Esophageal candida	Endoscopy	Oral nystatin + systemic amphoteracin-B in some refractory cases
Gastrointestinal Tract		
Duodenal ulceration	Upper GI series or endoscopy	Elective vagotomy and antrectomy
Colonic diverticulosis with symptoms	Barium enema	Elective colonic resection
Perirectal fistulae or abscess	Proctosigmoidoscopy	Internal sphincterotomy, unroofing and drainage
Lungs and Pleural Cavity		
Pulmonary infiltrates	Chest x-ray, bronchoscopy	Antibiotics if infection present
Pulmonary nodule	Initial observation via chest x-ray, consider bronchoscopy	
Enlarging pulmonary nodule, pulmonary cavity	Chest x-ray, chest tomography or CT, bronchoscopy with biopsy or transthoracic biopsy	Resection
Pulmonary effusion	Aspiration	Drainage and antibiotics if infection present

Skin and Soft Tissues		
Access sites	Site cultures	Remove, establish alternate access
Superficial skin abscess	Site cultures	Incision and drainage
Fungal skin lesions	Site cultures	Topical antifungal agents
Extremity ulcers	Site cultures, transcutaneous pO_2, consider arteriography	Antimicrobial agents, debridement, arterial bypass based on arteriogram, placement of allograft on opposite side
Genitourinary		
Kidneys, ureter, and bladder	Urine analysis and culture; IVP, voiding cystourethrogram, cystoscopy	Antibiotics if infection present. Bilateral nephrectomly and ureterectomy if persistent infection and/or significant reflux.
Genitalia	Exam	Antibiotics if infection present
Spleen	ABO determination	No splenectomy unless ABO incompatible donor-recipient pair; pneumococcal vaccination with or without splenectomy
General		
Hepatitis	Liver function studies; hepatitis B surface antigen + antibody; consider liver biopsy if evidence for chronic hepatitis	Hepatitis B vaccine if no serologic evidence of Hepatitis B
CMV	Viral serology	Consider CMV vaccine; utilize CMV − organs for CMV naive recipient if possible

435

gal prophylaxis should simultaneously be administered. Occasionally, patients may develop bone marrow suppression, presumably as a result of combined azathioprine and trimethoprim toxicity, but this problem may be resolved by reducing the dose of azathioprine. In a minority of cases, it is necessary to discontinue trimethoprim–sulfamethoxazole. The development of resistance to trimethoprim–sulfamethoxazole in the enteric flora of transplant patients has been reported, and these resistant organisms can cause significant systemic infection.[343] In general, however, the risk of such infection developing is probably outweighed by the overall prophylactic benefit. This management strategy will obviously require continual reassessment.

Wound Infection

In many early studies, wound infection rates in renal transplant patients were reported to be as high as 20% to 50%. Today, however, most series report a 0 to 3% incidence.[50,140,146,159,174,198,219,234,266,334] Wound infections may be either superficial or may involve the deep perigraft tissues. The incidence of systemic sepsis, mycotic aneurysm formation, graft loss, and patient death is markedly increased when either type of wound infection occurs, but lethal consequences are more common in the presence of a deep wound infection. A number of factors have been shown to predispose to wound infection in renal transplant patients and these include: urine leak, urinary tract infection (especially in the presence of renal allograft dysfunction), perinephric hematoma, reopening of the transplant wound for reasons other than infection, open drainage of the wound, and contamination of the allograft itself. Other predisposing factors include the presence of diabetes mellitus and cadaveric organ transplantation. Superficial infection in the wound itself also predisposes patients undergoing allograft nephrectomy to deep wound infection as well as systemic sepsis, and the procedure should be delayed until the local infection can be eradicated by local treatment.[50]

The diagnosis of wound infection in the transplant patient may often be difficult because these patients frequently develop an infected seropurulent collection rather than a thick, creamy purulent wound fluid. Fever may or may not be present, and there may be no elevation of the white blood cell count. Pain in the wound or flank may be the first sign of either a periallograft hematoma or urine leak with a concomitant wound infection. In this difficult situation, ultrasonography or computerized tomography (CT) with needle aspiration are often diagnostic. In fact, even a superficial wound infection can be diagnosed by ultrasonography.[176] This test combined with aspiration is often less costly than the added morbidity that attends the prolonged healing subsequent to opening a noninfected wound in a patient receiving high doses of corticosteroids.

Some patients will develop a fulminant deep wound infection that ruptures through into the peritoneal cavity causing peritonitis (see below). Unfortunately, the cause of the infection is often obscure when this occurs. Occasionally, a small urinary leak will mimic a wound infection. In those patients in whom negative cultures are obtained from a wound fluid collection, a vigorous attempt should be made to identify urinary tract disruption. This can be accomplished by the administration of methylene blue or indigo carmine intravenously and observing the wound fluid for presence of the dye. A cystogram, percutaneous nephrostogram, or radionuclide excretion study with collection and simultaneous scanning of the perirenal area, bladder, and measurement of radioactivity in the wound fluid output may be helpful in localizing the leak. In some cases, all of these methods are required to diagnose this problem. Unfortunately, those patients who present with such a problem often subsequently develop a deep wound infection.

Reduction of the formerly high wound infection rates that were reported has been accomplished by the concomitant use of prophylactic systemic and topical antimicrobial agents, as well as improvements in technique so that technical errors leading to urinary leakage, hematoma formation, and wound contamination are avoided.[140, 146, 152, 159, 234, 317, 318, 323] Drainage of the renal transplant wound is not indicated and should not be performed. The use of antimicrobial agents in this clean or clean–contaminated setting is warranted because of the high risk of the immunosuppressed host to infection. Antimicrobial agents should be administered so that tissue levels are present at the time of the incision. Repeated doses are often not necessary during the course of the operation due to slow clearance in the anephric patient, and, although we administer two post operative doses, the evidence that this further decreases the wound infection rate is lacking.

When intra-abdominal bleeding occurs after renal transplantation or allograft nephrectomy, it is frequently due to the presence of a deep transplant wound infection. Aggressive deep wound infections may occur early and cause suture line disruption but may also lead to mycotic aneurysm formation with rupture occurring weeks to months after transplantation.[160, 240, 298, 302, 304, 316] Several authors have demonstrated that in this situation arterial ligation is the safest approach to the control of immediate and subsequent bleeding and may be undertaken without extremity ischemia.[160, 240] In the presence of a deep wound infection, the allograft should be removed, and immunosuppression should be discontinued.

In the majority of cases, contamination of the allograft has not been associated with an increased incidence of complications. There are, however, several reports in which cadaver organ contamination was followed by severe wound infection and mycotic aneurysm formation post-transplantation. *Pseudomonas* species, in particular, appear to predispose to this type infection.[229, 332] It is often not possible, however, to obtain bacterial culture results prior to transplantation to avoid transplantation of contaminated donor organs. This is particularly true of cardiac, hepatic, and pancreatic transplantation, where limiting the organ preservation time is crucial. When positive cultures from the donor organ are obtained, a short (3- to 5-day) course of antimicrobial agents to which the organism is sensitive seems prudent.[8, 33, 73, 190, 300]

Hepatic, pancreatic, and cardiac transplant patients with more normal renal clearance mechanisms should receive antimicrobial agents more frequently during the procedure than uremic renal transplant patients. Sternal wound infections in cardiac transplant patients represent difficult management problems, which may require pedicle flaps in order to achieve adequate soft tissue coverage of the sternal defect.[247] Patients undergoing either hepatic or pancreatic transplantation should receive broad-spectrum antimicrobial agents, which are active against both aerobic and anaerobic pathogens, due to the possibility of enteric and biliary contamination during both the organ harvest and the transplant procedure.

Intra-abdominal Infection

When an intra-abdominal process develops in the immunosuppressed patient, the symptoms are often minimal or absent, and the resultant mortality may be extremely high. The usual paradigms the clinician uses when formulating a clinical opinion frequently require alteration for this group of patients. A catastrophic intra-abdominal event in a transplant patient may be caused by a variety of disease processes involving the gastrointestinal tract or the graft itself in the case of renal, hepatic, and pancreas allograft recipients. Management thus requires a high index of suspicion that an intra-abdominal process is present, and a vigorous attempt to establish rapidly the diagnosis and institute appropriate therapy (Fig. 19-3).

Gastrointestinal complications after transplantation occur frequently (6% to 37% incidence) and may involve either the upper or lower gastrointestinal tract, each of which may be involved in several different ways.[90, 168, 171, 201, 208, 306, 347] Gastroduodenal ulceration has been estimated to occur with a 4% to 12% incidence after renal transplantation and may lead to either bleeding or perforation. Although corticosteroid therapy has been most commonly implicated in the etiology of gastrointestinal ulceration after transplantation, hypercalcemia due to tertiary hyperparathyroidism has also been incriminated, occurring in a small number of patients with normal renal function.[280] More recently, it has been suggested that CMV infection may play a role in the development of gastroduodenal ulceration in this population. In fact, patients may develop CMV-induced ulceration of both the upper and lower gastrointestinal tract simultaneously.[58]

A wide range of mortality has been reported (1% to 42%) when gastroduodenal ulceration or perforation occurs in the transplant patient, and many authors believe that a history of symptoms attributable to ulcer disease warrants evaluation prior to transplantation.[2, 11, 45, 54, 72, 91, 101, 170, 191, 210, 239, 249, 278, 281, 286, 299, 310, 335, 345] Not all patients who develop upper gastrointestinal ulceration after transplantation, however, have a prior history of ulcer disease,[114, 170] and pretransplantation screening is thus not entirely predictive of a proclivity toward gastrointestinal bleeding post-transplantation. It does serve, however, to identify those patients at very high risk for bleeding after transplantation.

An elective operation prior to transplantation seems reasonable in those patients in whom a significant ulcer history or in whom active ulceration unresponsive to medical therapy exists and appears to reduce the incidence of post-transplantation bleeding.[91, 170, 239, 278, 299, 310, 324] Spanos and co-workers demonstrated that a resective procedure (vagotomy and antrectomy) in those patients with active ulceration led to a lower incidence of post-transplant bleeding from ulcer disease, compared to vagotomy and pyloroplasty.[299]

Acute fulminant pancreatitis has been observed after renal transplantation and occurs with an incidence of 2% to 3%. The mortality, however, is extremely high (>50%).[46, 92, 236] The etiologic basis of post-transplantation pancreatitis is unclear, but

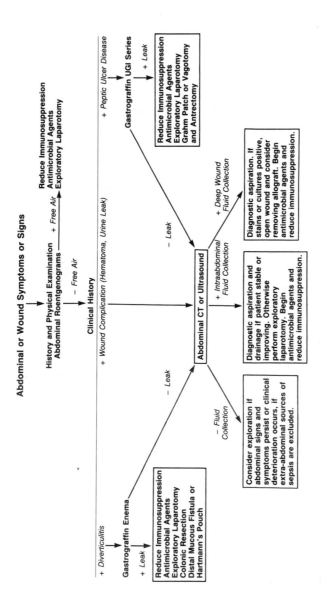

Figure 19–3.
Algorithm for the diagnostic evaluation of abdominal symptoms and signs occurring in a patient after organ transplantation.

steroids, azathioprine, hyperparathyroidism, and viral infections have all been implicated. Etiologic causes such as ethanolism and biliary tract disease have generally not been identified as significant predisposing factors, as they are in the general population. Patients typically die of persistent sepsis and multiple system organ failure. Graft pancreatitis may also occur in those patients undergoing pancreatic transplantation, may produce the systemic manifestations of severe pancreatitis, and can be associated with intra-abdominal sepsis.

A variety of disease processes involving the colon have been described in transplant patients. Perforation of the colon is most commonly caused by diverticular disease in this population, accounting for 30% to 45% of cases.[5,49,56,151,230,279] There is no evidence that perforation occurs more frequently in this group of patients, although diverticular disease is thought to occur with increased frequency in patients undergoing hemodialysis, possibly because of chronic constipation or autonomic nervous system dysfunction. An increased incidence of diverticulosis has also been reported in patients with polycystic kidney disease.[56] Colonic perforation may also occur spontaneously. Spontaneous perforation may have a number of etiologies: ischemic injury, CMV, fecal impaction due to constipation, and immunosuppressive drugs (azathioprine, corticosteroids) have all been implicated.[1,5,56,112,151,311] Constipation may occur for a number of reasons after transplantation (*e.g.*, diabetic enteropathy, bedrest, persistent uremia, and antacid therapy). Immunosuppressive agents may reduce the tensile strength of the bowel wall and may deplete the bowel wall of lymphoid tissue as well, leading to bacterial invasion of the bowel wall with subsequent local infection and ischemia. Ischemic and necrotizing enterocolitis may also occur and lead to perforation.

The mortality of colonic perforation is over 40% in most series (range: 33% to 83%) and is related to the delay in diagnosis and extent of contamination of the peritoneal cavity at the time of exploration in the setting of an immunosuppressed host unable to deal effectively with intra-abdominal sepsis.[5,49,56,112,212,279] Alexander and co-workers have recently demonstrated that patients explored within 48 hr after the onset of symptoms had a more favorable prognosis than those explored after this time.[5] Remine and Melrath have shown that the mean time from onset of symptoms to laparotomy for bowel perforation in patients receiving <20 mg of steroids each day was 2 days, while it was 8 days in those receiving >20 mg.[269] While many patients present with abdominal pain or fever and chills, these symptoms are often vague, poorly localized, and occur without the presence of ileus, especially in those patients receiving larger doses of corticosteroids.

Establishing the diagnosis may be difficult in these patients, and obtaining a water-soluble contrast enema when the flat plate and upright roentgenograms of the abdomen do not demonstrate free air is imperative (see Fig. 19-3). CT scans or an ultrasonographic examination of the abdomen should also be obtained if the diagnosis is in question and intra-abdominal sepsis is suspected. These studies obviously should not be obtained in those patients with acute abdominal pain and evidence of a perforated viscus on routine roentgenographic studies of the abdomen. Surgical management consists of resection of the involved region of bowel and exteriorization of the proximal colonic segment with either exteriorization of the distal segment or creation of a Hartmann's pouch. Resection and primary anastomosis of the colon should not be performed.[5,49,56,112,212] Also, all feculent and infected material should be removed, and the abdomen should be copiously irrigated at the time of laparotomy, because the prognosis is much worse if free peritonitis without containment is found at the time of exploration.[5,56,134] Aerobic and anaerobic antimicrobial coverage should be begun prior to laparotomy and altered on the basis of clinical course in conjunction with culture and sensitivity reports. The growth of *Candida* or other fungal pathogens from the infected material mandates treatment with amphotericin B. Immunosuppression should be discontinued, except for maintenance levels of corticosteroids. Immunosuppressive therapy can be gradually reinstituted when it is clear that the patient will recover and no residual infection is present. The risk of rejection appears low in most patients with severe infection present. In renal transplant patients who develop intra-abdominal sepsis it is not necessary to remove the allograft, as opposed to patients with deep wound infections, which involve the allograft itself in most cases. In fact, the trauma of additional surgery or a second procedure may be detrimental in this setting.

Most authors feel that, although routine screening of all patients for diverticular colonic disease prior to transplantation is not productive, those patients with a history of symptoms compatible with diverticulitis should undergo barium enema examination and elective pretransplant colonic resection and primary anastomosis should significant diverticular disease be discovered, in order to avoid the occurrence of colonic perforation while on immunosuppressive therapy.[5,49,56,212,279]

Massive colonic bleeding can occur after transplantation but is only rarely due to diverticular disease.[48] Involvement of the large bowel with CMV or occasionally aspergillosis may lead to ulceration and massive hemorrhage.[96,148,246,311,344] Sutherland and co-workers reported 12 patients with bleeding ulcers, the majority of which were in the cecum.[311] CMV inclusion bodies were found in tissue from seven of the ulcers, and 10 of the 12 patients died. Colonoscopy and arteriography should be used to define the site of bleeding, and vasopressin therapy should be instituted. Operative resection should be undertaken only if the bleeding cannot be otherwise controlled. The mortality of this disease process is extremely high, due to the massive blood loss that can occur, as well as the severity of the often present multisystem CMV disease.

As described above, when intra-abdominal sepsis occurs in the transplant patient, it represents a lethal process with a high mortality. Hau and co-workers[121] and Pollak and co-workers[260] reported mortality rates of 66.6% and 78.5%, respectively. Gastrointestinal perforation or transplant wound sepsis accounted for the majority of cases in these series. Immunosuppression may reduce the ability of the normal peritoneal host defense systems (translymphatic clearance, phagocytosis and killing, sequestration) to reduce the bacterial inoculum. In many cases, this leads to diffuse, poorly contained infection. Abdominal pain may be minimal and poorly localized, and temperature or white blood cell count elevations may not occur. In some unfortunate patients, the diagnosis of peritonitis is made only at autopsy. Because of this fact, a concerted effort must be made to establish the diagnosis of intra-abdominal sepsis, as well as the underlying etiology, and decide on the best operative approach. Wounds must be left open when infection is found during the course of laparotomy, despite the poor ability of patients treated with steroids to heal wounds by secondary intention.

In pancreas transplant patients, the mortality is 27% when intra-abdominal infection occurs. In most cases, therapy entails removal of the transplanted pancreas and drainage of any infected collections, as well as copious irrigation and systemic antimicrobial agents. Hesse and co-workers have demonstrated that in this particular group of patients gram-positive, gram-negative, and fungal pathogens all occur frequently.[130]

Bacterial Pneumonia

Bacterial pneumonia occurs within the first several months after transplantation and represents an important cause of lethality after transplantation.[35, 122, 123, 199, 293] Moore and co-workers, however, have reported an extremely low mortality (2%) in renal transplant patients.[215] After the immediate period following transplantation, fungal, viral, or protozoan agents are causative, although pneumococcal pneumonia can also occur in the late post-transplant period. Fever, malaise, and cough are common presenting symptoms of any type of pulmonary infections, although these may be absent in the immunosuppressed patient. As with other infections, bacterial pneumonia occurs more frequently in recipients of cadaver allografts and often occurs in relation to a treated rejection episode. Sputum cultures are rarely diagnostic, and an aggressive approach to obtain the diagnosis should be undertaken (Fig. 19-4). Bronchoscopy with use of a covered brush to avoid contamination from the upper respiratory tract is to be recommended. Empiric antimicrobial therapy based on the initial microbiologic results (Gram's, potassium hydroxide, Giemsa, methenamine silver, Ziehl-Neelsen stains) should then be instituted. Gram-positive organisms such as staphylococci and streptococci as well as gram-negative nosocomial pathogens are responsible for these infections.

Legionella pneumophila and *micdadei* infections occur with increased frequency after transplantation, and patients may present with high fever, nonproductive cough, dyspnea, and diffuse pneumonia or occasionally a lung abscess. In many cases, a source within the hospital environment has been identified, although infection can also occur sporadically.[22, 75, 89, 104, 106, 196, 202, 276, 320, 325] Patients should undergo bronchoscopy, although the diagnosis may be difficult because the Gram's stain is often negative. Cultures and direct immunofluorescence, however, will substantiate the diagnosis. An increase in systemic antibody titers can also be diagnostic. Patients in whom the diagnosis is even suspected should receive parenteral erythromycin, perhaps in combination with rifampin. Relapse can occur even after prolonged antimicrobial therapy.[276] In a hospital environment in which this agent is prevalent, erythromycin prophylaxis has been shown to be effective in reducing the infection rate due to this organism.[325]

Recipients of both heart and heart–lung allograft develop pulmonary infection with high frequency, bacterial pathogens being the most common organisms isolated.[40, 61, 110, 241] Dummer and co-workers reported a 28% incidence of bacterial pneumonia in cardiac transplant patients.[77] While initial series reported a high incidence (32%) of all infectious complications, with fungal infections predominating after cardiac transplantation, series in which patients have received lessened immunosuppressive therapy have noted a lower incidence of infection.[24, 61, 110, 214, 241] Some authors

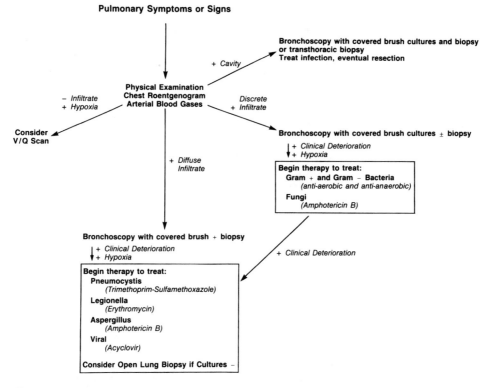

Figure 19–4.
Algorithm for the diagnostic evaluation of pulmonary symptoms and signs occurring in a patient after organ transplantation.

have postulated that fungal infections may be less frequent when cyclosporine is used.[76–78]

It has been postulated that the donor lung may be a reservoir for a wide variety of microbial species, and that cardiopulmonary dysfunction after transplantation may also predispose to these infections. A high frequency of positive cultures from the donor trachea has been demonstrated. The diagnosis of infection in these patients requires an aggressive approach, but colonization of the lower respiratory tract often makes the decision to treat difficult. Transtracheal aspiration, early bronchoscopy, and early empiric broad-spectrum antimicrobial agents are appropriate in many cases.[40]

Bacterial Sepsis

The majority of episodes of bacterial sepsis occur in the early period after transplantation, a wide range of incidence (10% to 41%) being reported. The majority are caused by infection at a specific site, although in some cases that occur during profound leukopenia translocation of bacteria across the bowel may occur. In renal transplant patients the most common site of infection is either the urinary tract or a wound. Bacterial infection of the lung also represents an important source of sepsis. Recipients of cadaver organs, patients undergoing therapy for rejection, and leukopenia have all been identified as important etiologic factors in the pathogenesis of sepsis.[9,186,188,198,232,266,272,336]

Gram-negative bacteria have become increasingly frequent nosocomial pathogens over the last several decades and are presently responsible for the majority of bacteremic episodes in transplant patients. The attendant sequelae of infections due to these organisms—septic shock, multiple system organ failure, and death—represent a significant cause of post-transplantation mortality. The manipulation or perturbation of various aspects of host defenses that transplant patients undergo predispose to these infections. Although many different organisms cause this form of sepsis, *Escherichia coli* predominates in overall frequency. Also common are isolates of *Klebsiella, Enterobacter,* and *Serratia,* while *Pseudomonas* bacteremia is somewhat less common. Sepsis due to *Proteus, Providencia, Acinetobacter, Aeromonas, Citrobacter, Achromobacter, Salmonella, Shigella, Bacteroides,* and numerous other organisms also has been reported. When gram-negative bacterial sepsis and shock occur in patients with no underlying disease, the mortality is significant (10% to 20%), and in immunosuppressed patients mortality is extremely high (>30%).[4,9,27,42,43,84,135,154,155,166,183,186,188,223,224,231,232,248,270,295,298,326,336,349] The use of routine treatment modalities such as antimicrobial agents, hemodynamic monitoring, aggressive fluid resuscitation, and metabolic support in the intensive care unit setting has reduced, but not eliminated the severe consequences of this disease process. In the transplant patient with suspected sepsis, empiric antimicrobial therapy should be administered, and a source should be sought. Extended spectrum penicillin or cephalosporin agents in combination with an aminoglycoside should be administered. If intra-abdominal sepsis is suspected, agents with activity directed against anaerobes should also be administered.

Experimental evidence has shown that antibody directed against endotoxin may ameliorate the lethal effects of sepsis, and such antibody preparations may eventually prove of benefit in septic transplant patients in whom this disease is extremely lethal.[79–82] Several investigators have demonstrated a reduction in mortality when anti-gram-negative bacterial human antiserum was administered to septic patients, but this has not been a universal finding.[23,162,185,351] Several clinical trials are currently in progress to determine the efficacy of either polyclonal or monoclonal antibody preparations directed against endotoxin in reducing the lethal effects of gram-negative bacterial infection and sepsis.

Fulminant sepsis also occurs with increased frequency (2% to 4% incidence) after splenectomy and during splenic dysfunction (*e.g.,* sickle cell disease, lymphoma) and is typically caused by encapsulated organisms such as *Streptococcus pneumoniae, Neisseria meningitidis,* and *Hemophilus influenza.*[237,285,350] A defect in various opsonins (IgG, properdin, tuftsin) seen after splenectomy has been postulated to contribute to the occurrence of such overwhelming infections.[55] Passive transfer of antipneumococcal antibody was once used in pneumococcal infection due to the lack of suitable antimicrobial agents and an inability to isolate specific bacterial antigens as immunogens.

More recently, a polyvalent pneumococcal vaccine has undergone extensive clinical testing. The currently available vaccine contains 23 serotypes, which represent the most common strains encountered. The vaccine is administered once, either subcutaneously or intramuscularly. Not all patients respond to each pneumococcal serotype in the polyvalent vaccine, and overwhelming sepsis has been reported even after vaccination.[39] Thus, while pneumococcal vaccination has been demonstrated to produce effective antibody titers in normal and asplenic patients, the response is often poor in patients with underlying malignancy and in those patients receiving chemotherapy and irradiation.[7,132] Also, the exact timeframe in which booster injections of vaccine will be required is not established. Current evidence, however, indicates a distinct trend in reducing septic complications by vaccination.[32,163,284,287] Because of the low morbidity of vaccination, it is therefore appropriate that all splenectomized patients should receive the polyvalent pneumococcal vaccine and antimicrobial prophylaxis. Controlled trials have not been performed with either penicillin or trimethoprim–sulfamethoxazole prophylaxis, however, and antibiotic resistant isolates of the pneumococcus have become more frequent recently.[195] Lifelong antimicrobial prophylaxis does require patient compliance, and some clinicians recommend that the asplenic individual self-administer antibiotics only if chills, fever, or other symptoms of infection appear.

Splenectomy was initially performed prior to or at the time of renal transplantation after it was demonstrated that patients would tolerate larger doses of azathioprine without severe leukopenia. Several reports have demonstrated that splenectomy does not enhance overall patient or graft survival and, in fact, predisposes to a higher incidence of infectious complications. Several reports have demonstrated that splenectomized transplant recipients are at increased risk for severe infection due to encapsulated organisms such *Streptococcus pneumoniae* and *Hemophilus influenza,* and patients who undergo this procedure should receive pneumococcal vaccination prior to splenectomy and prophylactic antibiotics subsequently.[3,31,34,127,147,172,252,265,283,312] We use trimethoprim–sulfamethoxazole for this purpose, as well as for urosepsis prophylaxis. We currently vaccinate all patients prior to transplantation, even if they will not be undergoing splenectomy. Vaccination is without significant risk in this immunosuppressed population. For these reasons, most centers have abandoned routine pretransplant splenectomy, reserving it for those patients in whom ABO mismatched organs are being transplanted.

Infections Due to Listeria

Listeria monocytogenes can cause meningitis or cerebritis, as well as bacteremia and pneumonia in transplant patients.[15,93,99,137,143,233,303] This organism is an intracellular parasite, cell-mediated immunity being required for killing. Stamm and co-workers[303] reported an overall mortality of 26% following *Listeria* infection, with disease outside of the central nervous system (CNS) having a better prognosis than meningeal infection. Any patient who presents with even vague neurologic symptoms (*e.g.,* headache) should undergo a complete evaluation, including a lumbar puncture (Fig. 19-5). Even a presumptive diagnosis of listerial meningitis demands empiric antimicrobial therapy due to the high mortality. Antimicrobial therapy consists of the

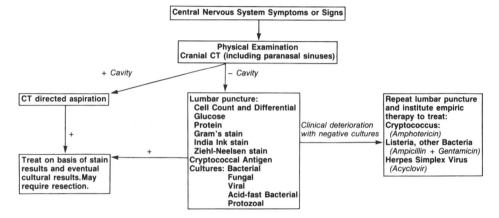

Figure 19–5.
Algorithm for the diagnostic evaluation of central nervous system symptoms and signs occurring in a patient after organ transplantation.

combined administration of a penicillin, such as ampicillin, with an aminoglycoside. We see this disease infrequently, probably because the majority of our patients receive trimethoprim–sulfamethoxazole, penicillin, or erythromycin prophylaxis.

Nocardial and Mycobacterial Infections

Nocardia asteroides is a true bacterium that causes disease primarily in the immunocompromised host. The typical presentation is that of some form of pulmonary infection, but joint and skin disease, ocular disease, and disseminated infection with sepsis and formation of brain abscesses are also frequent.[17,21,38,150,178,211,228,242,294] A spectrum of pulmonary disease from lung nodules to diffuse pneumonia has been described. A correlation between initial nocardial infection and subsequent mycobacterial disease has also been noted.[294] The diagnosis of pulmonary disease is made by way of bronchoscopy. Treatment consists of high-dose sulfisoxazole or trimethoprim––sulfamethoxazole. Even with therapy, the mortality is over 50% in most published series. We very rarely see this disease, and then only in patients who have not been receiving trimethoprim–sulfamethoxazole due to drug allergy or noncompliance.

Mycobacterial infections occurring in transplant patients assume a wide variety of forms. Isolated pulmonary disease, locally invasive pleuropulmonary disease, granulomatous hepatitis, gastrointestinal disease, bone and monoarticular joint disease, brain abscesses, and miliary disease have all been described,[10,16,36,62,64,95,105,124,169,177,238,301] and transmission of disease by way of the donor organ has also been reported.[169,218,251] The mortality in our patients with mycobacterial infection was 25%.[177] The diagnosis should be established based on cultural and stain results, and therapy should be instituted on the basis of initial microbiologic specimen stain results. Multidrug therapy (*e.g.*, isoniazid, ethambutol, rifampin, streptomycin, cycloserine) is often required, because drug-resistant, atypical mycobacteria in extrapulmonary sites are more often responsible for infection in this group of patients than in the normal population.[36,64,105,124,169,177,301] Isoniazid prophylaxis of high-risk ethnic groups, such as Native Americans and Orientals, or patients with a previous history of significant exposure, a positive tuberculin skin test, and inadequate subsequent treatment or prophylaxis is somewhat controversial, but is what we recommend in many cases. We observe patients receiving isoniazid carefully for any evidence of liver dysfunction. Reactivation disease can probably be avoided in most cases by adequate treatment if the diagnosis can be established prior to transplantation.

FUNGAL INFECTION

Fungal infection occurs with increased frequency in transplanted patients, presumably due to an unrestricted depression of cell-mediated immunity. Fungal infections are often difficult to diagnosis, both because the organisms are slow growing, leading to difficulties in obtaining cultural evidence of infection, and because they often occur in concert with other viral and bacterial pathogens. There are, however, well-known clinical presentations of these infections in the transplant patient on which the clinician may rely. In many cases, empiric therapy is justified based on solely a clinical diagnosis, because the morbidity of these infections is often over 50%. Commonly encountered infections are caused by opportunistic fungi belonging to the genera *Candida, Aspergillus, Cryptococcus, Torulopsis, Histoplasma, Coccidioides, Mucor, Rhizopus,* and *Tinea.* Occasionally, other soil fungi may also cause infections in transplant patients.[6,120,153,216,328,348] In the immediate post-transplant period, fungi occur in concert with other microbes in heavily immunosuppressed patients. Later, these organisms more often cause lethality as sole agents in a particular host.

Aspergillosis

Both *Aspergillus* species and *Legionella* species have been associated with epidemics that can often be traced to a common source. Aspergillosis often occurs subsequent to periods of construction, because the spores are commonly encountered in the soil and may be carried in the air.[14,161,167] *Aspergillus niger, fumigatus,* and *flavus* can all cause infection in immunosuppressed patients. Infection can involve the lung, upper respiratory tract, oropharyngeal region, ear, sinuses, skin and soft tissue, and CNS.[113,161,167,211,222,328,341] Preexisting pulmonary cavities with subsequent invasion by fungi and formation of an aspergilloma or fungus ball has been the classic description of this disease but is now seen less commonly due to more extensive pretransplant evaluation of these patients (see Table 19-1).

Patients more commonly develop a diffuse pneumonia with patchy infiltrates on chest roentgenograms, although consolidation (with or without cavitation) of a particular pulmonary lobe or segment may resemble the roentgenographic appearance of a bacterial pneumonia (Fig. 19-6).[341] Fever, malaise, nonproductive cough, pleuritic pain, dyspnea, and hemoptysis can all be presenting symptoms. Endocarditis, blood

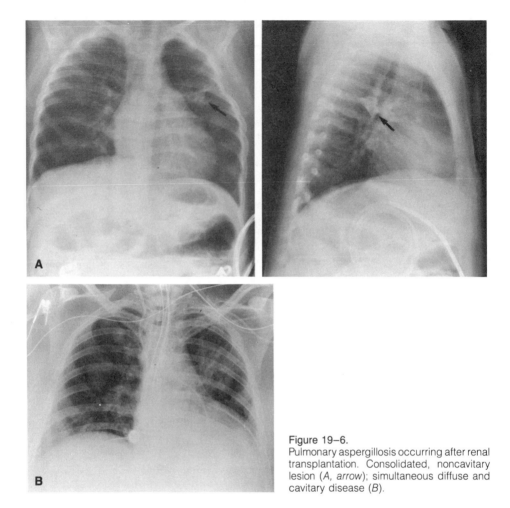

Figure 19–6.
Pulmonary aspergillosis occurring after renal transplantation. Consolidated, noncavitary lesion (*A, arrow*); simultaneous diffuse and cavitary disease (*B*).

vessel invasion with pulmonary infarction and embolization with widespread dissemination of fungal elements, and disseminated intravascular coagulation can all occur.[69, 165, 181, 184, 222, 329, 331] CNS involvement can also occur as an extremely insidious process with the development of a fungal brain abscess (see Fig. 19-5).[25, 26, 111] Few patients survive once this latter diagnosis is made.[222, 330, 341] The diagnosis of pulmonary aspergillosis should be established based on clinical presentation, as well as bronchoscopic stains and cultures. These organisms are frequent contaminants from the oropharynx and also are within the environment of many microbiology laboratories, leading to difficulty in establishing the diagnosis in some cases. Therapy with systemic amphotericin B should be instituted based on even a presumptive diagnosis. Patients with severe infections should also receive 5-fluorocytosine and rifampin. Unless clinical deterioration occurs, patients with cavitary disease should undergo an initial antifungal treatment period, following which resection of the involved pulmonary segment should occur. Cerebral abscesses should be diagnosed with CT and aspiration if possible and treated in similar fashion with long-term amphotericin B and eventual resection if feasible. We have, however, successfully treated a patient with a large lesion in the dominant cerebral hemisphere with drainage and intracavitary and systemic amphotericin alone (Fig. 19-7). Our experience indicates that deep fungal infections such as these require long-term systemic amphotericin B therapy with a total dose between 2 and 3 g.

Candida

Candida species (*albicans, tropicalis, parapsilosis,* and so forth) and *Torulopsis glabrata* are encountered frequently in immunosuppressed patients, but occur typically as saprophytes of the integument and mucous membranes. In heavily immunosuppressed patients, especially those with indwelling catheters, aggressive local and systemic infection can develop.[57, 138, 144, 236, 328] Prophylaxis with oral antifungal agents is warranted, especially during periods of maximal immunosuppression, uncontrolled diabetes, or during antibacterial antimicrobial therapy. High-dose oral nystatin (10^6 units every 4 to 6 hr), amphotericin B, ketoconazole, and miconazole all are efficacious. We rarely use ketoconazole in patients receiving cyclosporine, however, due to the sometimes dramatic increase in cyclosporine levels that can occur.

Invasive *Candida* infection may be difficult to diagnose but requires immediate treatment with systemic amphotericin B and 5-fluorocytosine. The diagnosis may be established through cultural evidence that indicates bloodstream invasion with or without a primary source, cultures from a normally sterile region of the body, evidence of chorioretinitis on ophthalmologic exam, positive cultures from several sites simultaneously including areas where this organism is not normally found, or any combina-

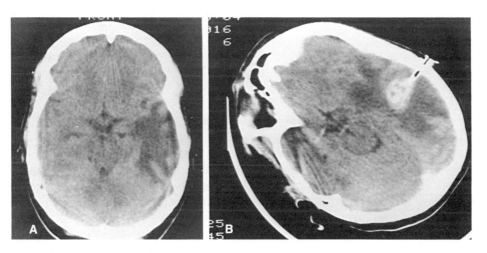

Figure 19–7.
Cerebral aspergillosis with formation of a brain abscess diagnosed by computerized tomography (*A*) with subsequent aspiration (*B*).

tion of the above. Treatment of *Candida* urinary tract infections with amphotericin B topically (by way of continuous bladder irrigation) is acceptable as first line therapy, but persistent fever or lack of response requires reevaluation and consideration of systemic antifungal therapy.

Cryptococcosis

Cryptococcus neoformans is an encapsulated fungus that causes pulmonary and CNS infection often in concert, as well as widespread cutaneous infection in immunosuppressed hosts.[125,138,142,319,338,339] Pulmonary disease may be very insidious and may produce mild fever, malaise, nonproductive cough, or no symptoms whatsoever. CNS disease may present as malaise, fever, or headache, either alone or in combination. While more specific neurologic signs may occur, focal deficits are rare. Any patient with pulmonary cryptococcosis should undergo lumbar puncture (see Fig. 19-5). High protein content, low glucose, and a mild lymphocytic leukocytosis are typical findings. India ink preparations may demonstrate the organism in the cerebral spinal fluid (CSF), but tests for CSF cryptococcal antigen and peripheral antibody may also be helpful in establishing the diagnosis.

Therapy consists of combined amphotericin B and 5-fluorocytosine. The total dose of amphotericin B that should be administered is not established, but a total dose of 1 to 1.5 g is recommended by many authors. Lack of clinical response should instigate reevaluation and a repeat lumbar puncture. The latter test should be performed again at the termination of therapy.

Other Fungal Infections

Histoplasma capsulatum can cause both pulmonary and disseminated disease in the immunosuppressed host.[67,138] The disease is most common, however, in endemic areas, such as the Mississippi River Valley. It can produce skin lesions, which resemble erythema nodosum, and recognition of these lesions may be a key to the diagnosis. *Coccidioides immitis* may produce disease in healthy or immunosuppressed persons who inhale the highly infective arthrospores in an endemic region.[59,282] The transplant patient may develop mild pulmonary disease, but disseminated cases have also been reported. Treatment of either disease consists of the long-term administration of systemic amphotericin B.

Phycomycoses due to *Mucor* and *Rhizopus* species can produce locally destructive rhinocerebral infections, which are very difficult to eradicate (Fig. 19-8).[94,108,115,255,346] CNS involvement is common and often fatal.[255] Treatment consists of reducing immunotherapy, local surgical excision, and long-term systemic amphotericin B. Unfortunately, relapse is common due to the locally aggressive nature of these infections. Other soil fungi can also cause lethal pulmonary and CNS infections in transplant patients. Some organisms, however, such as *Tinea* species and other dermatophytes cause widespread skin lesions but rarely cause disseminated disease or death. In some cases, however, it is necessary to resort to systemic antifungal therapy in order to treat even such superficial infections.

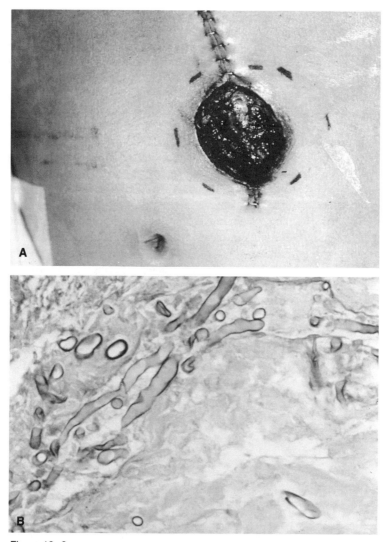

Figure 19–8.
Mucor wound infection in a liver transplant patient (*A*) in which nonseptate hyphae were seen microscopically within the tissue (*B*, 120×, hematoxalin and eosin). The wound was widely excised and the patient received systemic amphotericin B. (Courtesy of Drs. P. Andreone and N. Asher)

PROTOZOAN AND PARASITIC INFECTIONS

Pneumocystis carinii is a protozoan organism that causes pulmonary infection in immunosuppressed patients. Cough, tachypnea, and mild fever are common presenting symptoms and signs, and severe hypoxia is often present. Bilateral diffuse alveolar and interstitial pneumonia is seen on the chest roentgenogram. The diagnosis must be rapidly established by way of bronchoscopy and, in some cases, open lung biopsy due to the high attendant mortality (see Fig. 19-4). Treatment consists of parenteral trimethoprim–sulfamethoxazole, even if the diagnosis is presumptive. We very rarely see this disease, and then only in patients who have not been receiving trimethoprim–sulfamethoxazole due to drug allergy or noncompliance.[20,118,158]

Toxoplasma gondii can cause a mononucleosis syndrome in healthy patients, while in the immunosuppressed patient severe neurologic symptoms are most frequent. In transplant patients, the disease is frequently lethal, causing necrotizing encephalitis, myocarditis, or pneumonitis, but it is extremely difficult to diagnose. Transmission from the donor organ can occur, and *Toxoplasma* naive patients are more prone to develop infection if they receive an organ from a donor with evidence of previous infection due to this agent. Presumably for this reason, this disease is more common in cardiac allograft recipients, because heart tissue may contain more cysts than other organs. Histologic evidence from endocardial biopsy in cardiac allograft recipients or from lymph nodes in other groups of patients mandates therapy with pyrimethamine and sulfadiazine.[129,182,187,204,244,273,274]

Parasitic infections are more common in allograft recipients in tropical environments, although bacterial and fungal pathogens still predominate.[66] *Strongyloides stercoralis* infection is perhaps the most common and can produce skin, pulmonary, and visceral manifestations, the latter two of which can be lethal.[205,327] Schistosomiasis, malaria, cryptosporidiosis, amebiasis, and other parasitic infections have also been reported in renal transplant patients.[63,197,340,342] We have diagnosed and treated *Enterobius vermicularis* and *Taenia saginata* infections in several patients.

REFERENCES

1. Aguilo JJ, Zincke H, Woods JE, et al. Intestinal perforation due to fecal impaction after renal transplantation. J Urol 1976;116:153.
2. Ahonen J, Eklund B, Lindfors O, et al. Peptic ulceration in kidney transplantation. Proc Eur Dial Transplant Assoc Eur Ren Assoc 1977;14:396.
3. Alexander JW, First MR, Majeski JA, et al. The late adverse effect of splenectomy on patient survival following cadaveric renal transplantation. Transplantation 1984;37:467.
4. Alexander JW, Stinnett JD, Ogle CK, et al. A comparison of immunologic profiles and their influence on bacteremia in surgical patients with a high risk of infection. Surgery 1979;86:94.
5. Alexander P, Schuman E, Vetto RM. Perforation of the colon in the immunocompromised patient. Am J Surg 1986;151:557.
6. Alsip SG, Cobbs CG. *Pseudallescheria boydii* infection of the central nervous system in a cardiac transplant recipient. South Med J 1986;79:383.
7. Ammann AJ, Schiffman G, Addiego JE, et al. Immunization of immunosuppressed patients with pneumococcal polysaccharide vaccine. Rev Infect Dis 1981;3:S160.
8. Anderson CB, Haid SD, Hruska KA, et al. Significance of microbial contamination of stored cadaver kidneys. Arch Surg 1978;113:269.
9. Anderson RJ, Schafer LA, Olin DB, et al. Septicemia in renal transplant recipients. Arch Surg 1973;106:692.
10. Anuras S, Piros J, Bonney WW, et al. Liver disease in renal transplant recipients. Arch Intern Med 1977;137:42.
11. Archibald SD, Jirsch DW, Bear RA. Gastrointestinal complications of renal transplantation. 1. The upper gastrointestinal tract. Can Med Assoc J 1978;119:1291.

12. Armstrong JA, Evans AS, Rao N, et al. Viral infections in renal transplant recipients. Infect Immunol 1976;14:970.
13. Arora KK, Karalakulasingam R, Raff MJ, et al. Cutaneous herpes-virus hominis (type 2) infection after renal transplantation. JAMA 1974;230:1174.
14. Arrow PM, Andersen RL, Mainous PD, et al. Pulmonary aspergillosis during hospital renovation. Am Rev Respir Dis 1978;118:49.
15. Ascher NL, Simmons RL, Marker S, et al. *Listeria* infection in transplant patients. Arch Surg 1978;113:90.
16. Ascher NL, Simmons RL, Marker S, et al. Tuberculous joint disease in transplant patients. Am J Surg 1978;135:853.
17. Avram MM, Nair SR, Lipner HI, et al. Persistent nocardemia following renal transplantation. JAMA 1978;239:2779.
18. Balfour HH Jr, Sachs GW, Welo P, et al. Cytomegalovirus vaccine in renal transplant candidates: progress report of a randomized, placebo-controlled, double-blind trial. Birth Defects 1984;20:289.
19. Balfour HH Jr, Slade MS, Kallis JM, et al. Viral infections in renal transplant donors and their recipients: a prospective study. Surgery 1977;81:487.
20. Ballardie FW, Winearls CG, Cohen J, et al. *Pneumocystis carinii* pneumonia in renal transplant recipients—clinical and radiographic features, diagnosis and complication of treatment. Q J Med 1985;233:729.
21. Barmeir E, Mann JH, Marcus RH. Cerebral nocardiosis in renal transplant patients. Br J Radiol 1981;54:1107.
22. Bauling PC, Weil III R, Schroter PJ. *Legionella* lung abcess after renal transplantation. J Infect 1985;11:51.
23. Baumgartner JD, McCutchan JA, Van Melle G, et al. Prevention of gram-negative shock and death in surgical patients by antibody to endotoxin core glycolipid. Lancet 1985;i:59.
24. Baumgartner WA, Reitz BA, Oyer PE. Cardiac homotransplantation. Curr Probl Surg 1979;16:1.
25. Beal MF, O'Carroll P, Kleinman GM, et al. Aspergillosis of the nervous system. Neurology 1982;32:473.
26. Bennett JE, Centeno RS, Bentson JR, et al. CT scanning in rhinocerebral mucormycosis and aspergillosis. Neuroradiology 1981;140:383.
27. Berk MR, Meyers AM, Cassal W, et al. Non-typhoid *Salmonella* infections after renal transplantation. A serious clinical problem. Nephron 1984;37:186.
28. Berne TV, Fitzgibbons TJ, Silberman H. The effect of hepatitis B antigenemia on long-term success and hepatic disease in renal transplant recipients. Transplantation 1977;24:412.
29. Betts RF. Cytomegalovirus infection in transplant patients. Prog Med Virol 1982;28:44.
30. Bia MJ, Andiman W, Gaudio K, et al. Effect of treatment with cyclosporine versus azathioprine on incidence and severity of cytomegalovirus infection posttransplantation. Transplantation 1985;40:610.
31. Boice JL. Pneumococcal infection in bone marrow transplant recipients. Ann Intern Med 1979;92:571.
32. Bolan G, Broome CV, Facklam RR, et al. Pneumococcal vaccine efficacy in selected populations in the United States. Ann Intern Med 1986;104:1.
33. Bore PJ, Basu PK, Rudge CJ, et al. Contaminated renal allografts. Arch Surg 1980;115:755.
34. Bourgault AM, Van Scoy RE, Wilkowske CJ, et al. Severe infection due to *Streptococcus pneumoniae* in asplenic renal transplant patients. Mayo Clin Proc 1979;154:123.
35. Bowie DM, Marrie TJ, Janigan DT, et al. Pneumonia in renal transplant patients. Can Med Assoc J 1983;128:1411.
36. Branger B, Gouby A, Oules R, et al. *Mycobacterium haemophilum* and *Mycobacterium xenopi* associated infection in a renal transplant patient. Clin Nephrol 1985;23:46.
37. Briggs JD, Hamilton DNH, MacSween RNM, et al. Infectious mononucleosis, herpes simplex infection, and diffuse lymphoma in a renal transplant recipient. Transplantation 1978;25:227.
38. Britt RH, Enzmann DR, Remington JS. Intracranial infection in cardiac transplant recipients. Ann Neurol 1981;9:107.
39. Brivet F, Herer B, Fremaux A, et al. Fatal post-splenectomy pneumococcal sepsis despite pneumococcal vaccine and penicillin prophylaxis. Lancet 1984;2:356.
40. Brooks RG, Hofflin JM, Jamieson SW, et al. Infectious complications in heart–lung transplant recipients. Am J Med 1985;79:412.
41. Brown CB, Nicholls AJ, Edward N, et al. Hyperimmune immunoglobulin therapy for cytomegalovirus infections in renal transplant patients. Proc Eur Dial Transplant Assoc Eur Ren Assoc 1983;20:271.
42. Bryan CS, Reynolds KL, Brenner ER. Analysis of 1,186 episodes of gram-negative bacteremia in non-university hospitals. The effects of antimicrobial therapy. Rev Infect Dis 1983;5:629.

43. Bryant RE, Hood AF, Hood CE, et al. Factors affecting mortality of gram-negative rod bacteremia. Arch Intern Med 1971;127:120.
44. Burgos-Calderon R, Pankey GA, Figeroa JE. Infection in kidney transplantation. Surgery 1971;70:334.
45. Burleson RL, Kronhaus RJ, Marbarger PD, et al. Cimetidine, posttransplant peptic ulcer complications, and renal allograft survival. Arch Surg 1982;117:933.
46. Burnstein M, Salter D, Cardella C, et al. Necrotizing pancreatitis in renal transplant patients. Can J Surg 1982;25:547.
47. Canafax DM, Simmons RL, Sutherland DER, et al. Early and late effects of two immunosuppressive drug protocols on recipients of renal allografts: results of the Minnesota randomized trial comparing cyclosporine versus antilymphocyte globulin-azathioprine. Transplant Proc 1986;18:192.
48. Carlton PK, Whelchel JD. Massive colonic diverticular hemorrhage in a transplant patient. Am Surg 1978;44:159.
49. Carson SD, Krom RAF, Uchida K, et al. Colon perforation after kidney transplantation. Ann Surg 1978;188:109.
50. Chapman TP, Helling TS. Identification of factors responsible for wound infection following allograft nephrectomy. Am Surg 1985;51:446.
51. Chatterjee SN, Payne JE, Bischel MD, et al. Successful renal transplantation in patients positive for hepatitis B antigen. N Engl J Med 1974;291:62.
52. Cheeseman SH, Rubin RH, Stewart JA, et al. Controlled clinical trial of prophylactic human-leukocyte interferon in renal transplantation; effects on cytomegalovirus and herpes simplex infections. N Engl J Med 1979;30:1345.
53. Cheeseman SH, Stewart JA, Winkle S, et al. Cytomegalovirus excretion 2–14 years after renal transplantation. Transplant Proc 1979;11:71.
54. Chisholm GD, Mee AD, Williams G, et al. Peptic ulceration, gastric secretion, and renal transplantation. Br Med J 1977;1:1630.
55. Chu DZJ, Nishioka K, El-Hagin T, et al. Effects of tuftsin on postsplectomy sepsis. Surgery 1985;97:701.
56. Church JM, Braun WE, Novick AC, et al. Perforation of the colon in renal homograft recipients. Ann Surg 1986;203:69.
57. Clift RA. Candidiasis in the transplant patient. Am J Med 1984;77:34.
58. Cohen EB, Komorowski RA, Kauffman HM, et al. Unexpectedly high incidence of cytomegalovirus infection in apparent peptic ulcers in renal transplant recipients. Surgery 1985;97:606.
59. Cohen IM, Galgiani JN, Potter D, et al. Coccidioidomycosis in renal replacement therapy. Arch Intern Med 1982;142:489.
60. Condie RM, OReilly RJ. Prevention of cytomegalovirus infection by prophylaxis with an intravenous, hyperimmune, native, unmodified cytomegalovirus globulin. Randomized trial in bone marrow transplant recipients. Am J Med 1984;76:134.
61. Copeland JG, Mammana RB, Fuller JK, et al. Heart transplantation: four years experience with conventional immunosuppression. JAMA 1984;251:1563.
62. Coutts II, Jegarajah S, Stark JE. Tuberculosis in renal transplant recipients. Br J Dis Chest 1979;73:141.
63. Cruz I, Mody V, Callendar C, et al. Malaria infection in transplant recipient. J Natl Med Assoc 1978;70:105.
64. Cruz N, Ramirez-Muxo O, Bermudez R, et al. Pulmonary infection with *M. kansasii* in a renal transplant patient. Nephron 1980;26:187.
65. Cuvelier R, Pirson Y, Alexandre GPJ, et al. Late urinary tract infection after transplantation: prevalence, predisposition and morbidity. Nephron 1985;40:76.
66. Date A, Vaska K, Vaska PH, et al. Terminal infections in renal transplant patients in a tropical environment. Nephron 1982;32:253.
67. Davies SF. Disseminated histoplasmosis in renal transplant recipients. Am J Surg 1979;137:686.
68. Degos F, Degott C, Bedrossian J, et al. Is renal transplantation involved in post-transplantation liver disease? Transplantation 1980;29:100.
69. Demicco DD, Reichman RC, Violette EJ, et al. Disseminated aspergillosis presenting with endophthalmitis. Cancer 1984;53:1995.
70. Dienstag JL, Werner BG, McLane MF, et al. Absence of antibodies to HTLV-III in health workers after hepatitis B vaccination. JAMA 1985;254:1064.
71. Dienstag JL, Werner BG, Polk BF, et al. Hepatitis B vaccine in health care personnel: safety, immunogenicity, and indicators of efficacy. Ann Intern Med 1984;101:34.
72. Doherty CC, McGeown MG. Prevention of upper gastrointestinal complications after kidney transplantation. Proc Eur Dial Transplant Assoc Eur Ren Assoc 1978;15:361.

73. Doig RL, Boyd PJR. *Staphylococcus aureus* transmitted in transplanted kidneys. Lancet 1975; 2:243.

74. Douglas RG, Anderson MS, Weg JG, et al. Herpes simplex virus pneumonia. JAMA 1969;210:902.

75. Dowling JN, Pasculle AW, Frola FN, et al. Infections caused by *Legionella micdadei* and *Legionella pneumophila* among renal transplant recipients. J Infect Dis 1984;149:703.

76. Dresdale AR, Drusin RE, Lamb J, et al. Reduced infection in cardiac transplant recipients. Circulation 1985;72:237.

77. Dummer JS, Bahnson HT, Griffith BP, et al. Infections in patients on cyclosporine and prednisone following cardiac transplantation. Transplant Proc 1983;15:2779.

78. Dummer JS, Hardy A, Poorsattar A, et al. Early infections in kidney, heart and liver transplant recipients on cyclosporine. Transplantation 1983;36:259.

79. Dunn DL, Bogard WC, Cerra FB. Efficacy of type specific and cross reactive murine monoclonal antibodies directed against endotoxin during experimental sepsis. Surgery 1985;98:283.

80. Dunn DL, Ewald DC, Chandan N, et al. A single murine monoclonal antibody provides cross-genera protection during murine gram-negative sepsis. Arch Surg 1986;121:58.

81. Dunn DL, Ferguson R. Immunotherapy of gram negative bacterial sepsis: enhanced survival in a guinea pig model by use of rabbit antiserum to *Escherichia coli* J-5. Surgery 1982;92:212.

82. Dunn DL, Mach PA, Condie RM, et al. Anti-core endotoxin F(ab')₂ equine immunoglobulin fragments protect against lethal effects of gram negative bacterial sepsis. Surgery 1984;96:440.

83. Dunn DL, Matas AJ, Fryd DS, et al. Association of concurrent herpes simplex virus and cytomegalovirus with detrimental effects after renal transplantation. Arch Surg 1984;119:812.

84. DuPont HL, Spink WW. Infections due to gram-negative organisms: an analysis of 860 patients with bacteremia at the University of Minnesota Medical Center, 1958–1966. Medicine 1969;48:307.

85. Dusheiko G, Song E, Bowyer S, et al. Natural history of hepatitis B virus infection in renal transplant recipients—a fifteen-year follow-up. Hepatology 1983;3:330.

86. Eickhoff TC. Infectious complications in renal transplant recipients. Transplant Proc 1973;5:1233.

87. Eickhoff TC, Olin D, Anderson RJ. Current problems and approaches to diagnosis of infection in renal transplant recipients. Transplant Proc 1972;4:693.

88. Elliot WC, Houghton DC, Bryant RE, et al. Herpes simplex type 1 hepatitis in renal transplantation. Arch Intern Med 1980;140:1656.

89. England AC, Fraser DW, Plikaytis BD, et al. Sporadic legionellosis in the United States: the first thousand cases. Ann Intern Med 1981;94:164.

90. Faro RS, Corry RJ. Management of surgical gastrointestinal complications in renal transplant recipients. Arch Surg 1979;114:310.

91. Feduska NJ, Amend WJC, Vincenti F, et al. Peptic ulcer disease in kidney transplant recipients. Am J Surg 1984;148:51.

92. Fernandez JA, Rosenberg JC. Post-transplantation pancreatitis. Surg Gynecol Obstet 1976;143:795.

93. Finkelstein FO, Bastl C, Schiff M, et al. *Listeria* sepsis immediately preceding renal transplant rejection. JAMA 1976;235:844.

94. Fisher J, Tuazon CU, Geelhoed GW. Mucormycosis in transplant patients. Am Surg 1980;46:315.

95. Forslund T, Laasonen L, Hockerstedt K, et al. Tuberculosis of the colon in a kidney transplant patient. Acta Med Scand 1984;215:181.

96. Foucar E, Mukai K, Foucar K, et al. Colon ulceration in lethal cytomegalovirus infection. Am J Clin Pathol 1981;76:788.

97. Friedman HM, Grossman RA, Plotkin SA, et al. Relapse of pneumonia caused by cytomegalovirus in two recipients of renal transplants. J Infect Dis 1979;139:465.

98. Fryd DS, Peterson PK, Ferguson RM, et al. Cytomegalovirus as a risk factor in renal transplantation. Transplantation 1980;30:426.

99. Gantz NM. *Listeria* infection in renal transplant recipients. JAMA 1976;235:1326.

100. Gardner SD, Mackenzie EFD, Smith C, et al. Prospective study of the human polyomaviruses BK and JC and cytomegalovirus in renal transplant recipients. J Clin Pathol 1984;37:578.

101. Garvin PJ, Carney K, Castaneda M, et al. Peptic ulcer disease following transplantation: the role of cimetidine. Am J Surg 1982;144:545.

102. Gentry LO, Zelufff BJ. Diagnosis and treatment of infection in cardiac transplant patients. Surg Clin North Am 1986;66:459.

103. Glenn J. Cytomegalovirus infections following renal transplantation. Rev Infect Dis 1981;3:1151.

104. Goldstein JD, Keller JL, Winn WC, et al. Sporadic legionellaceae pneumonia in renal transplant recipients. Arch Pathol Lab Med 1982;106:108.

105. Gombert ME, Goldstine EJC, Corrado ML, et al. Disseminated *Mycobacterium marinum* infection after renal transplantation. Ann Intern Med 1981;94:486.

106. Gombert ME, Josephson A, Goldstein EJC, et al. Cavitary Legionnaires' pneumonia: nosocomial infection in renal transplant recipients. Am J Surg 1984;147:402.

107. Greenberg MS, Cohen G. Oral infection in immunosuppressed renal transplant patients. Oral Surg 1977;43:879.

108. Gribetz AR, Chuang MT, Burrows L, et al. Rhizopus lung abscess in renal transplant patient successfully treated by lobectomy. Chest 1980;77:102.

109. Griffin PJA, Salaman JR. Urinary tract infections after renal transplantation: do they matter? Br Med J 1979;1:710.

110. Griffith BP, Hardest RL, Bahnson HT. Powerful but limited immunosuppression for cardiac transplantation with cyclosporine and low-dose steroid. J Thorac Cardiovasc Surg 1984;87:35.

111. Grossman RI, Cavis KR, Taveras JM, et al. Computed tomography of intracranial aspergillosis. J Comput Assist Tomogr 1981;5:646.

112. Guice K, Rattazzi LC, Marchioro TL. Colon perforation in renal transplant patients. Am J Surg 1979;138:43.

113. Gustafson TL, Schaffner W, Lavely GB, et al. Invasive aspergillosis in renal transplant recipients: correlation with corticosteroid therapy. J Infect Dis 1983;148:230.

114. Haffner JF, Jakobsen A, Flatmark AL. Upper gastrointestinal bleeding in renal transplant recipients: the role of prophylactic gastric surgery. World J Surg 1983;7:738.

115. Hammer GS, Bottone EJ, Hirschman SZ. Mucormycosis in a transplant recipient. Am J Clin Pathol 1975;64:389.

116. Hamshere RJ, Chisolm GD, Shackman R. Late urinary-tract infection after renal transplantation. Lancet 1974;2:793.

117. Hanto DW, Frizzera G, Purtilo DT, et al. Clinical spectrum of lymphoproliferative disorders in renal transplant recipients and evidence for the role of Epstein-Barr virus. Cancer Res 1981;41:4253.

118. Hardy AM, Wajszczuk CP, Suffredini AF, et al. *Pneumocystis carinii* pneumonia in renal-transplant recipients treated with cyclosporine and steroids. J Infect Dis 1984;149:143.

119. Harnett GB, Bucens MR, Clay SJ, et al. Acute haemorrhagic cystitis caused by adenovirus type 11 in a recipient of a transplanted kidney. Med J Aust 1982;13:565.

120. Harris LF, Dan BM, Lefkowitz LB, et al. Paecilomyces cellulitis in a renal transplant patient: successful treatment with intravenous miconazole. South Med J 1979;72:897.

121. Hau T, Van Hook EJ, Simmons RL, et al. Prognostic factors of peritoneal infections in transplant patients. Surgery 1978;84:403.

122. Haverkos HW, Dowling JN, Pasculle AW, et al. Diagnosis of pneumonitis in immunocompromised patients by open lung biopsy. Cancer 1983;52:1093.

123. Hedemark LL, Kronenberg RS, Rasp FL, et al. The value of bronchoscopy in establishing the etiology of pneumonia in renal transplant recipients. Am Rev Respir Dis 1982;126:981.

124. Heironimus JD, Winn RE, Collins CB. Cutaneous nonpulmonary *Mycobacterium chelonei* infection. Successful treatment with sulfonamides in an immunosuppressed patient. Arch Dermatol 1984;120:1061.

125. Hellman RN, Hinrichs J, Sicard G, et al. Cryptococcal pyelonephritis and disseminated cryptococcosis in a renal transplant recipient. Arch Intern Med 1981;141:128.

126. Henry ML, Sommer BG, Ferguson RM. Beneficial effects of cyclosporine compared with azathioprine in cadaveric renal transplantation. Am J Surg 1985;140:533.

127. Henslee J, Bostrom B, Weisdorf D, et al. Streptococcal sepsis in bone marrow transplant patients. Lancet 1984; Vol. 1, 393.

128. Hepatitis B vaccine. Health and Public Policy Committee, American College of Physicians. Ann Intern Med 1984;100:149.

129. Herb HM, Jontofsohn R, Loffler HD, et al. Toxoplasmosis after renal transplantation. Clin Nephrol 1977;8:529.

130. Hesse UJ, Sutherland DER, Simmons RL, et al. Intra-abdominal infections in pancreas transplant recipients. Ann Surg 1986;203:153.

131. Hilfenhaus J, Moser H, Herrmann A, et al. Herpes simplex virus subunit vaccine: characterization of the virus strain used and testing of the vaccine. Dev Biol Stand 1982;52:321.

132. Hilleman MR, Carlson AJ Jr, McLean AA, et al. *Streptococcus pneumoniae* polysaccharide vaccine: age and dose responses, safety, persistence of antibody, revaccination, and simultaneous administration of pneumococcal and influenza vaccines. Rev Infect Dis 1981;3:S31.

133. Hillis WD, Hillis A, Walker G. Hepatitis B surface antigenemia in renal transplant recipient. Increased mortality risk. JAMA 1979;242:329.

134. Himal HS, Wise DJ, Cardella C. Localized colonic perforation following renal transplantation. Dis Colon Rectum 1983;26:461.

135. Hodgin UG, Sanford JP. Gram-negative rod bacteremia: an analysis of 100 patients. Am J Med 1965;39:952.

136. Hogan TF, Borden EC, McBain JA, et al. Human polyomavirus infections with JC virus and BK virus in renal transplant patients. Ann Intern Med 1980;92:373.

137. Holden FA, Kaczmer JE, Kinahan CC. Listerial meningitis and renal allografts. Postgrad Med 1980;68:69.

138. Howard RJ, Simmons RL, Najarian JS. Fungal infections in renal transplant recipients. Ann Surg 1978;188:598.

139. Hoy WE, Kissel SM, Freeman RB, et al. Altered patterns of posttransplant urinary tract infections associated with perioperative antibiotics and curtailed catheterization. Am J Kidney Dis 1985;6:212.

140. Hoy WE, May AG, Freeman RB. Primary renal transplant wound infections. NY State J Med 1981;81:1469.

141. Hurley JK, Greenslade T, Lewy PR, et al. Varicella-zoster infections in pediatric renal transplant recipients. Arch Surg 1980;115:751.

142. Iacobellis FW, Jacobs MI, Cohen RP. Primary cutaneous cryptococcosis. Arch Dermatol 1979;115:984.

143. Isiadinso OA. *Listeria* sepsis and meningitis. JAMA 1975;234:842.

144. Jones JM, Glass NR, Belzer FO. Fatal *Candida* esophagitis in two diabetics after renal transplantation. Arch Surg 1982;117:499.

145. Jorgensen F, Olsen H. Urinary tract infection in renal transplantation and the value of antibiotic treatment. Clin Nephrol 1973;1:297.

146. Judson RT. Wound infection following renal transplantation. Aust NZ J Surg 1984;54:223.

147. Julia A, Acebedo G, Jornet J, et al. Spontaneous pneumococcal peritonitis: late infection after bone-marrow transplantation. N Engl J Med 1985;312:587.

148. Kinder RB, Jourdan MH. Disseminated aspergillosis and bleeding colonic ulcers in renal transplant patient. J R Soc Med 1985;78:338.

149. Kirkman RL, Strom TB, Weir MR, et al. Late mortality and morbidity in recipients of long-term renal allografts. Transplantation 1982;34:347.

150. Kirmani N, Tuason CM, Ocuin JA, et al. Extensive cerebral nocardiosis cured with antibiotic therapy alone. J Neurosurg 1978;49:924.

151. Koep LJ, Peters TG, Starzl TE,. Major colonic complications of hepatic transplantation. Dis Colon Rectum 1979;22:218.

152. Kohlberg WI, Tellis VA, Bhat DJ, et al. Wound infections after transplant nephrectomy. Arch Surg 1980;115:645.

153. Kolbeck PC, Makhoul RG, Bollinger RR, et al. Widely disseminated *Cunninghamella* mucormycosis in a adult renal transplant patient: case report and review of the literature. Am J Clin Pathol 1984;83:747.

154. Kreger BE, Craven DE, Carling PC, et al. Gram-negative bacteremia: III. Reassessment of etiology, epidemiology and ecology in 612 patients. Am J Med 1980;68:332.

155. Kreger BE, Craven DE, McCabe WR: Gram negative bacteremia. IV. Reevaluation of clinical feature and treatment in 612 patients. Am J Med 1980;68:344.

156. Krieger JN, Brem AS, Kaplan MR. Urinary tract infection in pediatric renal transplantation. Urology 1980;15:362.

157. Krieger JN, Tapia L, Stubenbord WT, et al. Urinary infection in kidney transplantation. Urology 1977;9:130.

158. Kuller J, First MR, D'Achiardi R, et al. *Pneumocystis carinii* pneumonia in renal transplant recipients. Am J Nephrol 1982;2:312.

159. Kyriakides GK, Simmons RL, Najarian JS. Wound infections in renal transplant wounds: pathogenetic and prognostic factor. Ann Surg 1975;182:770.

160. Kyriakides GK, Simmons RL, Najarian JS. Mycotic aneurysms in transplant patients. Arch Surg 1976;111:472.

161. Kyriakides GK, Zinneman HH, Hall WH, et al. Immunologic monitoring and aspergillosis in renal transplant patients. Am J Surg 1976;131:246.

162. Lachman E, Pitsoe SB, Gaffin SL. Anti-lipopolysaccharide immunotherapy in management of septic shock of obstetric and gynaecological origin. Lancet 1984;i:981.

163. LaForce FM, Eickhoff TC. Pneumococcal vaccine: the evidence mounts. Ann Intern Med 1986;104:110.

164. L'age-Stehr J, Schwarz A, Offermann G, et al. HTLV-III infection in kidney transplant recipients. Lancet 1985;2:1361.

165. Langlois RP, Flegel KM, Meakins JL, et al. Cutaneous aspergillosis with fatal dissemination in a renal transplant recipient. Can Med Assoc J 1980;120:673.

166. Ledingham IM, McCardle CS: Prospective study of the treatment of shock. Lancet 1978;i:1194.

167. Lentino JR, Rosenkranz MA, Michaels JA, et al. Nosocomial aspergillosis. Am J Epidemiol 1982;116:430.

168. Lerut J, Lerut T, Gruwez JA, et al. Surgical gastro-intestinal complications in 277 renal transplantations. Acta Chir Belg 1980;79:383.

169. Lichtenstein IH, MacGregor RR. Mycobacterial infections in renal transplant recipients: report of five cases and review of the literature. Rev Infect Dis 1983;5:216.

170. Linder MM, Kosters W, Rethel R. Prophylactic gastric operations in uremic patients prior to renal transplantation. World J Surg 1979;3:501.

171. Lindstrom BL, Lindfors O, Eklund B, et al. Surgical complications in 500 kidney transplantations. Proc Eur Dial Transplant Assoc Eur Ren Assoc 1977;14:353.

172. Linnemann CC. Risk of pneumococcal infections in renal transplant patients. JAMA 1979;241:2619.

173. Linnemann CC Jr, First MR, Alvira MM, et al. Herpesvirus hominis type 2 meningoencephalitis following renal transplantation. Am J Med 1976;61:703.

174. Lobo PI, Rudolf LE, Krieger JN. Wound infections in renal transplant recipients—a complication of urinary tract infections during allograft malfunction. Surgery 1982;92:491.

175. Lopez C, Simmons RL, Mauer M, et al. Role of virus infections in immunosuppressed renal transplant patients. Transplant Proc 1973;5:803.

176. Lorber MI, Campbell DA, Konnak JW, et al. Etiology and management of early and late peritransplant infections. J Urol 1981;127:870.

177. Loveras J, Peterson PK, Simmons RL, et al. Mycobacterial infections in renal transplant recipients. Seven cases and a review of the literature. Arch Intern Med 1982;142:888.

178. Lovett IS, Houang ET, Burge S, et al. An outbreak of *Nocardia asteroides* infection in a renal transplant unit. Q J Med 1981;198:123.

179. Luby JP, Burnett W, Hull AR, et al. Relationship between cytomegalovirus and hepatic function abnormalities in the period after renal transplant. J Infect Dis 1974;129:511.

180. Luby JP, Ramirez-Ronda C, Rinner S, et al. A longitudinal study of varicella-zoster virus infections in renal transplant recipients. J Infect Dis 1977;135:659.

181. Luce JM, Ostenson RC, Springmeyer SC, et al. Invasive aspergillosis presenting as pericarditis and cardiac tamponade. Chest 1979;76:703.

182. Luft BJ, Noat Y, Araujo FG, et al. Primary and reactivated *Toxoplasma* infection in patients with cardiac transplants. Clinical spectrum and problems in diagnosis in a defined population. Ann Intern Med 1983;99:27.

183. McCabe WR, Jackson GG. Gram-negative bacteremia. Arch Intern Med 1962;110:847.

184. McClellan SL, Komorowski RA, Farmer SG, et al. Severe bleeding diathesis associated with invasive aspergillosis in transplant patients. Tranplantation 1985;39:406.

185. McCutchan JA, Wolf JL, Ziegler EJ, et al. Ineffectiveness of single-dose human antiserum to core glycolipid (*E. coli* J5) for prophylaxis of bacteremic, gram-negative infections in patients with prolonged neutropenia. Schweiz Med Wochenschr 1983;113S:40.

186. McDonald JC, Ritchy RJ, Fuselier PF, et al. Sepsis in human renal transplantation. Surgery 1971;69:189.

187. McGregor CGA, Fleck DG, Nagington J, et al. Disseminated toxoplasmosis in cardiac transplantation. J Clin Pathol 1984;37:74.

188. McHenry MC, Braun WE, Popowniak KL, et al. Septicemia in renal transplant recipients. Urol Clin North Am 1976;3:647.

189. Mahon FB, Malek GH, Uehling DT. Urinary tract infection after renal transplantation. Urology 1973;1:579.

190. Majeski JA, Alexander JW, First MR, et al. Transplantation of microbially contaminated cadaver kidneys. Arch Surg 1982;117:221.

191. Margolis DM, Saylor JL, Geisse G, et al. Upper gastrointestinal disease in chronic renal failure. Arch Intern Med 1978;138:1214.

192. Marker SC, Ascher NL, Kalis JM, et al. Epstein-Barr virus antibody responses and clinical illness in renal transplant recipients. Surgery 1979;85:433.

193. Marker SC, Howard RJ, Simmons RL, et al. Cytomegalovirus infection: a quantitative prospective study of 320 consecutive renal transplants. Surgery 1981;89:600.

194. Marker SC, Simmons RL, Balfour HH Jr. Cytomegalovirus vaccine in renal allograft recipients. Transplant Proc 1981;13:117.

195. Markman M, Mannisi J, Dick JD, et al. Sulfamethoxazole–trimethoprim-resistant pneumococcal sepsis. JAMA 1982;248:3011.
196. Marshall W, Foster RS, Winn W. Legionnaires' disease in renal transplant patients. Am J Surg 1981;141:423.
197. Martiniz AJ. Acanthamoebiasis and immunosuppression. J Neuropathol 1982;41:548.
198. Masur H, Cheigh JS, Stubenbord WT. Infection following renal transplantation: a changing pattern. Rev Infect Dis 1982;4:1208.
199. Mattson K, Edgren J, Kuhkback B. Pulmonary infections after renal transplantation. Ann Clin Res 1979;11:63.
200. Meakins JL. Clinical importance of host resistance to infection in surgical patients. Adv Surg 1981;15:225.
201. Meech PR, Hardie IR, Hartley CJ, et al. Gastrointestinal complications following renal transplantation. Aust NZ J Surg 1979;49:621.
202. Mehta P, Patel JD, Milder JE. *Legionella micdadei* (Pittsburgh pneumonia agent): two infections with unusual clinical features. JAMA 1983;249:1620.
203. Meignier B, Roizman B. Herpes simplex virus vaccines. Antiviral Res 1985;1:S259.
204. Mejia G, Leiderman E, Builes M, et al. Transmission of toxoplasmosis by renal transplant. Am J Kidney Dis 1983;2:615.
205. Meyers AM, Shapiro DJ, Milne FJ, et al. *Strongyloides stercoralis* hyperinfection in a renal allograft recipient. 1976;50:1301.
206. Meyers JD. Prevention and treatment of cytomegalovirus infections with interferons and immune globulins. Infection 1984;12:143.
207. Meyers JD, Wade JC, Shepp DH, et al. Acyclovir treatment of varicella-zoster virus infection in the immunocompromised host. Transplantation 1984;37:571.
208. Meyers WC, Harris N, Stein S, et al. Alimentary tract complications after renal transplantation. Ann Surg 1979;190:535.
209. Michel RP, Guttmann RD, Knaak J, et al. Antilymphocyte globulin in renal transplantation. Nephrotic syndrome and infection as possible complications. Arch Surg 1975;110:90.
210. Milito G, Taccone-Gallucci M, Brancaleone C, et al. Assessment of the upper gastrointestinal tract in hemodialysis patients awaiting renal transplantation. Am J Gastroenterol 1983;78:328.
211. Mills SA, Seigler HF, Wolfe WG. The incidence and management of pulmonary mycosis in renal allograft patients. Ann Surg 1975;182:617.
212. Misra MK, Pinkus GS, Birtch AG, et al. Major colonic diseases complicating renal transplantation. Surgery 1973;73:942.
213. Montgomerie JZ, Bacroft DMO, Croxson MC, et al. Herpes simplex virus infection after renal transplantation. Lancet 1969;2:867.
214. Montgomery JR, Barrett FF, Williams TW. Infectious complications in transplant patients. Transplant Proc 1973;5:1239.
215. Moore FD, Kohler TR, Strom TB, et al. The declining mortality from pneumonia in renal transplant patients. Infect Surg 1983;2:13.
216. Morales LA, Gonzalez ZA, Santiago-Delpin EA. Chromoblastomycosis in a renal transplant patient. Nephron 1985;40:238.
217. Morduchowicz G, Pitlik SD, Shapira Z, et al. Infections in renal transplant recipients in Israel. Isr J Med Sci 1985;21:791.
218. Mourad G, Soulillou J, Chong G, et al. Transmission of *Mycobacterium tuberculosis* with renal allografts. Nephron 1985;41:82.
219. Muakkassa WF, Goldman MH, Mendez-Picon G, et al. Wound infections in renal transplant patients. J Urol 1983;130:17.
220. Murphy JF, McDonald FD, Dawson M, et al. Factors affecting the frequency of infection in renal transplant recipients. Arch Intern Med 1976;136:670.
221. Murray HW, Knox DL, Green WR, et al. Cytomegalovirus retinitis in adults. Am J Med 1977;63:574.
222. Murray HW, Moore JO, Luff RD. Disseminated aspergillosis in a renal transplant patient: diagnostic difficulties re-emphasized. Johns Hop Med J 1975;137:235.
223. Mussche MM, Lameire NH, Ringoir SMG. *Salmonella typhimurium* infections in renal transplant patients. Nephron 1975;15:143.
224. Myerowitz RL, Medeiros AA, O'Brien TF. Recent experience with bacillemia due to gram-negative organisms. J Infect Dis 1971;124:239.
225. Myerowitz RL, Stalder H, Oxman MN, et al. Fatal disseminated adenovirus infection in a renal transplant recipient. Am J Med 1975;59:591.

460

226. Najarian JS, Fryd DS, Strand M, et al. A single institution randomized prospective trial of cyclosporine versus azathioprine–antilymphocyte globulin for immunosuppression in renal allograft recipients. Ann Surg 1985;201:142.

227. Naraqi S, Jackson GG, Janasson O, et al. Prospective study of prevalence, incidence, and source of herpesvirus infections in patients with renal allografts. J Infect Dis 1977;136:531.

228. Natas OB, Willassen Y. Lung infection caused by *Nocardia asteroides* in a renal transplant patient. Scand J Infect Dis 1983;15:317.

229. Nelson PW, Delmonico FL, Tolkoff-Rubin NE, et al. Unsuspected donor *Pseudomonas* infection causing arterial disruption after renal transplantation. Transplantation 1984;37:313.

230. Nghiem DD, Corry RJ. Colorectal perforation in renal transplant recipients. Am Surg 1983;49:554.

231. Nicholls A, Edward N, Catto GR. Staphylococcal septicaemia, endocarditis, and osteomyelitis in dialysis and renal transplant patients. Postgrad Med J 1980;56:642.

232. Nielsen HE, Korsager B. Bacteremia after renal transplantation. Scand J Infect Dis 1977;9:111.

233. Niklasson P, Hambraeus A, Lundgren G, et al. *Listeria* encephalitis in five renal transplant recipients. Acta Med Scand 1978;203:181.

234. Novick A. The value of intraoperative antibiotics in preventing renal transplant wound infections. J Urol 1980;125:151.

235. Oliveira DBG, Winearls CG, Cohen J, et al. Severe immunosuppression in a renal transplant recipient with HTLV-III antibodies. Transplantation 1986;1:260.

236. Olivero JJ, Lozano J, Duki WN. Acute pancreatitis, pancreatic pseudocyst, and *Candida* peritonitis in recipient of a kidney transplant. South Med J 1976;69:1619.

237. O'Neal BJ, McDonald JC. The risk of sepsis in the asplenic adult. Ann Surg 1981;194:775.

238. Ortuno J, Teruel JL, Marcen R, et al. Primary intestinal tuberculosis following renal transplantation. Nephron 1982;31:59.

239. Owens ML, Passaro E Jr, Wilson SE, et al. Treatment of peptic ulcer disease in the renal transplant patient. Ann Surg 1977;186:17.

240. Owens ML, Wilson SE, Maxwell JG, et al. Major arterial hemorrhage after renal transplantation. Transplantation 1979;27:285.

241. Oyer PE, Stinson EB, Jamieson SW, et al. Cyclosporine-A in cardiac allografting: a preliminary experience. Transplant Proc 1983;15:1247.

242. Panijayanond P, Olsson CA, Spivack ML, et al. Intraocular nocardiosis in a renal transplant patient. Arch Surg 1972;104:845.

243. Pass RF, Long WK, Whitley RJ, et al. Productive infection with cytomegalovirus and herpes simplex virus in renal transplant recipients: role of source of kidney. J Infect Dis 1978;137:556.

244. Pass RF, Morris RE, Shaw JF, et al. Ocular toxoplasmosis after renal transplantation. South Med J 1981;74:1033.

245. Pass RF, Whitley RJ, Whelchel JD, et al. Identification of patients with increased risk of infection with herpes simplex virus after renal transplantation. J Infect Dis 1979;140:487.

246. Patel NP, Corry RJ. Cytomegalovirus as a cause of cecal ulcer with massive hemorrhage in a renal transplant recipient. Am Surg 1980;46:260.

247. Pearl SN, Weiner MA, Dibbell DG. Sternal infection after cardiac transplantation; successful salvage utilizing a variety of techniques. J Thorac Cardiovasc Surg 1982;83:632.

248. Peces R, Fernandez F, Perez F, et al. *Salmonella enteritidis* infection in renal transplant recipients. Nephron 1985;41:122.

249. Perrott CAV, Botha JR, Meyers AM, et al. Peptic ulceration in the renal transplant patient. S Afr Med J 1981;59:253.

250. Peters C, Peterson P, Marabella P, et al. Continuous sulfa prophylaxis for urinary tract infection in renal transplant recipients. Am J Surg 1983;146:589.

251. Peters T, Reiter CG, Boswell RL. Transmission of tuberculosis by kidney transplantation. Transplantation 1984;38:514.

252. Peters TG, Williams JW, Harmon HC, et al. Splenectomy and death in renal transplant patients. Arch Surg 118:795.

253. Peterson PK, Balfour HH Jr, Fryd DS, et al. Fever in renal transplant recipients: causes, prognostic significance and changing patterns at the University of Minnesota Hospital. Am J Med 1981;71:345.

254. Peterson PK, Balfour HH Jr, Marker SC, et al. Cytomegalovirus disease in renal allograft recipients. A prospective study of the clinical features, risk factors and impact on renal transplantation. Medicine 1980;59:283.

255. Peterson PK, Dahl MV, Howard RJ, et al. Mucormycosis and cutaneous histoplasmosis in a renal transplant recipient. Arch Dermatol 1982;118:275.

256. Peterson PK, Ferguson R, Fryd DS, et al. Infectious diseases in hospitalized renal transplant recipients: a prospective study of a complex and evolving problem. Medicine 1982;61:360.
257. Pirson Y, Alexandre GPJ, vanYpersele de Strihou C. Long-term effect of HBs antigenemia on patient survival after renal transplantation. N Engl J Med 1977;296:194.
258. Plotkin SA, Smiley ML, Friedman HM, et al. Prevention of cytomegalovirus disease by Towne strain live attenuated vaccine. Birth Defects 1984;20:271.
259. Plotkin SA, Smiley ML, Friedman HM, et al. Towne-vaccine-induced prevention of cytomegalovirus disease after renal transplants. Lancet 1984;1:528.
260. Pollak R, Hau T, Mozes MF. The spectrum of peritonitis in renal transplant recipients. Am Surg 1985;51:617.
261. Prat V, Horcickova M, Matousovic K, et al. Urinary tract infection in renal transplant patients. Infection 1985;13:207.
262. Preiksaitis JK, Rosno S, Grumet C, et al. Infections due to herpesviruses in cardiac transplant recipients: role of the donor heart and immunosuppressive therapy. J Infect Dis 1983;147:974.
263. Prince AM, Szmuness W, Mann MK, et al. Hepatitis B immune globulin: final report of a controlled multicenter trial of efficacy in prevention of dialysis-associated hepatitis. J Infect Dis 1978; 137:131.
264. Quinnan GV Jr, Delery M, Rook AH, et al. Comparative virulence and immunogenicity of the Towne strain and a nonattenuated strain of cytomegalovirus. Ann Intern Med 1984;101:478.
265. Rai GS, Wilkinson R, Taylor RM, et al. Adverse effect of splenectomy in renal transplantation. Clin Nephrol 1978;9:194.
266. Ramos E, Karmi S, Alongi SV, et al. Infectious complication in renal transplant recipients. South Med J 1980;73:751.
267. Ramsey DE, Finch WT, Birtch AG. Urinary tract infections in kidney transplant recipients. Arch Surg 1979;114:1022.
268. Recommendations for protection against viral hepatitis. Recommendation of the Immunization Practices Advisory Committee. Centers for Disease Control, Department of Health and Human Services. Ann Intern Med 1985;103:391.
269. Remine SG, Melrath DC. Bowel perforation in steroid treated patients. Ann Surg 1980;192:581.
270. Romer FK, Nielsen HE, Christensen CK, et al. Bacterial infections after renal transplantation. Dan Med Bull 1980;27:266.
271. Rubin RH, Cosimi AB, Hirsch MS, et al. Effects of antithymocyte globulin on cytomegalovirus infection in renal transplant recipients. Transplantation 1981;31:143.
272. Rubin RH, Wolfson JS, Cosimi AB, et al. Infection in the renal transplant recipient. Am J Med 1981;70:405.
273. Ruskin J, Remington JS. Toxoplasmosis in the compromised host. Ann Intern Med 1976;84:193.
274. Ryning FW, McLeod R, Maddox JC, et al. Probable transmission of *Toxoplasma gondii* by organ transplantation. Ann Intern Med 1979;90:47.
275. Sachs GW, Simmons RL, Balfour HH Jr. Cytomegalovirus vaccine: persistence of humoral immunity following immunization of renal transplant candidates. Vaccine 1984;2:215.
276. Sanders KL, Walker DH, Lee TJ. Relapse of legionnaires' disease in a renal transplant recipient. Arch Intern Med 1980;140:833.
277. Saral R, Burns WH, Prentice HG. Herpes virus infections: clinical manifestations and therapeutic strategies in immunocompromised patients. Clin Haematol 1984;13:645.
278. Sarosdy MF, Saylor R, Dittman W, et al. Upper gastrointestinal bleeding following renal transplantation. Urology 1985;26:347.
279. Sawyer OI, Garvin PJ, Codd JE, et al. Colorectal complications of renal allograft transplantation. Arch Surg 1978;113:84.
280. Saylor RP, Sarosdy MF, Wright LF, et al. Hypercalcemia-induced upper gastrointestinal bleeding after renal transplantation. Urology 1984;24:337.
281. Schiessel R, Starlinger M, Wolf A, et al. Failure of cimetidine to prevent gastroduodenal ulceration and bleeding after renal transplantation. Surgery 1981;90:456.
282. Schroter GPJ, Bakshandef K, Husberg BS, et al. Coccidioidomycosis and renal transplantation. Transplantation 1977;23:485.
283. Schroter GPJ, West JC, Weil R. Acute bacteremia in asplenic renal transplant patients. JAMA 1977;237:2207.
284. Schwartz JS. Pneumococcal vaccine: clinical efficacy and effectiveness. Ann Intern Med 1986;96:208.
285. Schwartz PE, Strieoff S, Mucha P, et al. Post-splenectomy sepsis and mortality in adults. JAMA 1982;248:2279.

286. Schweizer RT, Bartus SA. Gastroduodenal ulceration in renal transplant patients. Conn Med 1978;42:85.
287. Shapiro ED, Clemens JD. A controlled evaluation of the protective efficacy of pneumococcal vaccine for patients at high risk of serious pneumococcal infections. Ann Intern Med 1984;101:325.
288. Simmons RL. Personal communication, 1986.
289. Simmons RL, Balfour HH Jr, Lopez C, et al. Infection in immunosuppressed transplant recipients. Surg Clin North Am 1975;55:1419.
290. Simmons RL, Canafax DM, Fryd DS, et al. New immunosuppressive drug combinations for mismatched related and cadaveric renal transplantation. Transplant Proc 1986;18:76.
291. Simmons RL, Lopez C, Balfour HH Jr, et al. Cytomegalovirus: clinical virological correlations in renal transplant recipients. Ann Surg 1974;180:623.
292. Simmons RL, Matas AJ, Ratazzi LC, et al. Clinical characteristics of the lethal cytomegalovirus infection following renal transplantation. Surgery 1977;82:537.
293. Simmons RL, Uranga VM, LaPlante ES, et al. Pulmonary complications in transplant recipients. Arch Surg 1972;105:260.
294. Simpson GL, Stinson EB, Egger MJ, et al. Nocardial infections in the immunocompromised host: a detailed study in a defined population. Rev Infect Dis 1981;3:492.
295. Singer C, Kaplan MH, Armstrong D. Bacteremia and fungemia complicating neoplastic disease: a study of 364 cases. Am J Med 1977;62:731.
296. Skinner GR, Woodman C, Hartley C, et al. Early experience with "antigenoid" vaccine Ac NFU1(S-) MRC towards prevention or modification of herpes genitalis. Dev Biol Stand 1982;52:333.
297. Smiley ML, Wlodaver CG, Grossman RA, et al. The role of pretransplant immunity in protection from cytomegalovirus disease following renal transplantation. Transplantation 1985;40:157.
298. Smith EJ, Milligan SL, Filo RS. *Salmonella* mycotic aneurysm after renal transplantation. South Med J 1981;74:1399.
299. Spanos PK, Simmons RL, Rattazzi LC, et al. Peptic ulcer disease in the transplant recipient. Arch Surgery 1974;109:193.
300. Spees EK, Oakes DD, Reinmuth B. Experiences with cadaver renal allograft contamination before transplantation. Br J Surg 69:482.
301. Spence RK, Dafoe DC, Rabin G, et al. Mycobacterial infections in renal allograft recipients. Arch Surg 1983;118:356.
302. Squifflet J-P, Pirson YD, Dardenne AN, et al. Mycotic aneurysm of renal graft artery: diagnosis by ultrasonography. Urology 1983;22:212.
303. Stamm AM, Dismukes WE, Simmons BP, et al. Listeriosis in renal transplant recipients: report of an outbreak and review of 102 cases. Rev Infect Dis 1982;4:665.
304. Starnes HF, McWinnie DK, Bradley JA, et al. Delayed major arterial hemorrhage after transplant nephrectomy. Transplant Proc 1984;16:1320.
305. Starr SE, Glazer JP, Friedman HM, et al. Specific cellular and humoral immunity after immunization with live Towne strain cytomegalovirus vaccine. J Infect Dis 1981;143:585.
306. Steed DL, Brown B, Reilly JJ, et al. General surgical complications in heart and heart–lung transplantation. Surgery 1985;98:739.
307. Stevens CE, Alter HJ, Taylor PE, et al. Hepatitis B vaccine in patients receiving hemodialysis. Immunogenicity and efficacy. N Engl J Med 1984;311:496.
308. Stiller CR. The Canadian multicenter transplant study group. A randomized clinical trial of cyclosporine in cadaveric renal transplantation. N Engl J Med 1983;309:809.
309. Straus SE, Rooney JF, Sever JL, et al. NIH Conference. Herpes simplex virus infection: biology, treatment, and prevention. Ann Intern Med 1985;103:404.
310. Stuart FP, Reckard CR, Schulak JA, et al. Gastroduodenal complications in kidney transplant recipients. Ann Surg 1981;194:339.
311. Sutherland DER, Chan FY, Foucar E, et al. The bleeding cecal ulcer in transplant patients. Surgery 1979;86:386.
312. Sutherland DER, Fryd DS, So SKS, et al. Long-term effect of splenectomy versus no splenectomy in renal transplant patients. Transplantation 1984;38:619.
313. Sutherland DER, Fryd DS, Strand M, et al. Results of the Minnesota randomized, prospective trial of cyclosporine versus azathioprine–antilymphocyte globulin for immunosuppression in renal allograft recipients. Am J Kidney Dis 1985;3:456.
314. Szmuness W, Stevens CE, Harley EJ, et al. Hepatitis B vaccine. Demonstration of efficacy in a controlled clinical trial in a high-risk population. N Engl J Med 1980;303:833.
315. Thomsen OF, Hansen HE. Bacteriuria and renal infection in kidney transplant recipients. Acta Pathol Microbiol Immunol Scand 1977;85:449.

316. Thukral R, Mir AR, Jacobson MP. Renal allograft rupture: a report of three cases and review of the literature. Am J Nephrol 1982;2:15.
317. Tillegard A. Renal transplant wound infection: the value of prophylactic antibiotic treatment. Scand J Urol Nephrol 1984;18:215.
318. Tilney NL, Strom TB, Vineyard GC, et al. Factors contributing to the declining mortality rate in renal transplantation. N Engl J Med 1978;299:1321.
319. Tipple M, Haywood H, Shadomy, et al. Cryptococcosis in renal transplant patients. Proc Deal Trans For 1976;6:13.
320. Tobin J O'H, Dunnill MS, French M, et al. Legionnaires' disease in a transplant unit: isolation of the causative agent from shower baths. Lancet 1980;2:118.
321. Tolkoff-Rubin NE, Cosimi AB, Russell PS, et al. A controlled study of trimethoprim–sulfamethoxazole prophylaxis of urinary tract infection in renal transplant recipients. Rev Infect Dis 1982;4:614.
322. Toussaint C, Dupont E, Vanherweghem JL, et al. Liver disease in patients undergoing hemodialysis and kidney transplantation. Adv Nephrol 1979;8:269.
323. Townsend TR, Rudolf LE, Westervelt FB, et al. Prophylactic antibiotic therapy with cefamandole and tobramycin for patients undergoing renal transplantation. Infect Control 1978:1:93.
324. van Roermund HP, Tiggeler RG, Berden JH, et al. Cimetidine prophylaxis after renal transplantation. Clin Nephrol 1982;18:39.
325. Vereerstraeten P, Stolear J-C, Schoutens-Serruys E, et al. Erthromycin prophylaxis for legionnaires' disease in immunosuppressed patients in a contaminated hospital environment. Transplantation 1986;41:52.
326. Vincenti F, Amend WJ, Feduska NJ, et al. Septic arthritis following renal transplantation. Nephron 1982;30:253.
327. Vishwanath S, Baker RA, Mansheim BJ. *Strongyloides* infection and meningitis in an immunocompromised host. Am J Trop Med Hyg 1982;31:857.
328. Wajszczuk CP, Dummer JS, Ho M, et al. Fungal infections in liver transplant recipients. Transplantation 1985;40:347.
329. Walsh TJ, Bulkley BH. *Aspergillus* pericarditis: clinical and pathologic features in the immunocompromised patient. Cancer 1982:49:48.
330. Walsh TJ, Hier DB, Caplan LR. Aspergillosis of the central nervous system: clinicopathological analysis of 17 patients. Ann Neurol 1985;18:574.
331. Walsh TJ, Hutchins GM. *Aspergillus* mural endocarditis. Am J Clin Pathol 1978;71:640.
332. Walsh TJ, Zachary JB, Hutchins GM, et al. Mycotic aneurysm with recurrent sepsis complicating posttransplant nephrectomy. Johns Hop Med J 1977;141:85.
333. Walter S, Pedersen FB, Vejlsgaard R. Urinary tract infection and wound infection in kidney transplant patients. Br J Urol 1975;47:513.
334. Walter S, Poulsen LR, Friedberg M, et al. The influence of wound drainage on the infection rate in kidney transplant patients. Br J Urol 1978;50:160.
335. Walter S, Thorup-Andersen J, Christensen U, et al. Effect of cimetidine on upper gastrointestinal bleeding after renal transplantation: a prospective study. Br Med J 1984;289:1175.
336. Wardle EN. Endotoxinemia in renal transplant recipients. Clin Nephrol 1975;3:31.
337. Washer GF, Schroter GPJ, Starzl TE, et al. Causes of death after kidney transplantation. JAMA 1983;250:49.
338. Watson AJ, Russell RP, Cabreja RF, et al. Cure of cryptococcal infection during continued immunosuppressive therapy. Q J Med 1985;217:169.
339. Watson AJ, Whelton A, Russell RP. Cure of cryptococcemia and preservation of graft function in a renal transplant recipient. Arch Intern Med 1984;144:1877.
340. Weeden D, Hopewell JP, Moorhead JF, et al. Schistosomiasis in renal transplantation. Br J Urol 1982;54:478.
341. Weiland D, Ferguson RM, Peterson PK, et al. Aspergillosis in 25 renal transplant patients. Ann Surg 1983;198:622.
342. Weisburger WR, Hutcheon DF, Yardley JH, et al. Cryptosporidiosis in an immunosuppressed renal-transplant recipient with IgA deficiency. Am J Clin Pathol 1979;72:473.
343. Wells CL, Podzorski RP, Peterson PK, et al. Incidence of trimethoprim–sulfamethoxazole-resistant Enterobacteriaceae among transplant recipients. J Infect Dis 1984;150:699.
344. West JC, Armitage JO, Mitros FA, et al. Cytomegalovirus cecal erosion causing massive hemorrhage in a bone marrow transplant recipient. World J Surg 1982;6:251.
345. Williams G, Castro JE. Cimetidine in the treatment of peptic ulceration following renal transplantation. Br J Surg 1979;66:510.
346. Wilson CB, Siber GR, O'Brien TF, et al. Phycomycotic gangrenous cellulitis. Arch Surg 1976;111:532.

464

347. Wood RP, Shaw BW Jr, Starzl TE. Extrahepatic complications of liver transplantation. Semin Liver Dis 1985;5:377.

348. Young CN, Meyers AM. Opportunistic fungal infection by *Fusarium oxysporum* in a renal transplant patient. Sabouraudia 1979;17:219.

349. Young LS, Stevens P, Kaijser B. Gram-negative pathogens in septicaemic infections. Scand J Infect Dis 1982;31:78.

350. Zarrabi MH, Rosner F. Serious infections in adults following splenectomy for trauma. Arch Intern Med 1984;144:1421.

351. Ziegler EJ, McCutchan JA, Fierer J, et al. Treatment of gram-negative bacteremia and shock with human antiserum to a mutant *Escherichia coli.* N Engl J Med 1982;307:1225.

20

○　　○　　○　　●　　●　　●

INFECTION IN
TRAUMA SURGERY

J. Wayne Meredith
Donald D. Trunkey

Trauma is a serious public health problem in the United States; it annually accounts for more than 145,000 deaths and the loss of more potential years of life than any other disease. There is a trimodal distribution of death following trauma. Approximately 50% of deaths occur within minutes of the accident. These patients die primarily from lacerations of the brain, brain stem, spinal cord, aorta, and rupture of the myocardial chambers. The second death peak occurs within hours of the injury, usually due to head injury (epidural, subdural, and intracerebral hematomas) or hemorrhage from major viscera or blood vessels. The third death peak constitutes approximately 20% of the total deaths and occurs days or weeks after the injury. The great majority of late deaths (78%) are due to sepsis and multiple organ failure.[6]

Although most infectious complications after trauma cluster in the latter phase of patient management (*i.e.,* days to weeks following injury), prevention of these events begins on arrival to the trauma center and must continue throughout the patient's hospitalization. Prevention of infection requires an understanding of the factors that predispose the trauma patient subsequently to develop infection or

466

multiple organ failure. It also requires appropriate treatment of the patient's injuries and compulsive management of the patient in the postoperative supportive care phase.

EFFECTS OF TRAUMA
THAT PREDISPOSE TO INFECTION

The Effects of Trauma on the Immune System

Traumatic shock and resuscitation have profound effects on the patient's immune system, which subsequently affect the ability to ward off infection. In most patients these effects are healthy and contribute to the patient's recovery; however, the severely injured patient may develop defects in the immune response that contribute to subsequent infection. An understanding of the immune system and of the effects trauma has on it is important in understanding the subsequent development of infection. For convenience, Fauci has divided the immune system into the nonspecific and the specific immune systems.[24] Although there is considerable overlap between the two systems, separating them greatly facilitates their discussion (Table 20-1).

Nonspecific Immune Response

The nonspecific immune system mediates a general inflammatory response to injury and provides for removal of destroyed and devitalized cells and bacteria. It

Table 20–1
Elements of the Immune System

NONSPECIFIC	SPECIFIC
Barrier mechanisms	Cellular
Skin	T lymphocytes
Mucous membranes	Helper/suppressor
Cellular	Effector/amplifier
Neutrophils	B lymphocyte
Macrophage	Monocytes
Eosinophils	Facilitory/inhibition
Humoral	Humoral
Complement system	Lymphokines/monokines
Coagulation system	Interleukins I, II
Fibrinolytic system	PGE_2
	Cachectin

includes the neutrophils and the macrophages as well as elements of the coagulation cascade, the complement cascade, and other plasma proteins.

The neutrophil is one of the major classes of phagocytic cells. Proper neutrophil function requires chemotaxis, phagocytosis, and intracellular killing. Decreased neutrophil chemotaxis has been well documented following trauma.[13,63] This appears to be related to a cellular defect of the polymorphonuclear neutrophil leukocytes (PMN) as well as to a serum inhibitory factor directed at the PMN. Both of these alterations occur early following injury.[51,60] Another step in neutrophil function is engulfment of the invading organism, phagocytosis, a complex process that requires interaction of various segments of the specific and nonspecific immune systems. Trauma causes alteration in several of the phagocytic processes, including decreased antibody production, increased complement system activity, and changes in macrophage function, each of which results in impairment of phagocytic ability. Once the neutrophil has ingested the microorganism, it must retain the ability to kill it. Neutrophil intracellular killing function does not appear to be depressed following hemorrhage or trauma,[23] although there is evidence of a defect in intracellular killing following burns.[2]

The macrophage is a pivotal cell in the inflammatory response and acts as a mediator of both the specific and nonspecific immune systems. Within the nonspecific immune system, the macrophage acts both as a phagocytic cell, subject to the same alterations as is the neutrophil, and as a director of the inflammatory response. The macrophage also plays a role in the regulation of the coagulation-fibrinolytic system. The macrophage/monocyte produces both plasminogen activator and tissue thromboplastin, or causes the endothelial cell to produce these substances. Plasminogen activator acts to convert plasminogen to plasmin and thus promotes fibrinolysis, while tissue thromboplastin activates the extrinsic system of coagulation by combining with factor VII. Victims of major trauma exhibit transient decreases in plasminogen activator production by macrophages. Sustained decreases in production correlate with septic complications.[64]

Another important element of the nonspecific immune system is the complement cascade. The complement system represents a series of powerful, rapidly acting plasma glycoproteins. These are mostly enzymatic proteins synthesized by the liver and by macrophages, and they exist in a nonactive state in normal plasma. Activation of the complement system results in a rapidly multiplying cascade pattern analogous to the coagulation cascade. Complement can be activated by either the classical or alternate pathway. The classical pathway is activated by the antigen–antibody complex. The alternate pathway, or properdin pathway, is initiated by the cleavage of C-3 into C-3A and C-3B. This can be initiated by certain proteases released from the destruction of cells or by components of host cell membranes or of bacterial cell walls (endotoxin). Activated complement or elements of the complement cascade cause chemotaxis of phagocytic and inflammatory cells, capillary permeability and smooth muscle contraction, as well as opsonization of antigen. Trauma causes an activation of complement. The degree of complement activation varies directly with injury severity.[47] If injury is very severe, as in burns or major crush type injuries, the activation of complement can be so exaggerated as to be pathologic. If the devitalized tissue is not removed, it stimulates a constant release of biologically active complement components (*e.g.,* C-3A, C-5A), which, on reaching the systemic circulation, cause vascular permeability and PMN aggregation and uncontrolled activation of the inflammatory response resulting in distant tissue damage and possibly multiple organ failure.[3, 12, 36]

An important but frequently overlooked element of the nonspecific immune system is the integrity of the patient's skin and mucous membranes. Alterations in the integument are obvious after direct trauma or burns. Alterations in GI barriers are less intuitively obvious, however; recent evidence shows that with shock and trauma and with prolonged absence of enteral feedings there is a breakdown of the integrity of the gut mucosal barrier.[32, 74, 77, 84] This alteration of mucosal integrity allows bacteria and/or their by-products, such as endotoxin, to enter the portal bloodstream. West and co-workers have shown that exposure of Kupffer's cells to endotoxin or killed *Escherichia coli* results in an initial rise followed by a profound depression of protein synthesis in its neighbor hepatocyte.[93, 94] Others have reported a significant proportion of multiple organ failure patients in whom no site of infection or bacteremia are ever identified.[10, 12] A breakdown in gut mucosal barrier has been postulated in these patients as a mechanism for the formation of multiple organ failure. It seems to be preventable by early administration of enteral nutrition,[32, 84] which may preserve the integrity of the mucosal barrier and IGA synthesis.

Specific Immune Response

The specific immune system is composed of the macrophages and two classes of lymphocytes, one originating in the thymus called T cells and the other a bursa equivalent or B cell. Immunocompetence requires a complex interaction among these three cellular elements of the specific immune system and their mediators (the interleukins, monokines, and lymphokines). One of the results of this interaction is the production of specific antibody by the B or bursa equivalent cells. The bursa equivalent cells are so named because they are analogous to cells originating in the bursa of Fabricius found in the chicken. No analogous structure has been identified in humans, although Peyer's patches have been suggested. B cells constitute about 15% of peripheral blood lymphocytes and are found primarily in the lymph nodes, spleen, and bone marrow. B cells and their derivatives, the plasma cells, produce immunoglobulins, which have specific activity against microorganisms.

The lymphocytes that differentiate under thymic influence are termed T cells. These constitute approximately 80% of peripheral blood lymphocytes. Using monoclonal antibody techniques, subsets of T lymphocytes can be identified by the presence of specific antigens on their surfaces. T cells with the OKT-4 marker are designated helper T cells. Helper T cells can be activated by a complex interaction among T cell, antigen, and a macrophage/monocyte. Upon activation, the helper T cell stimulates differentiation and activation of B cells as well as the clonal expansion of other specific helper T cells, the enhancement of macrophage/monocyte activity, and the production of various cytokines. T cells with the OKT-8 membrane marker are designated suppressor cells and regulate the specific immune system. Overall immune competence in part depends on the balance between helper and suppressor T cells. Recent studies have shown a depression of total T-cell numbers as well as a depression of helper cell-to-suppressor cell ratios following trauma. The degree of depression varies directly with the injury severity score. Greater than 50% depression is significantly associated with the occurrence of sepsis.[72]

The third essential cellular element in the specific immune system is the monocyte/macrophage. At least two classes of these cells have been identified, the facilitory macrophage and the inhibitory macrophage. The facilitory macrophage engulfs antigen, which leads to the expression of a specific class 2 HLA antigen on the cell surface. This antigen is termed the immune response antigen (IA). The presentation by the macrophage of foreign antigen and IA to the T cell is required for proper T-cell activation. The facilitory macrophage also produces the cytokine interleukin-1, also called endogenous pyrogen. This substance has the systemic effects of producing fever and activating the acute phase response. Interleukin-1 is also a potent stimulus for the synthesis and release of the cytokine interleukin-2 from T lymphocytes, which, in turn, is required for the rapid proliferation, clonal expansion, of specific B and helper T lymphocytes.

The inhibitory monocyte/macrophage produces the monokine prostaglandin E-2 (PGE-2), which negatively regulates interleukin-1 production and the expression of IA antigen and inhibits T-cell proliferation directly.

Trauma causes defects in macrophage function at several levels. Mitogen responsiveness, as measured by response to phytohemagglutinin (PH-A), has been shown to be depressed following injury. This identifies a defect in the interaction between macrophage and T cell, which, when sustained, correlates with septic complications.[64] A preponderance of inhibitory macrophages and T suppressor cells have also been identified in post-traumatic and splenectomy patients.[65] Other workers have identified a defect in the presentation of immune antigen to helper T cells by macrophages in burned mice, which is corrected by administration of interleukin-1.[49] This finding may be due to a preponderance of inhibitory macrophages that produce PGE-2, thus inhibiting interleukin-1 production by the facilitory macrophage. Other alterations in macrophage function include changes in macrophage production of plasminogen activator and tissue thromboplastin. The production of plasminogen activator has been shown to be depressed following trauma while the macrophage production of tissue thromboplastin has been shown to be augmented. Both of these findings when persistent are associated with septic complications.[66] Depressed macrophage migration responsiveness has also been identified[4] and is caused by circulating activated complement factors C-5A and C-3A. This depression of chemotaxis reaches a maximum at 5 to 7 days following injury and gradually reverts to normal during the second week after injury.

In summary, shock and tissue injury cause activation of inflammation, which includes a nonspecific and a specific response. In most instances of mild or moderate injury, the inflammatory response is well controlled and contributes to healing and clearance of infection. For reasons that are not completely understood yet, the severely injured patient may develop defects in the immune system, which, in turn, contribute to sepsis in the host and become part of the pathophysiology of sepsis and multiple organ failure. This usually occurs relatively late in the postinjury period (1 to 3 weeks). Obviously, other factors predispose to failure of specific organ systems or to multiple organ failure syndrome.

Factors Predisposing to Post-Traumatic Pulmonary Insufficiency

Respiratory failure is a frequent cause of death in trauma patients who survive beyond the first 48 hr post injury. Several factors resulting from injury or resuscitation predispose the patient to subsequent respiratory failure. Soft tissue and organ injury cause activation of the nonspecific inflammatory response. This causes an influx of inflammatory cells and activation of the complement and coagulation cascade systems. Hypotension and shock cause sludging in the microcirculation and further accumulation of platelets, debris and microemboli. When resuscitation is begun, these products are released back into the circulation. The first microcirculatory bed they meet is the lung. These products of tissue degradation and platelet emboli lodge in the pulmonary microcirculation where they can activate the complement system.[76] This, in turn, leads to chemotaxis and activation of neutrophils, which produces a local, pulmonary, nonspecific inflammatory response resulting in direct endothelial damage.[29,37] These factors may serve to set the stage for subsequent pulmonary failure.

The concept of preventing post-traumatic pulmonary insufficiency by administration of colloid solutions during resuscitation is erroneous. Tranbaugh and co-workers have studied severely traumatized patients and found little evidence to support the thesis of early increased capillary permeability in this setting.[89] Their patients were resuscitated with crystalloid solutions to a euvolemic state, and they found no increase in extravascular lung water. This finding is supported by the work of Demling,[17] who in animal models found only a small increase in pulmonary capillary permeability, which was easily accommodated by increased lymphatic flow and is not associated with any increase in lung weight. In fact, Tranbaugh and co-workers found that significant increases in extravascular lung water, a measure of pulmonary capillary permeability, do not occur in the traumatized patient until 7 to 21 days following injury and are usually associated with systemic or pulmonary sepsis.[89] Many authors have reported the association between sepsis and pulmonary failure, both as a part of the multiple organ system failure syndrome and as a single organ system failure.[12,54] The exact mechanism of pulmonary injury during sepsis has not been concisely defined, but substantial evidence indicates activation of the nonspecific inflammatory response as a consequence of the ongoing infection.

Factors Predisposing to Renal Failure

Post-traumatic renal insufficiency became recognized as an important entity during World War II. The morbidity and mortality continued through the Korean War, but since then, with improvement in fluid resuscitation, it is becoming less common. The mortality, however, remains high. The causes and mechanisms are still debated. Certainly, hypotension and hypovolemia are causative or contributory elements in most patients with this syndrome. Tubular precipitation with sludging and mechanical blockage have all been implicated, although the exact mechanisms are not clearly defined. Hemoglobinuria and myoglobinuria secondary to crush injuries, massive burns, prolonged limb ischemia or hemolytic transfusion reactions also cause or contribute to renal failure in the trauma patient. Pigmenturia should be treated by appropriate volume replacement, maintenance of generous urine output, and by administration of sodium bicarbonate to alkalize the urine and prevent crystallization.

During resuscitation, the trauma patient is potentially exposed to various nephrotoxic drugs, including aminoglycosides, cephaloridine, or methoxyflurane (general anesthesia). Most of these agents can be avoided, especially in this phase of management, and every effort should be made to do so. Most late renal failure is associated with an administration of nephrotoxic agents or with the onset of sepsis or multiple organ failure syndrome.

DEFINITIVE TREATMENT OF INJURIES

The most important factor predisposing to infection in the trauma patient is the injury itself, which may result in a loss of skin integrity, tissue devitalization, and exogenous or endogenous contamination. Appropriate treatment is essential and entails removal of devitalized tissue, cleansing of all contamination, and repair of the injuries in such a manner as to ensure proper healing and eliminate further contamination. A complete discussion of all possible injuries is not within the scope of this discussion. We will, therefore, confine our comments to a few selected injuries of particular interest.

Head Injuries

Head injuries are a common occurrence in our automobile-oriented society and account for nearly half of the deaths from blunt trauma.[6] CNS infection is a very serious albeit uncommon complication from head injury. Most post-traumatic CNS infections resulting from head trauma occur following open injuries. These include compound skull fractures, basilar skull fractures, and penetrating injuries. A skull fracture is compound if there is an associated scalp laceration. All too frequently these scalp lacerations are sutured without proper exploration or irrigation and debridement. Jennett found this to be the most common reason for a patient to be referred to a neurosurgeon with an established infection.[42] It usually occurs in patients with little or no alteration of consciousness, leaving the primary physician less suspicious for skull fracture and head injury. All scalp lacerations should be explored for fracture or debris and should then be irrigated thoroughly and debrided prior to closure.

Another type of open fracture is the basilar skull fracture, which results in a CSF leak. The leak may be into the sinuses (frontal, ethmoid, maxillary, or sphenoid) or into the ear. CSF otorrhea usually resolves spontaneously within 1 to 2 weeks and leads to meningitis less commonly than does CSF rhinorrhea.[57] Cerebrospinal fluid rhinorrhea should be treated expectantly for 2 to 3 weeks, and, if drainage persists, the fistula should be closed surgically. Meningitis develops in up to 25% of patients with CSF rhinorrhea.[42] The role of prophylactic antibiotics in this entity is controversial, although penicillin prophylaxis is a common practice. Probably the best data are included in a randomized control study by Ignelzi and VanderArk[40] which did not show any benefit from prophylactic antibiotics. In fact, their results suggested those patients placed on antibiotics merely developed organisms resistant to the antibiotic coverage.

Thoracic Injuries

In most patients with chest trauma, tube thoracostomy will be the definitive management for both hemothorax and pneumothorax. The critical factor in preventing subsequent empyema is complete reexpansion of the lung and obliteration of any space between the visceral and parietal pleuras. This cannot be overemphasized. The pleural surfaces can overcome contamination if there is a visceroparietal pleural apposition. If the lung cannot be completely reexpanded by a single chest tube, an explanation must be sought. Improper tube placement or improper suction are the most common culprits and require mechanical correction or placement of another chest tube. Massive air leaks should alert the surgeon to consider bronchial disruption and perform early bronchoscopy. An occasional cause of failure to reexpand the lung completely is persistent blood in the pleural space. Some authors advocate early thoracotomy and evacuation of clots in these patients.[38] We agree in principle that the pleural space must be evacuated and the visceral and parietal pleuras must be opposed. In actual practice, this is rarely an indication for thoracotomy in and of itself. The motion of the lung and diaphragm and the nature of the pleural surfaces promote early autolysis of clot in the pleural space. Most patients who have sufficient bleeding to overcome this thrombolytic tendency have sufficient bleeding to require thoracotomy for control of hemorrhage. Clotted hemothorax is preventable with adequate chest drainage, as shown by Wilson and co-workers.[95] Of 452 patients with traumatic hemothorax, no patient was operated on with the sole indication being retained clot. In 290 of these patients, complete drainage was achieved by tube thoracostomy. In another 118, there was incomplete drainage by the chest tube, although 78 of these had minimal residuals and recovered uneventfully. Forty patients had significant residual hemothorax; of these, 21 required thoracentesis or late chest tube insertion, and 6 developed empyema.

Abdominal Injuries

The spillage of gastrointestinal tract contents into the peritoneal cavity greatly increases the risk of postoperative infection; therefore, the proper management of these injuries is critical. Delays in diagnosis or missed injuries result in serious intra-abdominal infection and account for many of the late mortalities from abdominal trauma. These complications and deaths are totally avoidable by prompt thorough exploratory celiotomy within a few hours of injury.

Liver Injuries

The liver is the most commonly injured organ in patients with penetrating trauma and the second most commonly injured organ following blunt trauma. The immediate concern in most liver injuries is control of hemorrhage, which usually can be achieved easily with suture repair, cautery, or topical hemostatic agents. In more severe injuries, hemostasis may be accomplished by packing, hepatotomy with suture ligation of bleeding points, or by resection of the injured segments.[11,27,67,73] Occasionally, selective hepatic artery ligation is required. Hepatic vein injuries are particularly difficult to manage, and a variety of techniques are available to isolate the vena-cava blood flow, although results with any of these techniques remain suboptimal.

The nature of the injury and interventions required for control of hemorrhage lead to an incidence of intra-abdominal sepsis as high as 40% in patients with serious liver trauma (Table 20-2). There is great potential for dead space formation following hepatic resection, as well as potential for development of a hematoma by continued oozing from raw liver surfaces. There may be residual devitalized liver tissue as well. These factors, combined with the potential for bile leakage and the frequency of contamination by associated hollow viscus injuries, contribute to the formation of intra-abdominal abscess. Prevention of this infection requires attention to each of the above factors. Dead space can be prevented by avoidance of liver resection when possible.[11,27,67,73] If the liver injury is extensive and involves both lobes, we currently recommend management by packing of the hepatic injury to obtain hemostasis and to allow resuscitation in the intensive care unit (ICU) until coagulopathy, hypothermia, and metabolic acidosis can be corrected. The patient is then returned to the operating room, where the packing is removed and the injury is reinspected. Debridement of devitalized tissue is then performed, and meticulous hemostasis is obtained by direct suture ligature of bleeding points. Bile leakage is controlled in a similar manner. Potential dead space within deep crevices in the liver can be filled by placing a vascularized pedicle of omentum within the injury as described by Stone and Lamb.[88] At this time, thorough irrigation of the abdominal cavity is again performed, and inspection of associated injuries is also permitted.

Most liver lacerations can be managed without draining.[67] The principle is to

Table 20–2
Intra-abdominal Infection in Severe Hepatic Injuries

	MORTALITY (%)	INFECTION (%)	SEPTIC DEATHS (%)
Moore[67]	39	15.8	5.3
Pachter[72]	5.3	4	0
Feliciano[27]	10	40	10
Carmona[11]	12	29	6

drain bile, not blood. In serious injuries where it is suspected that intrahepatic biliary ducts will postoperatively leak significant quantities of bile, draining is required. This drainage should be through a separate stab wound using a large, soft sump tube and a closed technique.[28] Most liver injuries do not fall into this category, however, and are best managed without drainage.

Spleen Injuries

Splenic injury is common and, until recently, has been routinely treated by splenectomy. The recognition of the syndrome of overwhelming postsplenectomy sepsis in 1952[48] has led to the development of new understanding of the role of the spleen in host resistance and an emphasis on maintaining splenic function despite splenic injury.

It is now recognized that splenectomy is associated with numerous defects in the immune system. One of its most important immune functions is the clearance and processing of circulating antigens. The spleen receives a generous blood supply, 5% of cardiac output, 90% of which passes through the splenic sinuses where it comes in contact with splenic macrophages. Whereas, the liver will clear circulating bacteria that are opsonized, the spleen is required for efficient removal of those bacteria that are poorly opsonized, especially encapsulated organisms. The asplenic patient, therefore, may retain near-normal resistance to previously encountered organisms, which induce an amnastic response but will be susceptible to infection, occasionally fulminant, by newly encountered organisms.

Interaction among antigen, macrophages, and lymphocytes is also required for the development of an antibody response. The asplenic patient exhibits depressed levels of IgM and defective switching from an IgM to an IgG response.[55]

Loss of opsonization from poor antibody production may be compounded by the depression of circulating tuftsin and properdin levels following splenectomy. Tuftsin is a circulating tetrapeptide that stimulates motility and phagocytic activity of PMN, through an interaction with PMN-bound leukokinin. Properdin acts to initiate the alternate pathway of complement. Levels of both tuftsin and properdin are depressed in asplenic patients, but both are also produced by other organs, potentially lessening the significance of this depression.

The immune compromise resulting from splenectomy predisposes the patient to subsequent infection. The clinical significance of this predisposition was described by King and Shumacker[48] in 1952 and termed overwhelming postsplenectomy infection (OPSI) by Diamond[19] in 1969. This syndrome is characterized by an abrupt onset with a mild or absent prodrome followed by a florid bacteremia and fulminant course from apparent good health to coma or death in less than 24 hr. The syndrome occurs more frequently in children but may occur at any age. Most instances of OPSI occur within 2 years of splenectomy, but cases have been reported decades after splenectomy.[80] The risk of OPSI depends somewhat on the underlying condition requiring splenectomy.[22] The lowest risk group is the trauma patient[61] in whom the risk of postsplenectomy infection is 0.5% to 1%, which nonetheless represents a 50-fold increase over the population at large.

The most effective mechanism for preventing postsplenectomy infection is avoiding splenectomy. Many splenic injuries can be easily managed with splenic preservation. Small capsular tears can be managed by local hemostatic means, and more severe injuries can be managed by splenorrhaphy techniques.[21] Approximately 50% to 60% of splenic injuries can be managed by local hemostatic measures or splenic repair.[26,50,71] In those patients in whom splenorrhaphy is not possible, either due to the severity of the injury or instability of the patient due to other injuries, other methods must be used to minimize the risk of postsplenectomy sepsis. None of these other measures is as effective, however, as an intact spleen.

The first of these other measures to have been considered is iatrogenic splenosis. It has been shown that small fragments of spleen can be transplanted to the lesser sack, omentum, or abdominal wall. These fragments will grow and elicit blood supply from surrounding tissues. It appears, however, that a critical mass of spleen and a critical blood flow to the splenic tissue are required for preservation of the immunologic effects of the spleen. These transplanted, "born again spleen," fragments lack sufficient mass and sufficient blood supply to perform this function. Splenosis as an alternative to splenic preservation cannot be recommended.

Postoperatively, patients undergoing splenectomy should receive pneumococcal vaccine (Pneumovax). This is a polyvalent vaccine to pneumococcal polysaccharide of 14 pneumococcal serotypes. A newer vaccine containing 23 serotypes, which is active against 95% of the serotypes associated with pneumococcal infection, is now available. For many reasons, these vaccinations provide incomplete protection against overwhelming postsplenectomy sepsis. Pneumovax confers incomplete protection against all types of pneumococci, does not produce specific antibody in all immunized patients, and has not prevented pneumococcemia in some immunized patients.[26] Furthermore, OPSI is caused by pneumococcus in only 50% of cases. Oral penicillin prophylaxis may be indicated in infants but is not indicated in adults.

Duodenum Injuries

Duodenal injuries can be treacherous, especially if there is a delay in diagnosis, and even with prompt and appropriate operation may be associated with intra-abdominal infectious complications in as many as 26% of patients (Table 20-3). An

Table 20-3
Intra-abdominal Infection in Duodenal Injuries

	MORTALITY (%)	INFECTION (%)	SEPTIC DEATHS (%)
Ivatury[41]	25	26	9.5
Levison[53]	18.3	18.3	8.6
Stone[86]	13	16	1.6–3.7

476

extensive Kocher maneuver is required for adequate examination and mobilization of the duodenum. In this manner, the duodenum should be visually examined from the pylorus to the ligament of Treitz. The management of the injury will depend on its nature. Penetrating wounds without much devitalization may be closed primarily. When combined with biliary ductal injuries or pancreatic injuries, the surgeon must be more creative. The repair must involve suturing only viable, healthy tissue and preferably reconstruction of the biliary, pancreatic, and gastrointestinal tracts. Eighty percent of penetrating injuries and 45% of blunt injuries to the duodenum can be managed by debridement and primary repair.[53] Severe crush injuries of the duodenum and head of the pancreas may require pancreatoduodenectomy. This injury is rare, however, and most duodenal injuries can be managed without this extensive surgery. Other options include serosal patches, Roux-en-Y duodenal jejunostomies, pyloric exclusion, or Berne duodenal diverticulization.[8, 14, 20, 21, 53, 86, 91] The surgeon must be prepared to manage the duodenal injury by any of these methods.

Duodenal injuries should be decompressed by use of a retrograde tube placed through the jejunum or an antegrade tube placed through a gastrostomy. The retrograde tubes give the advantage of allowing feeding jejunostomy to be performed with the same loop of jejunum.[53, 86] The use of drains is somewhat controversial. Our policy is to avoid drainage of the duodenal closure itself.[53] Stone and Fabian also report excellent results without the use of drains.[86]

Pancreas Injuries

Failure to recognize pancreatic injuries significantly increases the morbidity and mortality of this injury.[85] The retroperitoneal location of the pancreas may prevent the diagnosis of some pancreatic injuries by peritoneal lavage, which can be recognized with CT scanning of the abdomen.[25] However, no nonoperative diagnostic maneuver can recognize all pancreatic injuries or totally excluded pancreatic injury. Smego and co-workers[85] have classified pancreatic injuries as grade one: contusion or hematoma; grade two: minor capsular and parenchymal disruption; grade three: major ductal injury; and grade four: severe crush. A critical feature in preventing subsequent pancreatic fistula or abscess is in recognizing ductal injury. The likelihood of ductal injury increases in higher grade injuries. Ductal injuries should be suspected if there is severe maceration or complete transection of the pancreas as well as laceration of more than half of the thickness of the pancreas, a central perforation of the pancreas, or direct visualization duct injury. Using a strict protocol of thorough pancreatic visualization and distal pancreatic resection in patients with ductal injuries, Smego and co-workers[85] report a pancreas-related mortality of 3% in 72 consecutive patients with pancreatic injuries (Table 20-4). Delay in diagnosis contributed to both deaths. These results are admirable, and their duplication requires a high index of suspicion, compulsive search for injury, and aggressive treatment.

Colon Injuries

During World War II, surgeons recognized that exteriorization of colon wounds by colostomy resulted in a striking reduction in mortality and morbidity. There was

Table 20–4
Intra-abdominal Infection in Pancreatic Injuries

	MORTALITY (%)	INFECTION (%)	SEPTIC DEATHS (%)
Smego[85]	29	6.7	6.9
Jones[44]	20	18.1	4.7
Graham[33]	16.3	8	6–8

further reduction in complications of colon injury observed during the Korean conflict.[81] Recently, several authors have reported satisfactory results with selected primary repair (Table 20-5). In 1979, Stone and Fabian[87] reported a randomized prospective study of 268 patients with colon injuries. Patients who had preoperative shock, massive hemorrhage, multiple organs injured, significant contamination, delay to surgery, or destructive wounds received mandatory colostomy. The remaining patients were randomized between colostomy and primary repair. Patients randomized to primary repair had better results than patients randomized to colostomy. Primary repair also resulted in a shorter hospital stay and decreased cost, not including cost of reoperation for colostomy closure. Primary repair has been favorably reported by others.[1,30,68] Subsequently, several authors have reported extending the indications for primary repair to include patients requiring resection of the right colon with primary anastomoses. We recommend primary repair only of simple lacerations not associated with multiple injuries, bleeding, significant contamination, or shock. We favor end ileostomy and mucous fistula formation for right colon injuries requiring resection, and end colostomy and mucous fistula for other colon injuries requiring resection. Colon injuries should not be drained.[87]

Rectal injuries are a subset of colon injuries. They should be treated by a proximal totally diverting colostomy, presacral drainage, and irrigation of the fecal contents from the rectum if the rectal wound has been repaired.

Table 20–5
Intra-abdominal Infection in Colon Injuries

	MORTALITY (%)	INFECTION (%)	SEPTIC DEATHS (%)
Flint[30]	16	24.8	6
Adkins[1]	3.6	7.1	1.8
Stone[87]	7.5	28	1.1

POSTOPERATIVE CARE

Prevention of Infection in Patients with Head Injury

Patients with severe head trauma are commonly slow in recovering and often require prolonged ICU support. During this phase, they are susceptible to the same nosocomial infections as any other ICU patients. In addition, these patients may have intracranial pressure (ICP) monitors in place for variable periods of time. Mayhall and co-workers[62] in a prospective study found that 11% of patients treated with ventricular ICP monitors developed ventriculitis or meningitis. They believed the risk of infection to be directly related to the duration of catheterization, although Kanter and Weiner[46] found the risk to be diminished after the sixth day.[46] There was no difference in patients treated with prophylactic antibiotics versus patients without. Aucoin[4] found the subarachnoid screw was associated with the lowest infection rate, followed by the subdural cup catheter and the ventriculostomy. Use of bacitracin flush solutions increased the risk of infection, and prophylactic antibiotics had no significant benefit. Aseptic technique must be strictly observed not only in the insertion of the monitor, but in the irrigation, zeroing, and other manipulations required for day to day maintenance.

In addition to the problems posed by disruptions in cranial integrity, the head injury patient also poses special problems related to level of consciousness. The comatose patient is susceptible to pressure sores, which may serve as a source of sepsis. This complication is preventable by frequently turning the patient and using water mattresses or similar devices to distribute pressure evenly. Obtunded patients are also predisposed to aspiration of gastric contents. In this patient population, the combination of depressed gag reflexes and the requirement for long-term nutritional support make aspiration an all too frequent occurrence. The risk of aspiration can be minimized by elevating the head of the bed and by feeding distal to the pylorus whenever possible, such as through a feeding jejunostomy (placed at the time of exploratory laparotomy) or by a transnasal Dobhoff type feeding tube. Continuous infusion is preferable to bolus feedings.

Prevention of Thoracic Infections in the Trauma Patient

Patients with thoracic trauma are prone to develop serious infections. Walker and co-workers[92] studied 310 consecutive patients with thoracic trauma and found 33% of those who survived greater than 5 days developed a thoracic infection. Seventy-one percent of deaths in these patients were due to systemic sepsis. Factors contributing to an increased risk of infection include blunt chest injury and prolonged endotracheal intubation. Patients with blunt chest trauma and flail chest can often be managed without ventilator support if given careful fluid management, pulmonary toilet, and close observation.[78, 90] Flail chest has three physiologic components. The most obvious, impaired chest wall mechanics, is usually the least significant of the three, although in some patients primary stabilization of rib fractures is indicated. The second physiologic component, pulmonary contusion, underlies many flail chest injuries, and its severity largely determines prognosis. Pulmonary contusion represents blood and edema in the pulmonary parenchyma about which little can be done. Pulmonary contusion results in an intrapulmonary shunt and hypoxia of variable degree. Ventilatory support should be instituted if respiratory failure ensues (Table 20-6). Fluid overload must be avoided. The third component of flail chest is a painful chest wall injury, which causes splinting and discourages deep breathing, coughing, and effective pulmonary toilet—common precursors of pneumonia. Judicious use of narcotics, intercostal nerve blocks, or epidural narcotic analgesics can be effective in either avoiding intubation or getting the patient off the ventilator, by improving pulmonary toilet. The latter modality significantly increases vital capacity and inspiratory force and provides pain relief, which is necessary for good coughing and deep breathing.[59]

Another important modality in the prevention of pulmonary infection is early mobilization of the patient. This requires early immobilization of long bone fractures. We recommend fracture fixation on admission if the patient's condition permits. If the patient is hemodynamically unstable, hypothermic, or demonstrates coagulopathy, he or she should be taken to the ICU and these problems should be corrected. The patient can then be returned to the operating room for fracture fixation within 12 to 36 hr. Early fixation of fractures has been shown to result in fewer deaths from remote multiple organ failure[32] and a significantly decreased incidence of pulmonary failure, fracture complications, positive blood cultures, and decreased narcotic requirements[12,31,84] (Table 20-7).

Prevention of Urinary Tract Infections

The urinary tract is especially prone to infection during the recovery phase from trauma. Chronic indwelling Foley and/or suprapubic catheters associated with the ICU milieu make colonization of the urinary tract common. The classic criteria for making the diagnosis of urinary tract infection, growth of greater than 10^5 organisms per milliliter of urine, should be tempered with clinical judgment prior to the institution of

Table 20–6
Indications for Mechanical Ventilation

PARAMETER	NORMAL	VENTILATOR INDICATED
Respiratory rate	12–20/min	>35/min
PCO_2	35–40 torr	>50 torr
Vital capacity	65–70 ml/kg	<10–15 ml/kg
Inspiratory force	> −60 cm H_2O	< −30 cm H_2O
Shunt	<5%	>15%

Table 20–7
Early Fracture Fixation versus Femur Traction

PARAMETER	EARLY FIXATION	10 DAYS TRACTION PRIOR TO FIXATION	30 DAYS TRACTION
ICU Days	7.5	15	27
Days on ventilator	3.4	9.7	21
Days febrile	3.8	8.8	13
% Patients with + blood culture	5%	40%	66%
% Fracture complications	4.2%	15.7%	75%

(Data from Seibel R, LaDuca J, Hassett JM, et al. Blunt multiple trauma (155 36), femur traction, and the pulmonary failure-septic state. Ann Surg 1985;202:283.)

antibiotics, which may promote overgrowth of more virulent organisms and cannot prevent colonization. Invasive infection, however, must be treated with antibiotics. Every effort must be made to discontinue catheter drainage as early as feasible.

TREATMENT OF INFECTIONS

CNS Infections

Treatment of post-traumatic meningitis is by intravenous antibiotics and closure of CSF fistulas if they persist. Osteomyelitis of the skull requires systemic antibiotics and aggressive debridement of devitalized bone.[5] Subdural and epidural empyemas can present as life-threatening space-occupying masses and are treated with craniotomy and drainage and debridement of devitalized tissue. Mortality for subdural empyema remains high.[5]

Pneumonia and Empyema

Occasionally, despite appropriate preventive measures, thoracic infection will develop in the severely injured patient. When this occurs, early diagnosis and appropriate treatment are essential. The diagnosis of pneumonia is difficult in the multiple trauma patient but may be made with the demonstration of: (1) a clinical picture of infection, (2) new pulmonary infiltrate on chest x-ray, and (3) properly obtained sputum specimen that demonstrates many polymorphonuclear white blood cells and a predominant organism. Pneumonia is treated by administration of appropriate antibiotics based on sputum and Gram's stain culture results. Occasionally, the patient will require bronchoscopy for removal of inspissated mucous plugs and to ensure there is no foreign body, such as a tooth or a blood clot, left in the bronchial tree.

Empyema in the trauma patient has an incidence of 4% to 5% in severely traumatized patients.[9] Predisposing factors include contamination of the pleural cavity, controlled mechanical ventilation, chest injuries, and high dose corticosteroids. *Staphylococcus aureus* is the most common organism, but gram-negative organisms have an increasing prevalence and account for nearly one half of isolates. If recognized early, most empyemas can be treated successfully by appropriate antibiotics and tube thoracostomy drainage. If recognized late or if adequate drainage cannot be obtained, rib resection and drainage will be required. Decortication to release trapped lung can be performed once infection has been cleared.[38]

Intra-abdominal Infections

The incidence of intra-abdominal infection following abdominal trauma varies considerably with the type of trauma (penetrating versus blunt) and the organs injured.[70] The risk of infection is significantly increased with left colon injuries, with presence of shock on arrival, with increased age of the patient, and as the number of injured organs increases.[87] If a patient who has had an abdominal injury appears septic, the presence of an intraperitoneal abscess should be assumed until proven otherwise. Ultrasonography and computerized tomography are useful, with CT scan having a better sensitivity and specificity. Both modalities can be used to drain selected abscesses,[83] but surgical drainage is still the gold standard. We recommend reexploration through a midline abdominal wound with a thorough exploration of the abdomen and dependent drainage of all abscess cavities. Appropriate antibiotics should be based on Gram's stain and subsequent cultures. An aminoglycoside for aerobic gram-negatives and clindamycin, chloramphenicol or metronidazole for anaerobic organisms are chosen. If the patient's condition does not improve within 6 to 12 hr, residual septic foci should be suspected and sought out.

IATROGENIC INFECTIONS

Commonly, the severely traumatized patient will spend days to weeks in an ICU setting. This is a microbiologically hostile environment for an immunosuppressed patient with deficiencies in his intrinsic host defense mechanisms. Schimpff and co-workers[82] report a 60% incidence of nosocomial infections in trauma patients staying in the ICU 5 days or more. Furthermore, in a later study from the same institution[10] more than 82% of infections that occurred were nosocomial in origin. These were related to the various catheters and lines used for monitoring and therapy of the critically ill patients. These included infections from venous and arterial catheters, ICP monitors, empyema and pneumonia, sinusitis, and urinary tract infections. The most common single organism was *Staphylococcus aureus*, but this was outnumbered 2 to 1 by gram-negative infections.[10]

ICP monitors play an ever-increasing role in the management of patients with head injury and elevated ICP. The information they provide is valuable, but it is not without cost. ICP monitors have been associated with an 11% incidence of CNS infection.[4] Mayhall and co-workers[62] found an overall 9% incidence of infection associated with ICP monitors with an increasing risk of infection if the monitors are left in longer than 5 days. This increases to a 42% incidence of infection by day 11. These authors recommend careful surveillance of aseptic technique during insertion and maintenance of catheters as well as limiting irrigation of the system and replacing the catheter if it is needed longer than 5 days. Other authors[44] suggest frequent changes of catheters may increase risk of infection. The administration of corticosteroids to control intracranial hypertension is common, yet the data to support its effectiveness are contradictory. Demaria and co-workers[16] studied 197 consecutive patients with multiple trauma to define the infectious complication of corticosteroids. All deaths that occurred 5 or more days after injury were caused by sepsis and all occurred in steroid recipients. The study also showed that 47.5% of steroid-treated early survivors developed infectious complications, whereas only 14.5% of patients without steroids did so. Until further evidence demonstrating a clear-cut advantage in mortality from head injury is available, we do not recommend the use of steroids for this purpose.

Walker and co-workers[92] report a 33% incidence of thoracic infections (pneumonia and empyema) in patients with thoracic trauma. Seventy-one percent of their late deaths were caused by systemic sepsis. These authors report pulmonary infection was significantly increased following prolonged endotracheal intubation. Another study[57] suggests early colonization of tracheostomy tubes by various means, but most notably the hands of attending personnel. Clearly, aseptic technique in the management of endotracheal and tracheostomy tubes is essential as well as handwashing between patients. Another source of pulmonary sepsis is the endotracheal tube, and the patient should be extubated as early as clinically possible. Caplan and co-workers[10] reported a high incidence (10% of nosocomial infections) of empyema associated with tube thoracostomy. Most of these were tubes placed late in the patient's course and were associated with prolonged endotracheal intubation, corticosteroids, aspiration pneumonia, and prior respiratory infection. Similarly, there are numerous reports of infection related to intravenous lines, Foley catheters, and other tubes and monitoring devices associated with managing the trauma patient.[10,18,82] The trauma team must strive to remove the IV cutdowns and other invasive lines that are placed in emergency situations and under questionable aseptic technique early in the patient's course. If they are still needed, replace them with lines placed under more ideal circumstances. The use of drains should be minimized. Drains should not be used for the drainage of blood or hematoma in the trauma patient, rather they should be used for drainage of pus or contaminated body fluids.

PROPHYLACTIC ANTIBIOTICS

The proper use of prophylactic antibiotics has been shown to be useful in the prevention of wound infection, especially in elective surgery. However, the injudicious use of broad-spectrum antibiotics in the trauma patient merely alters the host flora and represents a loss of one of the patient's host defenses. The use of prophylactic antibiotics will be discussed by types of injury.

Head Injury

The use of prophylactic antibiotics in head injuries remains controversial. Most investigators agree that minor traumatic wounds do not benefit from prophylactic antibiotics.[39,79] Ignelzi and VanderArk[40] demonstrated no benefit from prophylactic antibiotics in patients with basilar skull fractures. Their results further suggest that the patient who receives antibiotics develops gram-negative organisms resistant to the antibiotics the patient is receiving. This is certainly consistent with the injudicious use of prophylactic antibiotics in other regions of the body.

Another controversial area is the treatment of compound fractures of the cranium. Multiple studies designed to show the efficacy of antibiotics have not done so. The rationale for their use falls back on the orthopedic surgery literature; specifically the paper by Patzakis and co-workers.[75] This may or may not be a valid assumption, and it is our feeling that there are insufficient data to make a rational decision.

Maxillofacial Injuries

In general, maxillofacial injuries do not require prophylactic antibiotics.[35] Exceptions would be destructive wounds or particularly untidy wounds. There may be instances where cosmetic considerations override optimal surgical management such as delayed primary closure. In these cases, prophylactic antibiotics may be warranted to optimize primary closure. Controlled randomized studies have not provided scientific evidence to support such management, however. Injuries to the neck do not require prophylactic antibiotics.

Thorax Injuries

Prophylactic antibiotics as an adjunctive treatment measure in injuries of the chest is controversial. The study most often quoted is that of Grover and co-workers[35] who, in a double-blind prospective study, showed that patients treated with clindamycin had lower incidences of radiographic pneumonia, fever, and positive pleural and wound cultures. It should be noted, however, that fever and radiographic pneumonia are not necessarily clinically significant. Even from a cost–benefit analysis, argument for prophylactic antibiotics is marginal. Statistical significance was not achieved in Grover's study between the antibiotic-treated and placebo groups.

More recently, a double-blind study conducted by LoCurto and co-workers[56] showed that patients having a tube thoracostomy performed for trauma had less infectious complications when treated prophylactically with cefoxitin as compared with placebo. It should be pointed out, however, that 30% of those patients who had tube thoracostomy treated with placebo had wound infections, which is much higher than would be expected.

In contrast, a study performed by LeBlanc and Tucker[52] showed no statistical difference when patients were randomized between antibiotics and placebo. It is our feeling that antibiotics should be used only when there is gross contamination of the pleural cavity by rupture of a hollow viscus such as the esophagus or contamination of the pleural cavity by gastric or bowel contents and associated violation of the diaphragm.

Abdominal Injuries

Most surgeons are agreed that trauma to the abdominal viscera causing contamination by small bowel or colon requires therapeutic use of antibiotics and not prophylaxis.[15, 35, 45, 67, 69, 70] Multiple studies show higher incidence of wound and intraperitoneal infectious complications when antibiotics are withheld. When antibiotics are used with peritoneal toilet and delayed primary wound closure, infectious complications can be kept to a minimum. Antibiotics should be started as soon after the injury as possible and preferably before surgery. The use of antibiotics for solid visceral injuries has not proven efficacious in prospective randomized clinical trials.

Fractures

The most frequently cited randomized study showing the efficacy of antibiotics in compound fractures was reported in 1974 by Patzakis and co-workers[75] who showed that control patients had an infection rate of 13.9%, while patients treated with penicillin and streptomycin had a 9.7% infection rate, and patients receiving cephalothin had a significantly lower infection rate of 2.3%. Most orthopedic surgeons use prophylactic antibiotics for compound fractures.

A more recent study by Bergman[7] classified wounds as grades 1, 2, and 3 based on degree of soft tissue associated injury; grade 3 being the worst. Grade 1 wounds, which had minimal soft tissue lesions, showed no statistical difference between saline and antibiotic. Grades 2 and 3 wounds, however, were best managed with antibiotics, and statistical significance was achieved. We believe this study emphasizes that not all compound fractures need to be treated with antibiotics. It further reemphasizes the principles of wound irrigation, debridement, and delayed primary closure of wounds; still the gold standard for treatment for traumatic wounds.

SUMMARY

In summary, infection is a common cause of death in trauma patients who survive more than 5 days. The trauma patient has changes in both his specific and nonspecific immune systems, which can become pathologically exaggerated and lead to multiple organ failure or produce immunosuppression and predispose to infection. Errors in technique or judgment in management of the patient's injuries will often result in postoperative infectious complications. All injuries must be recognized and appropriately treated in a timely fashion. Catheters, tubes, and drains should be used when indicated, realizing they serve as an important source of potential infection. These invasive devices should be removed as early as practical. Similarly, prophylactic antibiotics must be administered only when indicated and for a short course. Constant, meticulous attention to the details of patient management, as in all of surgery, will be rewarded by improved results and lower infection rates.

REFERENCES

1. Adkins RB Jr, Zirkle PK, Waterhouse G. Penetrating colon trauma. J Trauma 1984;24:491.
2. Alexander JW. Immunity, nutrition and trauma: an overview. Acta Chir Scand [Suppl] 1985;522:141.
3. Antrum RM, Solomkin JS. Monocyte dysfunction in severe trauma: evidence for the role of C5a in deactivation. Surgery 1986;100:29.
4. Aucoin PJ. Intracranial pressure monitors: epidemiologic study of risk factors and infections. JAMA 1986;80:369.
5. Bakay L, Glasauer FE. Head injury. Boston: Little, Brown & Co., 1980.
6. Baker CC, Oppenheimer L, Stephens B, el al. Epidemiology of trauma deaths. Am J Surg 1980;140:144.
7. Bergman BR. Antibiotic prophylaxis in open and closed fractures. A controlled clinical trial. Acta Orthop Scand 1982;53:57.
8. Berne CJ, Donovan AJ, White EF, et al. Duodenal "diverticulization" for duodenal and pancreatic injury. Am J Surg 1974;127:503.
9. Caplan ES, Hoyt NJ, Rodriguez A, et al. Empyema occurring in the multiply traumatized patient. J Trauma 1984;24:785.
10. Caplan ES, Joshi M, Hoyt N, et al. Changing patterns of infection and infection-related mortality in 10,308 multiply-traumatized patients over a 7 year period. J Trauma 1986;26:670.
11. Carmona RH, Peck DZ, Lim RC Jr. The role of packing and planned re-operation in severe hepatic trauma. J Trauma 1984;24:779.
12. Carrico CJ, Meakins JL, Marshall JC, et al. Multiple-organic-failure syndrome. Arch Surg 1986;121:196.
13. Christou NV, Meakins JL. Neutrophil function in surgical patients: two inhibitors of granulocyte chemotaxis associated with sepsis. J Srug Res 1979;26:355.
14. Cocke WM Jr, Meyer KK. Retroperitoneal duodenal rupture. Proposed mechanism, review of literature and report of a case. Am J Surg 1964;108:834.
15. Dellinger EP, Wertz MJ, Lennard ES, et al. Efficacy of short-course antibiotic prophylaxis after penetrating intestinal injury. Arch Surg 1986;121:23.
16. DeMaria EJ, Reichman W, Kenny PR, et al. Septic complications of corticosteroid administration after central nervous system trauma. Ann Surg 1985;202:248.
17. Demling RH, Niehaus G, Will JA. Pulmonary microvascular response to hemorrhagic shock, resuscitation, and recovery. J Appl Physiol 1979;46:498.
18. Deutschman CS, Wilton PB, Sinow J, et al. Paranasal sinusitis: a common complication of nasotracheal intubation in neurosurgical patients. Neurosurgery 1985;17:296.
19. Diamond LK. Splenectomy in childhood and the hazard of overwhelming infection. Pediatrics 1969;43:886.
20. Donovan AJ, Hagen WE. Traumatic perforation of the duodenum. Am J Surg 1966;111:341.
21. Ein SH, Shandling B, Simpson JS, et al. Nonoperative management of traumatized spleen in children: how and why. J Pediatr Surg 1978;13:117.
22. Eraklis AJ, Filler RM. Splenectomy in childhood: a review of 1413 cases. J Pediatr Surg 1972;7:382.
23. Esrig BC, Frazee L, Stephenson SF, et al. Predisposition to infection and neutrophil function following hemorrhagic shock. Rev Surg 1976;33:431
24. Fauci AS. Host defense mechanisms against infection. Kalamazoo, MI: Current Concepts/Scope Publications, Upjohn Company, 1978.
25. Federle MP, Crass RA, Jeffrey RB, et al. Computed tomography in blunt abdominal trauma. Arch Surg 1982;117:645.
26. Feliciano DV, Bitondo CG, Mattox KL, et al. A four-year experience with splenectomy versus splenorrhaphy. Ann Surg 1985;201:568.
27. Feliciano DV, Mattox KL, Jordan GL Jr. Intra-abdominal packing for control of hepatic hemorrhage: a reappraisal. J Trauma 1981;21:285.
28. Fischer RP, O'Farrell KA, Perry JF Jr. The value of peritoneal drains in the treatment of liver injuries. J Trauma 1978;18:393.
29. Flick MR, Perel A, Staub NC. Leukocytes are required for increased lung microvascular permeability after microembolization in sheep. Circ Res 1981;48:344.

30. Flint LM, Vitale GC, Richardson JD, et al. The injured colon: relationships of managment to complications. Ann Surg 1981;193:619.

31. Goldstein A, Phillips T, Sclafani SJA, et al. Early open reduction and internal fixation of the disrupted pelvic ring. J Trauma 1986;26:325.

32. Grois RJA, Gimbrère JSF, van Niekerk JLM, et al. Early osteosynthesis and prophylactic mechanical ventilation in the multitrauma patient. J Trauma 1982;22:895.

33. Graham JM, Mattox KL, Jordan GL Jr. Traumatic injury of the pancreas. Am J Surg 1978;136:744.

34. Grover FL, Richardson JD, Fewel JG, et al. Prophylactic antibiotics in the treatment of penetrating chest wounds. A prospective double-blind study. J Thorac Cardiovasc Surg 1977;74:528.

35. Guglielmo BJ, Hohn DC, Koo PJ, et al. Antibiotic prophylaxis in surgical procedures. A critical analysis of the literature. Arch Surg 1983;118:943.

36. Heideman M. The role of complement in trauma. Acta Chir Scand [Suppl] 1985;522:233.

37. Hohn DC, Meyers AJ, Gherini ST, et al. Production of acute pulmonary injury by leukocytes and activated complement. Surgery 1980;88:48.

38. Hood RM. Surgical diseases of the pleura and chest wall. Philadelphia: WB Saunders, 1986.

39. Hutton PAN, Jones BM, Law DJW. Depot penicillin as prophylaxis in accidental wounds. Br J Surg 1978;65:549.

40. Ignelzi RJ, VanderArk GD. Analysis of the treatment of basilar skull fractures with and without antibiotics. J Neurosurg 1975;43:721.

41. Ivatury RR, Nallathambi M, Gaudino J, et al. Penetrating duodenal injuries. Analysis of 100 consecutive cases. Ann Surg 1985;202:153.

42. Jennett B, Miller JD. Infection after depressed fracture of skull. Implications for management of nonmissile injuries. J Neurosurg 1972;36:333.

43. Jennett WB. Management of head injuries. Philadelphia: FA Davis, 1981 (Contemporary Neurology, 20).

44. Jones RC. Management of pancreatic trauma. Am J Surg 1985;150:698.

45. Jones RC, Thal ER, Johnson NA, et al. Evaluation of antibiotic therapy after penetrating abdominal trauma. Ann Surg 1985;201:576.

46. Kanter RK, Weiner LB. Ventriculostomy-related infections (letter). N Engl J Med 1984;311:987.

47. Kapur MM, Jain P, Gidh M. The effect of trauma on serum C3 activation and its correlation with injury severity score in man. J Trauma 1986;26:464.

48. King H, Shumacker HB Jr. Splenic studies. I. Susceptibility to infection after splenectomy performed in infancy. Ann Surg 1952;136:239.

49. Kupper TS, Green DR, Durum SK, et al. Defective antigen presentation to a cloned T helper cell by macrophages from burned mice can be restored with interleukin-1. Surgery 1985;98:199.

50. Lange D, Zaret P, Meroltti G, et al. The use of absorbable mesh in splenic trauma. J Trauma 1986;26:678.

51. Lanser ME, Brown GE, Mora R, et al. Trauma serum suppresses superoxide production by normal neutrophils. Arch Surg 1986;121:157.

52. LeBlanc KA, Tucker WY, Prophylactic antibiotics and closed tube thoracostomy. Surg Gynecol Obstet 1985;160:259.

53. Levison MA, Petersen SR, Sheldon GF, et al. Duodenal trauma: experience of a trauma center. J Trauma 1984;24:475.

54. Lewis FR Jr, Blaisdell FW, Schlobohm RM. Incidence and outcome of posttraumatic respiratory failure. Arch Surg 1977;112:436.

55. Llende M, Santiago-Delpín EA, Lavergne J. Immunobiological consequences of splenectomy: a review. J Surg Res 1986;40:85.

56. LoCurto JA Jr, Tischler CD, Swan KG, et al. Tube thoracostomy and trauma—Antibiotics or not? J Trauma 1986;26:1067.

57. Lowbury EJL, Thom BT, Lilly HA, et al. Sources of infection with *Pseudomonas aeruginosa* in patients with tracheostomy. J Med Microbiol 1970;3:39.

58. MacGee EE, Cauthen JC, Brackett GE. Meningitis following acute traumatic cerebrospinal fluid fistula. J Neurosrug 1970;33:312.

59. Mackersie RC, Shackford SR, Hoyt DB, et al. Continuous epidural fentanyl analgesia: ventilatory function improvement with routine use in the treatment of blunt chest injury (Abst). J Trauma 1986;26:679.

60. Maderazo EG, Albano SD, Woronick CL, et al. Polymorphonuclear Leukocyte migration abnormalities and their significance in seriously traumatized patients. Ann Surg 1983;198:736.

61. Malangoni MA, Dillon LD, Klamer TW, et al. Factors influencing the risk of early and late serious infection in adults after splenectomy for trauma. Surgery 1984;96:775.

62. Mayhall CG, Archer NH, Lamb VA, et al. Ventriculostomy-related infections: a prospective epidemiologic study. N Engl J Med 1984;310:552.
63. Meakins JL, McLean APH, Kelly R, et al. Delayed hypersensitivity and neutrophil chemotaxis: effect of trauma. J Trauma 1978; 18:240.
64. Miller CL. Secondary immunodeficiency in burns and after surgical trauma. Clin Immunol Allergy 1981;1:641.
65. Miller CL, Baker CC. Development of inhibitory macrophage (Ø) after splenectomy. Transplant Proc 1979;11:1460.
66. Miller SE, Miller CL, Trunkey DD. The immune consequences of trauma. Surg Clin North Am 1982;62:167.
67. Moore FA, Moore EE, Seagraves A. Nonresectional management of major hepatic trauma. An evolving concept. Am J Surg 1985;150:725.
68. Nallathambi M, Ivatury R, Rohman M, et al. Penetrating colon injuries: exteriorized-repair vs loop colostomy. J Trauma 1986;26:680.
69. Nelson RM, Benitez PR, Newell MA, et al. Single-antibiotic use for penetrating abdominal trauma. Arch Surg 1986;121:153.
70. Nichols RL, Smith JW, Klein DB, et al. Risk of infection after penetrating abdominal trauma. N Eng J Med 1984;311:1065.
71. Oakes DD. Splenic trauma. Curr Probl Surg 1981;18:346.
72. O'Mahony JB, Palder SB, Wood JJ, et al. Depression of cellular immunity after multiple trauma in the absence of sepsis. J Trauma 1984;24:869.
73. Pachter HL, Spencer FC, Hofstetter SR, et al. Experience with the finger fracture technique to achieve intra-hepatic homostasis in 75 patients with severe injuries of the liver. Ann Surg 1983;197:771.
74. Pardy BJ, Spencer RC, Dudley HAF. Hepatic reticuloendothelial protection against bacteremia in experimental hemorrhagic shock. Surgery 1977;81:193.
75. Patzakis MJ, Harvey JP Jr, Ivler D. The role of antibiotics in the management of open fractures. J Bone Joint Sur 1974;56A:532.
76. Pietra GG, Rüttner JR, Wüst W, et al. The lung after trauma and shock—fine structure of the alveolar-capillary barrier in 23 autopsies. J Trauma 1981;21:454.
77. Rhodes RS, Depalma RG, Robinson AV. Intestinal barrier function in hemorrhagic shock. J Surg Res 1973;14:305.
78. Richardson JD, Adams L. Flint LM. Selective management of flail chest and pulmonary contusion. Ann Surg 1982;196:481.
79. Roberts AHN, Teddy PJ. A prospective trial of prophylactic antibiotics in hand lacerations. Br J Surg 1977;64:394.
80. Robinette CD, Fraumeni JF Jr. Splenectomy and subsequent mortality in veterans of the 1939–1945 war. Lancet 1977;2:127.
81. Sanders RJ. Management of colon injuries. Surg Clin North Am 1963;43:457.
82. Schimpff SC, Miller RM, Polakavetz S, et al. Infection in the severely traumatized patient. Ann Surg 1974;179:352.
83. Sclafani SJ, Goldstein AS, Shaftan GW. Interventional radiology—an alternate approach to operative drainage of post traumatic abscesses. J Trauma 1984;24:299.
84. Seibel R, LaDuca J, Hassett JM, et al. Blunt multiple trauma (ISS 36), femur traction, and the pulmonary failure-septic state. Ann Surg 1985;202:283.
85. Smego DR, Richardson JD, Flint LM. Determinants of outcome in pancreatic trauma. J Trauma 1985;25:771.
86. Stone HH, Fabian TC. Management of duodenal wounds. J Trauma 1979;19:334.
87. Stone HH, Fabian TC. Management of perforating colon trauma. Randomization between primary closure and exteriorization. Ann Surg 1979;190:430.
88. Stone HH, Lamb JM. Use of pedicled omentum as an autogenous pack for control of hemorrhage in major injuries of the liver. Surg Gynecol Obstet 1975;141:92.
89. Tranbaugh RF, Elings VB, Christensen J, et al. Determinants of pulmonary interstitial fluid accumulation after trauma. J Trauma 1982;22:830.
90. Trinkle JK, Richardson JD, Franz JL, et al. Management of flail chest without mechanical ventilation. Ann Thorac Surg 1975;19:355.
91. Vaughan GD III, Frazier OH, Graham DY, et al. The use of pyloric exclusion in the management of severe duodenal injuries. Am J Surg 1977;134:785.
92. Walker WE, Kapelanski DP, Weiland AP, Patterns of infection and mortality in thoracic trauma. Ann Surg 1985;201:752.

93. West MA, Keller GA, Cerra FB, et al. Killed *Escherichia coli* stimulates macrophage-mediated alterations in hepatocellular function during the vitro coculture: a mechanism of altered liver function in sepsis. Infect Immun 1985;49:563.

94. West MA, Keller GA, Hyland BJ, et al. Hepatocyte function in sepsis: Kupffer cells mediate a biphasic protein synthesis response in hepatocytes after exposure to endotoxin or killed *Escherichia coli.* Surgery 1985;98:388.

95. Wilson JM, Boren CH Jr, Peterson SR, et al. Traumatic hemothorax: is decorticated necessary? J Thorac Cardiovasc Surg 1979;77:489.

21

○   ○   ○   ◦   ●   ◦

UROLOGIC INFECTIONS IN SURGICAL PATIENTS

John N. Krieger

The great majority of infectious complications in urologic patients are no different than infections occurring in patients on other surgical services. The infecting microorganisms are similar and the metabolic and immunologic consequences of systemic infections are identical to those discussed in other chapters of this book. These observations raise an important question, "Why do we need a chapter on urologic aspects of surgical infections?"

Urology has been recognized as a distinct surgical subspecialty since the time of Hippocrates because of the special considerations necessary for successful treatment of diseases affecting the genitourinary tract. From the standpoint of surgical infectious diseases, it has long been recognized that certain dramatic urinary tract infections, such as perinephric abscess or Fournier's gangrene, may be difficult to diagnose or involve multiple organ systems and, thus, may require the expertise of both the urologist and the general surgeon. Recent studies have also demonstrated that the urinary tract is an important portal of entry for organisms causing less dramatic

490

infections which are associated with considerable morbidity because they are exceedingly common.

The purpose of this chapter is to provide a brief overview of urologic causes and consequences of genitourinary tract infections in surgical patients. Emphasis will be placed on the most common infections seen in surgical practice, hospital-acquired urinary tract infections. Consideration will be given to our own recommendations for prevention of these common infections. Finally, we will review some of the more dramatic, but fortunately uncommon, urinary tract infections.

HOSPITAL-ACQUIRED URINARY TRACT INFECTIONS

There are at least two distinct approaches to the question of hospital-acquired urinary tract infections in surgical patients, the epidemiologist's approach and the practicing surgeon's approach. The hospital epidemiologist points to the estimated one million hospital-acquired, or nosocomial, urinary tract infections which occur per year in the U.S. and observes that 60% of such infections occur on surgical services.[4,22] These infections certainly contribute to excess morbidity and costs for the overall population of surgical patients.[6,13] In contrast, most practicing surgeons are unimpressed by such theoretical arguments and have difficulty recalling specific instances where nosocomial urinary infections had a significant adverse impact on individual patients. Both viewpoints have merit: the problem is that few studies have approached the issue of hospital-acquired urinary tract infections in terms relevant to most clinical surgeons.

We carried out a series of studies to determine the clinical significance of the urinary tract as a source of infectious complications in hospitalized patients. Initially we had three major questions, "How common are hospital-acquired urinary tract infections? How much do these infections add to hospital costs? Most importantly, how often do patients with nosocomial urinary infections suffer major adverse consequences, such as secondary bloodstream or postoperative wound infections?"

INCIDENCE AND ECONOMIC COSTS OF HOSPITAL-ACQUIRED URINARY TRACT INFECTIONS

Since 1972, hospital-wide surveillance has been performed on a routine basis for the entire inpatient population at the University of Virginia Hospital.[42,43] An infection control practitioner visits every inpatient unit on a weekly basis to review each patient's nursing care plan. Charts of high risk patients are identified based on diagnoses, operations, procedures or length of hospitalization. The charts of these high-risk patients are then examined in detail. This method was found to have a high sensitivity for identification of hospital-acquired infections, when compared to prospective review of all patient charts, but to require significantly less time expenditure by the infection control practitioners.

A uniform set of definitions was used to identify patients with nosocomial infections.[22] An infection was considered to be hospital-acquired if it was neither present nor incubating when the patient was admitted to the hospital. Diagnosis of a urinary tract infection was based on growth in culture of more than 100,000 colony-forming units in a symptomatic patient. A hospital-acquired urinary tract infection was considered to be present if the patient had a previous negative culture, normal urinalysis or an admission culture positive for a different organism.

Our initial problem was to determine the overall incidence and treatment patterns for nosocomial urinary tract infections. We could then make crude estimates of their economic impact.

Prospective surveillance of 121,907 total patients admitted to the hospital during a 71-month period documented 3,024 nosocomial urinary tract infections.[22] The annual attack rate varied between 2.0 and 3.1 nosocomial urinary tract infections per 100 hospital admissions and did not vary significantly during the study period. Of particular interest, 59% of these infections occurred in patients on surgical services. Most nosocomial urinary tract infections were caused by aerobic gram-negative rods, particularly *Escherichia coli* (24%) and *Pseudomonas aeruginosa* (Fig. 21-1).

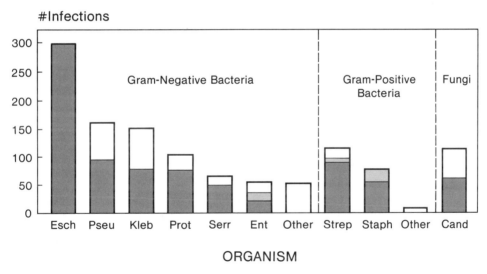

Figure 21-1.
Microbiology of 1,233 nosocomial urinary tract infections. Organisms are classified by genus and most common species. Gram-negative bacteria include ■, *Escherichia (Esch) coli, Pseudomonas (Pseu) aeruginosa, Klebsiella (Kleb), K. pneumoniae, Proteus (Prot) mirabilis, Serratia (Serr) marcescens, Enterobacter (Ent) cloacae* and ▓, *E. aerogenes.* Gram-positive bacteria include ■, *Streptococcus (Strep) faecalis and Staphylococcus (Staph) epidermis,* and ▓ *Staph. aureus.* Fungi include ■, *Candida (Cand) albicans.* □, other species in each genus. Overall, gram-negative rods caused 74% of infections, gram-positive cocci caused 16% and fungi caused 10%. (JN Krieger, Nosocomial urinary tract infections: secular trends. J Urol, volume 130, 103, © by Williams & Wilkins, 1983)

In a theoretical context, it may be interesting to speculate on whether antibiotic treatment is necessary for all patients with nosocomial bacteriuria. Certain limited observations favor this approach. For example, in some high risk populations, such as renal transplant recipients, the urinary tract may be the source of organisms causing postoperative wound sepsis or bloodstream infections.[2,25,28] On the other hand, it is possible to argue against routine treatment of hospital-acquired urinary tract infections. Most patients, particularly those with catheter-associated infections, do well without antibiotics once the catheter has been removed.[26] Furthermore, routine antibiotic treatment of hospital-acquired bacteriuria has not been demonstrated to reduce either patient symptoms or secondary complications in any carefully controlled study. Routine antibiotic therapy has been associated with emergence of antibiotic-resistant bacteria.[24,26] In practice, however, such hypothetical considerations often bear little resemblance to everyday medical practice.

To evaluate clinical treatment patterns, all 1,233 urinary tract infections which occurred during the final 23 months of the study were evaluated in detail.[22] We were surprised to find that only one patient did not receive antimicrobial therapy. The clinical records of 779 patients (63%) clearly documented that antimicrobial drugs were ordered specifically for treatment of hospital-acquired urinary tract infections (Fig. 21-2). All of the remaining patients received treatment for other infections or for unspecified reasons.

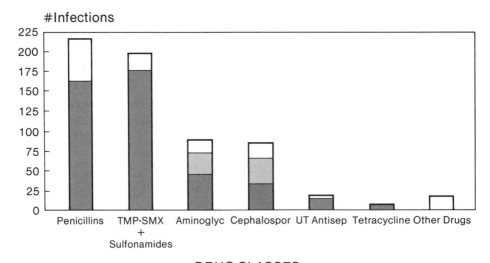

DRUG CLASSES

Figure 21–2.
Specific treatment of 779 nosocomial urinary tract infections. Drugs are organized by class and most common drugs. ■, ampicillin (*penicillins*), trimethoprim-sulfamethoxazole (*TMP-SMX + sulfonamides*), tobramycin (*Aminoglyc*), cephalexin (*Cephalospor*), nitrofurantoin (*UT Antisep*) and hydrochloride (*Tetracycline*). ▧, gentamicin (*Aminoglyc*) and cephalothin (*Cephalospor*). □, other drugs in each class. (JN Krieger, Nosocomial urinary tract infections: secular trends. J Urol, volume 130, 104 © by Williams & Wilkins, 1983)

We then evaluated the economic impact of hospital-acquired urinary tract infections in this patient population. A minimal estimate was obtained by adding the costs of the nine most frequently prescribed drugs for specific treatment of urinary tract infections. In an earlier study of surgical patients in our hospital patients with nosocomial urinary tract infections spent an average of two additional days in the hospital compared to case-matched controls who did not develop urinary infections.[13] Therefore, we also included the cost of extra hospital days. Based on this analysis, hospital-acquired urinary tract infections contributed at least $17,000.00 per month to hospital costs (over $200,000.00 per year). This is obviously a conservative estimate including only a portion of antibiotic usage but excluding all added physician and laboratory charges.

SERIOUS COMPLICATIONS OF HOSPITAL-ACQUIRED URINARY TRACT INFECTIONS

Epidemiologic estimates of the overall incidence and cost of hospital-acquired urinary tract infections impress hospital administrators, third party carriers and government bureaucrats. Numbers alone have less impact on surgeons, who are primarily concerned with the care of individual patients. From a practicing physician's standpoint, the risk for developing serious complications of nosocomial bacteriuria is much more important than the additional cost of antibiotics or hospital days. Surprisingly few studies have directly addressed the risk for significant complications of hospital-acquired bacteriuria. We used a mainframe computer to organize our database to study two serious consequences of nosocomial urinary infections, secondary bloodstream infections and postoperative wound infections.

BLOODSTREAM INFECTIONS MAY RESULT FROM HOSPITAL-ACQUIRED URINARY TRACT INFECTIONS

Development of life-threatening bloodstream infections is the most serious complication of nosocomial urinary tract infections.[8, 11, 30, 31, 35] These infections may be associated with a 40% mortality, which increases to approximately an 80% mortality if the patient is unstable hemodynamically.

To assure 100% sensitivity for detection of bloodstream infections, laboratory based surveillance was instituted of all bloodstream isolates in addition to review of nursing care plans and patient records.[23] Diagnosis of an episode of nosocomial bacteremia required a positive blood culture in a patient hospitalized for at least 24 hours and who had no clinical evidence of bacteremia on admission to the hospital. Determination of the importance of such isolates was made by the patient's physicians, who prescribed antibiotic therapy specifically for treatment of the infection. In order for a bloodstream infection to be considered to be secondary to a hospital-acquired urinary infection, it had to fulfill three criteria: both infections were caused by the identical organism; the urinary infection was documented prior to or on the same day as the bloodstream infection; and there was no evidence for a different primary site of infection.

During the 23-month study period, 40,718 patients were admitted to the hospital and 1,233 hospital-acquired urinary tract infections were identified by routine surveillance. Although 297 patients had both nosocomial urinary tract infections and nosocomial bloodstream infections, only 33 infections met the strict criteria for bloodstream infections secondary to nosocomial urinary tract infections.[23] Therefore, the attack rate for secondary bloodstream infections was at least 2.7 per 100 patients with nosocomial bacteriuria.

Review of the organisms responsible for these infections demonstrated that patients with nosocomial urinary infections caused by *Serratia marcescens* were at significantly higher risk for development of secondary bloodstream infections (16 per 100 patients) than patients infected with other nosocomial urinary pathogens (less than 4.3 per 100 patients, p 0.05).

Extensive statistical analyses were carried out to identify particular characteristics of patients with nosocomial urinary tract infections which placed them at especially high-risk for development of secondary bloodstream infections. Men with hospital-acquired urinary tract infections developed secondary bacteremia twice as often as women (p < 0.05). This finding is most likely a reflection of the high prevalence of structural genitourinary tract abnormalities among middle aged men. Neither age nor race was a significant risk for development of secondary bloodstream infections. Attention was directed to multiple other risk factors (Table 21-1). Genitourinary tract

Table 21–1
Risk Factors in Surgical Patients with Hospital-Acquired Urinary Tract Infections (UTIs)

RISK FACTOR	# UTIs (%) (n = 864)	# POSTOPERATIVE WOUND INFECTIONS SECONDARY TO NOSOCOMIAL BACTERIURIA (%) (n = 6)	# POSTOPERATIVE WOUND INFECTIONS (%) (n = 592)
Genitourinary manipulation*	774 (89.6)	6 (100)	55 (9.3)
Disease of nervous system or sensory organs*	293 (33.9)	3 (50)	43 (7.3)
Neoplasm	129 (14.9)		91 (15.4)
Genitourinary disease	117 (13.5)		82 (13.9)
Accidents and trauma	70 (8.1)	2 (33.3)	61 (10.3)
Endocrine disease	67 (7.8)		41 (6.9)
Immune deficiency	40 (4.6)		26 (4.4)
Circulatory disease	39 (4.5)	2 (33.3)	16 (2.7)
Congenital disease	10 (1.2)		13 (2.2)
Musculoskeletal disease	2 (0.2)	1 (16.7)	1 (0.2)

*Indicates significant difference, P < 0.01.

manipulation, especially catheterization, was by far the most frequent procedure, occurring in 86% of all patients with nosocomial urinary infections and in 73% of patients with secondary bloodstream infections. No other outstanding risk factors were identified which predicted which patients with nosocomial urinary tract infections were at particular risk for developing secondary bloodstream infections.

HOSPITAL-ACQUIRED URINARY TRACT INFECTIONS CAUSE WOUND INFECTIONS IN SURGICAL PATIENTS

By definition, a postoperative wound infection can only occur after an operation. For this reason the causes of surgical wound infections are especially relevant to surgeons. Many studies have been carried out to determine factors which influence the risk for development of a surgical wound infection. Previous studies have emphasized factors such as extent of preoperative contamination, nutritional status, use of antibiotics, preoperative skin preparation, and so forth. However, little attention has been given to the role of urinary tract infections in the genesis of postoperative wound sepsis. For this reason, we decided to estimate the minimal proportion of postoperative wound infections which complicate nosocomial urinary tract infections.

Prospective surveillance of 20,024 consecutive patients admitted to surgical services was used to identify patients with nosocomial infections during the 23-month study.[21] A simple definition was chosen for a postoperative wound infection: presence of pus at an incision, with the exception of minor stitch abscesses. The surgical wound infection was considered to be secondary to a hospital-acquired urinary tract infection if it met the following criteria: both infections were caused by the identical organism; the wound infection was documented subsequent to the onset of bacteriuria; and there was no evidence for a different primary focus of infection. If more than one organism was isolated from a wound, the predominant bacterium was considered to be the etiologic agent. Wound infections caused by enteric organisms in patients who had gastrointestinal tract operations were considered to arise from organisms originating in the intestine, not the urinary tract. Heavily contaminated wounds, such as burns, were excluded from analysis because they were considered to be infected on admission to the hospital.

A total of 864 nosocomial urinary tract infections were identified through prospective surveillance. This represented a rate of 4.2 hospital-acquired urinary infections per 100 surgical admissions.[21] During the same period there were 592 postoperative wound infections for a rate of 3.0 per 100 surgical admissions. One hundred fifteen patients had both nosocomial bacteriuria and surgical wound infections, but only six patients met the strict criteria for postoperative wound infections secondary to hospital acquired urinary tract infections (Fig. 21-3). These six patients had undergone operations by surgeons from five different subspecialities including: General Surgery, Orthopedic Surgery, Obstetrics and Gynecology, Thoracic and Cardiovascular Surgery, and Urology. However, one third of the purulent surgical wounds were never cultured. Frequently, the laboratory did not report both genera and

% OF TOTAL

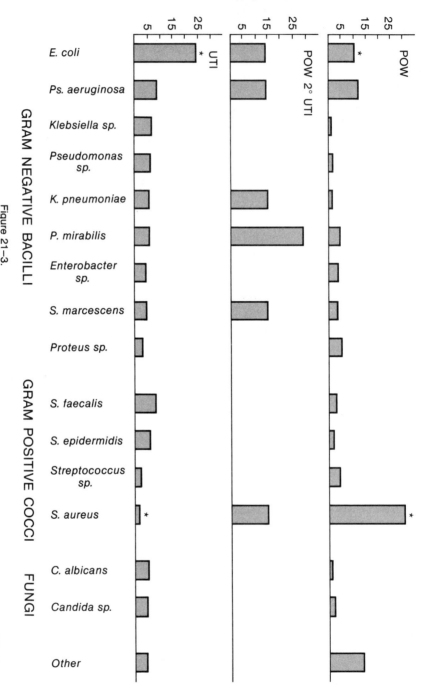

GRAM NEGATIVE BACILLI   GRAM POSITIVE COCCI   FUNGI

Figure 21-3.
Microbiology of 841 hospital-acquired urinary tract infections, *UTi*; 592 postoperative wound infections, *POW*, and six postoperative wound infections secondary to nosocomial bacteriuria, *POW 2° UTi*. Asterisk (*) Indicates significant differences, P < 0.01. (Krieger JN. Nosocomial urinary tract infections. Surg Gynecol Obstet 1983; 156:313-318. By permission of Surgery, Gynecology & Obstetrics)

species of organisms isolated from surgical wounds. Only 178 of the 592 surgical wound infections had adequate microbiologic data to be evaluated according to the criteria for secondary wound infections. Thus, at least 3.4% of evaluable surgical infections were caused by the hospital-acquired urinary tract organisms. The attack rate for secondary wound infections was 2.3 per 100 surgical patients with hospital-acquired bacteriuria.

We found that two potential risk factors for development of secondary wound sepsis were outstanding: genitourinary tract manipulation, particularly catheterization, and diseases of the nervous system and sensory organs (Table 21-2). We also found that hospital-acquired bacteriuria was more common in men than in women (1.3 : 1.0, $p < 0.05$), and that patients with nosocomial bacteriuria were older (mean 45 years) than patients with surgical wound infections (mean 34 years, $p < 0.001$). These findings are consistent with the high prevalence of obstructive uropathy in older men and the fact that many older patients did not have surgery, yet, due to their age, were more likely to develop bacteriuria. Patients with hospital-acquired urinary infections or secondary wound sepsis were more likely to have multiple risk factors than patients with surgical wound infections alone ($p < 0.04$).

In a statistical sense it is not meaningful to assess the added costs due to the

Table 21–2
Patients with Nosocomial Urinary Tract Infections (UTIs) and Patients with Bacteremia Secondary to Nosocomial UTIs

DIAGNOSIS OR PROCEDURE	% PATIENTS WITH UTI ONLY ($n = 1233$)	% PATIENTS WITH BACTEREMIA SECONDARY TO UTI ($n = 33$)	P^*
Genitourinary manipulation	83.4 (1028)	72.7 (24)	0.038
Disease of nervous system or sensory organs	27.6 (340)	9.1 (3)	0.015
Genitourinary disease	15.2 (187)	18.2 (6)	NS
Neoplasm	14.1 (174)	15.2 (5)	NS
General surgery	13.5 (166)	21.2 (7)	NS
Endocrine disease	10.7 (132)	9.1 (3)	NS
Trauma	8.8 (109)	9.1 (3)	NS
Immune deficiency	6.0 (74)	6.1 (2)	NS
Circulatory disease	3.9 (48)	9.1 (3)	NS
Congenital disease	1.4 (17)	0	†
Musculoskeletal disease	0.2 (3)	0	†
Pregnancy	0	0	†

Note: Diagnoses and procedures were categorized according to the International Classification of Diseases.
*Determined by χ^2 analysis.
†Numbers of cells obtained were insufficient for evaluation.

small size of this group of patients with surgical wound sepsis secondary to nosocomial urinary tract infections. However, from a clinical standpoint, these patients with secondary wound infections experienced considerable morbidity. Four additional operations were necessary in these six patients including: removal of an infected hip prosthesis, secondary closure of a abdominal wound dehiscience, laparotomy and drainage of a subhepatic abscess, and irrigation and debridement of an infected hip socket.

OVERVIEW OF THE IMPORTANCE OF NOSOCOMIAL URINARY TRACT INFECTIONS IN SURGICAL PATIENTS

Acquisition of an infection while a patient is hospitalized for a different reason causes unnecessary morbidity and expenditure of health care resources. We used prospective surveillance of over 120,000 consecutive hospital admissions to obtain minimal estimates of the human and economic costs which occur as a direct consequence of nosocomial urinary tract infections, the most common hospital-acquired infections. While nosocomial infections, such as pneumonias, bloodstream or postoperative wound infections, often produce dramatic manifestations; nosocomial urinary tract infections contribute insidiously to hospital costs through excess usage of antibiotics, increased length of hospitalization plus added laboratory and physician costs. Using very conservative criteria we estimated that hospital-acquired urinary tract infections added at least $1,000,000.00 to a single hospital's costs during this study and continue to add over $200,000.00 per year.

On occasion hospital acquired bacteriuria may result in serious complications. Rigid criteria were used to determine the minimal risk for two serious complications, secondary bloodstream infections and postoperative wound infections. The attack rate was 2.7 secondary bloodstream infections per 100 patients with nosocomial bacteriuria and 2.3 secondary surgical wound infections per 100 patients with nosocomial bacteriuria. Therefore, at least 5 per 100 patients with hospital-acquired urinary infections had one of these serious complications.

LIFE-THREATENING GENITOURINARY TRACT INFECTIONS

A complete review of the diagnosis, pathophysiology and treatment of life-threatening genitourinary tract infections is beyond the limited scope of this chapter. The metabolic and pathophysiologic events common to sepsis of many origins are thoroughly discussed in other sections of this book. There are two unique syndromes of urinary tract origin with which the general surgeon should be familiar, Fournier's gangrene, perinephric abscess, pyonephrosis, acute bacterial prostatitis, and urosepsis. We will briefly consider critical aspects of these clinical syndromes.

FOURNIER'S GANGRENE

In 1883, a French dermatologist named Fournier described a fulminating gangrenous condition affecting the male genitalia.[10] There were three distinguishing characteristics of the syndrome: absence of predisposing conditions, abrupt onset in a previously healthy young man and rapid progression. A wide variety of names have been applied to this condition during the last century, including necrotizing fasciitis of the genitalia,[3] synergistic gangrene of the scrotum and penis,[9] polymicrobial genital gangrene,[39] and necrotizing perineal infection,[19] among others. During this time the clinical definition of Fournier's gangrene has been expanded to include patients ranging in age from neonates to the elderly, patients experiencing a more gradual onset of disease and patients with varied predisposing conditions.[1,17]

Characteristically, patients experience swelling and erythema of the genitalia accompanied by fever, chills and malaise. On physical examination, necrosis of the genitalia may be impressive (see Fig. 21-4) and crepitus may be apparent, due to the presence of subcutaneous gas. The inflammatory and necrotic process may extend along fascial planes superiorly to the axillae and inferiorly to the perineal body.[17,37] Often a feculent odor is apparent.

Predisposing conditions are now recognized in most patients with Fournier's gangrene. These conditions include systemic diseases, particularly diabetes; genitourinary tract diseases, especially urethral stricture, trauma or infection; and gastrointestinal tract diseases, most often perirectal abscess.[17,37,41] The infecting microorganisms are usually a combination of both aerobic gram-negative rods, aerobic gram-

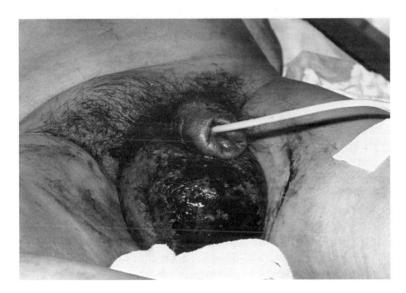

Figure 21–4.
Clinical presentation of an acute case of Fournier's gangrene in a patient with severe urethral stricture disease.

500

positive cocci and strict anaerobes, particularly Bacteroides species and, occasionally, Clostridia.

A high mortality rate, up to 45%, has been reported in recent reports of Fournier's gangrene.[17,37] Early, aggressive treatment offers the best chance for cure. Both aerobic and anaerobic cultures should be obtained prior to institution of broad-spectrum antibiotic coverage using drugs effective against aerobic gram-negative rods, aerobic gram-positive cocci and anaerobes should be instituted promptly. Surgery is indicated in all cases. Radical debridement of devitalized tissues is recommended by most authorities.[9,17,37] However, one recent report of four patients advocated much more limited debridement plus placement of through-and-through drains.[18] In our experience, limited procedures may be effective in occasional cases but patients with the full-blown syndrome are best managed by aggressive debridement of devitalized tissues. One additional therapeutic measure that has been recommended is the use of hyperbaric oxygen.[34] Although there have been no controlled trials of this mode of therapy, it may be reasonable to employ this measure as an adjunct to established techniques if facilities are available for this mode of therapy.

PERINEPHRIC ABSCESS

By definition, a perinephric abscess is located between the renal capsule and Gerota's fascia. The route of infection is believed to be either from hematogenous seeding from another focus of infection or from renal extension from an ascending urinary tract infection.[33,36,40] Since the advent of antibiotic therapy both the bacteriology and the most common route of infection have changed dramatically. Historically, *Staphylococcus aureus* was the most common organism and most infections were thought to arise as secondary foci from skin lesions. Gram-negative rods are currently the most common pathogens and the most common route now appears to be ascent of bacteria from the lower urinary tract. However, the high mortality attributable to these infections has remained essentially unchanged despite the availability of effective antibiotics. Recent series have reported mortality rates of 50% or more.[33,36,40]

Delay in diagnosis is the major reason for the persistently high mortality associated with perinephric abscess. Characteristically, patients are followed for weeks after they develop fever and unilateral flank pain. Other common complaints are abdominal pain, chills and dysuria and dehydration. Presence of diabetes or urinary tract calculi, particularly "struvite," or infection, stones are important predisposing factors for development of perinephric abscess.

Once the diagnosis of perinephric abscess is considered, the diagnostic evaluation and therapy are usually straightforward. The conventional radiographic evaluation included a plain film of the abdomen, intravenous pyelogram and, perhaps, retrograde pyelography. Newer radiographic techniques, particularly ultrasonography and computerized tomography, have greatly ease and accuracy of diagnosis of this condition.[15,16,44] Although antibiotics are useful to control sepsis and to prevent the spread of infection, drainage is the primary therapy. This may be accomplished by percutaneous methods in selected cases.[15] Open surgery is clearly indicated for large abscesses, multilocular abscesses or in the presence of a nonfunctioning kidney, which indicates the need for nephrectomy.

UROSEPSIS

Urosepsis is a generic term which is used to describe the combination of a bloodstream infection plus hemodynamic instability when the primary focus of infection is in the urinary tract. This syndrome may occur in two conditions with which the general surgeon should be familiar, pyonephrosis and acute bacterial prostatitis.

Pyonophrosis.

Patients with pyonephrosis usually present with symptoms of pyelonephritis in an obstructed, hydronephrotic, upper urinary tract. This condition is exactly analogous to acute suppurative cholangitis. The kidney is obstructed by stone, clot, sloughed papilla, fungus ball, tumor or a congenital abnormality. An acute infectious process, proximal to the obstruction, results in production of pus under pressure, rapid renal destruction and sepsis. In approximately 50% of cases the kidney is nonfunctioning and in many other instances it has markedly reduced function.[5]

Once the possibility of pyonephrosis has been considered, diagnosis is straightforward, using ultrasonography as the imaging procedure of choice. Prompt drainage is imperative. This may be accomplished by retrograde passage of a ureteral catheter, percutaneous placement of a nephrostomy catheter or open surgery as appropriate. Additional therapeutic measures include use of broad-spectrum antibiotics and other supportative measures.

Acute Bacterial Prostatitis.

Prostatitis syndromes cause tremendous morbidity among adult men.[20,32,38] The overwhelming majority of these patients are managed as outpatients and are of little concern to surgeons other than urologists. On occasion, however, inpatients on other surgical services may present with sepsis but the source is not apparent.

Acute bacterial prostatitis is one diagnostic consideration which is frequently overlooked in this situation. There may be a history of traumatic catheterization or forcible removal of the catheter by the patient. Almost invariably these patients have an indwelling transurethral catheter and they are often obtunded. Thus, eliciting genitourinary tract symptoms may be difficult or impossible. Frequently, the urine is grossly infected.

The problem is that the catheter is obstructing the drainage of infected prostatic secretions through the urethra. Use of appropriate antibiotics alone is rarely sufficient to control the infection. Removal of the urethral catheter is the critical aspect of therapy. If the patient requires bladder drainage, then placement of a suprapubic cystotomy tube is the procedure of choice.[20,38]

STRATEGIES FOR AVOIDING GENITOURINARY TRACT INFECTIOUS COMPLICATIONS IN SURGICAL PATIENTS

Surgeons are most easily interested in dramatic syndromes, such as Fournier's gangrene, urosepsis and pyonephrosis. Fortunately these are uncommon. Because of the life-threatening nature of these conditions emphasis is placed on prompt diagnosis and therapy—usually surgery. There is little that can be done to prevent these impressive genitourinary tract infections.

This chapter has emphasized the importance of hospital-acquired urinary tract infections for three reasons. First, these are the most common hospital-acquired infections. Second, nosocomial urinary tract infections are associated with significant, if seldom dramatic, morbidity. Third, a number of measures are available which may reduce the incidence of hospital acquired infections.

Preoperative Screening for Urologic Diseases.

Without question the most efficient and cost-effective strategy for prevention of infectious genitourinary tract problems is preoperative treatment of the urologic disorders. This is especially important for patients who require use of prosthetic materials (*i.e.*, heart valves, marlex, total hip replacement, and so forth.) because such patients are at risk for infection of their prostheses.

Preoperative screening for potential urinary tract disorders rarely needs to be elaborate and seldom requires urologic consultation. Several pertinent questions about past or current genitourinary tract problems, particularly following previous operations, and a directed physical examination will reveal many potential problems. In our experience this limited evaluation is commonly omitted by busy surgeons.

Laboratory studies are helpful in selected cases. Preoperative urinalysis is routine on most surgical services. It is a good idea to obtain this study in the office or several days prior to surgery. If the urinalysis is abnormal there will be time to repeat the urinalysis or to obtain a culture and initiate treatment of bacteriuria prior to surgery. In older men with a history of obstructive voiding problems it is our practice to obtain a preoperative uroflow study to assess the severity of obstruction.[7,14] In patients with significant urologic disorders or in those with a history of problems following previous surgery, preoperative urologic consultation may be prudent.

Prevention of Urinary Tract Infections in Hospitalized Patients.

Because dramatic complications of hospital-acquired urinary tract infections are uncommon, any individual surgeon will see few patients with secondary bacteremias or surgical wound sepsis. Prevention of these complications depends on reducing the incidence of nosocomial urinary infections and on identifying patients with hospital-acquired bacteriuria who are at especially high risk for complications.

The Clear Implication of Our Own Studies Is That We
Must be Certain of Our Indications for Genitourinary
Tract Manipulation.

Routine catheterization of surgical patients should be avoided. When necessary, indwelling bladder catheters require meticulous care. Maintenance of sterile, closed drainage is mandatory.[12,27,29] During the last decade a number of methods have been advocated to reduce the incidence of urinary tract infections in patients with indwelling catheters but none has been proven to be superior to scrupulous maintenance of sterile, closed drainage. Catheters should be kept in place for the minimal necessary time.

Despite our best efforts, nosocomial urinary tract infections will occur in some surgical patients. By careful analysis of risk factors we identified certain groups of patients at especially high risk for serious secondary complications.

Patients with nosocomial bacteriuria caused by *S. marcescens* were at high risk for development of secondary bloodstream infections. Older men, patients with diseases of the nervous system or sensory organs, and patients with multisystem diseases were at especially high risk for development of nosocomial bacteriuria and secondary surgical wound infections. Vigorous efforts to eliminate predisposing factors, treat the urinary tract infection, and careful observation for development of potential complications are especially indicated in such high risk patients.

REFERENCES

1. Alders N. Scrotal gangrene in a newborn baby. Arch Dis Child 1954;29:160.
2. Anderson RJ, Schafer LA, Olin DB, et al. Septicemia in renal transplant recipients. Arch Surg 1973;106:692.
3. Bahlman JCM, Fourie IJvH, Arndt TCH. Fournier's gangrene: necrotizing fasciitis of the male genitalia. Br J Urol 1982;55:85.
4. Centers for Disease Control. National Nosocomial Infections Study Report (6-month Summaries), 1977. Atlanta: US Dept of Health & Human Services, Public Health Service, November 1979.
5. Coleman BG, Arger PH, Mulhern CB, et al. Pyonephrosis: sonography in the diagnosis and management. Am J Roentgenol 1981;137:939.
6. Dixon RE. Effect of infections on hospital care. Ann Intern Med 1978;80:749.
7. Drach GW, Layton TN, Binard WJ. Male peak urinary flow rate: relationships to volume voided and age. J Urol 1979;122:210.
8. duPont HL, Spink WW. Infections due to gram-negative organisms: an analysis of 860 patients at the University of Minnesota Medical Center, 1958–1966. Medicine (Baltimore) 1969;48:307.
9. Flanigan AC, Kursh ED, McDougal WS, et al. Synergistic gangrene of the scrotum and penis secondary to colorectal disease. J Urol 1978;119:369.
10. Fournier AJ. Gangrene foudroyante de la verge. Semaine Med 1883;3:345.
11. Freid MA, Vosti KL. The importance of underlying disease inpatients with gram-negative bacteremia. Arch Intern Med 1968;121:418.
12. Garibaldi RA, Burke JP, Dickman ML, et al. Factors predisposing to bacteriuria during indwelling urethral catheterization. N Engl J Med 1974;291:215.
13. Givens CD, Wenzel RP. Catheter-associated urinary tract infections in surgical patients: a controlled study of the excess morbidity and costs. J Urol 1980;124:646.
14. Gould FK, Freeman R. Prediction of post-operative urinary tract infection in men undergoing cardiac surgery by measurement of urine flow. Br Med J 1984;288:286.

504

15. Haaga JR, Weinstein AJ. CT guided aspiration and drainage of abscesses. Am J Roentgenol 1980;135:1187.
16. Hoddick WJ, Jeffrey RB, Goldberg HI, et al. CT and sonography of severe renal and perirenal infections. Am J Roentgenol 1983;140:517.
17. Jones RB, Hirschman JV, Brown GS, et al. Fournier's syndrome: necrotizing subcutaneous infection of the male genitalia. J Urol 1979;122:279.
18. Kearney GP, Carling PC. Fournier's gangrene: an approach to its management. J Urol 1983;130:695.
19. Kovalcik PJ, Jones J. Necrotizing perineal infections. Am J Surg 1983;49:163.
20. Krieger JN. Prostatitis syndromes: pathophysiology, differential diagnosis, and treatment. Sex Transm Dis 1984;11:100.
21. Krieger JN, Kaiser DL, Wenzel RP. Nosocomial urinary tract infections cause wound infections postoperatively in surgical patients. Surg Gynecol Obstet 1983;156:313.
22. Krieger JN, Kaiser DL, Wenzel RP. Nosocomial urinary tract infections: secular trends, treatment and economics in a university hospital. J Urol 1983;130:102.
23. Krieger JN, Kaiser DL, Wenzel RP. Urinary tract etiology of bloodstream infections in hospitalized patients. J Infect Dis 1983;148:57.
24. Krieger JN, Levy-Zombek E, Scheidt A, et al. A nosocomial epidemic of antibiotic-resistant *Serratia marcescens* urinary tract infections. J Urol 1980;124:498.
25. Krieger JN, Tapia L, Stubenbord WT, et al. Urinary infection in kidney transplantation. Urology 1977;9:130.
26. Kunin CM. Detection, prevention and management of urinary tract infections. 3rd ed. Philadelphia: Lea & Febiger, 1979.
27. Kunin CM, McCormack RC. Prevention of catheter-induced urinary-tract infections by sterile closed drainage. N Engl J Med 1966;274:1156.
28. Lobo PI, Rudolf LE, Krieger JN. Wound infections in renal transplant recipients: a complication of urinary tract infections during allograft malfunction. Surgery 1982;92:491.
29. Maki DG, Hennekens CH, Bennett JU. Prevention of catheter-associated urinary tract infection. JAMA 1972;221:1270.
30. McCabe WR, Jackson GC. Gram-negative bacteremia. 1. Etiology and ecology. Arch Intern Med 1962;110:847.
31. McGowan JE, Parrot PL, Duty VP. Noscomial bacteremia: potential for prevention of procedure-related cases. JAMA 1977;237:2727.
32. Meares EM Jr, Stamey TA. Bacteriologic localization patterns in bacterial prostatitis and urethritis. Invest Urol 1968;5:492.
33. Merimsky E, Feldman C. Perinephric abscess: report of 19 cases. Int Surg 1981;66:79.
34. Riegels-Nielsen P, Hesselfeldt-Nielsen J, Bang-Jensen E, et al. Fournier's gangrene: five patients treated with hyperbaric oxygen. J Urol 1984;132:918.
35. Roberts FJ. A review of positive blood cultures: identification and source of microorganisms and patterns of sensitivity to antibiotics. Rev Infect Dis 1980;2:329.
36. Salvatierra O, Bucklew WB, Morrow JW. Perinephric abscess: A report of 71 cases. J Urol 1967;98:296.
37. Spirak JP, Resnick MI, Hampel N, et al. Fournier's gangrene: report of 20 cases. J Urol 1984;131:289.
38. Stamey TA. Pathogenesis and treatment of urinary tract infections. Baltimore: Williams & Wilkins, 1980.
39. Thadepalli H, Rao B, Datta NK, et al. Polymicrobial genital gangrene (Fournier's gangrene): clinical, microbiologic and therapeutic features. J Natl Med Assoc 1982;74:273.
40. Thorley JD, Jones SR, Sanford JP. Perinephric abscess. Medicine (Baltimore) 1974;53:441.
41. Walker L, Cassidy MT, Hutchison AG, et al. Fournier's gangrene and urethral problems. Br J Urol 1984;56:509.
42. Wenzel RP, Osterman CA, Hunting KJ, et al. Hospital-acquired infections. 1. Surveillance in a university hospital. Am J Epidemiol 1976;103:251.
43. Wenzel RP, Osterman CA, Hunting KJ, et al. Hospital-acquired infections. 2. Infection rates by site, service and common procedures in a university hospital. Am J Epidemiol 1976;104:645.
44. Wolverson MK, Jannadharao B, Sundaram M, et al. CT as a primary method in evaluating intraabdominal abscess. Am J Roentgenol 1979;133:1089.

22

○   ○   ○   ●   ●   ●

MEDIATORS
OF INFLAMMATION

Roger W. Yurt

Although maintenance and/or restitution of homeostasis is a basic principle of surgery, it has only been in recent years that the tissue hormones or inflammatory mediators have been appreciated for their role in the response to tissue injury and infection. In addition, it has become clear that the theory espoused by Cannon in 1926 applies to the mediator pathways. From this perspective, the inflammatory mediators are, in fact, a component of a finely tuned response to both endogenous and exogenous perturbation of an organism. At the tissue level, the mediators can be seen to function as hormones to modulate the cellular response to minor injury, while systemic manifestations of mediator activation frequently are a consequence of uncontrolled or unbalanced response to greater injury.

The recognition of the participation of the mediator systems in the maintenance of homeostasis[17] is based on the observation that each cascade is controlled by inhibitors, inactivators, or by mechanisms to limit the expression of the active mediators. Experimental documentation of this theory is difficult because most currently available techniques are not sufficiently sensitive to measure microcirculatory and cellular changes *in vivo*. Thus, it has been necessary to study these pathways *in vitro* or to correlate systemic manifestations with quantitative measurement of plasma

Table 22–1
Preformed and Generated Mediators From Cascades and Cells Involved in Injury and Infection

CELL/CASCADE	PREDOMINANT PRODUCTS
Mast Cell	Histamine, enzymes, chemotaxins, PGD_2, LTD_4, LTC_4, PAF, heparin, oxygen radicals
Macrophage	TNF, IL-1, tissue factor, plasminogen activator, PGE_2, LTB_4, PAF, oxygen radicals, lysozyme[72]
Endothelial Cell	Prostacyclin, PGE, cyclic AMP, angiotensin converting enzyme
Neutrophil	Oxygen radicals, enzymes, PGE, LTB_4, PAF, lactoferrin lysozyme
Coagulation	Thrombin, fibrin fragments, kallikrein, bradykinin, plasmin
Angiotensin	Angiotensin II
Complement	C3a, C5a, C3b, C3e, "attack sequence"

levels or effects on circulating cells. Nevertheless, it seems reasonable to view the systemic manifestations of injury as an exaggerated or uncontrolled response of pathways that under minimal perturbation serve to maintain homeostasis.

In this context, surgically induced or accidental injury and infection have a commonality in that they all appear to elicit a dose-related inflammatory mediator response. It is the intent here to examine the inflammatory mediators from the standpoint of mechanism of activation, inherent activity, and control of the action of the mediators. The sources of mediators will be reviewed under the major topics of plasma cascades and cell-derived mediators. The major products of activation of these pathways are listed in Table 22-1.

PLASMA CASCADES

The substrates and enzymes (usually proenzymes) of these cascades are, in general, found in the circulation. However, activation of the cascades may be initiated by cellular products, tissue damage, foreign materials, bacteria, or other cascades.

Coagulation

Coagulation may be initiated by way of the intrinsic (Hageman factor-dependent) or extrinsic (tissue factor) pathways. Primary activation of the Hageman factor-dependent (HF-dependent) pathway has greater potential with regard to mediator production because the kinin-generating and fibrinolytic pathways may also be initiated once Hageman factor is cleaved. Damaged endothelium, exposed collagen,[74] negatively charged surfaces, and lipopolysaccharides[71] activate this pathway. In addition, tissue enzymes[76] and proteases from circulating cells, such as neutrophil elastase,[121] can initiate the intrinsic pathway of coagulation.

The plasma proenzyme, prekallikrein, is converted to active kallikrein by inter-action of a trimolecular complex of kininogen, kallikrein, and Hageman factor.[20] Kallikrein, which itself has chemoattractant activity for neutrophils,[57] cleaves kinin-ogen to yield the vasoactive and pain-inducing peptide bradykinin. Secondary activa-tion of the complement cascade may occur because kallikrein has been shown to generate complement protein Cls from Clr.[22] In addition, the plasmin generated by way of the fibrinolytic pathway cleaves Cls *in vitro.*[83]

A role for these pathways after injury and during infection is supported by the observation that elastase is present in bronchoalveolar lavage fluid in patients suffer-ing from adult respiratory distress syndrome (ARDS).[101] It is likely that pulmonary mast cells are activated in the process as well because bradykinin has been shown to activate mast cells *in vitro.*[52]

Complement

The complement cascade may be initiated by way of the classical pathway, which is primarily an immune mechanism of activation whereas activation by way of the alternative pathway is primarily a nonimmune initiation. It appears that the alterna-tive pathway of activation is the cascade most often activated after injury and sepsis. Burn injury appears to activate complement by way of this pathway.[47] Microbial polysaccharides such as zymosan from yeast,[81] lipopolysaccharides from gram-nega-tive bacteria[40,65] and teichoic acid from pneumococci[122] initiate complement activa-tion by way of the alternative pathway. This sequence is continuously being activated in normal persons but is immediately interrupted by the action of BlH and C3bINA on active C3b. Surfaces that contain sialic acid, such as human cells, promote the process of inhibition of the pathway, whereas surfaces that are relatively deficient in sialic acid, such as foreign cells and the polysaccharides listed above, facilitate continued activa-tion of the pathway.[30] This primitive recognition process thereby facilitates lysis or opsonization of foreign or damaged tissue and bacteria. Additional mechanisms of secondary activation of the complement pathway include cleavage of C3 by plasmin that is generated in the coagulation cascade or by way of plasminogen activator release from macrophages. Tryptic enzymes, such as those released from the human mast cell, have also been shown to activate the complement system.[94]

The activation of the complement cascade can lead to cell lysis, opsonization of particulate substances, and generation of biologically active peptides. When the terminal components of the cascade are activated, a molecular complex is formed that leads to penetration of the cell membrane and subsequent lysis of the cell. C3b that is deposited on surfaces facilitates phagocytosis of the particle by macrophages, mono-cytes, and neutrophils by way of their C3b receptors. The biologically active peptides, C3a and C3b, cause mast cell degranulation. C5a is also a potent chemoattractant for neutrophils and, at high concentrations, can cause neutrophil degranulation. An additional cleavage product of C3, C3e, appears to mobilize neutrophils from the bone marrow.

The generation of C5a in a local area of injury or infection promotes attraction of neutrophils. However, on a systemic level, C5a appears to cause a generalized activa-tion of neutrophils, which may either sensitize or deactivate the cell[134] and may lead to localization in noninjured tissues.[105] It is possible that such global effects may participate in distant organ injury and increase susceptibility to infection. Activation of the complement cascade, sufficient to cause substantial mediator generation, may not be detected by gross methods of measurement of complement components. This relates to the potency of the mediators as well as to the rapid replacement of components that are consumed.[35]

Renin–Angiotensin System

A neutral peptide mediator, generated by the action of a neutrophil enzyme on a plasma substrate, has been shown to be identical to angiotensin II (AII). More recently, the substrate has been identified as angiotensinogen and the enzyme as cathepsin G.[123] AII was generated when this enzyme was released during neutrophil phagocytosis in *in vitro* studies.[108] Furthermore, enzymes isolated from human skin, mast cells,[124] endothelial cells, and macrophages[98] have the capacity to convert angiotensin I (AI) to AII. It, therefore, appears that AII can be generated by renal-independent mechanisms, at sites of injury, by the direct action of the neutrophil enzyme and indirectly through circulating active renin, which converts angiotensinogen to AI with subsequent cleavage of AI to AII (Fig. 22-1).[127] AII not only causes intense arteriolar vasoconstriction[80] but also increases vascular permeability.[86] Interaction with the activated HF-dependent system would counterbalance the response by way of kallikrein. Such a mechanism has been proposed[95] in the kidney and may occur on a local level. Not only does kallikrein generate bradykinin, but it converts prorenin to renin

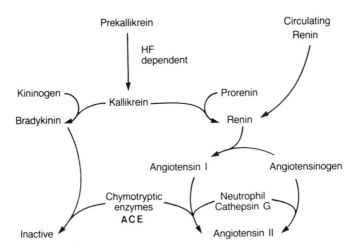

Figure 22–1.
Schematic representation of renin-dependent and renin-independent generation of angiotensin II. Modified from Yurt (127). (Yurt RW. Chemical mediators in injury. In: Shires GT, ed. Fluids, electrolytes and acid bases. New York: Churchill Livingstone, Inc. In press)

and provides an additional pathway for AII generation. The chymotryptic enzymes that have been shown to generate AII[124] have also been shown to destroy the activity of bradykinin.

CELL-DEPENDENT MEDIATOR GENERATION

The recognition in the early 1970s that changes in membrane function occur after hemorrhagic shock[97] has led to the observation that sodium, potassium, calcium, and water balance are perturbed in a variety of tissues after injury and during sepsis.[96] Although it has yet to be demonstrated that such changes are initiated by chemical messengers or that they affect immune function after injury, preliminary evidence suggests that at least one macrophage product, cachectin or tumor necrosis factor (TNF), can lead to a depression in transmembrane potential difference similar to that observed previously.[111] Initial data showing a relative loss of transmembrane potential in neutrophils after injury[29] support the importance of these changes. Clearly extra- and intracellular cation flux, particularly calcium, plays a significant role in cellular activation[43] and changes in membrane potential.[36]

The mechanisms of specific receptor-mediated cellular activation appear to have a common basis in most systems studied. Neurons,[5,16] mast cells,[49] neutrophils[100] and lymphocytes[21] all have been shown to respond to exogenous stimuli through an adenyl cyclase-dependent mechanism. A more detailed evaluation of the neutrophil activation sequence appears to be consistent with early events in neuron activation as described by Schramm and Selinger.[93] In the neutrophil, initial mobilization of calcium parallels the formation of a complex of a nucleotide regulatory protein, N protein, with the receptor–ligand complex.[68] The N protein subsequently binds to guanosine triphosphate (GTP) and then dissociates into stimulatory and inhibitory N proteins. Studies with pertussis toxin, which appears to interact with the N protein, suggest that this pathway is essential for the process to proceed[6] to the activation of phospholipase C. Phospholipase C enhances the conversion of phosphatidyl inositol to inositol triphosphate (IP$_3$) and diacylglycerol.[31] Additional calcium mobilization is initiated by IP$_3$ leading to phospholipase A$_2$ activation and arachidonic acid release while diacylglycerol participates in protein kinase C activation.[67] This sequence appears to be essential for subsequent generation of lipid-based mediators.

The morphologic correlate of lipid metabolism appears to be membrane rearrangement with a "pinching off" of lipid components as documented in studies of the mast cell.[62] These cell membrane events appear to be the initial steps in the production of prostaglandins, the slow reacting substance (SRS) compounds, and platelet-activating factor. The arachidonic acid liberated during activation or supplied by extracellular sources may be metabolized by way of the cyclooxygenase pathway to prostaglandins or by lipoxygenase to the leukotrienes.[91]

When arachidonic acid is metabolized by cyclooxygenase, a cascade is initiated that generates several biologically active compounds, including the short-lived endoperoxides (PGG and PGH$_2$). The classic prostaglandins (PGF$_2$, PGE$_2$, and PGD$_2$), thromboxane A_2, and prostacyclin may also be produced. The generation of these rapidly metabolized products is blocked by the nonsteroidal anti-inflammatory drugs. Because the products of this pathway have a short half-life, it is anticipated that their activity is primarily expressed in the local environment of the cell. In the early phase after injury, PGE_2,[39] as well as the endoperoxides,[44,115] enhance vasodilation and vasopermeability, and potentiate pain. On the other hand, PGE_2 also appears to possess anti-inflammatory activity, because it decreases leukocyte metabolism, phagocytosis, and lymphocyte function. Prostacyclin, the major cyclooxygenase product in blood vessel walls,[15] inhibits platelet aggregation and causes vasodilation. These effects are counterbalanced by the opposing activity of thromboxane A_2.[45,46]

A variety of biologically active products are generated by the action of lipoxygenase on arachidonate. The final products of the pathway vary among different cells (see Table 22-1), and there appears to be a mechanism, through differential enzyme activation, for shunting precursor lipid to or away from this pathway.[51] Lipoxygenase generates HPETE (hydroperoxy-6,8,11,14-eicosatetranoic acid) from arachidonic acid, which is converted to leukotriene A_4 (LTA_4). The SRS compounds, leukotrienes C_4, D_4, and E_4 are generated from LTA_4. In addition, leukotriene B_4 may be generated from LTA_4.[90] LTC_4, LTD_4, and LTE_4 cause bronchoconstriction, vasoconstriction, and edema formation.[27] The airway effects of the SRS compounds appear to be peripheral, rather than central[28] and, therefore, they affect compliance more than conductance in the lung. A product of 12-HPETE, 12-HETE, from platelets is a potent chemotactic agent for neutrophils.[42,112] Additional chemotactic activity is generated in this pathway in the form of LTB_4, which has activity toward the neutrophil comparable to that of C5a.[34,41] Furthermore, LTB_4 appears to augment natural cytotoxic cell activity[88] and to induce suppressor lymphocytes.[79,87] Neutrophils of patients who have sustained a burn injury have a time-related increased capacity to generate LTB_4.[14] *In vivo* injection studies, as well as the finding of increased levels of LTB_4 during inflammation, support a role for this mediator in the response to injury.[33]

Although steroids appear to induce the production of a phospholipase A_2 inhibitor[48] that would inhibit both pathways of arachidonic acid metabolism, selective inhibitors of the lipoxygenase pathway are not available for clinical use. Laboratory investigation has depended on a selective end-organ antagonist (FPL 55712) of SRS-A[82] and U-60,257, which appears to inhibit leukotriene production selectively.[4] The selective generation of prostaglandins and leukotrienes will be reviewed with regard to specific cell populations.

The lipid mediator, platelet-activating factor (PAF or PAF-acether), is also generated during activation of cells involved in the inflammatory response. This mediator, originally identified as a product of basophils[8] and mast cells,[114] is also produced by leukocytes,[7] macrophages,[69] neutrophils, platelets, and endothelial cells. Recent data indicate that lyso-PAF, the precursor of PAF, and arachidonic acid may originate from the same membrane phospholipid.[19,104] Furthermore, LTB_4 and PAF appear to be generated in parallel in stimulated neutrophils.[99] However, in this study, PAF was not released from the neutrophil, suggesting that PAF may be an intracellular mediator or a messenger between cells rather than an extracellular mediator.

The Neutrophil

Neutrophil function is reviewed in Chapter 23. The interactions of the neutrophil and its mediators, however, are mentioned briefly here. It appears that the lipid mediators, LTB_4, PAF, and 5-HETE, act on the neutrophil by way of a pathway that may be separable from the pathway of C5a and N-formyl-methionyl-leucyl-phenylalanine (FMLP) activation.[75] Although it appears that each mediator has a specific receptor on the neutrophil membrane, it is not clear whether the lipid products may exert some of their effects by a postreceptor mechanism. Such seems likely because LTB_4, PAF, and 5-HETE are not only activators but products of neutrophil activation as well.

Degranulation associated with phagocytosis of particulate matter or due to membrane perturbation by specific mediators leads to release of acid hydrolases, neutral proteases, and other granule-associated proteins. Additional products of activation include the oxygen derivatives—peroxide, superoxide anion, hydroxyl radicals, and singlet oxygen.[60] The predominant arachidonic acid metabolites in the neutrophil include thromboxanes and prostaglandins (predominantly PGE_2) and the chemotactic factor LTB_4.[9]

Products of other cell activation and the mediator cascades may act on the neutrophil. Kallikrein,[57] products of fibrinogen[59] and fibrin[102] cleavage have chemotactic activity. C5a, generated by complement activation, activates and modulates the activity of the neutrophil, and C5a may be cleaved from C5 by enzymes of the neutrophil.[119] Mast cell chemotactic factors appear to be specific for neutrophils.

Macrophage-Monocyte

The macrophage, previously identified for its phagocytic function, has more recently been recognized for the plethora of secretory mediators that it generates.[72] Like the mast cell, the macrophage resides at portals of entry of noxious substances, and, by virtue of its perivenular location, it is involved in most inflammatory processes. The reticuloendothelial system (RES) appears to be depressed after shock and trauma.[26,89,92] Conversely, agents that increase RES activity appear to improve resistance to experimentally induced shock. Although the RES appears to be depressed after injury, it is not clear whether this is due to depressed splenic and hepatic blood flow, mediator activity, circulating bacterial products such as endotoxin, or excessive particulate uptake by these cells.

Nathan has recently reviewed nearly 100 secretory products of the macrophage.[72] Many of these products, such as leukotriene B_4, reactive oxygen intermediates, PAF, and lysozyme, are produced by other cells as well. The more recently investigated products, IL-1 and TNF, appear to contribute significantly to injury and sepsis-induced inflammatory response. IL-1 or leukocytic pyrogen[77] appears to induce fever and regulate immune function by way of a PGE-dependent sequence.[25] The multiple effects on the neutrophil that were attributed to IL-1 have recently been reported to be due to contaminants, possibly TNF, in IL-1 preparations. Activities attributed to TNF include induction of shock,[110] neutrophil margination, and endo-thelial cell activation. Furthermore, TNF has been shown to cause a depression in cellular transmembrane potential both *in vivo* and *in vitro*.[111]

The multiplicity of macrophage-produced mediators provides pathways for this cell to interact with the coagulation and complement cascades as well as with neutrophils and lymphocytes.

Mast Cell

The variety and concentration of inflammatory mediators coupled with the likelihood that the cell will be activated by either direct injury or by way of other mediators place the mast cell at the center of injury-induced inflammatory responses. The mast cell is present in virtually every tissue studied and is prominent in skin and mucosal membranes.

As calculated by Yurt,[126] the mast cell mediator content of human skin alone exceeds that needed to cause cardiac arrest and proteolysis by 2000-fold. The content of heparin in these cells is estimated to be 100-fold greater than that needed to cause full anticoagulation. These mediators are released from preformed stores of granule-associated mediators. The granules, which have been partially reconstructed with rat components,[130] contain a core of macromolecular heparin proteoglycan[129] bound to enzyme, histamine, and additional mediators. The noncytolytic release of these media-tors may be caused by bradykinin, endotoxin, C3a, C5a, and cationic proteins from polymorphonuclear leukocytes (PMN).[126] Cytolytic damage to the cell, by traumatic injury, may also lead to the release of preformed mediators.[50,53] Once the granule is exposed to the external milieu, soluble mediators, such as histamine and eosinophil chemotactic factors,[10] are released into the microenvironment. However, a second step is required to dissociate the firmly bound residual mediator core[128] in rat mast cells. The mechanism of this second activation is not known, but it may depend on the oxidative cleavage of glycosidic bonds in the glycosaminoglycan side chains of heparin. Such has been postulated to occur when superoxide systems generate free radicals in adjacent phagocytosing neutrophils.[128]

After the generation and release of mast-cell mediators, both humoral and cellular responses occur. Histamine and the leukotrienes allow water, plasma protein, and additional mediators to enter tissues. The proteolytic activity of enzymes[61] and the anticoagulant activity of heparin[129] may participate in maintaining an open channel. This response may be modulated by the inhibitory activity of heparin toward complement[120] and other proteolytic enzymes.[128] Additional mediators, such as neu-trophil chemotactic factor (NCF),[3] lipid chemotactic factor (LCF),[113] and inflamma-tory factor[55] may participate in the migration of cells to the vicinity of injury. ECF-A[10] may attract eosinophils, which modulate the response through histaminase and arylsulfatase activity. Platelet-activating factor (PAF) from mast cells may activate platelets.[114] Although normal mast cells appear to predominantly produce prostaglan-din D_2[85] when arachidonic acid pathways are stimulated, SRS products are produced by stimulation with the calcium ionophore[125] and bone marrow-derived mast cells produce large amounts of LTC$_4$.[84] That LTD$_4$ is also produced by human lung mast cells[63] has recently been documented.

MODULATION OF
THE MEDIATOR RESPONSE

The final expression of initiation of the mediator systems depends on the extent of the activating stimulus, the presence of inhibitors of the pathway, specific inactivators of the mediator, interactions with other pathways, and the potency of the mediator itself. Currently available data relate primarily to studies of mediator cascades and cellular activation in isolated systems. One of the major regulatory mechanisms in cellular activation appears to depend on intracellular levels of the cyclic nucleotides.

The prostaglandins of the E series appear to decrease responsiveness, as shown by the inhibitory effect of PGE[54] on the release of histamine from mast cells through a rise in intracellular cyclic AMP. The anti-inflammatory activity of PGE$_2$ on macrophages appears to be related to the activation of adenylate cyclase; the extent and duration of the increase in cyclic AMP has been correlated with a depressed leukocyte function.[38] Prostaglandins E$_1$ and E$_2$ have been shown to stimulate cyclic AMP generation in human leukocytes,[12] an effect also confirmed with PGF$_2$.[103] Although epinephrine has been shown to increase intracellular cyclic AMP in leukocytes,[11] this beta-agonist effect has not been found to be significant in granulocytes.[64] For this reason, and based on additional data reported by Boxer and co-workers,[13] it appears that epinephrine-induced effects on marginated neutrophils may be caused by the increased cyclic AMP associated with the generation of the nucleotide from endothelium, rather than from the granulocyte itself. It is anticipated that changes in intracellular cyclic AMP will affect the expression of the glycoprotein (Mo1) associated with neutrophil adhesion.[2, 107] Other cell functions, such as phagocytosis, are not affected by increases in cyclic AMP; however, the degree of nitro blue tetrazolium (NBT) reduction was diminished by elevated cyclic AMP levels in those studies.[32] Additional mediators, such as histamine, appear to modulate cell function by affecting cyclic nucleotides, as in the inhibition of neutrophil chemotaxis by histamine.[78] Anderson and co-workers[1] have shown that histamine-induced depression of the chemotactic response was associated with increased intracellular levels of cyclic AMP. Conversely, when levels of cyclic AMP are depressed by norepinephrine, mediator release is enhanced in human lung fragments.[56] Furthermore, increases in cyclic GMP appear to enhance the release of mediator in this system.[56]

Additional evidence for the control of responses to mediators is based on the deactivation of neutrophils observed at subchemotactic doses of chemotaxin[73, 118] *in vitro* and *in vivo,* after tissue injury.[18] On the other hand, neutrophil function may be enhanced by appropriate doses of chemotaxin, or by less than 30% degranulation, as reported in studies of bactericidal activity and chemiluminescence[116] or chemotaxis,[37] respectively. Chemotactic factors also have been shown to regulate complement receptors on phagocytic cells.[30,58]

Even though it is well documented that glucocorticoids are increased after injury, the extent to which cellular activity is modulated is not well defined. Rabbit neutrophil responses to chemotactic factor have been shown to be depressed after exposure to glucocorticoids.[117] Corticosteroids have also been observed to enhance the activity of adenylate cyclase[24] and to attenuate beta-adrenergic receptors in neutrophils.[23] As previously indicated, steroids appear to induce a phospholipase A inhibitory protein that blocks arachidonic acid metabolism in neutrophils.[48]

CLINICAL MANIFESTATIONS OF THE INFLAMMATORY RESPONSE

Minor tissue injury and localized infections initiate a controlled response that is heralded by edema, erythema, localized vasodilation, and pain. This regulated humoral response usually proceeds to resolution of the process by the early chemotactic factor-induced infiltration of the tissue by neutrophils followed by delayed accumulation of macrophages (Table 22-2). However, major injury or progressive infection can lead to an uncontrolled local and systemic mediator response. Although host defenses are generally expected to be compromised in direct proportion to the extent of injury, the quantitative role of mediator systems after traumatic injury has not been well defined. This appears, in part, to be the result of a lack of opportunity to study mediator activity during the early phase of a major injury in patients. The very rapid changes in plasma concentrations of mast cell mediators after injury, in patients exposed to diverse stimuli[18,70] and in rats,[131] indicate that measurements need to be taken in the acute phase. Such early changes were also noted in the complement system of a rat injury model.[106] Studies of an animal model that document increased susceptibility to infection related to extent of burn injury[132] have provided a method that can be used to evaluate the relationship between the extent of injury and mediator activity. Within 4 hr after injury, the *in vivo* sensitivity of neutrophils to

Table 22–2
Sequence of Cellular and Cascade Response to Local Injury

SENTINEL CELLS	SECONDARY RESPONSE	TERTIARY RESPONSE
Mast cell	Neutrophil	Macrophage/monocyte
Macrophage		
Endothelial cell		
	Coagulation	Coagulation
	Complement	Complement
	Angiotensin	Angiotensin

FMLP had increased relative to the extent of injury, but their responsiveness to zymosan-activated serum was relatively depressed.[134] These *in vivo* studies also suggest that a multiplicity of factors are interacting to yield depressed host responses in the immediate postinjury period.

The extent of injury-related susceptibility to infection documented in these studies is likely related to the quantity of mediator released and the ability of control mechanisms to moderate the response. Data from burn-injury studies indicate that plasma histamine levels are proportional to the extent of injury[133] and are also related to the depth of injury.

Capillary leak, hypotension, decreased pulmonary compliance, depressed cellular immunity, and disorders of the complement, coagulation, and renin systems have all been observed after major injury. Although several mechanisms have been outlined that cause such changes, interestingly, activation of one system alone, the mast cell, could account for these sequelae of injury.[126] When the homeostatic mechanisms are perturbed to the extent that these disorders occur, intervention to control the exaggerated response is necessary.

Currently there are few data to support the clinical efficacy of pharmacologic intervention to control either mediator activation or the expression of mediator activity after injury. However, removal of the stimulus to mediator activation apparently leads to an improved outcome and likely to an improvement in host defense. Debridement of necrotic tissue removes the stimulus for further mediator activation and has been the standard approach to major injury. A renewed interest in the early removal of necrotic tissue, especially in a burn injury, has led to the appreciation that this approach can minimize the metabolic and inflammatory consequences of burn injuries[135] (for a detailed review, see Yurt, Ref 135). In an attempt to overcome the effects of an overwhelming release of mediator after a near-lethal burn injury, a second approach (*i.e.,* mediator removal) has been introduced. In these early studies,[66] it appeared that plasmapheresis does have a beneficial effect on cardiovascular stability and on the cellular immune response.

Laboratory investigations suggest that it may soon be found clinically useful to manipulate the mediator system. Complement depletion or the infusion of free-radical scavengers appears to minimize the early pulmonary sequelae of burn injury in rats.[105] A number of studies, such as those recently reported in a sheep model of lung injury,[109] suggest that pharmacologic manipulation of mediator release or expression may have clinical application. However, standard surgical approaches of early and rapid resuscitation, repair of injured tissue and organs, and the removal of nonviable tissue remain the primary approaches to moderating mediator release after injury.

ACKNOWLEDGMENTS

Supported in part by grants from the National Institutes of Health (2P50GM26145) and the Irma Hirschl Trust Career Scientist Award. This author gratefully acknowledges Sharon A. Joy for her assistance in the preparation of this chapter.

REFERENCES

1. Anderson RA, Glover A, Rabson AR. The *in vitro* effects of histamine and metiamide on neutrophil motility and their relationship to intracellular cyclic nucleotide levels. J Immunol 1977;188:1690.
2. Arnaout MA, Spits H, Terhorst C, et al. Deficiency of a leukocyte surface glycoprotein (LFA-1) in two patients with Mol deficiency: effects of cell activation on Mol/LAF-1 surface expression in normal and deficient leukocytes. J Clin Invest 1984;74:1291.
3. Austen KF, Wasserman SI, Goetzl EJ. Mast cell-derived mediators: structural and functional diversity and regulation of expression. In: Johansson S, Strandberg K, Uvans B, eds. Molecular and biological aspects of the acute allergic reaction. New York: Plenum Publishing, 1976:293.
4. Bach MK, Brashler JR, Smith HW, et al. 6,9-deepoxy-6,9 (phenylimino)-6,8 -prostaglandin I₁, (U-60,257), a new inhibitor of leukotriene C and D synthesis: *in vitro* studies. Prostaglandins 1982;23:759.
5. Batzri S, Selinger Z, Schramm M. Potassium ion release and enzyme secretion: adrenergic regulation by α- and β-receptors. Science 1971;174:1029.
6. Becker EL, Kermode JC, Naccache PH, et al. Pertussin toxin as a probe of neutrophil activation. Fed Proc 1986;45:2151.
7. Benveniste J. Platelet-activating factor, a new mediator of anaphylaxis and immune complex deposition from rabbit and human basophils. Nature 1974;249:581.
8. Benveniste J, Henson PM, Cochrane CG. Leukocyte-dependent histamine release from rabbit platelets. I. The role of IgE, basophils, and a platelet-activating factor. J Exp Med 1972;136:1356
9. Borgeat P, Samuelsson B. Arachidonic acid metabolism in polymorphonuclear leukocytes: effect of ionophore A23187. Proc Natl Acad Sci USA 1979;76:2147.
10. Boswell RN, Austen KF, Goetzl EJ. Intermediate molecular weight eosinophil chemotactic factors in rat peritoneal mast cells; immunologic release, granule association, and demonstration of structural heterogeneity. J Immunol 1978;120:15.
11. Bourne HR, Lehrer RI, Cline MJ, et al. Cyclic 3′,5′-adenosine monophosphate in the human leukocyte: synthesis, degradation, and effects on neutrophil candidacidal activity. J Clin Invest 1971;50:920.
12. Bourne HR, Melmon KL. Adenyl cyclase in human leukocytes: evidence for activation by separate beta adrenergic and prostaglandin receptors. J Pharmacol Exp Ther 1971;178:1.
13. Boxer LA, Allen JM, Baehner RL. Diminished polymorphonuclear leukocyte adherence. Function dependent on release of cyclic AMP by endothelial cells after stimulation of β-receptors by epinephrine. J Clin Invest 1980;66:268.
14. Braquet M, Ducousso R, Garay R, et al. Leukocyte leukotriene by secretion precedes anergy in burn injured patients. Lancet 1984;2(8409):976.
15. Bunting S, Gryglewski R, Moncada S, et al. Arterial wall generate from prostaglandin endoperoxides a substance (prostglandin X) which relays strips of mesenteric and coeliac arteries and inhibits platelet aggregation. Prostaglandins 1976;12:879.
16. Butcher FR, Putney JW. Regulation of parotid gland function by cyclic nucleotide and calcium. Advances in Nucleotide Research 1980;13:215.
17. Cannon WB. Some general features of endocrine influences of metabolism. Am J Med Sci 1926;171:1.
18. Center DM, Soter NA, Wasserman SI, et al. Inhibition of neutrophil chemotaxis in association with experimental angioedema in patients with cold urticaria: a model of chemotactic deactivation *in vivo*. Clin Exp Immunol 1979;35:112.
19. Chilton FH, Ellis JM, Olson SC, et al. 1-O-Alkyl-2-acyl-sn-glycero-3-phosphocholine: a common source of platelet-activating factor and arachidonate in human polymorphonuclear leukocytes. J Biol Chem 1984;259:12014.
20. Cochrane CG, Revak SD, Wuepper KD. Activation of Hageman factor in solid and fluid phases. J Exp Med 1973;138:1564.
21. Coffey RG, Hadden JW. Neurotransmitters, hormones, and cyclic nucleotides in lymphocyte regulation. Fed Proc 1985;44:112.
22. Cooper NR, Miles LA, Griffin JH. Activation of purified C1, the first complement component, by purified plasma kallikrein and plasmin (abstr). Thromb Haemost 1978;42:251.
23. Davies AO, Lefkowitz RF. *In vitro* desensitization of beta adrenergic receptors in human neutrophils. J Clin Invest 1983;71:565.
24. Davies AO, Lefkowitz RF. Corticosteroid-induced differential regulation of β-adrenergic receptors in circulating human polymorphonuclear leukocytes and mononuclear leukocytes. J Clin Endocrinol Metab 1980;51:599.

25. Dinarello CA, Marnoy SO, Rosenwasser LJ. Role of arachidonate metabolism in the immunoregulatory function of human leukocytic pyrogen/lymphocyte-activating factor/interleukin 1. J Immunol 1983;130:890.

26. Donovan AJ. The effect of surgery on reticuloendothelial cell function. Arch Surg 1967;94:247.

27. Drazen JM, Austen KF, Lewis RA, et al. Comparative airway and vascular activities of leukotrienes C1 and D *in vivo* and *in vitro*. Proc Natl Acad Sci USA 1980;77:4354.

28. Drazen JM, Lewis RA, Wasserman SI, et al. Differential effects of a partially purified preparation of slow reacting substance of anaphylaxis on guinea pig tracheal spirals and parenchymal strips. J Clin Invest 1979;63:1.

29. Duque RE, Phan SH, Hudson JL, et al. Functional defects in phagocytic cells following thermal injury. Am J Pathol 1985;118:116.

30. Fearon DT, Wong WW. Complement ligand–receptor interactions that mediate biological responses. Annu Rev Immunol 1983;1:243.

31. Feltner D, Smith RH, Marasco WA. Characterization of the plasma membrane bound GTPase from rabbit neutrophils: evidence for an N_i-like protein coupled to the formyl peptide, C5a, and leukotriene B_4 chemotaxis receptors. J Immunol 1986;137:1961.

32. Flyer RH, Finch SC. The effects of prostaglandin E_1 on human granulocyte metabolism during phagocytosis. Journal of Reticuloendothelial Society 1973;14:325.

33. Ford-Hutchinson AW. Leukotrienes: their formation and role as inflammatory mediators. Fed Proc 1985;44:25.

34. Ford-Hutchinson AW, Bray MA, Doig MV, et al. Leukotriene B_4, a potent chemokinetic and aggregating substance released from polymorphonuclear leukocytes. Nature 1980;286:264.

35. Frank MM. Complement in the pathophysiology of human disease. N Engl J Med 1987;316:1525.

36. Gallin JI, Durocher JR, Kaplan AP. Interaction of leukocyte chemotactic factors with the cell surface. I. Chemotactic factor-induced changes in human granulocyte surface charge. J Clin Invest 1975;55:967.

37. Gallin JI, Wright DG, Schiffman E. Role of secretory events in modulating human neutrophil chemotaxis. J Clin Invest 1978;62:1364.

38. Gemsa D. Stimulation of prostaglandin E release from macrophages and possible role in the immune response. Lymphokines 1981;4:335.

39. Gemsa D, Leser H, Seitz M, et al. Membrane perturbation and stimulation of arachidonic acid metabolism. Mol Immunol 1982;19:1287.

40. Gewurz H, Shin HS, Mergenhagen SE. Interactions of the complement system with endotoxic lipopolysaccharide: consumption of each of the six terminal complement components. J Exp Med 1968;128:1049.

41. Goetzl EJ, Pickett WC. Novel structural determinants of the human neutrophill chemotactic activity of leukotriene B_4. J Exp Med 1981;153:482.

42. Goetzl EJ, Woods JM, Gorman RR. Stimulation of human eosinophil and neutrophil polymorphonuclear leukocyte chemotaxis and random migration by 12-L-hydroxy-5,8,10,14-eicosatetraenoic acid. J Clin Invest 1977;59:179.

43. Goldstein IM, Hoffstein S, Gallin JI, et al. Mechanisms of lysosomal enzyme release from human leukocytes: microtubule assembly and membrane fusion induced by a component of complement. Proc Natl Acad Sci USA 1973;70:2916.

44. Hagermark O, Strandberg K, Hamberg M. Potentiating effect of prostaglandin E_2 and the prostaglandin endoperoxide PGH_2 on cutaneous responses in man. J Invest Dermatol 1976;22:266P.

45. Hamberg M, Samuelsson B. Prostaglandin endoperoxides. III. Novel transformation of arachidonic acid in human platelets. Proc Natl Acad Sci USA 1974;71:3400.

46. Hamberg M, Svensson J, Samuelsson B. Thromboxanes: a new group of biologically active compounds derived from prostaglandin endoperoxides. Proc Natl Acad Sci USA 1975;72:2994.

47. Heideman M, Kaijser B, Gelin LE. Complement activation and hematologic, hemodynamic, and respiratory reactions early after soft-tissue injury. J Trauma 1978;18:696.

48. Hirata F, Schiffman E, Venkatasubramanian K, et al. A phospholipase A_2 inhibitory protein in rabbit neutrophils induced by glucocorticoids. Proc Natl Acad Sci USA 1980;77:2533.

49. Holgate SI, Lewis RA, Austen KF. 3'5'-cyclic adenosine monophosphate-dependent protein kinase of the rat serosal mast cell and its immunologic activation. J Immunol 1980;124:2093.

50. Horokova Z, Beaven MA. Time course of histamine release and edema formation in the rat paw after thermal injury. Eur J Pharmacol 1974;27:305.

51. Humes JL, Sadowski S, Galavage M, et al. Evidence for two sources of arachidonic acid for oxidative metabolism by mouse peritoneal macrophages. J Biol Chem 1982;257:1591.

52. Johnson AR, Erdos EG. Release of histamine from mast cells by vasoactive peptides. Proc Soc Exp Biol Med 1973;42:1252.

53. Johnson AR, Moran NC. Interaction of toluidine blue and rat mast cells: histamine release and uptake and release of the dye. J Pharmacol Exp Ther 1974;189:221.

54. Kaliner M, Austen KF. Cyclic AMP, ATP, and reversed anaphylactic histamine release from rat mast cells. J Immunol 1974;112:664.

55. Kaliner M, Lemanske R. Inflammatory responses to mast cell granules. Fed Proc 1984;43:2846.

56. Kaliner M, Orange RP, Austen KF. Immunological release of histamine and slow reacting substance of anaphylaxis from human lung. IV. Enhancement by cholinergic and alpha adrenergic stimulation. J Exp Med 1972;136:556.

57. Kaplan AP, Kay AB, Austen KF. A prealbumin activator of prekallikrein. III. Appearance of chemotactic activity for human neutrophils by the conversion of human prekallikrein to kallikrein. J Exp Med 1972;135:81.

58. Kay AB. Complement receptor enhancement by chemotactic factors. Mol Immunol 1982;19:1307.

59. Kay AB, Pepper DS, Edward MR. Generation of chemotactic activity of leukocytes by the action of thrombin on human fibrinogen. Nature (New Biology) 1973;243:56.

60. Klebanoff SJ, Clark RA. In: The neutrophil: function and clinical disorders. New York: North-Holland, 1978;283.

61. Lagunoff D, Benditt EP. Proteolytic enzymes of mast cells. Ann NY Acad Sci 1963;103:185.

62. Lawson D, Raff MC, Gomperts B, et al. Molecular events during membrane fusion: A study of exocytosis in rat peritoneal mast cells. J Cell Biol 1977;72:242.

63. MacGlashan DW, Schleimer RP, Peters SP, et al. Generation of leukotrienes by purified human lung mast cells. J Clin Invest 1982;70:747.

64. MacGregor RR. Granulocyte adherence changes induced by hemodialysis, endotoxin, epinephrine, and glucocorticoids. Ann Intern Med 1977;86:35.

65. Marcus RL, Shin HS, Mayer MM. An alternate complement pathway: C3 cleaving activity, not due to C4,2a on endotoxic lipopolysaccharide after treatment with guinea pig serum; relation to properdin. Proc Natl Acad Sci USA 1971;68:1351.

66. McManus WF, Warden GO. Is there a role for plasmaphoresis/exchange transfusion in the treatment of the septic burn patient? J Trauma 1984;24(Suppl):S137.

67. Melloni E, Pontremoli S, Michetti M, et al. The involvement of calpain in the activation of protein kinase C in neutrophils stimulated by phorbol myristic acid. J Biol Chem 1986;261:4101.

68. Melnick D, Meshulam T, Aurelio M, et al. Activation of human neutrophils by monoclonal antibody PMN7C3: cell movement and adhesion can be triggered independently of the respiratory burst. Blood 1986;3:1388.

69. Mencia-Huerta JM, Benveniste J. Platelet-activating factor and macrophages. I. Evidence for the release from rat and mouse peritoneal macrophages and not from mastocytes. Eur J Immunol 1979;9:409.

70. Metzger WJ, Kaplan AP, Beaven MA, et al. Hereditary vibratory angioedema: confirmation of histamine release in a type of physical hypersensitivity. J Allergy Clin Immunol 1976;57:605.

71. Morrison DC, Cochrane CG. Direct evidence for Hageman factor (factor XII) activation by bacterial lipopolysaccharides. J Exp Med 1974;140:797.

72. Nathan CF. Secretory products of macrophages. J Clin Invest 1987;79:319.

73. Nelson RD, McCormack RT, Fiegel VD, et al. Chemotactic deactivation of human neutrophils: evidence for nonspecific and specific components. Infections and Immunology 1978;22:441.

74. Niewiarowski S, Bankowski E, Rogowicka I. Studies on the absorption and activation of Hageman factor (factor XII) by collagen and elastin. Thrombosis Diathesis and Haemorrhagica 1965;14:387.

75. O'Flaherty JT. Neutrophil degranulation: evidence pertaining to its mediation by the combined effects of leukotriene B_4, platelet-activating factor, and 5-HETE. J Cell Physiol 1985;122:229.

76. Oh-Ishi S, Uchida Y, Ueno A, et al. Bromelain, a thiol protease from pineapple stem, depletes high molecular weight kininogen by activation of Hageman factor (factor XII). Thromb Res 1979;14:665.

77. Oppenheim JJ, Stadler BM, Siraganian RP, et al. Lymphokines: their role in lymphocyte responses. Fed Proc 1982;41:257.

78. Patrone F, Dallegri F, Gianfranco L, et al. Reversal by cimetidine of histamine-induced inhibition of true chemotaxis in neutrophil polymorphonuclears. Res Exp Med (Berl) 1980;176:201.

79. Payan DG, Goetzl EJ. Specific suppression of human T lymphocyte function by leukotriene B. J Immunol 1983;131:551.

80. Peach MJ. Renin–angiotensin system: biochemistry and mechanisms of action. Physiol Rev 1977;57:313.

81. Pillemer L. Blum L, Lepow IH, et al. The properdin system and immunity. I. Demonstration and isolation of a new serum protein, properdin, and its role in immune phenomena. Science 1954;120:279.

82. Piper P, Vane J. The release of prostaglandins from lung and other tissues. Ann NY Acad Sci 1971;180:363.

83. Ratnoff OD, Naff GB. The conversion of C'ls to C'l esterase by plasmin and trypsin. J Exp Med 1967;125:337.

84. Razin F, Mencia-Huerta JM, Lewis RA, et al. Generation of leukotriene C₄ from a subclass of mast cells differentiated *in vitro* from mouse bone marrow. Proc Natl Acad Sci USA 1982;79:4665.

85. Roberts II J, Lewis RA, Lawson JA, et al. Arachidonic acid metabolism by rat mast cells. Prostaglandins 1978;15:717.

86. Robertson AL, Khairallah P. Effects of angiotensin II on the permeability of the vascular wall. In: Page IH, Bumpus FM, eds. Angiotensin. New York: Springer-Verlag, 1974:500.

87. Rola-Pleszczynski M, Borgeat P, Sirois P. Leukotriene B₄ induces human suppressor lymphocytes. Biochem Biophys Res Commun 1983;108:15.

88. Rola-Pleszcynski M, Gagnon L, Sirois P. Leukotriene B₄ augments human natural cytotoxic cell activity. Biochem Biophys Res Commun 1983;113:531.

89. Saba TM, Scovill WA. Effect of surgical trauma on host defense. Ann Surg 1975;7:71.

90. Samuelsson B. Leukotrienes: mediators of immediate hypersensitivity reactions and inflammation. Science 1983;220:568.

91. Samuelsson B, Hammarstrom S, Borgeat P. Pathways of arachidonic acid metabolism. Adv Inflamm Res 1979;1:405.

92. Schildt BE. Function of the RES after thermal and mechanical trauma in mice. Acta Chirurgia Scandinavia 1970;136:359.

93. Schramm M, Selinger Z. Message transmission: receptor controlled adenylate cyclase system. Science 1984;225:1350.

94. Schwartz LB, Bradford TR, Littman BH, et al. The fibrinolytic activity of purified tryptase from human lung mast cells. J Immunol 1985;135:2762.

95. Sealey JE, Atlas SA. Inactive renin: speculations concerning its secretion and activation. J Hypertension 1984;2(Suppl 1):115.

96. Shires GT. Principles and management of hemorrhagic shock. In: Shires GT, ed. Principles of Trauma Care. 3rd ed. New York: McGraw-Hill, 1985:3.

97. Shires GT, Cunningham JN, Baker CR, et al. Alterations in cellular membrane function during hemorrhagic shock in primates. Ann Surg 1972;176:288.

98. Silverstein E, Friedland J, Setton C. Angiotensin converting enzyme: induction in rabbit alveolar macrophages and human monocytes in culture. Adv Exp Med Biol 1979;121:149.

99. Sisson JH, Prescott SM, McIntyre TM, et al. Production of platelet-activating factor by stimulated human polymorphonuclear leukocytes. J Immunol 1987;138:3918.

100. Smolen JE, Korchak HM, Weissman G. Increased levels of cyclic adenosine-3, 5-monophosphate in human polymorphonuclear leukocytes after surface stimulation. J Clin Invest 1980;65:1077.

101. Spragg RG, Cochrane GG, McGuire WW. Enzymatic activity causing cleavage of Hageman factor system components in human bronchoalveolar lavage fluid (abstr). Am Rev Respir Dis 1980;122:279.

102. Stecher VJ. The chemotaxis of selected cell types to connective tissue degradation products. Ann NY Acad Sci 1975;256:177.

103. Stolc V. Restrained adenyl cyclase in human neutrophils: stimulation of cyclic adenosine-3′,5′-monophosphate formation and adenyl cyclase activity by phagocytosis and prostaglandins. Blood 1974;43:743.

104. Swendsen CL, Ellis JM, Chilton FH, et al. 1-0-Alkyl-2-acyl-sn-glycero-3-phosphocholine: a novel source of arkachidonic acid in neutrophils stimulated by the calcium ionophore A23187. Biochem Biophys Res Commun 1983;113:72.

105. Till GO, Beauchamp C, Menapace BS, et al. Oxygen radical dependent lung damage following thermal injury of rat skin. J Trauma 1983;23:269.

106. Till GO, Johnson JJ, Kunkel R, et al. Intravascular activation of complement and acute lung injury: dependence on neutrophils and toxic oxygen metabolites. J Clin Invest 1982;69:1126.

107. Todd RF, Arnaout MN, Rosin RE, et al. Subcellular localization of the large subunit of Mol, a surface glycoprotein associated with neutrophil adhesion. J Clin Invest 1984;74:1280.

108. Tonnesen MG, Klempner MS, Austen KF, et al. Identification of a human neutrophil angiotensin II-generating protease as cathepsin G. J Clin Invest 1982;69:25.

109. Traber DL, Adams T, Henriksen N, et al. Ibuprofen and diphenhydramine reduce the lung lesion of endotoxemia in sheep. J Trauma 1984;24:835.
110. Tracey KJ, Beutler B, Lowry SF, et al. Shock and tissue injury induced by recombinant human cachectin. Science 1986;234:470.
111. Tracey KJ, Lowry SF, Beutler B, et al. Cachectin/tumor necrosis factor mediates changes of skeletal muscle plasma membrane potentials. J Exp Med 1986;164:1368.
112. Turner SR, Tainer JA, Lynn WS. Biogenesis of chemotactic molecules by the arachidonate lipoxygenase system of platelets. Nature 1975;257:680.
113. Valone FH, Goetzl EJ. Immunologic release in the rat peritoneal cavity of lipid chemotactic and chemokinetic factors for polymorphonuclear leukocytes. J Immunol 1978;120:102.
114. Valone FH, Whitmer DI, Pickett WC, et al. The immunological generation of a platelet-activating factor and a platelet-lytic factor in the rat. Immunology 1979;37:841.
115. Vane JR. Prostaglandins as mediators of inflammation. In: Samuelsson B, Paoletti R, eds. Advances in prostaglandins and thromboxane research, vol 2. New York: Raven Press, 1976:791.
116. Van Epps DE, Garcia ML. Enhancement of neutrophil function as a result of prior exposure to chemotactic factor. J Clin Invest 1980;66:167.
117. Ward PA. The chemosuppression of chemotaxis. J Exp Med 1966;124:209.
118. Ward PA, Becker EL. The deactivation of rabbit neutrophils by chemotactic factor and the nature of the activatable esterase. J Exp Med 1968;127:693.
119. Ward PA, Hill JH. C5 chemotactic fragments produced by an enzyme in lysosomal granules of neutrophils. J Immunol 1970;104:535.
120. Weiler JM, Yurt RW, Fearon DT, et al. Modulation of the formation of the amplification convertase of complement, C3b, Bb, by native and commercial heparin. J Exp Med 1978;147:409.
121. Wiggins RC, Cochrane CG, McGuire WV. Hageman factor: mechanisms and consequences of activation. In: McConn R, ed. The role of chemical mediators in the pathophysiology of acute illness and injury. New York: Raven Press, 1982:1.
122. Winkelstein JA, Tomasz A. Activation of the alternative pathway by pneumoccocal cell wall teichoic acid. J Immunol 1978;120:174.
123. Wintroub BU, Klickstein LB, Kaempfer CE, et al. A human neutrophil-dependent pathway for generation of angiotensin II: purification and physiochemical characterization of the plasma protein substrate. Proc Natl Acad Sci USA 1981;78:1204.
124. Wintroub BU, Schechter NB, Lazarus GS, et al. Angiotensin I conversion by human and rat chymotryptic proteinases. J Invest Dermatol 1984;83:336.
125. Yecies LD, Wedner HJ, Johnson SM, et al. Slow reacting substance (SRS) from ionophore A23187-stimulated peritoneal mast cells of the normal rat. I. Conditions of generation and initial characterization. J Immunol 1979;122:2083.
126. Yurt RW. Role of the mast cell in trauma. In: Dineen P, Hildick-Smith G, eds. The surgical wound. Philadelphia: Lea & Febiger, 1981:37.
127. Yurt RW: Chemical mediators in injury. In: Shires GT, eds. Fluids, electrolytes, and acid bases, Clinics in Critical Care Medicine Series. New York: Churchill Livingstone, in press.
128. Yurt RW, Austen KF. Cascade events in mast cell activation and function. In: Berlin RD, Herrmann H, Lepow IH, et al. Molecular basis of biological degradative processes. New York: Academic Press, 1978:125.
129. Yurt RW, Leid RW, Austen KF, et al. Native heparin from rat peritoneal mast cells. J Biol Chem 1977;252:518.
130. Yurt RW, Leid RW, Spragg J, et al. Preparative purification of the rat mast cell chymase. Characterization and interaction with granule components. J Exp Med 1977;146:1405.
131. Yurt RW, Mason AD Jr, Pruitt BA Jr. Evidence against participation of mast cell histamine in burn edema. Surgical Forum 1982;33:71.
132. Yurt RW, McManus AT, Mason AD Jr, et al. Increased susceptibility to infection related to extent of burn injury. Arch Surg 1984;119:183.
133. Yurt RW, Pruitt BA. Baseline and post-thermal injury plasma histamine in rats: time, depth, and surface area related changes. J Appl Physiol 1986;60:1782.
134. Yurt RW, Pruitt BA. Decreased wound neutrophils and indiscrete margination in the pathogenesis of wound infection. Surgery 1985;98:191.
135. Yurt RW, Shires GT. Burns. In: Mandell G, Douglas RG, Bennett JE, eds. Principles and practices of infectious diseases. 3rd ed. New York: John Wiley & Sons, 1990:830.

23

○   ○   ○   ●   ●   ●

THE NEUTROPHIL

John D. Meyer
John Mihran Davis

The polymorphonuclear leukocyte (PMN) serves as the major effector of the nonspecific immune response in host resistance to infection. The most abundant cell in the circulation, its function in the phagocytosis and killing of microbes is essential in the localization and containment of infection in the tissues. The rapidity with which the neutrophil's response to infection occurs, long before the generation of specific humoral and cell-mediated responses, underscores the importance of this cell in the prevention of systemic infection by pathogenic bacteria. Host resistance to infection may thus be significantly altered by disorders resulting in decreased production or impaired performance of neutrophils; these conditions may arise from hereditary, acquired, or iatrogenic causes. Furthermore, the neutrophil may itself be contributory to tissue injury by way of release of granule enzymes or toxic oxygen products in a number of systemic disorders. Recognition of disordered neutrophil activity and its potential consequences in the surgical patient is useful in proper management of these patients. Neutrophil function, both in the intact host as well as in disordered states, will be examined in this chapter, followed by a review of changes in PMN function and the resultant effects on host resistance seen in a variety of surgical patients.

NEUTROPHIL DEVELOPMENT

The bone marrow is the sole site of PMN production in the normal human. Neutrophils are derived from pleuripotential stem cells in the marrow; these also give rise to the other cells of the granulocyte line, the basophil, eosinophil, and monocyte.[34] Granulocyte development in the marrow consists of a mitotic and a postmitotic phase, each of 4 to 7 days' duration.[38] The initial recognizable precursor of the neutrophil is the myeloblast, a cell approximately twice the size of the mature PMN, which contains numerous primitive ribosomes, mitochondria, and a Golgi apparatus.[33] Cell division and growth result in the formation of the larger promyelocyte. This cell contains a more prominant Golgi apparatus and rough endoplasmic reticulum. The nucleus is eccentrically placed and bean-shaped. This stage is notable for the formation of the numerous azurophil granules in the cytoplasm; these are described in greater detail below. Production of these granules terminates with the end of the promyelocytic phase. Subsequent mitosis results in reduction of azurophil granule concentration and production of the myelocyte. Specific or secondary granule formation is the hallmark of the myelocytic phase; accompanying changes include a reduction of cell size to 10 μ, reduction of mitochondrial and ribosomal numbers, and appearance of glycogen particles in the cytoplasm.[83] The nucleus becomes indented, and chromatin becomes more condensed. The mitotic phase of development ends with the completion of specific granule formation.

Morphologic maturation of the cell in the absence of further division occurs in the postmitotic phase, leading from the metamyelocyte through the "band," an immature neutrophil, to the mature PMN. The nucleus becomes increasingly segmented, with further condensation of nuclear material. A reduction in cellular organelles, including ribosomes, mitochondria, and the Golgi apparatus, continues while glycogen granules proceed to accumulate in the cytoplasm. Membrane deformability, motility, and phagocytic ability gradually increase during this stage.[38] A decrease in the negative surface charge of the neutrophil is noted during the postmitotic phase. This phenomenon results from loss of sialic acid from the cell surface and may represent a mechanism for release of cells from the marrow.[87] The postmitotic phase thus ends with the development of a complex cell capable of sustained movement, phagocytosis of foreign material, and microbicidal activity.

NEUTROPHIL KINETICS

Production of mature granulocytes in the bone marrow occurs at the rate of approximately 1.5×10^9 cells per kilogram body weight per day. Cells in the postmitotic phase, acquiring functional capabilities in the marrow, form the marrow granulocyte reserve, estimated at 8.8×10^9 cells per kilogram of body weight.[38] The normal neutrophil reserve in the marrow may thus contain 6 to 10 times the daily neutrophil requirement in normal subjects. Release of cells from the marrow, with concomitant depletion of reserves, is markedly enhanced in the presence of inflammatory or infectious stimuli; this phenomenon may be experimentally produced by the administration of endotoxin or etiocholanolone. Increased production and delivery of functional neutrophils must then occur in the face of increasing demand. Regulatory mechanisms responsible for the stimulation and release of cells have been attributed to several factors. Colony-stimulating factor (CSF), a glycoprotein elaborated by macrophages, peripheral blood monocytes, and stimulated lymphocytes, and found in normal serum and urine, is felt to be a primary stimulus for multiplication of stem cells and production of granulocytes.[65, 118] Bacteria or sources of bacterial products appear to be activators of production of CSF by macrophages and lymphocytes.[115] Increased neutrophil production results in reduction of bacterial load and removal of further stimulus for CSF production. Endotoxin may produce enhanced neutrophil release by way of a similar mechanism.

The total blood or intravascular neutrophil pool, comprised of cells released from the marrow into the circulation, may be divided into circulating and marginated subgroups. The marginated pool of cells is comprised of PMNs transiently sequestered along the endothelial surfaces of small veins; these cells are in equilibrium with the circulating pool. Landmark studies in the 1960s estimated the number of cells in the circulating and marginated pools at 300 million and 400 million cells per kilogram of blood, respectively.[10] The marginated pool may be released into the circulation through exercise or epinephrine infusion, while endotoxin will produce a transient increase in margination of circulating neutrophils.[151] A relatively short period of time is spent by the neutrophil in the circulation, with the average half-life of approximately 6 hr.

Chemotactic factors stimulating neutrophil aggregation and adherence to endothelial surfaces are believed responsible for PMN migration into the tissues. Leukocytes adherent to vessel walls extend pseudopodia between endothelial cells, following which the cell squeezes though the space,[83] a phenomenon termed *diapedesis.* Migration may be to areas of vascular injury, inflammation, or areas of direct contact with the external environment, such as the oral cavity, gastrointestinal tract, tracheobronchial tree, and cervical canal. Duration of neutrophil survival in extravascular tissues is unknown, although estimates range from 1 to 4 days.[33] Neutrophil distribution may be impaired in states in which the integrity of the vasculature is compromised, such as diabetes and peripheral vascular disease, contributing to the decreased resistance to local infection seen in these conditions.

NEUTROPHIL STRUCTURE

The mature neutrophil measures between 10 and 12 μ. The most striking features of this cell are the prominant multilobed nucleus, a feature shared with other constituents of the granulocyte line, and the marked abundance of cytoplasmic granules (see Table 23-1). Chromatin in the nucleus is condensed, and nucleoli are absent. The functional significance of the multilobed nucleus is not known. The mature neutrophil is functionally an end cell and is not capable of further cell division.

Table 23–1
Neutrophil Granule Contents

CLASS	AZUROPHILIC	SPECIFIC
Microbicidal enzymes	Lysozyme Myeloperoxidase	Lysozyme
Neutral serine proteases	Elastase Cathepsin G Proteinase 3	
Acid hydrolases	N-acetyl-β-glucosaminidase Cathepsins B & D β-glucuronidase β-glycerolphosphatase α-mannosidase	
Metalloproteases		Collagenase
Others	Bactericidal cationic proteins	Lactoferrin Vitamin B_{12}-binding proteins Cytochrome b Histaminase FMLP receptors

(Adapted from Falloon J, Gallin JI. Neutrophil granules in health and disease. J Allergy Clin Immunol 1986; 77:653.)

The granules visible within the cell may be divided into two major populations differing in content, morphology, and time of appearance during granulopoiesis. The azurophil, or primary, granules appear early in maturation during the promyelocyte stage.[13] These constitute approximately 25% to 30% of the granule population of the mature neutrophil, are highly electron-dense, and are relatively large, ranging from 0.5 to 0.8 μ.[14] With subsequent cell division of the promyelocyte to form the myelocyte, production of primary granules ceases and the specific or secondary granules appear.[13,14] These are smaller (0.5 μ) and less electron-dense than the azurophil granules; they are specific to the neutrophil, whereas azurophil granules of the promyelocyte are similar to those of the promonocyte.

Azurophil granules contain various microbicidal and hydrolytic enzymes and proteases consistent with a postulated lysosomal function in digestion of phagocytosed material and killing of ingested bacteria. The microbicidal activity of lysozyme derives from hydrolysis of N-acetylmuramyl-N-acetylglucosamine linkages in bacterial mucopeptide coats.[83,137] Myeloperoxidase functions in a halide-hydrogen peroxide bactericidal system whereby agents toxic to a variety of microorganisms are generated.[81,82] Additionally, it may play a role in the regulation of the phagocytosis-induced respiratory burst, which results in oxygen consumption and peroxide formation.[83] Degradation of phagocytosed material is performed by acid hydrolases and neutral serine proteases present in the granule.[20,51,61] Cationic neutral proteases have been shown to act on components of the complement system, inactivating the complement component C5a and thereby modulating inflammatory and chemotactic responses.[153,154] Elastase, a serine protease, may additionally enable neutrophils to penetrate tissue; its release may also play a role in the endothelial cell damage seen in the adult respiratory distress syndrome (ARDS).[108,149]

The specific granules also contain lysozyme as well as collagenase, lactoferrin, and vitamin B_{12} binding protein.[51] Lactoferrin has been shown to inhibit bacterial growth;[26,110] its bacteriostatic effects are believed to be secondary to chelation of iron essential for bacterial growth. A direct bactericidal action of lactoferrin has also been demonstrated, as well as a role in promotion of PMN adhesiveness and enhancement of hydroxyl radical production.[7,8,111] The function of the vitamin B_{12} binding proteins in the neutrophil remains unknown. Generation of the chemoattractant C5a by way of activation of the alternate complement pathway may be induced by specific granule contents,[154] serving to amplify the inflammatory response through complement activation and to enhance recruitment of neutrophils by way of generation of chemoattractants. Deactivation of C5a by azurophil granule contents, as noted above, may provide a means of down-regulation of this mechanism.

Specific granule contents, in contrast to those of the azurophil granules, are more accessible for extracellular release; spontaneous exocytosis of specific granules *in vitro* is enhanced by nonspecific adherence to surfaces and by migration in response to chemotactic agents.[153] Additionally, a role of the specific granule in modulation of cellular membrane receptors has been postulated. Plasma membrane receptors for the chemotactic peptide N-formyl-methionyl-leucyl-phenylalanine (FMLP) and the complement fragment C3b have been demonstrated to exist intracellularly and presumably within the specific granule membrane.[18,57] Degranulating stimuli[58] and exudation *in vivo*[160] result in both a preferential loss of specific granule contents and increased expression of receptors for FMLP and C3b. Assymetric distribution of FMLP receptors on activated neutrophil surfaces has been noted,[141] possibly a result of specific granule discharge at the leading edge of the cell during chemotaxis.[51] Thus in addition to its secretory function, the specific granule may be responsible in part for altering cell responsiveness to inflammatory or other activating stimuli.

The PMN membrane appears to be composed of a phospholipid bilayer with freely moveable membrane proteins inserted within, a structure termed the fluid-mosaic model.[128] The presence of specific binding sites for various humoral mediators, including the immunoglobulins IgG and IgA, the complement fractions C3b and C5a, and the chemoattractant FMLP, has been demonstrated on the neutrophil membrane.[9,28,96,136,150] Although homogeneously distributed throughout the resting cell membrane, certain classes of receptors demonstrate clustering at the leading edge of cells responding to a gradient of chemoattractant.[147] Evidence exists, as well, for the modulation of receptor numbers present on the membrane by way of exocytosis of specific granules. The fluidity of the plasma membrane of the neutrophil aids in the extension of pseudopodia and locomotion toward a chemotactic stimulus. Adjacent to the plasma membrane are microfilaments composed of actin and myosin polymers forming the contractile mechanism necessary for locomotion.[135,140]

Microtubules composed of tubulin dimers are also present in the neutrophil cytoplasm;[92] their function is believed to be orientation of the cell during movement and in organization of granules prior to degranulation.[76,93] Microtubule-mediated reorganization of membrane lipids and proteins may produce alterations in membrane viscosity, allowing extension of pseudopodia.[19] Further characterizing the mature neutrophil are a marked paucity of cytoplasmic organelles, including mitochondria and ribosomes, indicative of greatly diminished synthetic processes within the cell. These cells are rich in glycogen granules, which are distributed throughout the cytoplasm and serve as the primary energy source for neutrophil function.[126]

METABOLISM

The mature PMN in the resting state is metabolically dormant, with little energy demand or expenditure. As noted above, numerous glycogen granules are present within the cell; these provide the major substrate for glycolysis. Stimulation of the plasma membrane prior to ingestion of foreign particles is associated with a marked increase in metabolic activity and oxygen consumption by the phagocytosing neutrophil;[121,122] this event is termed the *respiratory or metabolic burst*. This phagocytosis-induced increase in oxygen consumption results in the formation of several toxic oxygen products, including superoxide anions, hydrogen peroxide, singlet oxygen, and hydroxyl radicals, all used in the killing of ingested bacteria.[83] The antimicrobial activity of these products is augmented by the presence of halide ions and myeloperoxidase. Initiation of the respiratory burst has been attributed to an NADPH oxidase associated with the plasma membrane and activated by way of stimulation of the membrane by foreign particles.[11,40] Evidence suggests the involvement of a cytochrome b electron transport system associated with the specific granules in the transfer of electrons from NADPH to oxygen, resulting in the formation of toxic oxygen products.[21] Glucose oxidation by way of the hexose monophosphate shunt is also markedly increased, rising to 20% to 40% of the total glucose utilization during phagocytosis.[139] This pathway results in the regeneration of NADPH, thereby renewing available substrate for formation of oxygen derivatives. The hexose monophosphate (HMP) pathway results in the formation of ribulose-5-phosphate and CO_2; *in vitro* stimulation of neutrophils in the presence of ^{14}C-labeled glucose provides a sensitive measure of the amplitude of the respiratory burst and hence of PMN microbicidal function.

Antioxidant systems within the cell are responsible for the degradation and detoxification of generated peroxide and superoxide not used in microbial killing. Cytoplasmic catalase and glutathione peroxidase catalyze the production of water from hydrogen peroxide. Superoxides are converted to peroxide through the action of superoxide dismutase, a reaction that may also occur spontaneously. Hydrogen peroxide elaborated by phagocytosing PMNs may also be secreted into the extracellular fluid where it may exert toxic effects on other cells, including tumors and host synovial tissues.[11,32]

Degranulation, which together with phagocytosis comprise the major energy-dependent functions of the neutrophil, appears to require energy derived from glycolysis.[83] Suppression of the HMP shunt yields no adverse effect on degranulation, while stimulation of the membrane by immune aggregates results in increased HMP shunt activity with no net increase in granule release. The demonstrated dissociation of the neutrophil respiratory burst and degranulation indicates that although the two events are usually concomitant, they are not intertwined nor is one a prerequisite for the other.

NEUTROPHIL FUNCTION

Neutrophil function in response to infection or inflammation is considered to be the sum of three components: chemotaxis, phagocytosis, and intracellular killing. These represent separate and distinct cellular processes and may be studied independently *in vitro* despite their interrelation in the host response to infection. Elucidation of these cellular events has been further facilitated by study of patients with functional PMN abnormalities. Each component of neutrophil function will be considered separately here, with reference to the overall scheme of neutrophil function (see Table 23-2).

Table 23–2
Disorders of Neutrophil Function in the Surgical Setting

Neutropenia	**Opsonic and Phagocytic Defects**
Cytotoxic therapy	Burns
Malnutrition	Rheumatoid arthritis
Drug-induced	Malnutrition
Autoimmune	Diabetes mellitus
Sequestration (hypersplenism)	Sickle cell disease
Burns (early)	Immature cells (leukemia, aplastic anemia)
Chemotactic Defects	**Intracellular Killing Defects**
Burns	Burns
Trauma	Severe infection
Severe infection	Trauma
Mutiple organ failure syndrome	Local anesthesia
Anesthesia	Corticosteroid therapy
Corticosteroid therapy	Diabetes mellitus
Diabetes mellitus	Malnutrition
Neonates	**Neutrophil Degranulation**
Rheumatoid arthritis	Burns
Uremia	Adult respiratory distress syndrome
Periodontitis	Severe infection
	Rheumatoid arthritis

Chemotaxis

Chemotaxis may be defined as the directed migration of cells in response to a concentration gradient of an attractant substance. The directed nature of this response distinguishes it from chemokinesis, an increase in random, nondirected movement. Both activities result in increased delivery of neutrophils to an inflammatory site.

Substances stimulating chemotaxis are varied and include products of cellular metabolism, complement fragments, bacterial products, and monokines.[38] Activation of the complement cascade by bacteria or bacterial products results in generation of the potent chemoattractant C5a. This factor has a very short half-life and is rapidly degraded to C5a desArg, which retains chemotactic activity through combination with a serum co-chemotaxin.[53, 113] As C5a desArg is rapidly formed from C5a, it is believed to be the most important, although less potent, *in vivo* chemoattractant when complement activation occurs. Amplification and modulation of the chemotactic response to complement-derived chemotactic factors may be performed by the neutrophil itself by way of granule contents, which activate generation of complement or degrade complement fragments.[153, 154]

The tripeptide FMLP has been shown to be chemotactic for neutrophils in minute concentrations. This substance is one of a series of synthetic compounds structurally related to chemotactically active products found in bacterial (*E. coli*) culture filtrates. Demonstration of specific binding of FMLP to receptors on the cell membrane has suggested a mechanism for detection and subsequent chemotaxis toward bacterial proteins having an analogous terminal sequence.[123, 124, 150] Furthermore, competitive inhibition studies using naturally occurring chemotactic factors in culture filtrates have indicated that these cell products share common receptor sites with the synthetic tripeptides; the receptors appear to be different from those for C5a. Biologically active lipids produced from arachidonic acid are potent mediators of numerous inflammatory responses, including chemotaxis. Prostaglandins and thromboxane A_2 may influence chemotaxis and neutrophil adherence.[54] Products of lipoxygenase metabolism of arachidonate, in particular leukotriene B_4 (LTB_4) and hydroxyeicosatetraenoic acid (HETE), appear to be the most potent of these inflammatory mediators. LTB_4 stimulates several neutrophil functions, including adherence, chemotaxis, and increased C3b receptor expression.[62, 63, 112] It may also serve to modulate responses to other chemotactic factors, such as FMLP, thereby providing a mechanism for cell recruitment in inflammatory responses.[56] Binding of LTB_4 to specific receptors on the neutrophil membrane has been demonstrated; this binding is not inhibited by FMLP or by C5a.[64] Kallikrein and some products of the fibrinolytic system may also stimulate PMN chemotactic activity.[37]

The means of transduction of the signal produced by chemotactic factor binding into stimulation of direct migration is unclear. Alterations in membrane potential, changes in flux of the divalent cations calcium and magnesium, and release of phosphoinositides from the membrane have been proposed as mechanisms whereby the chemotactic signal is translated into activity.[60, 129] Activation of protein kinase C, a mediator of protein phosphorylation, may be involved in control of polymerization of microtubules.[85] Cationic flux may also play a role in the generation of the contractile forces of locomotion by way of actin and myosin polymers. The great sensitivity of the chemotactic response is indicated by the apparent ability of the neutrophil to detect a gradient of chemotactic substance as small as 1% across the membrane surface from leading edge to tail[158] thus enabling it to move in a relatively direct manner toward an inflammatory source.

Intrinsic modulation of chemotactic responsiveness is performed by the neutrophil in response to its environment. Evidence exists for an intracellular pool of available FMLP receptors located on the membrane surfaces of specific granules.[103,105] Following exposure to degranulating stimuli, which produces a selective exocytosis of specific granules, a marked increase in the number of surface FMLP receptors was noted concomitant with a decrease in receptor affinity,[58] likely reflective of externalization of intracellular receptors. Additionally, exposure of neutrophils to chemotactic peptide results in a decrease in FMLP binding accompanied by irreversible association of peptide with the cell, indicative of internalization of bound ligand–receptor complexes.[142] The bacterial cell wall component, lipopolysaccharide, appears to modulate C5a and LTB_4 receptor sites and chemotactic responsiveness.[66] The effect of this regulation of receptor sites is to decrease neutrophil sensitivity at high concentrations of chemotactic factors and thereby maintain proper cell orientation when approaching an inflammatory focus.[159] As noted above, the specific and azurophil granules contain substances capable of generating and inactivating the complement component C5a;[154] oxidative inactivation of unbound chemotactic factors by stimulated neutrophils may also occur in the presence of high concentrations of mediators.[30,155] The neutrophil's ability to regulate its chemotactic responsiveness by way of membrane receptor changes and actions on local chemoattractants appears to play a substantial role in its inflammatory function.

Opsonization and Phagocytosis

Once at the site of infection, the neutrophil proceeds to opsonize, or prepare, invading bacteria prior to phagocytosis of the organism. Although the PMN is capable of ingesting unaltered bacteria, coating of microorganisms with opsonins greatly increases the efficiency of their recognition and ingestion by way of specific receptors on the PMN membrane. The major opsonins involved in *in vivo* phagocytosis by neutrophils are the complement component C3b and specific antibodies, primarily of the IgG class.[83] Additionally, nonspecific opsonizing proteins, including fibronectin and the acute phase reactant C-reactive protein, may serve to enhance phagocytosis by neutrophils. Binding of IgG to specific microbial antigens enables recognition of the Fc portion of the antibody by receptors on the PMN surface. Interaction of the bound antibody and receptor provides a signal for ingestion of the coated microorganism, and phagocytosis proceeds. Complement activation, which may occur by way of the classical or alternate pathways, generates C3, which is itself cleaved to C3b. This fragment is capable of attachment to bacterial cell walls, following which recognition and binding to specific neutrophil receptors occurs. Apparent differences exist between these two major opsonins in the extent to which ingestion is stimulated. Enhancement of particle binding to neutrophils occurs primarily by way of C3b opsonization, whereas ingestion is triggered by interaction of IgG-particle complexes with Fc receptors on the PMN.[48,94] Augmentation of the efficiency of IgG in stimulating ingestion occurs in the presence of bound C3b, thereby reducing the amount of immunoglobulin necessary for phagocytosis.[48]

Following recognition and binding of opsonized particles to the neutrophil membrane, phagocytosis proceeds rapidly. Cellular pseudopodia extend to surround the bound particle. Attachment of opsonin ligands on the particle surface to receptors on the extending pseudopodium occurs in a sequential fashion, enabling the membrane to circumferentially adhere to the entire particle.[69] The ingested particle is eventually fully enclosed in a vacuole surrounded by previously external cell membrane. Fusion of the engulfing pseudopodia forms a discrete closed phagosome. Activation of the respiratory burst, resulting in increased oxygen uptake by the neutrophil, is stimulated by binding and ingestion of foreign particles; the metabolic changes involved in this activation have been described previously.

Phagocytosis may be influenced by intracellular and environmental factors. Enhancement of ingestion by increased cyclic GMP and inhibition by elevated cyclic AMP levels have been demonstrated; beta-adrenergic agonists and theophylline experimentally diminish particle ingestion by way of this mechanism.[77] Alterations in phagocytosis may occur at extremes of pH, which might affect PMN function in the acidic local environment of an abcess cavity. Physiologic tonicity and temperature are required for optimum ingestion, as are calcium and magnesium.[114,140] The tetrapeptide tuftsin, an IgG fraction that binds to neutrophils, serves as an enhancer of phagocytosis, increasing it two to three times.[102]

Degranulation, although involved with bactericidal activity of the neutrophil, is initiated in association with ingestion. Release of granule constituents into the extracellular space may occur through a process termed *regurgitation during feeding*, in which lysosomal granules discharge into the phagosome before completion of closure or when the cell is in contact with foreign surfaces.[74] Contents may also be released directly into the external environment by way of exocytosis, a means of attacking extracellular substances or particles too large to ingest. Granule fusion with the completed phagosome and release of contents form a secondary lysosome, a mechanism important in bacterial killing and subsequent digestion. The azurophil granule, with its numerous microbicidal and digestive enzymes, is the major effector of this intracellular degranulation.

Intracellular Killing

Microbicidal activity and intracellular killing are initiated after formation of the phagocytic vacuole, and proceed by way of both oxygen-dependent and oxygen-independent mechanisms. The occurrence of these processes in the closed phagocytic vacuole is noteworthy, as it allows a high concentration of toxic substances within an enclosed space and minimizes potential toxicity to both the PMN itself and to neighboring cells.

Oxygen-dependent microbicidal systems may or may not require the enzyme myeloperoxidase (MPO). The MPO-independent systems involve the generation and release into the vacuole of toxic oxygen metabolites by way of the respiratory burst. These products, which include peroxide, superoxide, hydroxyl radicals, and singlet oxygen, may exert their microbicidal effects by way of initiation of oxidizing reactions in the bacterial cell wall.[11] Bactericidal pathways dependent on MPO require this enzyme as well as hydrogen peroxide and the presence of halide ions.[82,120] This system exerts its effect on ingested bacteria through probable halogenation and oxidation of cellular components.[83] The efficacy of this system is greatly reduced in the absence of any of the three components, as well as in the presence of the catalase produced by ingested bacteria, which diminishes available peroxide. Quantification of the cellular response in bacterial killing may be performed by measurement of O_2 uptake, or indirectly assessed by reduction of markers such as nitroblue tetrazolium (NBT) or by the chemoluminescence occurring upon formation of oxygen products.

Oxygen-independent microbicidal mechanisms are more specific and hence more limited in their range of activity.[38] The majority of components involved in this system are enzymatic and are released into the phagosome through fusion of intracellular granules; they include lysozyme, lysosomal hydrolases, lactoferrin, neutral proteases, and cationic proteins. The activities of these substances have been discussed previously; lysozyme, for example, is specific for the cell wall of sensitive bacteria, but lacks activity for gram-negative organisms, which are protected by mucopolysaccharide coats. Enhancement of the activity of these enzymes is achieved by reduction of the vacuole *p*H to approximately 6.0. The opsonins IgG and complement may further augment bacterial killing by non-oxygen dependent mechanisms through damage to cell walls and constituents.[80] Following killing of microorganisms, digestion occurs through the actions of acid hydrolases and perhaps other enzymes liberated from the primary granules.

Disorders of Neutrophil Function

Host susceptibility to infection may be vastly increased in conditions leading to disruption of neutrophil function. Such conditions may result from inherited, acquired, or iatrogenic causes. Neutrophil defects most commonly seen in the surgical setting stem predominantly from causes extrinsic to the PMN; recovery of normal function may occur, albeit slowly, once the disrupting stimulus has been removed or treated. In this section, we will review changes in neutrophil function resulting from a variety of clinical conditions and the resultant effects on host resistance; particular emphasis will be placed on those occurring in settings familiar to the surgeon.

Neutropenia

Quantitatively, neutropenia may be defined as a neutrophil count below 1500 cells/mm³. Severity of complications increases as the neutrophil count decreases; marked increases in the incidence of infection are seen at counts below 500 PMNs/mm³. Reduction of circulating neutrophils may be acquired or hereditary, with the former far more common. Acquired neutropenias most often result from cytotoxic therapy of malignancies or immunologic disorders. Drug reactions may also result in decreases in PMN count; chloramphenicol, sulfonamides, penicillins, cephalosporins, vancomycin, and phenothiazines all have been implicated as causative agents.[44,49] Silver sulfadiazine, used as an anti-infectious agent in burn therapy, has also been noted to produce acute neutropenic reactions.[79] An autoimmune phenomenon resulting in production of antibodies directed against neutrophils has been reported in some neutropenic patients.[23] Anti-neutrophil antibody production may result in sequestration of PMNs in the spleen, as may hypersplenism of other etiologies. Hereditary neutropenia may be seen in infantile genetic agranulocytosis, familial neutropenia, or cyclic neutropenia, in which hematopoiesis occurs in periodic cycles. Infectious complications in neutropenic patients are primarily a consequence of reduced PMN numbers rather than neutrophil dysfunction, although accompanying functional defects may be present in hereditary disorders or in immature cells released into the circulation after cytotoxic therapy. The clinical manifestations and consequences of immunosuppression, including neutropenia, are explored elsewhere in this volume.

Burns

Modern advances in cardiovascular and pulmonary resuscitation have substantially reduced the mortality associated with fluid and electrolyte disturbances in burn injury. Disruption of the normal skin barrier, however, exposes these patients to constant bacterial assault, which, despite improved microbial surveillance and topical chemotherapy, may progress from wound infection to systemic invasion and sepsis. The failure to control and contain infection after thermal injury is indicative of disruption of normal host defense mechanisms, including neutrophil function. The etiology of the neutrophil dysfunction seen in burns appears to be multifactorial, resulting in persistent neutrophil activation with consequent depression of normal activity.

Peripheral blood neutrophil counts exhibit a triphasic response following thermal injury. An increase of up to 300% is seen in the inital 24 hr post-burn; this is secondary to release of cells from both the marginated pool and postmitotic marrow reserve.[50] This is followed by slightly subnormal levels, with a nadir at about the third day. A slow increase in PMN count then occurs, stabilizing at approximately twice normal levels. Although neutrophil count in most patients conforms to this pattern, a subpopulation exhibits a paradoxic neutropenia, with a poor outcome in response to infection.[107] A decrease in granulocyte colony stimulating factor and the presence of an inhibitor of G-CSF have been demonstrated in these patients.[95,115] This paradoxical down-regulation of granulopoiesis in the face of incipient infection may be either secondary to direct bacterial toxicity or an attempt to minimize neutrophil-mediated tissue destruction resulting from generalized PMN activation.

A decrease in the chemotactic response of neutrophils of burn patients has been extensively documented.[15,36,55,70,148] The relationship of this diminished migratory response to the clinical course of the burn patient and to the occurrence of systemic infection is not clearly defined. Several studies demonstrate significant differences in chemotaxis in survivors versus nonsurvivors.[36,70,148] Although others have shown little correlation between response and outcome,[42] this may be in part reflective of the significant advances in burn therapeutics, including early excision of injured tissue, occurring within the last decade. A temporal relation between diminished chemotaxis and the onset of infection has been noted;[36] reduced migration correlated with extent of degranulation, indicating altered responsiveness after secretion of specific granules. The extent of burn injury appears to correlate inversely with the leukotactic response; accumulation of PMNs at the burn site was noted to be reduced in an experimental 60% total body surface area (TBSA) burn as compared to that seen in a 30% injury.[156] Additionally, increases in bacterial proliferation in burn wounds parallel decreases in chemotaxis over a 3-week period.[37] Diminution in chemotactic responsiveness in patients with thermal injury appears to reduce the effectiveness of containment of sepsis to the site of injury and increases the risk of disseminated infection.

Evidence of changes in the phagocytic ability of neutrophils following burn injury is less clear. Several studies have demonstrated unaltered[2] or increased[3] *in vitro* phagocytic ability in burn PMNs. Serum opsonic capacity was also noted to be normal or transiently depressed with a rapid return to normal early in the course of burn injury.[5, 41] Reports demonstrating decreased phagocytosis have implicated, to varying degrees, defects in specific or nonspecific opsonization.[5, 6, 43] These data suggest that circulating opsonic proteins such as fluid-phase C3b, present in high levels in burn patients, act to decrease phagocytic capacity of neutrophils.[109] Abnormalities of opsonic activity correlated with bacteremic episodes,[5, 6] suggesting failure of control of infection through diminished opsonization.

In contrast to the apparent maintenance of phagocytic ability, intracellular killing mechanisms demonstrate marked abnormalities during the course of thermal injury. Decreased chemoluminescence, oxygen radical production, and *in vitro* bacterial killing by neutrophils of burn patients have been noted.[3, 47] Suppression by burn plasma of oxygen radical production in normal cells also occurs, indicative of a plasma component contributing to PMN dysfunction. Defects in intracellular killing appear to be strongly associated with the onset of sepsis.[2, 3, 6, 41] Furthermore, analysis of immunologic profiles of these patients indicates that diminished microbicidal activity correlates most strongly with poor outcome.[5]

As might be expected from both the nature of burn injury and the defects in neutrophil function described above, the pathogens producing sepsis after burn injury are predominantly locally invasive organisms, which progress to bacteremia and generalized sepsis if invasion is unchecked. Failure of the PMN to migrate to the site of injury and to kill proliferating microbes effectively accounts for the inability to contain local invasion by bacteria. Thus, the major organisms producing burn wound infection are group A streptococci, staphylococci, gram-negative enteric bacilli, and invasive fungi,[68] all of which produce tissue invasion to various degrees. Sepsis resulting from these organisms reflects the breakdown of specialized neutrophil responses in control and containment of infection to the portal of entry.

The means by which alterations in neutrophil function and consequent depression of host resistance occur in these patients is the subject of extensive investigation. As noted previously, neutrophils possess mechanisms for intrinsic regulation of responsiveness; changes in this responsiveness occur following stimulation by a variety of substances. The *in vitro* phenomena of specific and nonspecific deactivation, whereby exposure to chemotaxins in low doses may enhance chemotaxis while producing a generalized blunting of response at higher doses,[106] appear to parallel changes in granulocyte function seen after thermal injury. Recent studies have demonstrated increased expression of neutrophil C3b receptors, accompanied by elevated C3a levels and diminished chemotaxis to complement fragments, occuring in burn patients.[99] Others have shown decreases in receptors and binding activity for the chemotaxin C5a following elevations in circulating levels of this mediator.[104, 134] Infusion of the chemotactic peptide FMLP in animals with an experimental burn produced increased susceptibility to infection and a shortened survival time, supporting the hypothesis that generation of endogenous chemotaxins after injury contributes to depression of host resistance.[157] The extensive complement activation that occurs in response to thermal injury may provide a source for abnormal systemic neutrophil stimulation with resultant alterations of PMN activity. Further evidence for the systemic activation of neutrophils is seen in their capacity to generate the inflammatory mediator leukotriene B_4. Marked increases in the *in vitro* production of this substance are seen within 6 hr of injury, followed by a depression in LTB_4 generation over the following several weeks.[24] This appears to parallel diminished chemotaxis to LTB_4[45] and may be indicative of down-regulation of neutrophil function in the face of prolonged stimulation. Derangement of normal neutrophil function after thermal injury thus appears to be effected by way of persistent and abnormal stimulation by inflammatory mediators; these effectors would, under less disruptive conditions, enhance host response to infection.

Sepsis, Trauma, and the Adult Respiratory Distress Syndrome

Acute bacterial infection, as would be expected, produces enhancement of neutrophil response mechanisms. Hyperactivity of chemotaxis, chemokinesis, NBT reduction, and chemoluminescence in the PMNs of patients with bacterial infection have been noted.[16, 75] Lipopolysaccharide, the major cell wall component of gram-negative bacteria, has been found to prime neutrophils for enhanced release of oxygen metabolites *in vitro*[71] and may stimulate increased arachidonic acid metabolism in neutrophils and macrophages *in vivo*,[1, 97] all indicative of neutrophil activation. This enhanced activity is reflective of stimulation of the nonspecific immune mechanisms of the neutrophil in response to acute bacterial challenge.

Paradoxically, however, patients with severe bacterial sepsis have been noted to exhibit diminished neutrophil function similar to that noted in patients with burns.[3, 6, 130] Depression of chemotaxis, superoxide production, and microbicidal activity, concomitant with increased degranulation of neutrophils, have been reported.[46, 131, 133] The temporal relationship between abnormalities of PMN function and clinical evidence of infection remains uncertain. Experimental data in which induction of moderately severe infection produced no demonstrable neutrophil abnormality indicates that PMN dysfunction proceeds and perhaps contributes to severe infection rather than resulting from it.[3] Documentation of an increase in recurrent infection with delayed recovery of normal neutrophil response in patients with intraperitoneal infections[130] and a correlation of periodic variations in PMN function with the onset of sepsis[2] provide further evidence for functional depression of these cells prior to early clinical signs of infection.

An increased incidence of infectious complications is seen in patients following severe trauma.[125] This predisposition to infection is indicative of diminished host response following injury. Elucidation of neutrophil function in these patients has revealed abnormalities in migratory function and oxygen metabolite production.[29,39,88] Decreases in chemoluminescence in normal neutrophils has been produced by the serum of trauma patients, reflecting depression of bactericidal ability by circulating factors.[86] Chemotactic abnormalities are maximal at 2 to 3 days post-injury and show a slow improvement thereafter.[89] This PMN migratory dysfunction correlates with anergy, development of sepsis, and increased mortality in trauma patients.[29]

Abnormalities of neutrophil function seen in sepsis and trauma likely stem from pathophysiologic mechanisms similar to those seen in burns. A depletion in components of the complement cascade is seen in serious gram-negative infection.[52] Increased plasma complement factors have been noted in sepsis[132,133] and trauma,[89] indicative of complement activation by infection or insult. Once activated, complement fragments are believed to modulate PMN function through down-regulation of responsiveness. This nonspecific deactivation of cellular function is similar to that proposed for changes in leukocyte responses after burn injury and appears to represent a common mechanism in response to abnormally increased stimulation by chemotaxins or other circulating mediators. Alterations in neutrophil function may also occur upon exposure to exogenous substances such as lipopolysaccharide, which modifies responses to C5a and LTB_4 after experimental infusion.[66,97] The humoral mediator cachectin-tumor necrosis factor (TNF), elaborated by macrophages in response to endotoxin challenge, may also play a substantial role in modulation of PMN function by way of stimulation of adherence, degranulation, and other activities.[84,127] Extensive complement activation may also predispose to bacteremic episodes through impairment of opsonization and reduced bacterial lysis.[73]

Recent investigation has established a strong link between the systemic neutrophil activation seen in severe infection, trauma, burns, and other critical illness, and the genesis of ARDS. Pathologic neutrophil accumulation observed in the lungs of affected patients strongly indicated a role for the PMN in mediating the destructive changes and increased alveolar-capillary permeability seen in this syndrome.[35] Specific findings implicating the neutrophil include the sequestration of PMN microemboli in the vasculature, release of neutrophil-derived proteases capable of damaging pulmonary tissue, and intra-alveolar presence of PMN proteases and oxidants.[27,78,108] Studies of neutrophil function in ARDS patients have demonstrated reduced chemotaxis,[59,132] an enhanced respiratory burst,[161] and marked degranulation,[59,72,132] all signs of PMN activation. Elevated plasma levels of the complement fragments C3a and C5a have been noted in ARDS[132] as well as increased alveolar LTB_4 levels in experimental models,[144] suggesting a role for these mediators in stimulation and possible recruitment of neutrophils to the lungs. Bacterial products themselves, endotoxins in particular, may also directly enhance granulocyte activation independent of their ability to activate complement.[25, 152] The final result of activation and recruitment of PMN in this manner is formation of cell aggregates in the lung vasculature, with increased neutrophil migration into the interstitium and alveolar space. Damage to the lung parenchyma, with resultant increased permeability and alveolar edema, occurs upon release of cytotoxic enzymes and oxygen metabolites produced by the neutrophil. The abnormal neutrophil responses occurring in ARDS appear as well to be those responsible for the dysfunction produced in other organs during the course of sepsis, trauma, or other severe illness. Termed the *multiple organ failure syndrome*,[27] this damage to the lungs, liver, kidneys, cardiovascular system, and other tissues appears to be a common end point of marked homeostatic disruptions arising from a variety of causes. Abnormal and persistent systemic neutrophil activation, the product of an enhanced or uncontrolled inflammatory response, appears to be a prime contributor to this organ damage.

Iatrogenic Dysfunction: Surgery, Anesthesia, and Pharmacologic Agents

Surgical intervention, with its consequent changes in host metabolic and homeostatic responses, might be expected to alter neutrophil activity. However, evidence from patients undergoing surgery has demonstrated no significant abnormalities of neutrophil function,[46, 145] or brief impairment with return to normal in 24 hr.[22] Postoperative depression of chemotaxis instead correlated with the onset of infection or other factors. Anesthesia, by contrast, induces a transient depression of chemotaxis during the immediate postoperative period.[100, 138] This resolves by the third day following surgery and does not appear related to infectious sequelae. Local anesthetic agents, such as tetracaine, have been shown to reduce neutrophil degranulation and superoxide generation in response to zymosan or activated serum, perhaps diminishing local inflammatory response in the area of use.[67]

Pharmacologic agents that may result in neutropenia were discussed previously. Effects on intrinsic PMN function are also produced by some types of drugs. Antiinflammatory therapy, including the use of corticosteroids and nonsteroidal antiinflammatory agents, results in a significant decrease in PMN adherence.[83, 146] A broad range of neutrophil activities, including chemotaxis, degranulation, and peroxide formation, are inhibited by corticosteroid administration;[83] this accounts in part for the diminished resistance to infection that accompanies use of these agents. Methylmethacrylate, a polymer used in joint-implantation surgery, appears to impair phagocytosis and killing by PMNs; this may serve to increase the risk of local infection after some orthopedic procedures.[116] Antibiotic therapy, while of undisputed value in the treatment of infection, may paradoxically alter inflammatory responses of neutrophils. Tetracycline, nafcillin, erythromycin, and sulfadiazine all produced *in vitro* inhibition of chemotaxis at high doses. Tetracycline additionally appears to produce alterations in generation or inactivation of chemotactic factors at lower doses.[90, 91] Treatment with antibiotics may thus alter normal host defense mechanisms, although demonstration of deleterious effects in the clinical setting is lacking.

Neutrophil Dysfunction in Systemic Disease

Disruptions of normal metabolism, nutrition, and other homeostatic mechanisms may exert significant effects on neutrophil activity. Abnormal function of the PMN may account for the increased incidence of infectious complications seen in some systemic disorders.

Diabetes mellitus is associated with diminished adherence, chemotaxis, phagocytosis, and intracellular killing.[101,143] Little correlation between chemotaxis and severity of disease has been noted; however, incubation of neutrophils from diabetic patients with glucose and insulin appears to restore normal migratory responses. Partial reversal of diminished phagocytosis by anti-diabetic therapy has also been achieved,[12] suggesting that PMN defects may bear some relation to insulin deficiency. Infection in diabetic patients may be due to this depression of function; in addition the vascular compromise seen in these patients may further inhibit delivery of leukocytes to tissue sites of inflammation or bacterial invasion.

Impairment of phagocytosis and microbicidal activity has been observed in protein-calorie malnutrition in human subjects. Diminished phagocytosis related directly to opsonin deficiency and reduction of complement components in malnourished patients. The defect in PMN-mediated killing is more difficult to define; both normal and decreased parameters (NBT reduction, HMP shunt activity) have been reported.[83] Many reports suggest that the primary host defect is the inability of apparently insignificant tissue injuries to heal properly, leaving open a source for constant bacterial contamination. This persistent low-grade bacterial stimulation may be responsible for many of the alterations in PMN activity seen in malnutrition. An absolute neutropenia was found to be present in many severely malnourished patients.[119] Infection in these patients may be reflective of both impairment of neutrophils and diminished available numbers. Furthermore, concomitant nutritional disorders, such as iron deficiency, may be responsible for reduction in microbicidal activity. Neutrophil dysfunction in hypermetabolic states (*e.g.,* burns) may be partially ameliorated by aggressive protein feeding and replacement, indicative of some nutritional role in altered cellular activity.[4] Acute reduction in caloric intake over a short period, an event occurring in most patients undergoing surgery, resulted in no significant variation in neutrophil function.[3] A relatively severe alteration in metabolism resulting from protein-calorie malnutrition or injury appears necessary for induction of disordered PMN activity through decreases in number, persistent bacterial stimulation, or direct effect of protein and nutrient deficiencies on the cell itself.

Diminished phagocytosis and defective opsonization may occur in rheumatoid arthritis as a consequence of rheumatoid factor ingestion by neutrophils. Development of septic arthritis in affected joints may result from reduced phagocytic activity in synovial fluid with high concentrations of rheumatoid factor. Ingestion of this substance by PMNs with regurgitation of granules during feeding results in the release of enzymes responsible for synovial tissue and cartilage destruction seen in rheumatoid arthritis. Additional clinical situations in which abnormal neutrophil responses have been noted are uremia,[17] periodontal disease,[31] and in the neonate;[98] all may predispose to varying extents to increased incidence or recurrence of infection.

This review of PMN function has attempted to outline the various mechanisms used in response to and control of infectious microorganisms by the neutrophil, as well as describing alterations in these mechanisms occurring in clinical settings familiar to the surgeon. In light of the predisposition to infection and organ failure that results from neutrophil dysfunction, an appreciation of these changes is valuable in proper anticipation and control of complications that may arise in the care of the critically ill patient.

REFERENCES

1. Aderem AA, Cohen DS, Wright SD, et al. Bacterial lipopolysaccharides prime macrophages for enhanced release of arachidonic acid metabolites. J Exp Med 1986;164:165.
2. Alexander JW, Dionigi R, Meakins JL. Periodic variation in the antibacterial function of human neutrophils and its relationship to sepsis. Ann Surg 1971;173:206.
3. Alexander JW, Hegg M, Altemeier WA. Neutrophil function in selected surgical disorders. Ann Surg 1968;168:447.
4. Alexander JW, Macmillan BG, Stinnett JD, et al. Beneficial effects of aggressive protein feeding in severely burned children. Ann Surg 1980;192:505.
5. Alexander JW, Ogle CK, Stinnett JD, et al. A sequential, prospective analysis of immunologic abnormalities and infection following severe thermal injury. Ann Surg 1978;188:809.
6. Alexander JW, Stinnett JD, Ogle CK, et al. A comparison of immunologic profiles and their influence on bacteremia in surgical patients with a high risk of infection. Surgery 1979;86:94.
7. Ambruso DR, Johnston RB. Lactoferrin enhances hydroxyl radical production by human neutrophils, neutrophil particulate fractions, and an enzymatic generating system. J Clin Invest 1981;67:352.
8. Arnold RR, Russell JE, Champion WJ, et al. Bactericidal activity of human lactoferrin: differentiation from the stasis of iron deprivation. Infect Immun 1982;35:792.
9. Aswanikumar SB, Corcoran B, Schiffman E, et al. Demonstration of a receptor on rabbit neutrophils for chemotactic peptides. Biochem Biophys Res Commun 1977;74:210.
10. Athens JW, Haab OP, Raab SO, et al. Leukokinetic studies. III. The distribution of granulocytes in the blood of normal subjects. J Clin Invest 1961;40:159.
11. Babior BM. Oxygen-dependent microbial killing by phagocytes. N Engl J Med 1978;298:659.
12. Bagade JD, Nielson KL, Bulger RJ. Reversible abnormalities in phagocytic function in poorly controlled diabetic patients. Am J Med Sci 1972;263:451.
13. Bainton DF, Farquhar MG. Origin of granules in polymorphonuclear leukocytes. Two types derived from opposite faces of the Golgi complex in developing granulocytes. J Cell Biol 1966;28:277.
14. Bainton DF, Ullyot JL, Farquhar MG. The development of neutrophilic polymorphonuclear leukocytes in human bone marrow. Origin and content of azurophil and specific granules. J Exp Med 1971;134:907.
15. Balch HH. Resistance to infection in burn patients. Ann Surg 1963;157:1.
16. Barbour AG, Allred CD, Solberg CO, et al. Chemoluminescence by polymorphonuclear leukocytes from patients with active bacterial infection. J Infect Dis 1980;141:14.
17. Baum J, Cestero RVM, Freemer RB. Chemotaxis of the polymorphonuclear leukocyte and delayed hypersensitivity in uremia. Kidney Int 1975;7(Suppl):147.
18. Berger M, O'Shea J, Cross AS, et al. Human neutrophils increase expression of C3bi as well as C3b receptors upon activation. J Clin Invest 1984;74:1566.
19. Berlin RD, Fera JP. Changes in membrane microviscosity associated with phagocytosis: effects of colchicine. Proc Natl Acad Sci USA 1977;74:1072.
20. Blendin J, Janoff A. The role of lysosomal elastase in the digestion of *Escherichia coli* proteins by human polymorphonuclear leukocytes. J Clin Invest 1976;58:971.
21. Borregard N, Heiple JM, Simons ER, et al. Subcellular localization of the b-cytochrome component of the human neutrophil microbicidal oxidase: translocation during activation. J Cell Biol 1983;97:52.
22. Bowers TK, O'Flahery J, Simmons RL, et al. Postsurgical granulocyte dysfunction: studies in healthy kidney donors. J Lab Clin Med 1977;90:720.
23. Boxer LA, Greenberg MS, Boxer GJ, et al. Autoimmune neutropenia. N Engl J Med 1975;293:748.

24. Braquet M, Lavaud P, Dormont D, et al. Leukocytic functions in burn-injured patients. Prostaglandins 1985;29:747.
25. Brigham KL, Meyrick B. Endotoxin and lung injury. Am Rev Respir Dis 1986;133:913.
26. Bullen JJ, Rogers HJ, Leigh C. Iron-binding proteins in milk and resistance to *Escherichia coli* infection in infants. Br Med J 1972;1:69.
27. Carrico CJ, Meakins JL, Marshall JC, et al. Multiple-organ-failure syndrome. Arch Surg 1986;121:196.
28. Chenoweth DE, Hugli TE. Demonstration of specific C5a receptor on intact polymorphonuclear leukocytes. Proc Natl Acad Sci USA 1978;75:3943.
29. Christou NV, McLean APH, Meakins JL. Host defense in blunt trauma: interrelationships of kinetics of anergy and depressed neutrophil function, nutritional status, and sepsis. J Trauma 1980;20:833.
30. Clark RA. Chemotactic factors trigger their own oxidative inactivation by human neutrophils. J Immunol 1982;129:2725.
31. Clark RA. Disorders of granulocyte chemotaxis. In: Gallin JI, Quie PG, eds. Leukocyte chemotaxis: methods, physiology, and clinical implications. New York: Raven Press, 1978:329.
32. Clark RA, Klebanoff SJ. Neutrophil mediated tumor cell cytotoxicity: role of the peroxidase system. J Exp Med 1975;141:1442.
33. Cline MJ. The white cell. Cambridge, MA: Harvard University Press,1975.
34. Cline MJ, Golde DW. Controlling the production of blood cells. Blood 1979;53:157.
35. Craddock PR, Hammerschmidt DE, White JG, et al. Complement (C5a) induced granulocyte aggregation *in vitro:* a possible mechanism of complement-mediated leukostasis and leukopenia. J Clin Invest 1977;60:260.
36. Davis JM, Dineen P, Gallin JI. Neutrophil degranulation and abnormal chemotaxis after thermal injury. J Immunol 1980;124:1467.
37. Davis JM, Gallin JI. Abnormal rabbit heterophil chemotaxis following thermal injury. An *in vivo* model of an abnormality in the chemoattractant receptor for f-met-leu-phe. Arch Surg 1987; in press.
38. Davis JM, Gallin JI. The neutrophil. In: Oppenheim JJ, Rosenstreich DL, Potter M, eds. Cellular functions in immunity and inflammation. New York: Elsevier North Holland, 1981:77.
39. Davis JM, Stevens JM, Peitzman A, et al. Neutrophil migratory activity in severe hemorragic shock. Circ Shock 1983;10:199.
40. DeChatelet LR, McPhail LC, Malliken D, et al. An isotopic assay for NADPH oxidase activity and some characteristics of the enzyme from human polymorphonuclear leukocytes. J Clin Invest 1975;55:714.
41. Deitch EA, Gelder F, McDonald JC. Sequential prospective analysis of the nonspecific host defense system after thermal injury. Arch Surg 1984;119:83.
42. Deitch EA, Gelder F, McDonald JC. Prognostic significance of abnormal neutrophil chemotaxis after thermal injury. J Trauma 1982;22:199.
43. Deitch EA, Gelder F, McDonald JC. The relationship between CIG depletion and peripheral neutrophil function in rabbits and man. J Trauma 1982;22:469.
44. DuComb L, Baldessarini RJ. Timing and risk of bone marrow depression by psychotropic drugs. Am J Psych 1977;134:1294.
45. Duhaney R, Meyer JD, Felsen D, et al. Human neutrophil chemotaxis to and generation of leukotriene B4 after burn injury. Manuscript in preparation, 1987.
46. Duigan JP, Collins PB, Johnson AH, et al. The association of impaired neutrophil chemotaxis with postoperative surgical sepsis. Br J Surg 1986;73:238.
47. Duque RE, Phan SH, Hudson JL, et al. Functional defects in phagocytic cells following injury. Am J Pathol 1985;118:116.
48. Ehlenberger AG, Nussenzweig V. The role of membrane receptors for C3b and C3d in phagocytosis. J Exp Med 1977;145:357.
49. Erslev AJ, Wintrobe MM. Detection and prevention of drug-induced blood dyscrasias. JAMA 1962;181:114.
50. Eurenius K, Broose RO. Granulocyte kinetics after thermal injury. Am J Clin. Pathol 1973;60:337.
51. Falloon J, Gallin JI. Neutrophil granules in health and disease. J Allergy Clin Immunol 1986;77:653.
52. Fearon DT, Ruddy J, Schur PH, et al. Activation of the properdin pathway of complement in patients with gram-negative bacteremia. N Engl J Med 1975;292:937.
53. Fernandez HN, Henson PM, Otani A, et al. Chemotactic response to human C3a and C5a anaphylotoxins. I. Evaluation of C3a and C5a leukotaxis *in vitro* and under stimulated *in vivo* conditions. J Immunol 1978;120:109.
54. Ferreira SH. Prostaglandins. In: Houck JC, ed. Chemical messengers of the inflammatory process. Amsterdam: Elsevier North Holland, 1979;113.

55. Fikrig SM, Karl SC, Suntharalingam K. Neutrophil chemotaxis in patients with burns. Ann Surg 1977;186:746.

56. Fletcher MP. Modulation of the heterogeneous membrane potential to n-formyl-methionyl-leucyl-phenylalanine (FMLP) by leukotriene B4: evidence for cell recruitment. J Immunol 1986;136:4213.

57. Fletcher M, Gallin JI. Human neutrophils contain an intracellular pool of putative receptors for the chemoattractant n-formyl-methionyl-leucyl-phenylalanine. Blood 1983;62:792.

58. Fletcher MP, Gallin JI. Degranulatory stimuli increase the availability of receptors on human neutrophils for the chemoattractant f-met-leu-phe. J Immunol 1980;124:1585.

59. Fowler AA, Fisher BJ, Centor RM, et al. Development of the adult respiratory distress syndrome: progressive alterations in neutrophil chemotactic and secretory processes. Am J Pathol 1984;116:427.

60. Gallin JI, Rosenthal AS. The regulatory role of divalent cations in human granulocyte chemotaxis: evidence for an association between calcium exchanges and microtubule assembly. J Cell Biol 1974;62:594.

61. Ginsburg I, Sela MN. The role of leukocytes and their hydrolases in the persistence, degradation, and transport of bacterial constituents in tissue. Relation to chronic inflammatory processes in staphylococcal, streptococcal, and mycobacterial infections and in chronic periodontal disease. CRC Crit Rev Microbiology 1976;4:249.

62. Goetzl EJ. Mediators of immediate hypersensitivity derived from arachidonic acid. N Engl J Med 1980;303:822.

63. Goetzl EJ, Pickett WC. The human PMN leukocyte chemotactic activity of complex hydroxy-eicosatetraenoic acids (HETEs). J Immunol 1980;125:1789.

64. Goldman DW, Goetzl EJ. Specific binding of leukotriene B4 to receptors on polymorphonuclear leukocytes. J Immunol 1982;129:1600.

65. Golde DW, Cline MJ. Identification of the colony stimulating cells in human blood. J Clin Invest 1972;51:2981.

66. Goldman DW, Enkel H, Gifford LA, et al. Lipopolysaccharide modulates receptors for leukotriene B4, C5a, and formyl-methionyl-leucyl-phenylalanine on rabbit polymorphonuclear leukocytes. J Immunol 1986;137:1971.

67. Goldstein IM, Lind S, Hoffstein S, et al. Influence of local anesthetics upon human polymorphonuclear leukocyte function *in vitro*. J Exp Med 1977;146:483.

68. Goodwin CW, Yurt RW. Epidemiology of burn wounds. In: Davis JM, Shires GT, eds. Host Defenses in Trauma and Surgery. New York: Raven Press, 1986:5.

69. Griffin FM Jr, Griffin JA, Leider JE, et al. Studies on the mechanism of phagocytosis. I. Requirements for circumferential attachment of particle-bound ligands to specific receptors on the macrophage plasma membrane. J Exp Med 1975;142:1263.

70. Grogan JB. Suppressed *in vitro* chemotaxis of burn neutrophils. J Trauma 1976;16:985.

71. Guthrie LA, McPhail LC, Henson PM, et al. Priming of neutrophils for enhanced release of oxygen metabolites by bacterial lipopolysaccharide. J Exp Med 1984;160:1656.

72. Hallgren R, Borg T, Venge P, et al. Signs of neutrophil and eosinophil activation in adult respiratory distress syndrome. Crit Care Med 1984;12:14.

73. Heideman M, Saravis C, Clowes GHA. Effect of nonviable tissue and abcesses on complement depletion and the development of bacteremia. J Trauma 1982;22:527.

74. Henson PM. The immunologic release of constituents from neutrophil leukocytes. I. The role of antibody and complement on non-phagocytosable surfaces or phagocytosable particles. J Immunol 1971;107:1535.

75. Hill HR, Gerrard JM, Hogan NA, et al. Hyperactivity of neutrophil leukotactic responses during active bacterial infection. J Clin Invest 1974;53:996.

76. Hoffstein ST. Intra- and extracellular secretion from polymorphonuclear leukocytes. In: Weissman G, ed. The cell biology of inflammation. Amsterdam: Elsevier North Holland, 1980:87.

77. Ignarro LJ, Lint TF, George WJ. Hormonal control of lysosomal enzyme release from human neutrophils. Effect of autonomic agents on enzyme release, phagocytosis, and cyclic nucleotide levels. J Exp Med 1974;139:1395.

78. Janoff A, White R, Carp H, et al. Lung injury induced by leukocytic proteases. Am J Pathol 1979;97:111.

79. Jarrett F, Ellerbe S, Demling R. Acute leukopenia during topical burn therapy with silver sulfadiazine. Am J Surg 1978;135:818.

80. Klebanoff SJ. Antimicrobial mechanisms in neutrophilic polymorphonuclear leukocytes. Semin Hematol 1975;12:117.

81. Klebanoff SJ. Myeloperoxidase: contribution to the microbicidal activity of intact leukocytes. Science 1970;169:1095.

82. Klebanoff SJ. Myeloperoxidase-halide-hydrogen peroxide anti-bacterial system. J Bacteriol 1968;95:2131.

83. Klebanoff SJ, Clark RA. The neutrophil: function and clinical disorders. New York: Elsevier North Holland, 1978.

84. Klebanoff SJ, Vadas MA, Harlan JM, et al. Stimulation of neutrophils by tumor necrosis factor. J Immunol 1986;136:4220.

85. Korchack HM, Vienne K, Rutherford LE, et al. Neutrophil stimulation: receptor, membrane, and metabolic events. Fed Proc 1984;43:2749.

86. Lanser ME, Mao P, Brown GE, et al. Serum-mediated depression of neutrophil chemiluminescence following blunt trauma. Ann Surg 1985;202:111.

87. Lichtman MA, Weed RI. Alteration of the cell periphery during granulocyte maturation: relationship to cell function. Blood 1972;39:301.

88. Madarazo EG, Albano SD, Woronick CL, et al. Polymorphonuclear leukocyte migration abnormalities and their significance in severely traumatized patients. Ann Surg 1983;198:736.

89. Madarazo EG, Woronick CL, Albano SD, et al. Inappropriate activation, deactivation, and probable autooxidative damage as a mechanism of neutrophil locomotory dysfunction in trauma. J Infect Dis 1986;154:471.

90. Majeski JA, Alexander JW. Evaluation of tetracycline in the neutrophil chemotactic response. J Lab Clin Med 1977;90:259.

91. Majeski JA, McClellan MA, Alexander JW. Effect of antibiotics on the *in vitro* neutrophil chemotactic response. Am Surg 1976;42:785.

92. Malavista SE, Bensch KG. Human polymorphonuclear leukocytes: demonstration of microtubules and effect of colchicine. Science 1967;156:521.

93. Malech HL, Root RK, Gallin JI. Structural analysis of human neutrophil migration: centriole, microtubule, and microfilament organization and function during chemotaxis. J Cell Biol 1977;75:666.

94. Mantovani B. Different roles of IgG and complement receptors in phagocytosis by polymorphonuclear leukocytes. J Immunol 1975;115:15.

95. McEuen DD, Ogawa M, Eurenius K. Myelopoeiesis in the infected burn. J Lab Clin Med 1977;89:540.

96. Messner RP, Jenlinck J. Receptors for human gamma G globulin on human neutrophils. J Clin Invest 1970;49:2165.

97. Meyer JD, Duhaney R, Hesse D, et al. Bolus infusion of endotoxin in man: altered granulocyte chemotaxis, complement activation, and leukotriene B4 generation. Manuscript in preparation, 1987.

98. Miller ME. Chemotactic function in the neonate: humoral and cellular aspects. Pediatr Res 1971;5:487.

99. Moore FD Jr, Davis C, Rodrick M, et al. Neutrophil activation in thermal injury as assessed by increased expression of complement receptors. N Engl J Med 1986;314:948.

100. Moudgil GC, Allan RB, Russel RJ, et al. Inhibition by anesthetic agents of human leukocyte locomotion towards chemical attractants. Br J Anaesth 1977;49:97.

101. Mount AG, Baum J. Chemotaxis of polymorphonuclear leukocytes from patients with diabetes mellitus. N Engl J Med 1971;284:621.

102. Najjar VA. Defective phagocytosis due to deficiencies involving tetrapeptide tuftsin. J Pediatr 1975;87:1121.

103. Neidel JE, Dolumatch BL. Cellular processing of the formyl peptide receptor. Agents Actions [Suppl] 1983;12:309.

104. Nelson RD, Chenoweth DE, Solomkin JS, et al. Cytotaxin receptors on human neutrophils: modulation of C5a receptor numbers. Agents Actions [Suppl] 1983;12:274.

105. Nelson RD, Fiegle VD, Chenoweth DE. Human neutrophil peptide receptors: mobilization mediated by phosphilipase. Am J Pathol 1982;107:202.

106. Nelson RD, McCormack RT, Fiegle VD, et al. Chemotactic deactivation of human neutrophils: evidence for nonspecific and specific components. Infect Immun 1978;22:441.

107. Newsome TW, Eurenius K. Suppression of granulocyte and platelet production by *Pseudomonas* burn wound infection. Surg Gynecol Obstet 1973;136:375.

108. Nuytinck JKS, Goris JA, Redl H, et al. Posttraumatic complications and inflammatory mediators. Arch Surg 1986;121:886.

109. Ogle JD, Ogle CK, Alexander JW. Inhibition of neutrophil function by fluid phase C3b of complement. Infect Immun 1983;40:967.

110. Oram JD, Reiter B. Inhibition of bacteria by lactoferrin and other chelating agents. Biochim Biophys Acta 1968;70:351.

111. Oseas R, Yang HH, Baehner RL, et al. Lactoferrin, a promotor of polymorphonuclear leukocyte adhesiveness. Blood 1981;57:939.

112. Palmblad J, Malmsten CL, Uden A-M, et al. Leukotriene B4 is a potent and stereospecific stimulator of neutrophil chemotaxis and adherence. Blood 1981;58:658.

113. Perez HD, Goldstein IM, Webster RO, et al. Enhancement of the chemotactic activity of human C5a des arg by an anionic peptide ("cochemotaxin") in normal serum and plasma. J Immunol 1981;126:800.

114. Peterson PF, Verhoef J, Quie PG. Influence of temperature on opsonization and phagocytosis of staphylococci. Infect Immun 1977;15:175.

115. Peterson V, Hansbrough J, Buerk C, et al. Regulation of granulopoiesis following severe thermal injury. J Trauma 1983;23:19.

116. Petty W. The effect of methylmethacrylate on bacterial phagocytosis and killing by human polymorphonuclear leukocytes. J Bone Joint Surg 1978;60:752.

117. Pruett TL, Chenoweth DW, Fiegel VD, et al. *Escherichia coli* and human neutrophils: effect of bacterial supernatant with hemolysin activity upon chemotaxin receptors. Arch Surg 1985;120:212.

118. Robinson WA. Granulocytosis in neoplasia. Ann NY Acad Sci 1979;230:212.

119. Rosen EU, Geefhuysen J, Anderson J. Leukocyte function in children with kwashiorkor. Arch Dis Child 1975;50:220.

120. Rosen H, Klebanoff SJ. Bactericidal activity of a superoxide anion-generating system. A model for the polymorphonuclear leukocyte. J Exp Med 1979;149:27.

121. Rossi F, Romeo D, Patriarca P. Mechanism of phagocytosis-associated oxidative metabolism in polymorphonuclear leukocytes and macrophages. J Reticuloendothel Soc 1972;12:127.

122. Sbarra AJ, Karnovsky ML. The biochemical basis of phagocytosis. I. Metabolic changes during the ingestion of particles by polymorphonuclear leukocytes. J Biol Chem 1959;234:1355.

123. Schiffman E, Corcoran BA, Aswanikumar S. Molecular events in the response of neutrophils to synthetic N-f-met chemotactic peptides: demonstration of a specific receptor. In: Gallin JI, Quie PG, eds. Leukocyte chemotaxis: methods, physiology and clinical implications. New York: Raven Press, 1978:97.

124. Schiffman E, Showell HJ, Corcoran BA, et al. The isolation and partial characterization of neutrophil chemotactic factors from *E. coli*. J Immunol 1975;114:1831.

125. Schimpff SC, Miller RM, Polakavetz S, et al. Infection in the severely traumatized patient. Ann Surg 1974;179:352.

126. Scott RB, Still WJS. Glycogen in human peripheral blood leukocytes. II. The macromolecular state of leukocyte glycogen. J Clin Invest 1968;47:353.

127. Shalaby MR, Aggarwal BB, Rinderknecht E, et al. Activation of human polymorphonuclear neutrophil functions by interferon and tumor necrosis factors. J Immunol 1985;135:2069.

128. Singer SJ, Nicolson GL. The fluid mosaic model of the structure of cell membranes. Cell membranes are viewed as two-dimensional solutions of oriented globular proteins and lipids. Science 1972;175:720.

129. Snyderman R, Goetzl EJ. Molecular and cellular mechanisms of leukocyte chemotaxis. Science 1981;213:830.

130. Solomkin JS, Bauman MP, Nelson RD, et al. Neutrophil dysfunction during the course of intraabdominal sepsis. Ann Surg 1981;194:9.

131. Solomkin JS, Cotta LA, Brodt JK, et al. Neutrophil dysfunction in sepsis. III. Degranulation as a mechanism for non-specific deactivation. J Surg Res 1984;36:407.

132. Solomkin JS, Cotta LA, Satoh PS, et al. Complement activation and clearance in acute illness and injury: evidence for C5a as a cell-directed mediator of the adult respiratory distress syndrome in man. Surgery 1985;97:668.

133. Solomkin JS, Jenkins MK, Nelson RD, et al. Neutrophil dysfunction in sepsis. II. Evidence for the role of complement activation products in cellular deactivation. Surgery 1981;90:319.

134. Solomkin JS, Nelson RD, Chenoweth DE, et al. Regulation of neutrophil migratory function in burn injury by complement activation products. Ann Surg 1984;200:742.

135. Southwick FS, Stossel TP. Contractile proteins in leukocyte function. Semin Hematol 1983;20:305.

136. Spiegelberg HL, Laurence DA, Henson P. Cytophilic properties of IgA to human neutrophils. Adv Exp Med Biol 1974;45:67.

137. Spitznagel JK, Shafer WM. Neutrophil killing of bacteria by oxygen-independent mechanisms: a historical summary. Rev Infect Dis 1985;7:398.

138. Stanley TH, Hill GE, Portas MR, et al. Neutrophil chemotaxis during and after general anesthesia and operation. Anesth Analg 1976;55:668.

139. Stjenholm RL, Manak RC. Carbohydrate metabolism in leukocytes. XIV. Regulation of pentose cycle activity and glycogen metabolism during phagocytosis. J Reticuloendothel Soc 1970;8:550.

140. Stossel TP. Phagocytosis. N Engl J Med 1974;290:717.

141. Sullivan SJ, Daukas G, Zigmond SH. Assymetric distribution of the chemotactic polypeptide receptor on polymorphonuclear leukocytes. J Cell Biol 1984;99:1461.

142. Sullivan SJ, Zigmond SH. Chemotactic peptide receptor modulation in polymorphonuclear leukocytes. J Cell Biol 1980;85:703.

143. Tan JS, Anderson JL, Watanakunakorn C, et al. Neutrophil dysfunction in diabetes mellitus. J Lab Clin Med 1975;85:26.

144. Taniguchi H, Taki F, Takagi K, et al. The role of leukotriene B4 in the genesis of oxygen toxicity in the lung. Am Rev Respir Dis 1986;133:805.

145. van Dijk WC, Venbrugh HA, Van Ryswyk REN, et al. Neutrophil function, serum opsonic activity, and delayed hypersensitivity in surgical patients. Surgery 1982;92:21.

146. Venezio FR, DiVincenzo C, Pearlman F, et al. Effects of the newer nonsteroidal anti-inflammatory agents, ibuprofen, fenoprofen, and sulindac, on neutrophil adherence. J Infect Dis 1985;152:690.

147. Walter RJ, Berlin RD, Oliver JM. Assymetric Fc receptor distribution on human PMN oriented in a chemotactic gradient. Nature 1980;289:724.

148. Warden GD, Mason AD, Pruitt B. Evaluation of leukocyte chemotaxis in vitro in thermally injured patients. J Clin Invest 1974;54:1001.

149. Weiss SJ, Regiani S. Neutrophils degrade subendothelial matrices in the presence of alpha₁ proteinase inhibitor: cooperative use of lysosomal proteinases and oxygen metabolites. J Clin Invest 1984;73:1297.

150. Williams LT, Snyderman R, Pike MC, et al. Specific receptor sites for chemotactic peptides on human polymorphonuclear leukocytes. Proc Natl Acad Sci USA 1977;74:1204.

151. Wolff SM, Rubenstein M, Mulholland JH, et al. Comparison of hematologic and febrile responses to endotoxin in man. Blood 1965:26:190.

152. Worthen GS, Haslett C, Smedley LA, et al. Lung vascular injury induced by chemotactic factors: enhancement by bacterial endotoxins. Fed Proc 1986;45:7.

153. Wright DG, Gallin JI. Secretory responses of human neutrophils: exocytosis of specific (secondary) granules by human neutrophils during adherence *in vitro* and during exudation *in vivo*. J Immunol 1979;123:285.

154. Wright DG, Gallin JI. Functional differentiation of neutrophil granules: generation of C5a by a specific (secondary) granule product and inactivation of C5a by azurophil (primary) granule products. J Immunol 1977;119:1068.

155. Yuli I, Snyderman R. Extensive hydrolysis of N-formyl-methionyl-leucyl-phenylalanine by human polymorphonuclear leukocytes. J Biol Chem 1986;261:4902.

156. Yurt RW, Pruitt BA. Decreased wound neutrophils and indiscrete margination in the pathogenesis of wound infection. Surgery 1985;98:191.

157. Yurt RW, Shires GT. Increased susceptibility to infection due to infusion of exogenous chemotaxin. Arch Surg 1987;122:111.

158. Zigmond S. Mechanisms of sensing chemical gradients by polymorphonuclear leukocytes. Nature 1974;249:450.

159. Zigmond SH. Consequences of chemotactic peptide receptor modulation for leukocyte orientation. J Cell Biol 1981;88:644.

160. Zimmerli W, Seligmann B, Gallin JI. Exudation primes human and guinea pig neutrophils for subsequent responsiveness to the chemotactic peptide n-formylmethionylleucylphenylalanine and increases complement component C3bi receptor expression. J Clin Invest 1986;77:925.

161. Zimmerman GA, Renzetti AD, Hill HR. Functional and metabolic activity of granulocytes from patients with adult respiratory distress syndrome: evidence for activated neutrophils in the pulmonary circulation. Am Rev Respir Dis 1983;127:290.

24

○　　○　　○　　●　　●　　○

RESPIRATORY DISTRESS SYNDROME IN ABDOMINAL SEPSIS

Philip S. Barie

The association of serious illness with catastrophic pulmonary failure has been made in numerous reports for more than a century. These reports began to appear with increasing frequency after World Wars I and II, but the concept of a discrete syndrome of acute respiratory failure developed only after Vietnam-era reports were analyzed. Interestingly, evidence for the development of such a syndrome in civilian populations developed contemporaneously, leading to the landmark report of Ashbaugh and colleagues[5] in 1967, which described the syndrome accurately and proposed the designation, adult respiratory distress syndrome (ARDS).

Despite this recognition, debate raged regarding the pathogenesis of the syndrome in a virtual vacuum of scientific investigation. Initial controversy over whether the observed pulmonary edema was acute heart failure from fluid overload was not settled until ARDS was associated with low or normal pulmonary vascular pressures after the development, in 1970, of the Swan-Ganz catheter.[130]

Complete clinical descriptions of the syndrome included hypoxemia refractory to oxygen therapy, exudative pulmonary edema fluid, progressive decreases in pulmonary compliance, and radiographic evidence of diffuse, bilateral, homogenous, interstitial pulmonary infiltrates. It was quickly recognized that the development of the syndrome was a catastrophe. The syndrome often developed in young, previously healthy persons whose underlying medical or surgical problem was often otherwise easy to manage. Mortality exceeded 50%, and recovery in survivors was protracted and complicated by a degree of permanent ventilatory insufficiency. Despite this recognition and well-informed speculation based largely from postmortem histologic examination, very little solid data regarding pathogenetic mechanisms or specific therapy was available, although valuable modalities for ventilatory support, in particular mechanical ventilation with positive end-expiratory pressure (PEEP),[117] were described soon after the appearance of the early definitive descriptions of the syndrome.

The "modern era" of understanding of ARDS probably began in 1975 with the description of an intact animal mammalian model suitable for study and experimental therapy of abnormal pulmonary transvascular fluid exchange.[127] This model and others have since been extensively validated and serve as the basis for the tremendous increases in understanding that have occurred in the past decade. Although innumerable injurious agents have been tested in these experimental systems, the recognition of gram-negative sepsis as an important precipitant of the syndrome has developed from both clinical and experimental observation. Clinical observations of remote organ failure in sepsis, sometimes of isolated respiratory failure,[137] but often of more than one organ system, also began to appear in the mid-1970s.[60] These reports often included patients with acute respiratory failure and led to the development of the parallel concept of multiple organ failure (MOF) syndrome.[31,47] Although ARDS may certainly develop as part of the MOF syndrome, ARDS may also develop as an isolated phenomenon, and the expression of the MOF syndrome in an individual patient may occasionally exclude ARDS.

RISK FACTORS FOR THE DEVELOPMENT OF ARDS

Although ARDS is now clearly recognized as a syndrome, this recognition was delayed for some time because of the apparently disparate causes of the syndrome. Early reports were numerous and consisted of small numbers of patients with many potential causes of the syndrome, with the result that the importance of certain risk factors remained unapparent. Even when specific disease processes were clearly associated with the development of ARDS, the relative risk associated with individual disease states remained unclear. This type of information was felt to be of critical importance, because ARDS is rare (overall incidence 0.1%) when examined in the context of all hospitalizations.[56] Effective intervention mandated the precise identification of patients at risk, because it became increasingly apparent from clinical experience and experimental evidence that specific therapy aimed at ARDS itself was very limited in scope and effectiveness, particularly if instituted only after the development of respiratory failure.[21] Retrospective and prospective surveys of patient populations at risk now allow precise determinations of the incidence of ARDS.

A number of disease processes may now be considered predisposing causes of ARDS on the basis of these data, although seldom does the incidence exceed 50%. In acute pancreatitis, for example, widely identified as an etiologic factor in ARDS,[6, 139] the incidence is approximately 8%. Other common causes include aspiration of gastric contents, massive blood transfusion, multiple fractures, and near-drowning.[107] Analyses such as these may be complicated by the fact that many of these risk factors may coexist in a single patient, as with the multiply injured patient who receives massive blood transfusions. It is clear that coexistent risk factors increase the risk of ARDS in an individual patient,[107] while simultaneously decreasing the likelihood of survival.[57]

Virtually all of these studies indicate that sepsis is among the leading risk factors for the development of ARDS. Two prospective studies have evaluated consecutive patients felt to be in high-risk groups for the development of ARDS in an attempt to determine the likelihood for developing the syndrome. Fowler and colleagues followed 993 patients during a period of 1 year.[56] The group consisted of all patients in any of eight predetermined high-risk groups, including cardiopulmonary bypass surgery, burns of any size, bacteremia with two or more positive blood cultures, massive transfusion (10 or more units within 48 hr), fracture (one or more long bones, or pelvic fracture, or both), disseminated intravascular coagulation, pneumonia requiring ICU care, or witnessed aspiration of gastric contents. Of these patients 68 (6.8%) developed ARDS. The likelihood of developing ARDS for any of these predisposing factors is displayed in Table 24-1. Of note, selection of these particular eight high-risk criteria missed 20 additional cases of ARDS that occurred in the institution during this period, meaning that these criteria successfully screened for 77% of ARDS cases. In this series, pulmonary aspiration was the most prevalent risk factor.

A similar prospective study was undertaken by Pepe and colleagues,[107] who also selected patients from eight high-risk groups to follow for the development of ARDS. Using different criteria to identify their high-risk groups (see Table 24-1), these investigators collected 136 patients over an 18-month period. In contrast to the study of Fowler and co-workers,[56] 46 patients in this study (34%) developed ARDS. While both studies clearly showed that the likelihood of ARDS increases in patients with multiple risk factors and showed comparable overall mortality from ARDS (65% versus 61%), a number of important differences besides the incidence of ARDS in patients at risk are worth consideration.

While Fowler and co-workers found pulmonary aspiration most likely to cause ARDS in their series, Pepe and colleagues found aspiration to be less likely than sepsis to cause ARDS. Sepsis led to ARDS in 38% of patients with sepsis as a single risk factor, while sepsis alone or in concert with other risk factors led to ARDS in 47% of cases.[107] In contrast, the overall incidence of ARDS after sepsis in the study of Fowler and

Table 24–1
Diagnostic Groups* Used for Prospective Analysis of Predisposition to ARDS

FOWLER ET AL[57]	INCIDENCE (%)	PEPE ET AL[107]	INCIDENCE (%)
Bacteremia	4	"Sepsis syndrome"	38
Aspiration	36	Aspiration	30
Multiple transfusions	5	Multiple transfusions	24
Fracture	5	Multiple fractures	8
Disseminated intravascular coagulation	22		
Pneumonia	12		
Burns	2		
		Pulmonary contusion	17
		Near-drowning†	
		Pancreatitis†	
		Shock†	

* Diagnostic groups were not identically defined for the two studies. Descriptions of differences may be found in the text.
† Insufficient total numbers of cases with this diagnosis as a sole risk factor to allow meaningful calculation of incidence.

colleagues was 8% of 331 patients with bacteremia, pneumonia, or presumed sepsis on clinical grounds. One potential explanation for this difference is the suprisingly low incidence of ARDS following bacteremia (3.8%) in this series in comparison to other data available in the literature.[49,76] The reason for this discrepancy is unclear.

Important methodologic differences may account for the differing results in these two studies. Possible causes for the divergence could include differences in patient populations as defined by the groups considered at high risk in each study, or could represent differences in the severity of illness in patient groups common to both studies. While Fowler and colleagues had only a 6.8% incidence of ARDS in their study group, their entrance criteria did identify 77% of all cases of ARDS developing during the period. In contrast, the selection criteria employed by Pepe and colleagues identified a 34% incidence of ARDS in their study population while their criteria identified only 42% of all cases of ARDS in their institution during the study period.

Fowler and colleagues included cardiopulmonary bypass surgery as one of their eight high-risk groups, despite the fact that ARDS after cardiopulmonary bypass surgery is rare[32] (see Table 24-1). Similarly, burns were included as a high-risk group in this study despite the fact that burns, in the absence of smoke inhalation injury or burn wound sepsis, do not appear to cause ARDS.[40] If these two criteria were eliminated (using only six), the incidence of ARDS in the at-risk group would increase to 9.3% from 5.8% while the study still detected 70% of all cases. The eight criteria selected by Pepe and colleagues may be more appropriate, because clinical sepsis without confirmatory bacteremia accounted for 9 of the 20 "missed" cases of ARDS in the study of Fowler and colleagues. If Fowler and co-workers had used seven of the eight diagnoses proposed by Pepe and colleagues (including presumed sepsis, near-drowning, pancreatitis, and pulmonary contusion, and not accounting for severity criteria), the incidence would have nearly doubled to 11.2% while 86.3% of all cases were identified.

Because modification of Fowler's diagnostic criteria to conform to Pepe's study keeps the overall incidence of ARDS low but identifies a larger proportion of all cases in their study, it seems likely that the diagnostic categories of Pepe and colleagues are appropriate but more stringently applied to account for the differences between these two studies. In fact, the criteria for inclusion in a diagnostic high-risk group appear to be much more stringent in the study of Pepe and co-workers.[107] For example, bacteremia without evidence of a deleterious systemic response such as metabolic acidosis or peripheral vasodilation did not meet the criteria for sepsis as defined by Pepe and colleagues, while bacteremia alone was sufficient criteria for inclusion according to Fowler. Furthermore, massive transfusion constituted 10 or more units of blood or packed erythrocytes within 12 hr according to Pepe, but within 48 hr for Fowler and colleagues. Diagnostic criteria for inclusion of fractures were also more stringently set by Pepe and co-workers. Had their inclusion criteria been set less stringently, the incidence of ARDS in the population at risk would undoubtedly have been lower, while the percentage of total cases identified by high-risk groups would have been higher. Even though sepsis was the most likely clinical entity to lead to ARDS in this series, Pepe and colleagues specifically excluded 11 cases of primary pneumonia and 40 other cases because of head injuries or portal hypertension where patients might have had reasons besides ARDS to develop respiratory failure. Because of these exclusions and the particularly strict criteria for sepsis used by Pepe and colleagues, it appears likely that the high incidence of sepsis leading to ARDS reported by Pepe in this study may be an underestimate.

It is certain from both of these studies that prospective assessment of risk for the development of ARDS depends on carefully selected criteria for diagnosis and severity.[122] Review of patient populations at highest risk suggests that systemic sepsis (bacteremia and altered hemodynamics) may be the most potent risk factor for the development of ARDS. Fowler and colleagues prospectively monitored all patients admitted to medical, surgical, and burn intensive care units at their institution over a 1-year period[57] using their eight previously defined high-risk groups.[56] In this study of 88 patients who developed ARDS, infection was considered etiologic in 44% of all patients with the syndrome.[57] Included in these 39 infected, predisposed cases were 10 patients with pneumonia, 9 patients with bacteremia, 9 patients with clinical sepsis without a documented source, and 11 additional patients with bacteremia or pneumonia as one of the multiple risk factors for the development of ARDS. Although it is not clear in this study how many cases of pneumonia were nonbacterial in origin, excluding all cases of pneumonia not associated with bacteremia still leaves 33% of ARDS cases due to sepsis. Twenty-two percent of cases of ARDS in this series were due to bacteremia from any source (18%, if the three cases of pneumonia associated with bacteremia are excluded), an overall incidence which was the highest for all risk factors in this series. Similarly, Bell and colleagues prospectively identified sepsis as the predisposing cause of ARDS in 30 out of 141 patients (21.3%),[8] making sepsis also the predominant cause of ARDS in their study. Twenty-seven of these 30 patients had a bacteremia (19%), an incidence nearly identical with that of Fowler and co-workers.[57] In contrast to the findings of Fowler and colleagues, two thirds of the septic patients developed ARDS in this series from primary pulmonary infections. Although these data confirm that sepsis is the leading cause of the syndrome as it develops, it cannot be inferred from these studies how likely septic patients are to develop ARDS, with or without bacteremia.

RISK OF ARDS FOLLOWING BACTEREMIA

Although sepsis is clearly the most common predisposing cause of ARDS, and septic patients appear likely to develop ARDS, the question of whether bacteremia alone is equally capable of causing ARDS remains to be examined. Clearly, all patients with bacteremia cannot be considered septic by usual criteria such as hypotension, acidosis, thrombocytopenia, or altered mental status, so examination of bacteremia as a specific risk factor appears to be valid. Kaplan and colleagues retrospectively reviewed 86 cases of gram-negative bacteremia characterized by two positive blood cultures in an attempt to answer this question.[76] Twenty cases of ARDS were identified, an incidence of 23%. This incidence is 200-fold greater than the overall incidence of ARDS in general hospital admissions, strongly suggesting that gram-negative bacteremia is a contributing factor in ARDS. Similarly, Fein and colleagues reviewed 116 consecutive patients with septicemia and found an overall incidence of 18%,[49] which is similar to the incidence described by Kaplan and colleagues. Of note, the Fein study included small numbers of patients with gram-positive bacteremia or fungemia in their evaluation. Seventeen of the 21 patients developing ARDS in this study did so following gram-negative bacteremia. The likelihood of developing ARDS after gram-negative bacteremia was 23%, virtually identical to the incidence reported by Kaplan and co-workers. Three patients of the 39 with gram-positive bacteremia developed ARDS, an incidence of 8%, while one of two patients with blood cultures positive for fungal organisms developed ARDS. Although occasional reports of ARDS from gram-positive organisms have appeared previously,[144] acute respiratory failure following fungal sepsis is rare. ARDS following anaerobic bacteremia must be rarer still, because cases were reported in neither of these two studies and reports are notably absent elsewhere in the literature.

Of note in both of these studies of bacteremia are the observations that both shock and thrombocytopenia increased the likelihood that bacteremia would lead to ARDS.[49, 76] When the results of these two studies are combined (Table 24-2), shock and bacteremia resulted in ARDS in 83% of cases, while thrombocytopenia complicating bacteremia led to the development of ARDS in 65% of cases. While there are almost no data to suggest that shock alone produces pulmonary injury in humans,[39] clinical and laboratory investigators have postulated that thrombocytopenia may directly result in acute lung injury.[56] However, an equally plausible possibility is that bacteremia complicated by septic shock and thrombocytopenia reflects a severe underlying infectious process highly likely to result in mortality. Fowler and colleagues have also noticed that persistent acidosis increases mortality from ARDS, further highlighting the deadly association of ARDS and generalized sepsis.[57]

Table 24–2
Influence of Bactermia-Associated Conditions on the Pathogenesis and Mortality of ARDS

BACTERMIA AND		ARDS	NO ARDS
Shock*	Kaplan et al[76]	13/20	5/64
	Fein et al[49]	21/21	12/95
	Totals	34/41 (83%)[‡]	17/159 (11%)
Thrombocytopenia[†]	Kaplan	11/16	18/45
	Fein	13/21	15/95
	Totals	224/37 (65%)[‡]	33/140 (24%)
Mortality	Kaplan	18/20	36/66
	Fein	17/21	33/95
	Totals	35/41 (85%)[‡]	69/161 (43%)

*Shock was defined as systolic blood pressure less than 90 mmHg (Kaplan), or less than 60 mm Hg (Fein).
†Thrombocytopenia was defined as platelets less than 100,000/mm³ in both studies.
‡$p < 0.001$ by χ^2 analysis of combined results.

NONBACTEREMIC SEPSIS AND ARDS

The relationship between documented bacteremia and patients who appear septic on clinical grounds must be examined, because some series of bacteremia have a low incidence of subsequent ARDS[56] while hemodynamic instability in association with bacteremia seems a particular predisposition to ARDS.[49, 76, 107] The question of whether sepsis in the absence of bacteremia can result in ARDS is of great importance because bacteremia may be transient and missed by culturing techniques, particularly in intra-abdominal abscesses or other closed space infections. Of equal importance are the observations that sepsis may result from exdotoxemia caused by gastrointestinal translocation of endotoxins derived from endogenous flora,[38] and that experimental acute lung injury follows subcutaneously administered endotoxin.[143] Fowler and colleagues identified equal numbers of cases of ARDS following bacteremic and nonbacteremic sepsis.[56]

Bell and colleagues noted that the presence of bacteremia before the development of ARDS had important implications for determining the source of the infection.[8] This information had a critical bearing on outcome in their series, because only 7 of 18 patients (39%) with bacteremia and an identifiable (and therefore surgically drainable) source of infection died, while there were no survivors among the nine patients with bacteremia from an unknown source (Table 24-3). Because it is clear that identification (and presumably surgical drainage) of infections causing bacteremia will favorably influence mortality from ARDS compared with either bacteremia from an inapparent source of nonbacteremic sepsis regardless of localization (see Table 24-3), it becomes of critical importance to identify sources of bacteremia promptly. Autopsy data from the study of Bell and colleagues revealed that the peritoneal cavity was the source of bacteremia in seven of the nine cases, all mortalities, where the source of bacteremia was inapparent antemortem.[8]

Table 24–3
Relationship of Identified Infection and Bacteremia to Mortality From ARDS

INFECTION SOURCE	BLOOD CULTURES	NUMBER	MORTALITY (%)
Identified	Positive	18	39
Identified	Negative	28	71
Unidentified	Negative	14	71
Unidentified	Positive	9	100

(Modified from Bell RC, Coalson JJ, Smith JD, et al. Multiple organ failure and infection in adult respiratory distress syndrome. Ann Intern Med 1983; 99:293.)

TEMPORAL RELATIONSHIP BETWEEN SEPSIS AND ARDS

Examination of the relationship between sepsis and ARDS would not be complete without considering whether the appearance of sepsis precedes or follows the development of clinical respiratory failure. Although gram-negative bacteremia clearly leads to ARDS in about 20% of cases, Bell and colleagues noted that nonbacteremic infections were as likely to develop after the onset of ARDS as before.[8] The development of a nonbacteremic infection following the onset of ARDS was predominantly pulmonary in origin. This finding is not surprising because pulmonary parenchymal necrosis occurs in ARDS.[81] Necrotic tissue may be a nidus for establishment of pulmonary infections. Nosocomial pulmonary infections are extremely common in critically ill patients, partly because the airway is persistently instrumented by endotracheal tubes and suction catheters, and also because pulmonary edema impairs bacterial clearance from the lung.[80] Of note, the subsequent development of pneumonia in nonbacteremic ARDS did not adversely influence mortality (66% in both groups).[8] Similar findings were recently reported by Montgomery and colleagues.[98] In this study, "sepsis syndrome" (hypotension, peripheral vasodilation, or unexplained metabolic acidosis in addition to a documented source of infection)[107] developed in 70% of patients with ARDS. Sepsis syndrome preceded ARDS in 13 patients; in the other 20 patients, sepsis developed as a complication of ARDS. An abdominal source of infection was most common (70%) in patients who had sepsis syndrome before the onset of ARDS while a pulmonary source was never implicated. In contrast, abdominal infections were uncommon sources (2 of 20, 10%) in those patients who acquired sepsis syndrome after ARDS. When ARDS preceded clinical sepsis, the source of infection was pulmonary in 75% (15 of 20) of cases. Furthermore, positive antemortem blood cultures were significantly more common in patients with nonpulmonary sources of sepsis (7 of 17) than in those with pulmonary sources (1 of 15).

The accumulated evidence indicates that sepsis is the most prevalent risk factor in patients at risk for ARDS[57, 107] and that gram-negative bacteremia, particularly if complicated by clinical sepsis (hypotension, vasodilation, acidosis or thrombocyto-penia),[49,76,98] poses an extreme risk both for development of ARDS and mortality therefrom. Identification and drainage of sources of bacteremia may decrease mortality from ARDS.[81] Intra-abdominal and other nonpulmonary sources of infection are more likely to cause bacteremia in patients with ARDS[98] while sepsis following ARDS is likely pulmonary in origin[8,98] and furthermore does not seem to influence mortality adversely. The data strongly point to the primacy of intra-abdominal infection in the pathogenesis of ARDS.

PATHOGENESIS OF ARDS CAUSED BY INFECTION

Infusion of live *Pseudomonas aeruginosa* bacteria into various experimental animals produces a characteristic picture qualitatively similar to the pulmonary pathophysiology seen in human ARDS.[26] The infusion of endotoxin derived from *Escherichia coli* also produces characteristic responses that are qualitatively and quantitatively virtually identical to those seen after infusion of live bacteria.[20] Endotoxins are lipopolysaccharide components of gram-negative bacterial cell walls, which are extremely active substances biologically and are the bacterial components presumed to cause acute lung injury as well as injury to other organs. Endotoxemia produces complex pulmonary abnormalities including changes in hemodynamics, vascular permeability, and lung mechanics.

The principal animal model for the study of endotoxin-induced acute lung injury is an unanesthetized sheep in which the efferent duct of the caudal mediastinal lymph node has been cannulated for the collection of pulmonary lymph.[127] Sheep are exquisitely sensitive to endotoxin, in that doses too small to cause shock can readily produce acute lung injury and death from respiratory failure.[48] Collection of pulmonary lymph allows direct assessment of pulmonary transvascular fluid and protein exchange. Because the functional abnormalities in this preparation—acute pulmonary edema with normal left atrial pressure, hypoxemia refractory to oxygen therapy and decreased lung compliance—are very similar to those described in human ARDS,[5] this preparation has received wide acceptance as a suitable animal model of the clinical syndrome.[22]

Pulmonary artery pressure and pulmonary vascular resistance increase markedly within minutes after beginning a sublethal endotoxin infusion.[20] Marked alterations in lung mechanics also accompany endotoxin infusion in sheep. In addition to the potent pulmonary vasoconstriction producing the pulmonary hypertension, intense bronchoconstriction causes large increases in airway resistance and decreases in pulmonary compliance.[125] The airway and vascular responses are temporally coincident both in onset and in resolution, attenuating markedly within 3 to 4 hr.[20,125] Arterial hypoxemia also occurs early, presumably due to ventilation–perfusion inequality from the marked vasoconstriction and bronchoconstriction. It is tempting to ascribe this hypoxemia to pulmonary edema formation, but the hypoxemia is established long before alterations in vascular permeability are detected.

Pulmonary microvascular endothelial integrity is assessed by the collection of pulmonary lymph.[127] Lymph protein clearance (a product of lymph flow and the ratio of lymph and plasma protein concentrations) is used as a marker of alterations in endothelial permeability,[20] which is assumed to be the pathophysiologic lesion for pulmonary edema formation. Endotoxemia in sheep causes a sustained increase in lung lymph protein clearance, which begins only after the vaso- and bronchoconstriction have begun to resolve.[20] If higher doses of endotoxin are given, there is a further decrease in lung compliance and hypoxemia becomes marked as pulmonary edema develops and fatal respiratory failure ensues.[48]

Endotoxin infusion produces striking structural damage to lung tissue, notably sequestration and damage to neutrophils in the pulmonary circulation.[72,88,89,94] Marked circulating leukopenia accompanies pulmonary hypertension during endotoxin infusion.[125] Increased numbers of granulocytes can be identified in the pulmonary microcirculation within 15 min after intravenous endotoxin.[94] Ultrastructural examination revealed that many of the granulocytes were activated or damaged, because both specific and azurophil granules were identified extracellularly. The leukocyte infiltration also included lymphocytes and monocytes, and shortly thereafter, occasional leukocytes could be identified migrating into the interstitual spaces between capillaries and alveoli. As time progressed beyond 1 hr, evidence of damage to capillary endothelium and type 1 (surfactant-producing) alveolar pneumocytes was apparent, and early interstitial edema formation could be identified.[94]

The striking early accumulation of granulocytes in the pulmonary microcirculation has led to the hypothesis that granulocytes may play a role in initiating or promoting the pulmonary response to endotoxin. However, there is ample evidence that endotoxin has direct effects on pulmonary endothelium, thereby rendering the endothelial cells no longer a barrier to fluid and protein flux. Endotoxins derived from various gram-negative bacteria clearly cause injury to endothelial monolayers *in vitro* as characterized by cellular detachment, prostacyclin production, and eventual cytolysis.[65,95,96,100] Ultrastructural changes in these *in vitro* systems appear within 30 min of incubation with endotoxin, and alterations in permeability can also be identified across the monolayer *in vitro*.[24]

Despite the finding that endotoxin may directly injure endothelial cells, endotoxin-induced lung injury is also neutrophil dependent. Neutrophils are not only sequestered but apparently activated in the pulmonary circulation by endotoxin, because lysosomal enzymes of neutrophil origin can be identified in pulmonary lymph. Furthermore, in the neutropenic sheep, the pulmonary hypertensive response to endotoxin is preserved, but the alterations in lung mechanics and vascular permeability are markedly attentuated.[67,69] However, other recent evidence has led to speculation that neutrophils may not directly initiate the injury process but rather may amplify or promote the process once initiated.[22] Neutrophil depletion attentuates but does not abolish endotoxin-related injury,[67,69] and pulmonary leukostasis induced by other potent chemotaxins (complement fragments generated by zymosan or cobra-venom factor) produces minimal pulmonary changes in comparison to endotoxin.[93,108] Therefore, the interaction of neutrophils with endotoxin-damaged endothelial cells may be the critical pathophysiologic feature. Endotoxin may prime neutrophils so that they become more responsive to an activation signal, producing increased amounts of superoxide anion and enzyme release.[66] Because oxygen radicals and proteases are proposed mediators of neutrophil-mediated endothelial injury (see following text), injury may be promoted by enhanced production of these cytotoxins. An alternate hypothesis is that direct endotoxin-induced endothelial injury may render endothelium particularly susceptible to the toxic products of neutrophils.[23]

Despite the evidence that endotoxemia causes thrombocytopenia in many mammalian species,[19,88,133] platelets are probably not important mediators of acute lung injury after endotoxin.[94,124] Although platelets are important sources of certain eicosanoid species (especially thromboxane A2, see below) which have been implicated in certain portions of the response to endotoxemia,[104] endotoxemia in platelet-depleted sheep is indistinguishable from endotoxemia in control animals.[124]

HUMORAL MEDIATORS OF LUNG INJURY IN SEPSIS

Complement

Endotoxin can activate complement, and fragments of activated complement (especially C5a) are chemotactic for neutrophils and can also activate neutrophils,[35] suggesting that the cascade of events following complement activation could be the basis of endotoxin-induced acute lung injury. However, an all-encompassing complement hypothesis appears to be an insufficient explanation based on the indirect evidence cited above. Infusion of endotoxin and plasma-containing activated complement are dissimilar, with faster resolution of leukopenia and pulmonary hypertension and modest alterations in permeability from activated complement. Endotoxin infusion into partially decomplemented animals does not prevent acute lung injury.[53] However, because only partial reduction of complement activity still results in generation of chemotactic activity in response to endotoxin,[53] the precise role of complement activation after endotoxemia remains hypothetical. If complement activation does prove to play a role, it may be through its chemotactic function, recruiting large numbers of neutrophils to a site of injury, and promotion of neutrophil adhesiveness to endothelial cells.[132]

Eicosanoids

Free arachidonic acid is released from endothelial cells in response to a number of noxious stimuli; arachidonic acid is substrate for the synthesis by many cell types of a large number of prostaglandin and prostaglandin-related compounds (eicosanoids) that appear to be important factors in the genesis of acute lung injury. The action of the cyclooxygenase and thromboxane synthesis enzyme systems leads to generation of the extremely potent vasoconstrictor and platelet aggregator thromboxane A_2 (TXA_2) by way of the short-lived cyclic endoperoxides PGG_2 and PGH_2. Although probably generated by a number of cell types, physiologically significant sources of thromboxane A_2 appear to derive from platelets and leukocytes.

Thromboxanes have received attention as mediators of sepsis and shock, because elevated plasma and lymph levels of thromboxane B_2 (TXB_2—the stable and biologically inactive metabolite of TXA_2) are consistently identified in experimental endotoxemia[34] and elevated plasma thromboxane levels have been identified in humans in septic shock.[112] Data on the precise role of thromboxane generation in cardiorespiratory dynamics in sepsis are mixed. Thromboxane products appear to mediate the early-phase bronchoconstriction and pulmonary hypertension phase of endotoxemia, because TXB_2 concentrations in plasma and lymph peak when pulmonary hypertension and abnormalities of lung mechanics are maximal.[104, 125] Furthermore, inhibitors of cyclooxygenase,[104] thromboxane synthesis,[1] and thromboxane receptor antagonists[3] all prevent the early-phase response. Although a small amount of data suggests that thromboxane synthetase inhibition may attentuate permeability changes and pulmonary edema formation after endotoxin,[25] the bulk of evidence indicates that thromboxane generation does not directly cause permeability changes[17, 25]

Prostacyclin (PGI_2), the other important cyclooxygenase product of arachidonic acid metabolism, is a potent vasodilator released from endothelial cells in large quantities in response to injury. Peak plasma and pulmonary lymph PGI_2 concentrations occur with peak TXB_2 concentrations early in the response to endotoxin, and generation of both is inhibited by the cyclooxygenase inhibitors which also inhibit the alteration in lung mechanics and pulmonary hypertension.[104, 125] PGI_2 is released by injured endothelial cells by a mechanism promoted by neutrophil adherence to endothelium,[96] but the physiologic role of PGI_2 in response to injury remains unclear. It is possible that local release of vasodilator mediators such as PGI_2 may promote restoration of ventilation–perfusion inequality caused by vaso- and bronchoconstriction or maintain local blood flow through small vessels partially occluded by microthrombi. PGl_2 infusion has been reported protective against lethal canine endotoxemia,[79] but salutary effects in the systemic circulation may not be referable to the pulmonary circulation.

Leukotrienes (LT) B_4, C_4, D_4 and E_4 are products of the action of lipoxygenases on arachidonic acid and are recognized to have potent physiologic effects. The key pathophysiologic consequences are vasoconstriction with consequent decreased cardiac output secondary to increased afterload,[52] bronchoconstriction and reduced lung compliance, with increased pulmonary vascular resistance,[51, 105] increased postcapillary venular permeability,[51, 110] and aggregation and activation of platelets and leukocytes.[55] It is quite likely that leukotrienes are important mediators of acute lung injury in sepsis. Elevated LTE_4 has been identified in plasma after endotoxemia[63] and LT precursors 5-hydroxyeicosatetraenoic acid (HETE) and 12-HETE have been identified in high concentrations in pulmonary lymph after endotoxemia.[104] These increases occur several hours after infusing endotoxin, after the early alterations in lung mechanics and hemodynamics have subsided, reaching highest concentrations in lymph as the increased permeability phase of the injury occurs. Neither of these two compounds are necessarily mediators of the response themselves but clearly reflect increased metabolic activity of the lipoxygenase pathway, although 12-HETE clearly is chemotactic for neutrophils.[135] Direct evidence of the role of lipoxygenase products as mediators of toxicity in sepsis is limited, but Brigham and colleagues have recently implied that LTB$_4$ concentrations increase markedly in lung lymph after endotoxin, reaching maximum values as leukopenia becomes most profound.[24] LTB$_4$ appears to mediate neutrophil adherence to endothelial cells, perhaps thereby accounting for the leukopenia.[71] A limited amount of data that either lipoxygenase inhibitors[82] or specific LT antagonists[33] reduce mortality from endotoxemia in rats provides further evidence, although direct evidence that specific interdiction of the lipoxygenase pathway ameliorates acute lung injury is lacking.

OXYGEN RADICALS AND PROTEASES

Superoxide anion, hydroxyl radical, and hydrogen peroxide are all generated by activated inflammatory cells and are clearly cytotoxic.[58, 78] Because endotoxin-induced acute lung injury has many features suggestive of an inflammatory response, attention has focused on possible influences of these mediators on lung injury in sepsis. Data from intact sheep indicate that both the antioxidant enzyme catalase[97] and the free-radical scavenger n-acetylcysteine attenuate both the early and late phase responses to endotoxin. Small amounts of endotoxin may "prime" neutrophils to produce larger amounts of both oxygen radicals and proteases when activated.[66] However, oxygen radicals may be generated by many cells independent of inflammation. Free-radical scavengers may attentuate the direct cytotoxicity of endotoxin on endothelial cells *in vitro* and PGI$_2$ production from cultured endothelium.[22]

Numerous proteases are released from activated inflammatory cells[78] and may also play a role in acute lung injury.[75, 131] Furthermore, increased proteolytic enzyme activity has clearly been documented in patients with ARDS.[87] There may be an important relationship between oxygen-radical generation and the balance between protease and antiprotease activity in acute lung injury. Oxygen radicals may inactivate antiproteases and thereby produce unopposed proteolytic enzyme activity with subsequent cytolysis.[30] Thus, oxygen-radical production could both directly cause injury as well as promote protease-induced injury. Antiproteases may be protective against direct endotoxin-induced endothelial cytotoxicity,[24] either by prevention of oxygen radical-induced promotion of proteolysis, or because some antiproteases also have antioxidant activity.[118]

MONONUCLEAR CELLS AND CYTOKINES

Although neutrophil sequestration and degranulation seem the predominant pathophysiologic event leading to acute lung injury after endotoxin, there is evidence that circulating mononuclear cells and cells derived from them do participate in the injury process. Pulmonary lymphocyte sequestration also occurs after endotoxin infusion,[94] and these lymphocytes appear to adhere to endothelium, degranulate and migrate to the interstitual spaces as do neutrophils. Endotoxin has long been known to stimulate B lymphocytes *in vitro,*[18] and elaboration of chemoattractant lymphokines may serve to regulate both lymphocyte and granulocyte traffic in the pulmonary inflammatory response.[22, 138] Direct evidence implicating lymphocytes is scarce, but intriguing. A striking reduction in the early endotoxin response occurs in sheep having prior T-lymphocyte depletion from chronic thoracic duct drainage.[16]

Monocytes are also more evident in lung tissue after endotoxemia,[94] so it may be reasonable to presume a key role for either tissue or alveolar macrophages in the production of acute lung injury. Endotoxin may stimulate alveolar macrophages to release leukotrienes,[85] oxygen-radical species, or proteases, all of which have been clearly implicated in the pathogenesis of lung injury. Endotoxin-stimulated alveolar macrophages can produce many substances that are chemotactic for neutrophils,[43, 46, 123] although it is unclear whether these monokines initiate neutrophil sequestration in the lungs or whether they are produced later in the inflammatory response.

Platelet-activity factor (1-0-alkyl-2-acetyl-sn-glyceryl-3-phosphorylcholine; PAF) is another putative mediator of acute lung injury in sepsis. A great deal of interest surrounds this mediator because it readily produces increased vascular permeability when injected subcutaneously.[73] Profound hypotension due to ventricular dysfunction occurs after intravenous injection,[44, 52] and PAF appears in circulating quantities sufficient to cause hypotension after intravenous endotoxin.[44] Furthermore, PAF release from various immune cells is enhanced in experimental bacterial peritonitis.[74] Despite the apparent association between infection and PAF generation, whether PAF may be considered a mediator of the endotoxin-induced alterations constituting acute lung injury remains unclear. It is logical that the lung could be a target organ because PAF is released from various cells found in the lungs, including endothelial cells, mast cells, alveolar macrophages, platelets, and neutrophils.[4, 28, 29] Specifically, PAF is synthesized by neutrophils during phagocytosis or after stimulation with C5a,[83] and exogenous PAF has been reported to produce neutrophil aggregation[27, 68] and neutrophil-dependent and -independent enhancement of vascular permeability.[86] PAF is also a very potent bronchoconstrictor and induces pulmonary superoxide production after inhalation.[136] Nonetheless, pretreatment with PAF antagonists counteracts the systemic hypotension caused by endotoxin,[44, 133] but does not appear to modify the striking changes in pulmonary hemodynamics or vascular permeability characteristic of endotoxin.[133] PAF has been infused into the same sheep model that has been extensively characterized for endotoxin infusion.[27] Similarly with endotoxin, PAF infusion causes leukopenia and pulmonary hypertension, although the latter is transient and readily reversible at the end of the infusion. In contrast, the increases in pulmonary transvascular protein clearance were minimal by comparision. Both the pulmonary hypertension and increased protein clearance were attentuated by prior cyclooxygenase inhibitors indicating that, like endotoxin, PAF induces cyclooxygenase-mediated pulmonary vasoconstriction. In striking contrast to endotoxin, pulmonary edema formation does not occur after PAF infusion. Although PAF has important *in vitro* effects (including possibly the expression of direct endotoxin-induced endothelial damage), the physiologic relevance of this mediator *in vivo* remains undefined.

Cachectin (tumor necrosis is factor-alpha, TNF) is a polypeptide hormone secreted in large amounts by endotoxin-activated macrophages[13] and to a lesser degree by circulating monocytes. Initial interest in TNF as a mediator of endotoxin shock developed when mice passively immunized against cachectin were protected from lethal endotoxemia.[14] When TNF is infused into rats in quantities similar to that produced endogenously during endotoxemia, hemoconcentration, shock, and metabolic acidosis supervene. Marked pulmonary damage is apparent, characterized by severe interstitial pneumonitis and intense pulmonary vascular leukostasis.[134] The mechanism by which this toxicity is expressed is unclear, but a number of possible pathogenetic mechanisms have been identified. TNF has profound effects on vascular endothelium and may be directly toxic to endothelial cells.[114] TNF may also mediate microvascular thrombosis by induction of endothelial procoagulant activity,[101] interleukin-1 production,[42,84] and changes in cellular morphology.[129] The release of interleukin-1 from monocytes and endothelial cells may be an important part of the response, because interleukin-1 promotes neutrophil adhesion and degradation.[46,123] However, TNF may also directly promote injury by activation of neutrophils, stimulating neutrophil adhesion to endothelial cells and enhancing phagocytosis.[61,116] This effect may occur in concert with interferon-gamma, which activates macrophages and stimulates oxygen-radical formation and phagocytic potential of these cells.[99] Interferon-gamma augments the production of TNF in response to endotoxin.[15,102]

TNF may be a critical mediator of endotoxin-induced shock and tissue injury because many of the previously identified mechanisms (neutrophil and macrophage activation, neutrophil adherence and phagocytosis, oxygen-radical production, endothelial morphologic changes, and many of the hemodynamic consequences) of endotoxemia may be traced back to TNF. Although it is not clear whether TNF can stimulate leukotriene biosynthesis directly, such a mechanism also seems possible because leukotrienes are derived from activated macrophages and neutrophils. As such a critical mediator, TNF becomes as inviting target for pharmacologic manipulation.[12] Specific neutralization of TNF and related cytokines may offer new options for therapy.

THERAPEUTIC STRATEGY IN ARDS

Reports of mortality exceeding 60% in series of patients with ARDS are commonplace, and mortality may approach 90% in patients with sepsis as the underlying cause of the respiratory failure.[49,76] With persistent reports of high mortality despite the tremendous increase in understanding of the pathophysiology of acute respiratory failure, it is not surprising that advances in the laboratory have thus far yielded little of clinical benefit. Important advantages may yet be derived from compounds such as eicosanoid antagonists or synthesis inhibitors or oxygen-radical scavengers. Initial attempts at immunomodulator therapy with E-series prostaglandins, which may decrease production as well as suppress neutrophil aggregation, chemotaxis, and activation, were met with enthusiasm[11,70] but could not be duplicated. Two important obstacles impede evaluation of new drugs for therapy of ARDS. Besides the fact that almost none of these investigational compounds have yet come to clinical trials, virtually all laboratory studies show efficacy only when the animals are treated before the injury has been established. Salutary effects are diminished or lost entirely when treatment of the established syndrome is modeled, again emphasizing the critical importance of identifying patients at risk at the earliest possible opportunity. In the absence of specific therapy, patient care in ARDS consists of sophisticated but supportive measures.

The clinical hallmarks of acute respiratory failure of many differing etiologies are indistinguishable, because the lungs respond stereotypically to a wide variety of insults. The classic syndrome consists of arterial hypoxemia, which is generally refractory to supplemental oxygen therapy; diffuse interstitial pulmonary edema, which eventually evolves to alveolar flooding and is characterized by low or normal pulmonary vascular pressures; and decreased lung volumes and lung compliance caused by destruction of surfactant-producing cells and subsequent atelectasis.[2, 64] Supportive therapy is directed at all three of these characteristics.

Oxygen therapy is the obvious solution for hypoxemia, but the hypoxemia of ARDS is often refractory to supplemental oxygen because the hypoxemia results not only from pulmonary edema and atelectasis but also from ventilation–perfusion inequality.[37] Effective ventilation of unperfused alveoli adds nothing to arterial oxygenation. Furthermore, oxygen in concentrations great enough to have an impact on oxygenation (greater than 50%) is clearly toxic, even to normal lungs.[41] Oxygen toxicity has many features indistinguishable from ARDS, perhaps because injury may be mediated by toxic oxygen-radical species in both insults. Although unproven, it is widely presumed that oxygen toxicity may be additive in ARDS. It is generally accepted that oxygenation should be maintained with as little oxygen as possible when supporting the patient with ARDS.

The mainstay of support for patients with acute respiratory failure is ventilation with PEEP.[117,128,141] PEEP ventilation addresses both the oxygenation and ventilation–perfusion inequality problems by increasing functional residual capacity, thereby restoring normal ventilation–perfusion relationships[111] and supporting adequate oxygenation using lower inspired oxygen concentrations.[118] Unfortunately, PEEP ventilation is not a panacea for acute respiratory failure. Prophylactic administration of PEEP does not prevent the development of clinical acute respiratory failure in patients at risk[126] and has not led to further decreases in overall mortality since its initial introduction despite extensive evaluations of how to best employ PEEP therapy.[117] Furthermore, the high levels (greater than 15 cm of water) of PEEP necessary to support oxygenation in severe acute respiratory failure have substantial intrinsic morbidity including barotrauma, such as pneumothorax, and potentially serious reductions of cardiac output.[117,141]

The profound hemodynamic alterations associated with PEEP therapy make careful fluid management extremely important, because increased pulmonary vascular pressures clearly worsen pulmonary edema when microvascular permeability is increased. Pulmonary hypertension is clearly a poor prognostic sign in acute respiratory failure,[145] so pulmonary vascular pressures should be minimized to prevent excessive morbidity and mortality from ARDS. Thus, a Swan-Ganz catheter[130] is required both for measurement of pulmonary vascular pressures and for collection of mixed venous blood for calculation of such variables as physiologic shunt and oxygen consumption. The choice of fluids to be administered was extremely controversial when ARDS was initially described and characterized, with colloid-containing fluids such as 5% or 25% albumin favored by some in the belief that increased plasma protein concentrations would diminish net transvascular fluid flux and thereby minimize pulmonary edema formation. This practice has proved questionable for a number of reasons, not the least of which are that hypoalbuminenia does not increase transvascular fluid flux experimentally, and that correlations between colloid oncotic pressure and pulmonary microvascular pressure are poor. Coupled with the observations that serum half-life of exogenously administered albumin is only a few hours and that transvascular fluid and protein movement are both clearly enhanced in the increased microvascular permeability state, which is pathognomonic for ARDS,[20] it is conceivable that extravascular fluid accumulation, particularly in the septic patient where the permeability defect may be generalized and not merely limited to the lungs, may actually be promoted by colloid administration. For these reasons, many investigators and clinicians prefer that crystalloid in the form of balanced salt solutions such as Ringer's lactate be used exclusively for the resuscitation of these patients. Fluid requirements may be large for these patients, both because extravascular fluid accumulation may be great and because plasma volume expansion may be necessary to counteract the low cardiac output state occasioned by PEEP therapy. Generalized edema formation is not of concern in these patients as long as pulmonary vascular pressures remain low, because hydrostatic and not oncotic forces are the principal determinant of pulmonary transvascular fluid and protein exchange.[20, 103, 106]

Treatment with high-dose intravenous corticosteroids has been a matter of intense interest for therapy both of septic shock[115] and acute lung injury associated with sepsis.[120] Glucocorticoids are no longer recommended therapy in septic shock[119] or acute lung injury. In theory, corticosteroids have a number of properties potentially very useful as therapy of sepsis-induced lung injury. Steroids appear to prevent the release of free arachidonic acid from endothelial cells,[54] inhibiting the generation of some cyclooxygenase and lipoxygenase products but not thromboxanes.[104] Moreover, steroids prevent pulmonary neutrophil sequestration both experimentally[7] and clinically[140] and also inhibit activation of both neutrophils and certain lymphocytes. The partial inhibition of arachidonate metabolism may explain why high doses of methylprednisolone given to sheep prior to endotoxin infusion markedly reduce permeability changes but have little effect on the antecedent pulmonary hypertension.[21] However, steroids do not influence the direct effects of endotoxin on endothelial cells,[24] raising the possibility that steroids may modify leukotriene-mediated interactions between neutrophils and endothelium.[24, 71]

Although experimental steroid pretreatment may be protective, clinical attempts to treat high-risk patients prophylactically have not been successful[141] and evidence that steroid treatment will favorably influence the established syndrome is scant.[120] Some evidence exists to suggest that steroid therapy may be detrimental.[36, 141] In particular, steroids seem to increase the incidence of nosocomial pneumonia in critically ill patients in general[36] and to increase markedly the infection rate in acute lung injury.[141] Because secondary pneumonias are a recognized major complication of ARDS even when corticosteroid therapy is not employed,[8,98] the need to avoid further nosocomial infectious morbidity caused by a drug of disproven benefit contraindicates steroid therapy of acute lung injury as well.

ACUTE LUNG INJURY AND MULTIPLE ORGAN FAILURE

It is well established that the mortality of acute respiratory failure associated with sepsis may approach 90%,[49,76] a figure that clearly exceeds the 60% mortality generally associated with ARDS from all causes. Because it is clear that the lung responds stereotypically to a wide variety of insults,[20,41,131] it may be that outcome is determined more by the underlying disease process than by the magnitude of the pulmonary dysfunction itself. In fact, ventilatory support of these patients has evolved to the point where inability to oxygenate a patient is an uncommon cause of death from respiratory failure,[92,98,109] with death usually attributable to the underlying disease process. Control of the focus of infection with adequate surgical debridement and drainage and adjuvant broad-spectrum antibiotic therapy is a critical feature of therapy of these patients.

Because death from unmanageable respiratory failure is unusual, disease processes elsewhere in the body also related to sepsis may be implicated as the cause of excess mortality. The development of sequential failure of multiple, seemingly disparate organ systems in association with acute respiratory failure may explain this phenomenon.[31,47] MOF syndrome is increasingly common, characterized by sequential failure of organ systems following trauma or sepsis. Up to 70% of cases of MOF are clearly related to sepsis, which may also be extra-abdominal in origin.[59,90,92] Mortality averages 75%, increasing as the number of involved organs increases.[59,90,91] If four or more organ systems are involved, survival is rare.[59,91] The syndrome may follow up to half of operations for intra-abdominal sepsis, and is now the predominant cause of death unrelated to trauma in surgical intensive care units.[31,59,90,92] Involved organs or systems may include the lungs, liver, kidneys, central nervous system (stupor or coma), gastrointestinal tract ("stress-induced" upper gastrointestinal hemorrhage), and coagulation (disseminated intravascular coagulation). Cardiac failure and the ubiquitous nutritional and metabolic derangements of sepsis are occasionally included in the definition.[92] Organs or systems may fail alone or in combination, and failure of a particular organ is not predictive of subsequent events.[62]

The pathogenesis of MOF is clearly complex and a matter of current debate,[31] although it is readily apparent that there is an important relationship with systemic infection and the humoral factors generated in sepsis. In addition to complement, arachidonate metabolites, oxygen species, and other mediators previously mentioned, one important hypothesis is the "gut" hypothesis. This hypothesis attempts to account for the fact that many patients who develop MOF appear septic but are not bacteremic,[8,31,107] suggesting that the source of sepsis may be indigenous flora resident in the gastrointestinal tract. Gastrointestinal tract function is profoundly altered in the critically ill, septic patient, with adynamic ileus, gastric mucosal ulcerations, acute acalculous cholecystitis and other alterations being commonplace. The mucosa of the normal gastrointestinal tract provides an effective barrier to bacteria and endotoxin, a basic function that may be lost in critical illness, resulting in translocation of endogenous bacteria and subsequent failure of host defenses.[38] Hepatocyte[77] and hepatic reticuloendothelial function[113] are likewise depressed, resulting in diminished intravascular clearance of bacteria and other circulating particulates. Maintenance of the normal barrier appears to depend in part on normal intestinal flora.[10] Gastrointestinal microflora are markedly altered in the critically ill,[45] and broad-spectrum antibiotic therapy may also promote translocation.[9]

Acute respiratory failure, sepsis, and the MOF syndrome are closely linked. Respiratory failure occurs early in the syndrome, usually within 72 hr of the precipitating event. The reason for the particular susceptibility of the lung is unclear, although the large pool of neutrophils normally marginated in the pulmonary circulation may be critically important. The early development of respiratory failure and the particular susceptibility of the lung to injury combine to make acute respiratory failure the most common single manifestation of MOF[59] so much that isolated respiratory failure due to sepsis (as opposed to other causes of ARDS) appears uncommon by comparison.

As with acute lung injury, therapy for MOF is empiric and supportive.[31] In addition to respiratory care, prophylaxis of gastrointestinal hemorrhage with antacids or H_2-receptor antagonists, adequate nutritional support, judicious employment of fluids, blood products, and cardiotonic agents, and dialysis (if necessary) characterize the current approach to the syndrome. Appropriate antibiotic therapy is an important adjunct, but an aggressive search for foci of infection is paramount.

Mortality from MOF is sufficiently high and the overall accuracy of localizing diagnostic studies is sufficiently imprecise that an increasing body of evidence suggests that the development of organ failure is a valid indication for abdominal exploration when an extra-abdominal source of infection (principally pneumonias) can be excluded.[50,91,121] In order to influence mortality favorably, abdominal reexploration must be undertaken before systemic consequences of sepsis, such as metabolic acidosis, peripheral vasodilation, or hypotension dependent on vasopressor support, supervene.[121] With this aggressive approach, positive findings at laparotomy are encountered in 80% of cases and overall mortality of MOF can be reduced to 30%[91] to 50%.[121] Despite the critical condition of these patients, operative mortality from a negative laparotomy may be as low as 18%,[91] fully justifying this aggressive approach.

REFERENCES

1. Anderegg K, Anzeveno P, Cook JA, et al. Effect of a pyridine derivative thromboxane synthetase inhibitor and its inactive isomer in endotoxin shock in the rat. Br J Clin Pharmacol 1983;18:725.
2. Andreadis N, Petty TL. Adult respiratory distress syndrome: problems and progress. Am Rev Respir Dis 1985;132:1344.
3. Armstrong RA, Jones RL, Wilson NH. Effect of the thromboxane receptor antagonist EP092 on endotoxin shock in the sheep. Prostaglandins 1985;29:703.
4. Arnoux B, Burand J, Rigand M, et al. Release of platelet activating factors (PAF-acether) and arachidonic acid metabolites from alveolar macrophages. Agents Actions 1981;11:555.

564

5. Ashbaugh DG, Bigelow DB, Petty TL, et al. Acute respiratory distress in adults. Lancet 1967; 2:319.
6. Barie PS, Tahamont MV, Malik AB. Prevention of increased pulmonary vascular permeability after pancreatitis by granulocyte depletion. Am Rev Respir Dis 1982;126:904.
7. Begley C, Ogletree M, Meyrick B, et al. Modification of pulmonary responses to endotoxemia in awake sheep by steroidal and non-steroidal antiflammatory agents. Am Rev Respir Dis 1984;130:1140.
8. Bell RC, Coalson JJ, Smith JD, et al. Multiple organ failure and infection in adult respiratory distress syndrome. Ann Intern Med 1983;99:293.
9. Berg RD. Promotion of the translocation of enteric bacteria from the gastrointestinal tracts of mice by oral treatment with pencillin, clindamycin, or metronidazole. Infect Immun 1981;33:854.
10. Berg RD, Owens WE. Inhibition of translocation of viable *Escherichia coli* from the gastrointestinal tracts of mice by bacterial antagonism. Infect Immun 1979;25:820.
11. Bernard G, Lucht W, Niedermeyer M, et al. Effect of n-acetylcysteine on the pulmonary response to endotoxin in awake sheep and upon *in vitro* granulocyte function. J Clin Invest 1984;73:1772.
12. Beutler B, Cerami A. Cachectin: more than a tumor necrosis factor. N Engl J Med 1987;316:379.
13. Beutler B, Mahoney J, Letrang N, et al. Purification of cachectin, a lipoprotein lipase-suppressing hormone secreted by endotoxin-induced RAW 264.7 cells. J Exp Med 1985;161:984.
14. Beutler B, Milsark IW, Cerami AC. Passive immunization against cachectin/tumor necrosis factor protects mice from lethal effect of endotoxin. Science 1985;229:869.
15. Beutler B, Tkacenko V, Milsark I, et al. Effect of gammainterferon on cachectin expression by mononuclear phagocytes: reversal of the endotoxin-resistance phenotype. J Exp Med 1986;164:1791.
16. Bohs CT, Fish JC, Miller TH, et al. Pulmonary vascular response to endotoxin in normal and lymphocyte-depleted sheep. Circ Res 1979;46:13.
17. Bowers R, Ellise E, Brigham K, et al. Effects of prostaglandin cyclic endoperoxides on the lung circulation of sheep. J Clin Invest 1979;63:131.
18. Bradley SG. Cellular and molecular mechanisms of action of bacterial endotoxins. Annu Rev Microbiol 1979;33:67.
19. Bredenberg CE, Taylor GA, Webb WR. The effect of thrombocytopenia on the pulmonary and systemic hemodynamics of canine endotoxic shock. Surgery 1980;87:59.
20. Brigham KL, Bowers R, Haynes J. Increased sheep lung vascular permeability caused by *E. coli* endotoxin. Circ Res 1979;45:292.
21. Brigham KL, Bowers RE, McKeen CK. Methylprednisolone prevention of increased lung vascular permeability following endotoxemia in sheep. J Clin Invest 1981;67:1103.
22. Brigham KL, Meyrick B. Endotoxin and lung injury. Am Rev Respir Dis 1985;133:913.
23. Brigham KL, Meyrick B. Granulocyte-dependent injury of pulmonary endothelium: a case of miscommunication. Tissue Cell 1984;16:137.
24. Brigham KL, Meyrick B, Bernard G, et al. Free radicals and arachidonic acid metabolites in endotoxin-induced pulmonary endothelial injury. In: Taylor AE, Matalon S, Ward P, eds. Physiology of oxygen radicals. Bethesda, MD: American Physiological Society, 1986:199.
25. Brigham K, Ogletree M. Effects of prostaglandins and related compounds on lung vascular permeability. Bull Eur Physiopathol Respir 1981;17:703.
26. Brigham KL, Woolverton WC, Blake LH, et al. Increased sheep lung vascular permeability caused by *Pseudomonas* bacteremia. J Clin Invest 1974;54:792.
27. Burhop KE, VanDerZee H, Bizios R, et al. Pulmonary vascular response to platelet-activity factor in awake sheep and the role of cyclooxygenase metabolites. Am Rev Respir Dis 1986;134:548.
28. Camussi G, Aglietta M, Coda R, et al. Release of platelet-activating factor and histamine. II. The cellular origin of human PAF: monocytes, polymophonuclear neutrophils and basophils. Immunology 1981;42:191.
29. Camussi G, Aglietta M, Malavosi F, et al. The release of platelet-activating factor from human endothelial cells in culture. J Immunol 1983;131:2397.
30. Carp H, Janoff A. *In vitro* suppression of serum elastase inhibiting capacity by reactive oxygen species generated by phagocytosing polymorphonuclear leukocytes. J Clin Invest 1979;64:793.
31. Carrico CJ, Meakins JL, Marshall JC, et al. Multiple-organ-failure syndrome. Arch Surg 1986;121:196.
32. Chenuneth ED, Cooper SW, Hogli TE, et al. Complement activation during cardiopulmonary bypass. Evidence of generation of C3a and C5a anaphylatoxins. N Engl J Med 1981;304:477.
33. Cook JA, Wise WC, Halushka PV. Protective effect of a selective leukotriene antagonist in endotoxemia in the rat. J Pharmacol Exp Ther 1985;235:470.
34. Cook JA, Wise WC, Halushka PV. Elevated thromboxane levels in the rat during endotoxemia. J Clin Invest 1980;65:227.

35. Craddock P, Hammerschmidt D, White J, et al. Complement (C5a)-induced granulocyte aggregation *in vitro:* a possible mechanism of complement mediated leukostasis and leukopenia. J Clin Invest 1977;60:260.

36. Craven DE, Kunches LM, Kilinsky V, et al. Risk factors for pneumonia and fatality in patients receiving continuous mechanical ventilation. Am Rev Respir Dis 1986;133:792.

37. Dantzker DR, Brook CJ, Dehart P, et al. Ventilation–perfusion distribution in the adult respiratory distress syndrome. Am Rev Respir Dis 1979;120:1039.

38. Deitch EA, Maejima K, Berg R. Effect of oral antibiotics and bacterial overgrowth on the translocation of the GI tract microflora in burned rats. J Trauma 1985;25:385.

39. Demling RH, Manohar M, Will JA, et al. The effect of plasma oncotic pressure on the pulmonary microcirculation after hemorrhagic shock. Surgery 1979;86:323.

40. Demling RH, Niehaus G, Perea A, et al. Effect of burn-induced hypoproteinemia on pulmonary transvascular fluid filtration rate. Surgery 1979;85:339.

41. Deneke SM, Fanburg BL. Normobaric oxygen toxicity of the lung. N Engl J Med 1980;303:76.

42. Dinarello CA. Interleukin-1 and the pathogenesis of the acute-phase response. N Engl J Med 1984;311:1413.

43. Dinarello CA, Cannon JC, Wolff SM, et al. Tumor necrosis factor (cachectin) is an endogenous pyrogen and induces production of interleukin-1. J Exp Med 1986;163:1433.

44. Doebber TW, Wu MS, Robbins JC, et al. Platelet activating factor (PAF) involvement in endotoxin-induced hypotension in rats. Studies with PAF receptor antagonist kadsurenone. Biochem Biophy Res Commun 1985;127:799.

45. DuMoulin GC, Hedley-White J, Paterson DJ, et al. Aspiration of gastric bacteria in antacid-treated patients: a frequent cause of postoperative colonization of the airway. Lancet 1982;1:242.

46. Dunn CJ, Fleminke WE. The role of interleukin-1 in the inflammatory response with particular reference to endothelial cell-leukocyte adherence. J Leukocyte Biol 1985;37:745.

47. Eiseman B, Beart R, Norton L. Multiple organ failure. Surg Gynecol Obstet 1977;144:323.

48. Esbenshade AM, Newman J, Lams P, et al. Respiratory failure after endotoxin infusion in sheep; lung mechanics and lung fluid balance. J Appl Physiol 1982;53:967.

49. Fein AM, Lippman M, Holtzman H, et al. The risk factors, incidence and prognosis of the adult respiratory distress syndrome following septicemia. Chest 1983;83:40.

50. Ferraris VA. Exploratory laparotomy for potential abdominal sepsis in patients with multiple-organ failure. Arch Surg 1983;118:1130.

51. Feuerstein G. Autonomic pharmacology of leukotrienes. J Auton Pharmacol 1985;5:149.

52. Feuerstein G, Hallenbeck JM. Prostaglandins, leukotrienes, and platelet-activating factor in shock. Annu Rev Pharmacol Toxicol 1987;27:301.

53. Flick MR, Horn JK, Hoeffel JM, et al. Reduction of total hemolytic complement activity with Naja haje cobra venom factor does not prevent endotoxin-induced lung injury in sheep. Am Rev Respir Dis 1986;133:62.

54. Flower RJ. Steroidal anti-inflammatory drugs as inhibitors of phospholipase A2. In: Galli C, Galli G, Poveillati G, eds. Advances in prostaglandin and thromboxane research. Vol. 3. New York: Raven Press, 1978;105.

55. Ford-Hutchison A, Bray M, Doig M, et al. Leukotriene B, a potent chemokinetic and aggregating substance releases from polymorphonuclear leukocytes. Nature 1980;286:264.

56. Fowler AA, Hamman RF, Good JT. Adult respiratory distress syndrome: risk with common predispositions. Ann Intern Med 1983;98:593.

57. Fowler AA, Hamman RF, Zerbe GO, et al. Adult respiratory distress syndrome, prognosis after onset. Am Rev Respir Dis 1985;132:472.

58. Freeman BA, Crapo JD. Biology of disease: free radicals and tissue injury. Lab Invest 1982;47:412.

59. Fry DE, Pearlstein L, Fulton RL, et al. Multiple system organ failure. The role of uncontrolled infection. Arch Surg 1980;115:136.

60. Fulton RL, Jones CE. The cause of post-traumatic pulmonary insufficiency in man. Surg Gynecol Obstet 1975;140:179.

61. Gamble JR, Harlan JM, Klebanoff SJ, et al. Stimulation of the adherence of neutrophils to umbilical vein endothelium by human recombinant tumor necrosis factor. Proc Natl Acad Sci USA 1985;82:8667.

62. Greenburg AG. Multisystem organ failure. Contemp Surg 1983;22:31.

63. Hagmann W, Denzlinger C, Keppler D. Production of peptide leukotrienes in endotoxic shock. FEBS Lett 1985;180:309.

64. Hallman M, Spragg R, Havell JH, et al. Evidence of lung surfactant abnormality in respiratory failure. J Clin Invest 1982;70:673.

65. Harlan JM, Harker LA, Reidy MA, et al. Lipopolysaccharide-mediated bovine endothelial cell injury *in vitro*. Lab Invest 1983;48:269.

66. Haslett C, Guthrie LA, Kopaniak MM, et al. Modulation of multiple neutrophil functions by preparative methods or trace concentrations of bacteria: lipopolysaccharide. Am J Pathol 1985;119:101.

67. Heflin AC, Brigham KL. Prevention by granulocyte depletion of increased vascular permeability of sheep lung following endotoxemia. J Clin Invest 1981;68:1253.

68. Henson PM. Platelet-activating-factor (PAF) as a mediator of neutrophil–platelet interactions in inflammation. Agents Actions 1981;11:545.

69. Hinson J, Hutchison A, Ogletree M, et al. Effect of granulocyte depletion on altered lung mechanics after endotoxemia in sheep. J Appl Physiol 1983;55:92.

70. Holcroft JW, Vassar MJ, Weber CJ. Prostaglandin E1 and survival in patients with the adult respiratory distress syndrome: a prospective trial. Ann Surg 1986;203:371.

71. Hoover RL, Karnovsky MJ, Austin KF, et al. Leukotriene B4 action on endothelium mediates augmented neutrophil/endothelial interaction. Proc Natl Acad Sci USA 1984;81:2191.

72. Horn RG, Collins RD. Fragmentation of granulocytes in pulmonary capillaries during development of the generalized Schwartzmann reaction. Lab Invest 1968;19:451.

73. Humphrey DM, McManus LM, Satouchi K, et al. Vasoactive properties of acetyl glyceryl ether phosphorylcholine. Lab Invest 1982;46:422.

74. Inarrea P, Gomez-Cambronero J, Pascual J, et al. Synthesis of PAF acether and blood volume changes in gram-negative sepsis. Immunopharmacology 1985;9:45.

75. Janoff A, White R, Carp H, et al. Lung injury by leukocyte proteases. Am J Pathol 1979;97:111.

76. Kaplan RL, Sahn SA, Petty TL. Incidence and outcome of the respiratory distress syndrome on survival of patients in respiratory failure. Arch Intern Med 1979;139:867.

77. Keller GA, West MA, Cerra FB, et al. Multiple systems organ failure: modulation of hepatocyte protein synthesis by endotoxin-activated Kupffer cells. Ann Surg 1985;201:87.

78. Klebanoff SJ. Antimicrobial mechanisms in neutrophilic polymorphonuclear leukocytes. Semin Hematol 1975;12:117.

79. Krausz MM, Utsunomiya T, Feuerstein G, et al. Prostacyclin reversal of lethal endotoxemia in dogs. J Clin Invest 1981;67:1118.

80. La Force FM, Mullane JF, Boehme RF, et al. The effect of pulmonary edema on antibacterial defenses of the lung. J Lab Clin Med 1973;82:634.

81. Lamy M, Fallat RJ, Koeniger E, et al. Pathologic features and mechanisms of hypoxemia in adult respiratory distress syndrome. Am Rev Respir Dis 1976;114:267.

82. Lefer AM. Eicosanoids as mediators of ischemia and shock. Fed Proc 1985;44:275.

83. Lewis RE, Granger HJ. Neutrophil-dependent mediator of microvascular permeability. Fed Proc 1986;45:109.

84. Libby P, Ordavas JM, Auger KR, et al. Endotoxin and tumor necrosis factor induce interleukin-1 gene expression in adult human vascular endothelial cells. Am J Pathol 1986;124:179.

85. Luderitz TH, Rietch L, Schade J. Release of leukotrienes from macrophages stimulated by lipopolysaccharide endotoxin. Immunology 1983;165:213.

86. Worthen GS, Goins AJ, Mitchel BC, et al. Platelet-activating factor causes neutrophil accumulation and edema of rabbit lungs. Chest 1983;83(S5):13.

87. McGuire WW, Spragg R, Cohen AB, et al. Studies on the pathogenesis of the adult respiratory distress syndrome. J Clin Invest 1982;69:543.

88. McKay DG, Margaretten W, Csavossy I. An electron microscopic study of the effects of endotoxin shock in rhesus monkeys. Surg Gynecol Obstet 1967;125:825.

89. McKay DG, Margaretten W, Csavossy I. An electron microscope study of the effects of endotoxin on the blood vascular system. Lab Invest 1966;15:1815.

90. Machiedo GW, LoVerme PJ, McGovern PJ, et al. Patterns of mortality in a surgical intensive care unit. Surg Gynecol Obstet 1981;152:757.

91. Machiedo GW, Tikelis J, Suval W, et al. Reoperation for sepsis. Am Surg 1985;51:149.

92. Manship L, McMillin RD, Brown JJ. The influence of sepsis and multisystem and organ failure on mortality in the surgical intensive care unit. Am Surg 1984;50:94.

93. Meyrick B, Brigham KL. Effect of a single infusion of zymosan activated plasma on the pulmonary microcirculation of sheep: structure–function relationships. Am J Pathol 1984;114:32.

94. Meyrick B, Brigham KL. Acute effects of *E. coli* endotoxin on the pulmonary microcirculation of unanesthetized sheep: structure:function relationships. Lab Invest 1983;48:458.

95. Meyrick B, Ryan US, Brigham KL. Direct effects of *E. coli* endotoxin on structure and permeability of pulmonary endothelial monolayers and endothelial layers of intimal explants. Am J Pathol 1986;122:140.

96. Meyrick BR, Workman M, Frazer M, et al. Endothelial prostacyclin production is a late event in granulocyte migration into bovine pulmonary artery intimal explants. Blood 1985;66:1379.

97. Milligan SA, Hoeffel J, Flick MR. Endotoxin-induced acute lung injury in unanesthetized sheep is prevented by catalase. Am Rev Respir Dis 1985;131:422.

98. Montgomery AB, Stager MA, Carrico CJ, et al. Causes of mortality in patients with the adult respiratory distress syndrome. Am Rev Respir Dis 1985;132:485.

99. Nathan CF, Prendergast TJ, Wiebe ME, et al. Activation of human macrophages: comparision of other cytokines with interferon-gamma. J Exp Med 1984;160:600.

100. Nawroth PP, Stern DM. Modulation of endothelial cell hemostatic properties by tumor necrosis factor. J Exp Med 1986;163:740.

101. Nawroth PP, Stern DM, Kaplan KL, et al. Prostacyclin production by perturbed bovine aortic endothelial cells in culture. Blood 1984;64:801.

102. Nedwin GE, Svedersky LP, Bringman TS, et al. Effect of interleukin-2, interferon-gamma, and mitogens on the production of tumor necrosis factors alpha and beta. J Immunol 1985; 135:2492.

103. Nylander WA, Hammon JW, Roselli RJ, et al. Comparison of the effects of saline and homologous plasma infusion on lung fluid balance during endotoxemia in the unanesthetized sheep. Surgery 1981;90:221.

104. Ogletree ML, Begley CJ, King GA, et al. Influence of steroidal and nonsteroidal anti-inflammatory agents on the accumulation of arachidonic acid metabolites in plasma and lung lymph after endotoxemia in awake sheep. Measurements of prostacyclin and thromboxane metabolites and 12-HETE. Am Rev Respir Dis 1986;133:55.

105. Ogletree M, Snapper J, Brigham K. Immediate pulmonary vascular and airway responses after intravenous leukotriene D4 injections in awake sheep. Physiologist 1982;25:275.

106. Parker RE, Wickersham NE, Roselli RJ, et al. Effects of hypoproteinemia on lung microvascular protein sieving and lung lymph flow. J Appl Physiol 1986;60:1293.

107. Pepe PE, Potkin RT, Holtman-Reus D, et al. Clinical predictors of the adult respiratory distress syndrome. Am J Surg 1982;144:124.

108. Perkowski SZ, Havill AM, Flynn JT, et al. Role of intrapulmonary release of eicosanoids and superoxide anion as mediators of pulmonary dysfunction and endothelial injury in sheep with intermittent complement activation. Circ Res 1983;53:574.

109. Pine RW, Wertz MJ, Lennard ES, et al. Determinants of organ malfunction and death in patients with intraabdominal sepsis. Arch Surg 1983;118:242.

110. Piper PJ. Pharmacology and biochemistry of leukotrienes. Eur J Respir Dis 1982;122:54.

111. Ralph DD, Robertson HT, Weaver LJ, et al. Distribution of ventilation and perfusion during positive end expiratory pressure in the adult respiratory distress syndrome. Am Rev Respir Dis 1985;131:54.

112. Reines HD, Halushka PV, Cook JA, et al. Plasma thromboxane concentrations are raised in patients dying with septic shock. Lancet 1982;2:174.

113. Saba TM, Jaffe E. Plasma fibronectin (opsonic glycoprotein): its synthesis by vascular endothelial cells and role in cardiopulmonary integrity following trauma as related to reticuloendothelial function. Am J Med 1980;68:577.

114. Sato N, Goto T, Haranak K, et al. Actions of tumor necrosis factor on cultured vascular endothelial cells: morphologic modulation, growth inhibition, and cytotoxicity. JNCI 1986;76:1113.

115. Schumer W. Steroids in the treatment of clinical septic shock. Ann Surg 1976;184:333.

116. Shalaby MR, Aggarwal BB, Rinderknecht E, et al. Activation of human polymorphonuclear neutrophil functions by interferon-gamma and tumor necrosis factors. J Immunol 1985;135:2069.

117. Shapiro BA, Cane RD, Harrison RA. Positive end-expiratory pressure therapy in adults with special reference to acute lung injury: a review of the literature and suggested clinical correlations. Crit Care Med 1984;12:127.

118. Shasby DM. Antioxidant activity of some antiproteases. Am Rev Respir Dis 1985;131:293.

119. Sheagren JN. Septic shock and corticosteroids. N Engl J Med 1981;305:456.

120. Sibbald WJ, Driedger AA, Finley RJ. High dose corticosteroids in the treatment of pulmonary microvascular injury. Ann NY Acad Sci 1982;384:496.

121. Sinanan M, Marci RV, Carrico CJ. Laparotory for intraabdominal sepsis in ICU patients: indications and outcome. Arch Surg 1984;119:652.

122. Skau T, Nystrom PO, Carlsson C. Severity of illness in intraabdominal infection. Arch Surg 1985;120:152.

123. Smith RJ, Bowman BJ, Spetiale SC. Interleukin-1 stimulates granule exocytosis from human neutrophils. J Leukocyte Biol 1985;317:746.

568

124. Snapper J, Hinson J, Hutchison A, et al. Effects of platelet depletion on the unanesthesized sheep's pulmonary response to endotoxin. J Clin Invest 1984;74:1782.

125. Snapper J, Hutchison A, Ogletree M, et al. Effects of cyclooxygenase inhibitors on the alterations in lung mechanics caused by endotoxemia in the unanesthesized sheep. Am Rev Respir Dis 1983;127:306.

126. Springer RP, Stevens PM. The influence of positive end-expiratory pressure on survival of patients in respiratory failure. Am J Med 1979;66:196.

127. Staub NC, Bland RD, Brigham KL, et al. Preparation of chronic lung lymph fistulas in sheep. J Surg Res 1975;19:315.

128. Stevens PM. General assessment and support of the adult respiratory distress syndrome. Ann NY Acad Sci 1982;384:477.

129. Stolpen AH, Guinan EC, Fiers W, et al. Recombinant tumor necrosis factor and immune interferon act singly and in combination to reorganize human vascular endothelial cell monolayers. Am J Pathol 1976;123:16.

130. Swan HJC, Ganz W, Forrester J. Catheterization of the heart in man with use of a flow-limited balloon-tipped catheter. N Engl J Med 1970;283:447.

131. Tahamont MW, Barie PS, Blumenstock FA, et al. Increased lung vascular permeability after pancreatitis and trypsin infusion. Am J Pathol 1982;109:15.

132. Tonnesen MG, Smedley LA, Henson PM. Neutrophil-endothelial cell interactions. Modulation of neutrophil adhesiveness induced by complement fragments C5a and C5a des arg and formyl-methionyl-leucyl-phenylalanine *in vitro*. J Clin Invest 1984;74:1581.

133. Toyofuku T, Kubo K, Kobayashi T, et al. Effects of ONO-6240, a platelet-activating factor antagonist, on endotoxin shock in unanesthesized sheep. Prostaglandins 1986;31:271.

134. Tracey KT, Beutler B, Lowry SF, et al. Shock and tissue injury induced by recombinant human cachectin. Science 1986;234:470.

135. Turner SR, Tainer JA, Lynn WS. Biogenesis of chemotactic molecules by the arachidonate lipoxygenase system of platelets. Nature 1975;257:680.

136. Vargaftig BB, Lefort J, Chignard M, et al. Platelet-activating factor induces a platelet-dependent bronchoconstriction unrelated to the formation of prostaglandin derivatives. Eur J Pharmacol 1980;65:185.

137. Vito L, Dennis RC, Weisal RD, et al. Sepsis presenting as acute respiratory failure. Surg Gynecol Obstet 1974;138:896.

138. Ward PA, Offen CD, Montgomery JR. Chemoattractants of leukocytes with special reference to lymphocytes. Fed Proc 1971;30:1721.

139. Warshaw AL, Richter JM. A practical guide to pancreatitis. Curr Prob Surg 1984;21(12):1.

140. Warshawski FJ, Sibbard WJ, Driedger AA, et al. Abnormal neutrophil–pulmonary interaction in the adult respiratory distress syndrome. Qualitative and quantitative assessment of pulmonary neutrophil kinetics in humans with *in vivo* 111-In neutrophil scintigraphy. Am Rev Respir Dis 1986;133:797.

141. Weigelt JA, Norcross JF, Borman KR, et al. Early steroid therapy for respiratory failure. Arch Surg 1985;536.

142. Weisman IM, Rinaldo JE, Rogers RM. Positive end-expiratory pressure in adult respiratory failure. N Engl J Med 1982;307:1381.

143. Wenger H, Wong C, Demling RH. Pulmonary dysfunction secondary to soft-tissue endotoxin. Arch Surg 1985;120:159.

144. Wiles JB, Cerra FB, Siegel JH, et al. The systemic septic response: does the organism matter? Crit Care Med 1980;8:55.

145. Zapol WM, Snyder MT. Pulmonary hypertension in severe acute respiratory failure. N Engl J Med 1977;296:476.

25

○ ○ ○ ● ● ●

GYNECOLOGIC INFECTION

William J. Ledger

There is no hope for a scientific formulation of treatment without an understanding of the microbiology of gynecologic infection. Rational medical therapy requires this basic information so that appropriate antibiotics can be selected by the responsible physicians. This point is particularly pertinent in the 1980s, for in the past decade our perspectives of the bacterial nature of gynecologic infections have expanded.

The past 10 years have been noteworthy because of the marked changes in the microbiologic understanding of gynecologic infection. Prior to this, major emphasis was placed on a "pathogen," a single species of bacteria causing disease. This view of infection emphasized such microbiologic correlations as *Neisseria gonorrhea* causing salpingitis[19] or *Escherichia coli* as the agent of sepsis in patients with life-threatening infected abortions.[27] This old theme of a single species of bacteria as the cause of the abnormal pelvic process has now been replaced by the more accurate description of pelvic infections resulting from the interaction of many different species of bacteria. Also, physician concern about the bacterial participants in infection has shifted from *Neisseria gonorrhea* and *Escherichia coli* to the gram-negative anaerobic rods; the familiar *Bacteroides fragilis,* and less commonly recognized species as *Bacteroides melaninogenicus, Bacteroides bivius,* and *Bacteroides disiens.* This new stress on anaerobic bacteria is based on a number of microbiologic observations. These include the findings that anaerobic bacteria can be recovered from the pelvic site of infection in the majority of cases,[30] these same bacteria are frequently isolated from the bloodstream of women with a bacteremia secondary to a pelvic site of infection,[15] and anaerobic bacteria are invariably isolated from the purulent contents of a pelvic abscess.[12] There are other new microbiologic emphases. Recent literature has indicated that *Chlamydia* can be isolated from many patients with gynecologic infections, particularly those women with salpingitis.[20] The microbiologic picture of pelvic infection that emerges is one that is more complicated and complex than we were aware of in the past. There are many species of organisms involved in individual infections, and many of the bacteria isolated are not the familiar names of the past.

The emphasis in the antibiotic treatment of pelvic infections has switched as well. Formerly, therapeutic intervention to modify the natural progression of disease seemed simple and direct. Physicians began treatment with penicillin and an aminoglycoside to cover aerobic pathogens. If patients did not improve, they were operated on to drain or remove a pelvic abscess, because physicians had been taught that there was no medical treatment for a pelvic abscess. It is apparent that this treatment philosophy was based on a limited view of the reality of pelvic infections and frequently was not in the patient's best interests. Today, there is much greater emphasis on initial therapy with other antibiotics including clindamycin, metronidazole, cefoxitin, or doxycycline, because of their activity against gram-negative anaerobes or *Chlamydia.* One significant clinical outcome of these new antibiotic strategies is that fewer patients fail treatment and develop a pelvic abscess that necessitates operative intervention. There are observed changes in clinical practice. Physician decisions in the operating room have been modified with a much greater emphasis on the conservation of pelvic organs. There are many reasons for this. Pelvic infections are less extensive because of better antibiotic therapy, but, in addition, because of the widespread availability of *in vitro* fertilization programs in which pregnancies can be achieved in patients who were infertile because of tubal damage that could not be reversed. The old justification for complete extirpation because of the inability of this type of patient to conceive is no longer true. The current theme in every operative decision is conservation of pelvic organs, if possible.

Despite these new advances in our understanding, large gaps still exist in the scientific base of understanding of pelvic infections. Much of this is related to problems of studying pelvic inflammation in the human. As physicians, we would like to know what bacteria are present at the site of infection when the patient first has symptoms, what bacteria are eliminated from soft tissue infection sites when patients are successfully treated with antibiotics, and which species remain at the focus of infection when the physician judges that the initial antibiotics have failed. This information is not available. We depend on empirical choices in most cases. When initial antibiotic choices fail to yield a cure, the next step is the prescription of other antibiotics that have different antibacterial coverage than the original selection.

Because of our inability to sample these internal sites of infection directly, the microbiologic information needed to broaden our knowledge of pelvic infections is not available in the human female. This missing gap in microbiologic information has led to the use of animal models to simulate soft tissue pelvic infections in the human. The model that has most influenced clinical practice was developed by Gorbach and Bartlett. In their studies a male rat was employed. A gelatin capsule was filled with rat feces mixed with barium sulfate and inserted into the peritoneal cavity of these animals. As the capsule subsequently dissolves, the peritoneal cavity is exposed to large numbers of aerobic and anaerobic bacteria that are present in the feces. These animals initially become acutely ill with peritonitis, have an associated bacteremia with gram-negative aerobes, and 40% die. The survivors recover for a few days and then become moribund again. When sacrificed, they are found to have intra-abdominal abscesses in which anaerobic bacteria are the predominant isolates. These intra-abdominal abscesses are not present in those animals dying of sepsis earlier in the course of infection. The investigators have characterized this pathologic process as a biphasic response to the multibacterial insult of the gelatin capsule filled with feces, an early onset phase with gram-negative aerobic sepsis and death, and a late onset phase of abscess formation in which anaerobes predominate.[34]

The beauty of this animal model is the ease with which it lends itself to study. The end points are unequivocal, death or intra-abdominal abscess formation. Antibiotic intervention can be employed to see if it modifies these easily measured end points, death from sepsis or intra-abdominal abscess formation.

Chemotherapy studies indicate that the rat's response to this massive bacterial insult can be modified. A combination of an antibiotic effective against gram-negative aerobes (gentamicin) and anaerobes (clindamycin) significantly reduces both the death rate from sepsis and subsequent formation of intra-abdominal abscesses. These results are better than those seen with the more traditional combination of penicillin and an aminoglycoside, and better results have also been achieved with those cephalosporins and penicillins with good activity against gram-negative aerobes and anaerobes[2] (Table 25-1).

Despite the impressive results of these animal studies, two important questions must be answered affirmatively before they can be applied to the human. Does this animal model of infection have any similarity with pelvic infections seen in the human? I believe the answer to this is a qualified yes. Early onset sepsis is seen in women with pelvic infections. The differences are that mortality from sepsis is rare and organisms other than gram-negative aerobes, particularly gram-positive aerobes and all anaerobes, can be recovered from the bloodstream of these women. Late onset abscess formation is seen in the human, and anaerobes are the most important isolates in these conditions. The second question involves the timing of the therapeutic intervention. In the animal model, if antibiotics are delayed more than 4 hr after the intraperitoneal insertion of the feces-filled capsule, they are not effective. In contrast in the human, the patient is neither evaluated by a physician nor are antibiotics prescribed until she has manifested some signs of infection, including fever, tachycardia, or pain. In some cases the early signs are so minimal that when the women first present to doctors, a pelvic abscess is already present. In order to evaluate clinical results with antibiotics in

Table 25–1
Outcome of Antibiotic Therapy Regimens

TREATMENT GROUPS	DEATH FROM SEPSIS	ABCESS	CURED
Untreated controls	108 of 295	87 of 187	0 of 295
	(37%)	(100%)	(0%)
Limited-spectrum antibiotics			
Aminoglycosides	4 of 97	91 of 93	2 of 87
	(5%)	(98%)	(2%)
Clindamycin	37 of 89	3 of 53	49 of 89
	(42%)	(6%)	(55%)
Traditional combination			
Penicillin and aminoglycoside	0 of 30	22 of 30	8 of 30
	(0 %)	(73%)	(27%)
Cephalosporins alone			
Cepalothin	8 of 50	4 of 42	38 of 50
	(16%)	(10%)	(76%)
Cefoxitin	0 of 30	2 of 30	28 of 30
	(0%)	(7%)	(93%)
New combinations			
Clindamycin and gentamicin	10 of 158	6 of 148	142 of 158
	(7%)	(5%)	(90%)

these different clinical situations, I have arbitrarily divided infections into two categories, those in which treatment was started at an early phase of infection and those in which the infection was already well-established when treatment was begun.[13] The results are noted in[13] Table 25-2. The successful treatment rate was much higher in women with early infections, and the number of patients requiring operative intervention for a cure was greater in well-established infections.

There are several important lessons for the clinician from this type of clinical analysis. Those patients first seen early in the evolvement of an infection are more likely to have a clinical cure with the antibiotics initially prescribed. Nearly all clinical trials with antibiotics involve patients with early infections. I am not critical of this. That is the way initial trials should be planned to assess the effectiveness of a new antibiotic agent. The physician investigator wants to gain some experience with the drug before using it in seriously ill patients. There is a caution. The discerning reader of the reports of these initial clinical trials should not take the results and then try to apply them to patients with more serious well-established infections. The failure rate with antibiotics will be greater in patients with well-established infections, and the numbers needing operative intervention will also be greater. Excellent results in clinical trials do not predict excellent results when more seriously ill patients are treated. A different set of studies is needed to determine effectiveness in well-established infections. There is another lesson from Table 25-2. Patients suspected of having a pelvic abscess are not automatic candidates for surgical intervention, because at least half of these patients with well-established infections respond to antibiotics alone. Medical therapy is important in these women.

Knowing this, two recent studies should influence physician strategies in patients with well-established infections. A major concern of physicians in these cases should be *Bacteroides fragilis,* particularly the encapsulated variety, which is so often an important factor in pelvic abscesses.[3] Initial antibiotic prescription must be directed toward the elimination of this organism from the site of infection. We are fortunate in the United States that a cooperative study has been underway using *Bacteroides fragilis* isolates from infections in patients across the country. In one laboratory, these isolates were subjected to tests of antibiotic susceptibility. The results are noted in Table 25-3 and document the resistance patterns of this species in

Table 25–2
Therapy Outcome in Early and Well-established Infections

STAGE OF INFECTION	TOTAL	NUMBER CURED (%)	SURGICAL INTERVENTION
Early	403	337 (83.6%)	26 (6.4%)
Well-established	98	47 (48%)	50 (51%)

Table 25–3
Resistance Rates of *Bacteroides fragilis* Group

ANTIMICROBIAL AGENT	% RESISTANT (1981)	% RESISTANT (1983)
Metronidazole	0	0
Chloramphenicol	0	0
Clindamycin	6	7
Cefoxitin	8	16
Piperacillin	12	8
Moxalactam	22	12
Cefotaxime	54	42
Cefoperazone	57	54
Teracycline	63	67
Cefamandole		92
Cefonacid		99
Cefuroxime		61

1981[32] and 1983.[31] Some comment is appropriate. In each of these 2 years, there were no resistant strains to either metronidazole or chloramphenicol. There were small shifts in the susceptibility patterns of other antibiotics. Clindamycin was stable, piperacillin had less resistance, while cefoxitin showed an increase. The vast majority of isolates to these three antibiotics were susceptible. In contrast, there were large numbers of isolates resistant to tetracycline. This is of historical interest because tetracycline was the drug of choice for *Bacteroides* in the 1960s.[18] Other drugs showed resistance. A number of third-generation cephalosporins, including cefoperozone, cefonacid, and cefuroxime, had unacceptably high rates of resistance. Their recent introduction into clinical practice does not make them more attractive choices. There were other lessons from these studies. Another important finding for the practitioner was the observation that resistance patterns varied greatly from hospital to hospital. In some of the participating hospitals, none of the strains of *Bacteroides fragilis* were resistant to cefoxitin, while in others more than 20% were resistant.[31] This means that it is entirely appropriate for the individual physician to demand that the laboratory periodically do accurate susceptibility testing of gram-negative anaerobic isolates to determine the characteristics of the anaerobes involved in infection.

Another important study evaluated the ability of individual antibiotics to reduce the numbers of *Bacteroides fragilis* in an environment simulating an abscess in which there was a high count of bacteria. The results are noted in Table 25-4. There were many parallels with the previous study of antibiotic resistance. Most agents with low rates of resistance were also effective in reducing bacterial numbers. Metronidazole was the most efficient agent in this model, followed closely by clindamycin and cefoxitin. Of special note is that in this high bacterial count environment, chloramphenicol with no resistant strains of *Bacteroides fragilis* fails to work, and abscess formation occurs.

Using the data from these studies, physicians treating patients with well-established pelvic infections should prescribe antibiotics that are effective against gram-

Table 25–4
Activity of Antibiotics Against *Bacteroides fragilis*

ANTIBIOTIC	REDUCTION IN BACTERIAL COUNTS + SEM
Metronidazole	6.7 ± 0.6
Clindamycin	5.0 ± 0.6
Moxalactam	3.8 ± 0.6
Cefoxitin	3.5 ± 0.6
Cefotaxime	1.1 ± 0.3
Carbenicillin	1.0 ± 0.3
Cephalothin	0.4 ± 0.2
Cefoperazone	0.1 ± 0.1

negative anaerobic bacteria. Items for consideration include antibiotic resistance as well as the ability of the antibiotic to reduce the high numbers of bacteria within an abscess. With the information available in Tables 25-3 and 25-4, one drug from a group that includes metronidazole, clindamycin, cefoxitin, or piperacillin would be appropriate. Many patients with well-established infections will respond to antibiotic therapy alone. In those patients who fail to respond to medical therapy, some form of operative intervention will be necessary. These operative decisions will vary with individual cases. Pelvic abscesses can be drained or removed in toto. There are increasing attempts to conserve pelvic organs. These well-established infections are difficult therapeutic problems. Fortunately, the majority of women with a pelvic infection will be seen early in the course of the infection. This is deservedly the most important consideration for therapeutic intervention.

Early Infections

Infected Abortions

Patients with an infected abortion are less frequently seen by physicians in the 1980s than they were in the three preceding decades. A number of events have contributed to this decline in incidence. The more widespread availability of better contraceptive techniques have reduced the number of women with unwanted pregnancies. More important, the easy access to physician-run pregnancy termination services has meant that women can have procedures performed with qualified physician supervision to end an unwanted pregnancy. These are not the clandestine operations of the past in which secrecy outweighed concerns about the possible aftermaths of infection. Easy entry to current medical services means that women can avoid long delays in getting the operation if they decide on this option. This is important because the later in pregnancy the termination is performed, the higher the subsequent infection rate. All of these trends have contributed to the clinical reality of both fewer and less serious infections following abortion.

Those few patients with infected abortions represent a low-risk population. They usually respond to antibiotics such as a penicillin, a cephalosporin, or chloramphenicol plus the operative removal of the intrauterine products of conception, the curettage. In fact, one recent review of this subject reported 97% of the patients were cured with this initial regimen, only 2% needed other antibiotics, and less than 1% had a pelvic abscess that required operative intervention.[13] These are phenomenal results, particularly in view of the fact that some of these women who are cured have an associated bacteremia with *Bacteroides* that is often resistant to penicillin and first-generation cephalosporins.[25] Chow and co-workers have suggested that these better than expected outcomes are related to the effectiveness of curettage in removing the nidus of infection and the ability of the uterus to cleanse itself of bacteria after the curettage had been performed.[6] In this clinical setting, host defense mechanisms seem more important than the choice of antibiotics. There is one potential cloud in this clear clinical sky. This emphasis on short-term therapeutic response in infected abortions ignores one important aspect of therapy. There are long-range implications because some women will have blocked tubes and be infertile as a result of these postabortal infections. This area demands further study. One report demonstrated that *Chlamydia* was recovered from many women with postabortal infections.[21] This pathogen is not susceptible to the penicillins and cephalosporins used frequently in these patients. Because of this, either tetracycline or clindamycin would be appropriate antibiotics to prescribe for those patients with a postabortal infection.

There are some patients with infected abortions who create special problems and concerns for the physician. These patients can require special diagnostic tests and closer surveillance. The more advanced the pregnancy is when the termination procedure is performed, the higher the infection rate is, but more severe infections are seen as well. There are at least two reasons for this. With these large uteri, there is a greater chance that all products of conception will not be removed by the termination procedure. In attempts to make the operative intervention complete, there is possibility that damage and/or perforation of the uterus may occur. In some of these instances, an extrauterine hematoma forms, which subsequently becomes infected. Physicians must be aware of this possibility, and this dictates a careful pelvic examination to determine if there are any extrauterine masses. If physical findings confirm this or there is a concern about retained tissue within the uterus, ultrasonography of the pelvis can be a helpful diagnostic test. When retained intrauterine products of conception are suspected, a repeat curettage should be performed after the patient has been started on antibiotics. In this situation, I prefer a combination of either clindamycin and gentamicin or cefoxitin with a tetracycline. If a uterine perforation is suspected, the treatment is usually observation with the same antibiotic coverage. There are clinical situations in which observation is not appropriate. If active intraperitoneal bleeding is suspected, if the uterine perforation has been recognized to occur laterally in which there is a possibility of uterine artery damage, or if the perforation has occurred with a functional suction apparatus, a laparotomy is required to evaluate the extent of pelvic organ and bowel damage as well as to control any active bleeding. The goal in all of these procedures is to preserve the pelvic organs, and the earlier the operative intervention is done, the more likely this will be achieved. Physician delay can be costly for the patient. Fortunately, the most severe infections of the past, an overwhelming clostridial sepsis that followed the use of necrotizing materials to achieve the termination, are rarely seen in the 1980s. There is another lesson for all of us. Any person, physician or layman, who places the rights of the fetus above those of the mother and is determined to eliminate pregnancy termination should be aware that one result of this policy will be a resurgence of serious pelvic infections. In some cases, these can require hysterectomy to eliminate the pelvic site of infection, and in others renal failure and death. Removal of the option of a safe termination of an unwanted pregnancy means that some desperate women will seek an abortion late in pregnancy outside of the closely regulated medical community.

Salpingitis

Salpingitis is the most important pelvic infection in nonpregnant women. There are a number of reasons for this judgment. There are large numbers of women who are afflicted with this problem. Some estimate that over a million women per year have this infection in the United States alone. These numbers by themselves would be cause for concern, but the dimensions of the problem become staggering when the medical impact of the residual effects of these infections are calculated. Some careful long-term studies have been done of women with a past history of salpingitis who subsequently attempt to become pregnant. A significant number of these women have residual tubal damage that prevents conception[36] (Table 25-5). The percentages increase with each subsequent episode of salpingitis and seem greater in women over the age of 24 than in younger women (see Table 25-5). This is an important outcome of a disease, because it eliminates an important life option for the victims. The focus in medicine should be to prevent this bad end result and not use all of our resources in dealing with the outcomes of infection. Medical advances are occurring. *In vitro* fertilization is exciting new technology that enables some of these women to become pregnant, an impossibility in the past. This is still complicated, expensive therapy.

The starting point for physician care of patients with salpingitis is an accurate and early diagnosis. A number of detailed and carefully thought out studies have modified our awareness of the presentation of patients with salpingitis. In the past, gynecologists stressed the spectra of signs, symptoms, and laboratory findings that patients should have so that physicians could accurately make the diagnosis. Patients with salpingitis had pelvic pain and a fever above 38°C; on pelvic examination they had bilateral adnexal swellings or masses; and these patients also had an elevated white blood cell count and sedimentation rate. The underlying philosophic concern when formulating these strict criteria was the fear that gynecologists would give antibiotics to patients with pelvic pain caused by such noninfectious problems as an ectopic pregnancy or the torsion of an adnexa. Obviously, women with this pathology would not respond to antibiotics, and the necessary operative intervention would be delayed while the physician awaited the patient's response to antibiotics. This attempt to develop diagnostic criteria was laudable. The problem was that this rigid set of requirements was not sensitive enough to differentiate patients who had salpingitis from those who did not. If these rigid standards were used, physicians would not diagnose and subsequently treat most patients with salpingitis. These concerns were confirmed by definitive studies using laparoscopy within 6 hr of admission in women with a clinical diagnosis of salpingitis. These laparoscopic evaluations yielded three groups of patients: those with salpingitis, those with other pelvic pathology, and those

Table 25–5
Percentage of Women with Infertility Because of Tubal Occlusion after
One, Two, Three or More Episodes of Salpingitis

NUMBER OF INFECTIONS	% POST SALPINGITIS INFERTILITY IN AGE GROUPS		
	15–24 yr	25–39 yr	Total
1	9.4	19.2	11.4
2	20.9	31.0	23.1
3 or more	51.6	60.0	53.9

with a normal pelvis. If we then use the criteria of pelvic pain, fever, adnexal masses, and abnormal peripheral blood studies in a comparison of patients found on laparoscopy to have salpingitis to those with a visually normal pelvis, a number of disturbing points become obvious[11] (Table 25-6). Pelvic pain did not differentiate women with salpingitis from those with a normal pelvis. It is true that a temperature above 38°C was present in significantly greater numbers of patients with salpingitis. The problem with this sign is that it is present in less than half of the women found at laparoscopy to have salpingitis. Patients with salpingitis had bilateral swelling or masses significantly more often than women with a normal pelvis. However, this criterion lacks sensitivity. Only one half of the women with salpingitis have this finding, while one quarter of the women found to have a normal pelvis on laparoscopy examination were thought to have these pelvic findings. Finally, an elevated sedimentation rate was more frequent in women with salpingitis. This observation lacks specificity. Although an elevated sedimentation rate was present in 75% of those women with salpingitis on laparoscopic examination, it was also present in 50% of women with a normal pelvis. These observations raise great doubts in my mind about the validity of clinicians rigidly employing these criteria to make the diagnosis of salpingitis. In an attempt to relax these diagnostic guidelines and enable physicians to make the diagnosis in more patients, new criteria for the diagnosis of salpingitis were published[9] (Table 25-7). I applaud these efforts because they do increase the numbers of women who will be diagnosed at an early stage of salpingitis. However, I am troubled by this listing because it is not the result of a long-term prospective study, but instead is the best guess of a committee determination. Without a database, there is no way to determine whether any of the criteria have more significance than any of the others. There are no studies on the specificity and sensitivity of these measures. In addition, there is increasing evidence from clinical studies that women who do not fulfill the formula for diagnosis in this latest schema have been found to have irreversible tubal damage from unsuspected salpingitis in the past.[24] My own requirements for diagnosis are much looser than noted in Table 25-7. I suspect salpingitis in any sexually active woman with pelvic pain. I do those tests that will be helpful in differentiating other causes of pain if this is indicated. For example, a pregnancy test can be helpful in women with a suspected early accident of pregnancy, and ultrasonography can be useful to deter-

Table 25–6
The Classic Signs and Laboratory Findings of Salpingitis Observed in Women with a Laparoscopic Diagnosis of Salpingitis and Those with a Normal Pelvis

CLASSIC SIGNS AND LABORATORY FINDINGS	SALPINGITIS PATIENTS	NORMAL PATIENTS	STATISTICAL SIGNIFICANCE
Acute pelvic pain	94	94	No
Fever above 38°C	41.3	19.6	Yes
Tender adnexal swelling or mass	49.4	24.5	Yes
Elevated sedimentation rate	75.9	52.7	Yes

Table 25–7
Criteria for the Diagnosis of Acute Salpingitis (Without Laparoscopy)

A. Three of the following signs or symptoms must be present:
   1. Lower abdominal pain and tenderness, with or without rebound tenderness.
   2. Cervical motion tenderness.
   3. Adnexal tenderness.
B. In addition, one or more of the following conditions must be present:
   1. Fever equal to or greater than 38°C.
   2. White blood cell count equal to or greater than 10,000/mm³.
   3. Inflammatory pelvic mass documented by clinical examination or sonogram or both.
   4. Culdocentesis reveals white blood cells and bacteria on Gram's stain of peritoneal fluid.
   5. Gram-negative intracellular diplococci found on Gram's stain of material from cervix.

---

mine a site of pregnancy or to confirm the presence of an adnexal mass. In the past, I have been enthusiastic about the use of needle culdocentesis to obtain peritoneal fluid from the afebrile patient suspected of having salpingitis. The presence of bacteria and white blood cells in this fluid indicated an intra-abdominal source of inflammation, and in most of the patients in which this test was employed the cause was usually an infected fallopian tube. I am currently less enthusiastic about this invasive diagnostic technique because of the patient discomfort associated with it. No matter how gently and skillfully I have done this procedure, all the patients have discomfort and none want it repeated. I still use it on occasion, but I have recently placed more emphasis on a vaginal smear. This is a noninvasive technique and is not uncomfortable. Westrom has noted that he has never had a patient with salpingitis on laparoscopic examination who did not have many inflammatory cells present on microscopic examination of the vaginal smear.[35] Clearly, vaginal inflammatory cells can be present in patients with local pathology such as cervicitis. There will be false-positive tests, but the absence of white cells in a vaginal smear of a patient with suspected salpingitis makes that diagnosis suspect to me. I treat many more women presenting with pelvic pain with antibiotics than I did in the past.

Although salpingitis is an important medical problem, there are few solid guidelines for therapy. This is unfortunate because this is such an important infection for women. Physicians would like to know what antibiotics are the most effective in preventing irreversible tubal damage, and these data are simply not available. There can be pitfalls in attempting to interpret the literature. For example, one recent compendium of retrospective studies showed that newer cephalosporins used alone had a statistically significant better cure rate (96.5% versus 83.6%) than penicilins or tetracyclines alone.[13] Before enthusiastically switching to these cephalosporin as the treatment of choice in patients with salpingitis, we have to factor in the observations of Sweet and co-workers.[29] These investigators did a follow-up study of patients with salpingitis successfully treated by all clinical measures with cefoxitin. To their dismay, they found many of these patients were culture positive for *Chlamydia* when an endometrial biopsy was used as the sample source for the culture. This is an important finding because *Chlamydia* can cause salpingitis, with the end result of blocked tubes and pelvic adhesion formation with minimal patient symptoms.[8] These patients treated with cefoxitin with an apparent clinical cure still had *Chlamydia* present, and this organism has the capability of causing tubal obstruction and pelvic adhesion formation. This observation has to be a consideration in the therapeutic strategies for these patients.

There are a number of important considerations for the physician taking care of the patient with suspected salpingitis. Pretreatment evaluation should include an endocervical culture for *Neisseria gonorrhea*. Although it is not a medical routine to date, an endometrial biopsy for a *Chlamydia* culture will be increasingly used in the future.[29] This technique has a higher yield of positive cultures than either an endocervical culture or the use of peritoneal fluid obtained by culdocentesis. The next sticking point for decision making is whether or not to admit these patients. Unfortunately, again, prospective studies have not been done to determine whether long-term treatment results are better when patients are admitted or treated as outpatients. Criteria for admission have been published and modified[28] (Table 25-8). There have been no prospective studies done to determine the accuracy of these guidelines, but one modification requires comment because it is so contrary to the policy on most gynecologic services. The newer guidelines do not favor admission for those patients with an elevated temperature as compared to those who are afebrile. An elevated

Table 25–8
Criteria for Admission of Patients to the Hospital for Treatment of Salpingitis

OLD	NEW (1982)	COMMENTS
1. The diagnosis is uncertain.	1. The diagnosis is uncertain.	1. Remains the same.
2. None.	2. Surgical emergencies such as appendicitis and ectopic pregnancy must be excluded.	2. New
3. A pelvic abcess is suspected.	3. A pelvic abcess is suspected.	3. Remains the same.
4. Upper peritoneal signs.	4. Severe illness precludes outpatient management.	4. Modified.
5. The patient is pregnant.	5. The patient is pregnant.	5. Remains the same.
6. Nausea and vomiting preclude oral antibiotics.	6. The patient is unable to follow or tolerate an outpatient regimen.	6. Modified.
7. Failure to respond to oral antibiotics within 48 hrs.	7. Patient has failed to respond to outpatient therapy.	7. Modified.
8. None.	8. Clinical followup after 48–72 hrs of antibiotic therapy cannot be arranged.	8. New
9. Temperature 38°C or higher.		9. Dropped.
10. Presence of an IUCD.		10. Dropped.

temperature is usually a factor favoring admission of the patient to the hospital. It is fortunate that this emphasis on the patient's being febrile has changed. Most patients with salpingitis in whom *Neisseria gonorrhea* is isolated are febrile. Compare this to the population pool of women with salpingitis in whom the majority are afebrile (see Table 25-6).[36] These febrile patients, culture positive for *Neisseria gonorrhea*, have been shown to usually respond to antibiotics and are the patients most likely to complete therapy with patent tubes.[37] The old emphasis on fever as a criteria for admission provided a hospital bed for the lowest-risk patient with the best possibility of a normal pelvis post treatment. This determination that the afebrile patient is a higher risk than the febrile patient with salpingitis flies in the face of our medical instincts, but is a fact. As many of these women as possible should be admitted to provide them the best opportunity for a long-term clinical care.

Definitive guidelines for the antibiotic treatment of patients with salpingitis have been provided by the Centers for Disease Control.[5] There is a familiar refrain in my criticism. These guidelines have been established without a prospective study to establish a database. They are based on justifiable concerns about *Neisseria gonorrhea*, particularly penicillin-resistant strains, and *Chlamydia trachomatis*. These are laudable. They would have more than theoretical weight if comparative studies had been done to confirm the effectiveness of the proposed regimens. I am particularly concerned about the outpatient treatment recommendations. The single shot of cefoxitin or the alternative antibiotics do not provide adequate treatment for gram-negative anaerobic bacteria, and neither does the long-term treatment with doxycycline. One dose of cefoxitin is not adequate, and too many strains of *Bacteroides fragilis* are resistant to doxycycline. I am concerned about the possibility of patients developing a pelvic abscess with this recommended regimen because I have seen such women on my service. An alternative approach would be to repeat the cefoxitin treatment over a number of days in an outpatient setting or to use oral metronidazole. The validity of these approaches will require prospective study.

There are a number of situations in the treatment of women with salpingitis in which operative intervention will be needed. Each is unique, and individual decisions need to be made. The patient with the intraperitoneal rupture of a tubo-ovarian abscess is a surgical emergency. There is evidence from older literature, before anaerobes were recognized as having the importance they do in pelvic abscesses, that delay in doing the surgery was accompanied by a higher mortality rate.[33] These patients can usually be easily recognized. They have a rigid abdomen, with diffuse peritoneal signs, and a pulse rate disproportionately high in comparison to the temperature. The presence of free intraperitoneal pus can be confirmed by a culdocentesis or a paracentesis. The treatment is surgical exploration, with lavage of the peritoneal cavity and the removal of pelvic organs. Fortunately, these cases are rarely seen now, and at least one factor is the greater awareness of gram-negative anaerobic bacteria by physicians when prescribing antibiotics for pelvic infections. The next category of patients who need operative exploration are those women who fail to respond to systemic antibiotics. Criteria change for the definition of failure. In 1987, the patient who is still markedly febrile after 72 to 96 hr of treatment and has shown no evidence of a response is a candidate for laparotomy. The guiding surgical philosophy in the care of these women is to do the least possible, compatible with the patient's long-term health. Unless a tubo-ovarian abscess is present, pelvic organs should be preserved. Even in the case of tubo-ovarian abscesses, at least one group has reported good results with aspiration of pus, and not surgical removal.[10] The final category is those patients who are taken to the operating room for intra-abdominal pathology and then are found to have acute salpingitis. This is a therapeutic morass for the uninitiated because these women have grossly abnormal pelvic findings and the natural reaction is to remove the diseased organs. Many of these inflamed fallopian tubes look much worse than the acutely inflamed appendix. Despite this appearance, removal of the tubes is not appropriate. These patients almost always will respond to systemic antibiotic therapy. The good surgeon should close the abdomen after getting cultures from the fimbria. No portion of the tube and uterus should be removed. These women will respond nicely to systemic antibiotics and have the chance for a pregnancy sometime in the future.

Hospital-Acquired Infections

The starting point for any discussion of hospital-acquired infection on the gynecology service is prevention. Clearly, prevention is a more laudable goal than the treatment of a postoperative infection. There have been two important foci on prevention. The first and most popular has been the use of prophylactic antibiotics. In gynecology, there has been widespread acceptance in the use of these antibiotics for vaginal hysterectomy, radical pelvic surgery, abdominal hysterectomy, reconstructive tubal surgery, and for hysterosalpingography. In these various clinical settings, prophylactic antibiotics have decreased both the frequency and severity of postoperative infections.

To provide a framework for the rational evaluation of the employment of prophylactic antibiotics, a number of guidelines have been proposed.[14] These can be a help to the physician trying to determine if prophylactic antibiotics should be used in an individual case or for a particular operation. Each guideline will be followed by a few explanatory statements:

1. The proposed operation should have a significant risk of postoperative site infections.—There are two components to this guideline. Operative site infection is important. If the problem on a gynecology service is pneumonia or urinary tract infections after pelvic surgery, systemic antibiotic prophylaxis is not the solution. The other component for discussion is the word significant. This usually implies frequency, for example, vaginal hysterectomy is frequently followed by a postoperative pelvic infection if prophylactic antibiotics are not employed. Infrequent infections can also be significant. For example, any infection following tubal reconstructive surgery would be a disastrous result for the patient involved.

2. The operation should be associated with endogenous bacterial contamination.—The bacterial contamination in most gynecologic

operations comes from the lower genital tract. Although surface preparation with an antiseptic solution prior to the operation will lower the number of bacteria, the count will increase again as more bacteria come to the surface of the vagina or from the endocervix. In one study, hot cautery of the cervix just prior to hysterectomy eliminated this source of contamination, and the postoperative infection rate was markedly reduced.[23]

3. The prophylactic antibiotic employed should have laboratory evidence of effectiveness against some of the contaminating microorganisms.—This is a vague guideline because the evidence with vaginal hysterectomy is that all prophylactic antibiotics are effective and have equivalent success rates. There may be variances among different antibiotics that were not picked up because the study population was too small, but, to date, there are no data to support the hypothesis that a broader spectrum antibiotic with good activity against gram-negative anaerobes will have better results in hysterectomy studies.

4. There should be clinical evidence of effectiveness of prophylatic antibiotics.—This is the bottom line for decision making. To date, there is unequivocal support from the literature for the use of prophylactic antibiotics in vaginal hysterectomy and radical pelvic surgery. There is a less than uniform favorable response to prophylactic antibiotics in abdominal hysterectomy. Some studies have shown no benefit, but it must be noted that no unfavorable results have been reported. A controlled prospective study has not been reported in patients undergoing reconstructive tubal surgery.

5. The prophylactic antibiotic should be present at the operative site sometime during the procedure.—This is a significant need. Burke demonstrated in the laboratory that systemic antibiotics were most effective when given just before or at the time of local bacterial contamination.[4] This has been borne out clinically as well. It is important that the physician prescribing prophylactic antibiotics be aware of the pharmacokinetics of the antibiotics prescribed. For example, one study of abdominal hysterectomy found morbidity increased when the procedure lasted 3 hr or more.[26] This long interval of time would mean an ineffective therapeutic level of antibiotic at the surgical site when the vagina, with its bacterial contamination, is opened near the end of the abdominal hysterectomy. There are two possible solutions. More frequent dosing at 1- to 2-hr intervals with short acting antibiotics until the operation is complete or the use of longer acting antibiotics such as cefazolin or cefotetan for the preoperative dose. Prospective studies with large numbers of patients will be needed to see if this improves results.

6. A short course of prophylaxis should be employed.—There are two components to this guideline. It works. This is important in these days of concern about medical costs. In addition, it avoids toxic effects of antibiotics related to long-term prophylaxis, such as pseudomembranous enterocolitis.[17]

7. First-line antibiotics should not be used for prophylaxis.—This is theoretically acceptable because we want our new broader spectrum or more effective agents saved for treatment and not used routinely for prophylaxis. To date, this has caused no problem, because there have not been better results with any single antibiotic agent used for prophylaxis in gynecology.

8. The benefits should outweigh the risks.—To date, major gynecologic surgery in which the vagina is part of the operative field seems safer with prophylactic antibiotics. Other individual indications, such as tubal reconstruction surgery, can be justified in individual cases.

Other preventive measures can lower postoperative infection. Cruse has demonstrated a number of components of preoperative and intraoperative care that result in a lower postoperative abdominal wound infection rate. Preoperatively, patients should not be shaved the night before surgery. Intraoperatively, plaster adhesive skin drapes should not be used, a hot cautery knife should not be employed, and drains should not be used in the operative wounds. There is some controversy about drains. One study had good results when closed suction drains were used in obese women, in which the site of exit of the drain was separate from the wound.[22] These findings should all be part of the preoperative planning in the gynecologic patients who need a laparotomy. Prevention is clearly a better strategy than the best of any therapeutic regimen. Despite all of these efforts, some patients will develop a postoperative infection and require treatment.

The cornerstone of care of the febrile postoperative gynecologic patient is to establish a diagnosis. Focusing on a site of infection makes any subsequent therapeutic efforts much more rational. There is no quick and easy fix on such patients. They require an initial thorough physical examination in an attempt to determine an infection site, and the commitment to repeat these examinations if the patient is not responding to the initial therapy prescribed. This must be stressed because the examination of these women for a postoperative site infection can be very difficult. There is much induration in the pelvic examination of the normal posthysterectomy patient, so that differentiation of normal postoperative response and pelvic cellulitis requiring antibiotics is difficult. Also, wound collections, either at the vaginal cuff or in the abdominal wound, may not be present at the examination with the initial temperature elevation, but they then become apparent later. In addition to the general and pelvic examination, other evaluations may be helpful. Complete blood counts to help to determine the extent of the operative and postoperative blood loss, and the evaluation of the white blood cell count and differential can focus attention on possibilities of diagnosis. A culture can be helpful later, if there is a failure of response to therapy, and a positive urine culture can be diagnostic and can direct therapy toward the urinary tract. If the patient has a mass on pelvic examination or has persistence of fever postoperatively, a number of very good and highly sophisticated imaging techniques can be employed to help determine the diagnosis.

The therapy of postoperative site infections is straightforward. They have the characteristics of mixed bacterial infections, in which anaerobic bacteria are very important. A constant focus in therapy is operative drainage of a collection. The patient with a vaginal cuff collection or an abdominal wound infection is better served by drainage rather than systemic antibiotics. In the patient with a postoperative pelvic infection, the therapy should be directed toward gram-negative anaerobic organisms. Clindamycin or metronidazole in combination with an aminoglycoside is a good choice, as well as a second-generation cephalosporin like cefoxitin or one of the newer penicillins, piperacillin or mezlocillin alone. Imipinem/cilastin also shows great promise. Most patients respond quickly to therapy. All of these antibiotics, alone or in combination, have some organisms that are not susceptible. The physician should be aware of these gaps; the persistently febrile patient may require an addition or change of antibiotics. One concern in the past with the persistently febrile patient was septic pelvic thrombophlebitis, which required heparin in addition to antibiotics.[16] With our increased awareness of the importance of gram-negative anaerobes in postoperative pelvic infections, the problem that seems initiated by anaerobic bacteria is seldom seen these days.

REFERENCES

1. Bartlett JG. Recent developments in the management of anaerobic infections. Rev Infect Dis 1983;5:235.
2. Bartlett JG, Louie TJ, Gorbach SL, et al. Therapeutic efficacy of 29 antimicrobial regimens in experimental intra-abdominal sepsis. Rev Infect Dis 1981;3:535.
3. Brook I. Encapsulated anaerobic bacteria in synergistic infections. Micro Rev 1986;50:452.
4. Burke JF. The effective period of preventive antibiotic action in experimental incisions and dermal lesions. Surgery 1961;50:161.
5. Centers for Disease Control. 1985 STD treatment guidelines. MMWR 1985;34(suppl):1S.
6. Chow AW, Marshall JE, Guze LB. A double blind comparison of clindamycin with penicillin plus chloramphenicol in treatment of septic abortion. J Infect Dis 1977;135:S35.
7. Cruse P. Wound infection surveillance. Rev Infect Dis 1981;3:374.
8. Gump DW, Gibson M, Ashikaga T. Evidence of prior pelvic inflammatory disease and its relationship to *Chlamydia trachomatis* antibody and intrauterine contraceptive device use in infertile women. Am J Obstet Gynecol 1983;146:153.
9. Hager WD, Eschenbach DA, Spence MR, et al. Criteria for diagnosis and grading of salpingitis. Obstet Gynecol 1983;61:113.
10. Henry-Suchet J, Solen A, Loffredo V. Laparoscopic treatment of tubo-ovarian abscesses. J Reprod Med 1984;29:579.
11. Jacobson , Westrom L. Objecturized diagnosis of acute pelvic inflammatory disease. Am J Obstet Gynecol 1969;105:1088.
12. Landers DV, Sweet RL. Tubo-ovarian abscess: Contemporary approach to management. Rev Infect Dis 1983;5:876.
13. Ledger WJ. Selection of antimicrobial agents for treatment of infections of the female genital tract. Rev Infect Dis 1983;5:598.
14. Ledger WJ, Gee C, Lewis WP. Guidelines for antibiotic prophylaxis in gynecology. Am J Obstet Gynecol 1975;121:1038.
15. Ledger WJ, Norman M, Geo C, et al. Bacteremia on an obstetric-gynecologic service. Am J Obstet Gynecol 1975;121:205.

16. Ledger WJ, Peterson EP. The use of heparin in the management of pelvic thrombophlebitis. Surg Gynecol Obstet 1970;131:1115.
17. Ledger WJ, Puttler OL. Death from pseudomembranous enterocolitis. Obstet Gynecol 1975;45:609.
18. Ledger WJ, Sweet RL, Headington JT. *Bacteroides* species as a cause of severe infections in gynecologic patients. Surg Gynecol Obstet 1976;133:837.
19. Lip J, Burgoyne X. Cervical and peritoneal bacterial flora associated with salpingitis. Obstet Gynecol 1966;28:561.
20. Mardh PA, Ripa T, Svenson L, et al. *Chlamydia trachomatis* infection in patients with acute salpingitis. N Engl J Med 1977;296:1377.
21. Moller BR, Ahrons S, Laurin J, et al. Pelvic infection after elective abortion associated with *Chlamydia trachomatis.* Obstet Gynecol 1982;59:210.
22. Morrow CP, Hernandez WL, Townsend DE, et al. Pelvic celiotomy in the obese patient. Am J Obstet Gynecol 1977;127:335.
23. Osborne NG, Wright RC, Dubay M. Pre-operative hot conization of the cervix: a possible method to reduce post-operative febrile morbidity following vaginal hysterectomy. Am J Obstet Gynecol 1979;133:374.
24. Rosenfeld DL, Seidman SM, Bronson RA, et al. Unsuspected chronic pelvic inflammatory disease in the infertile female. Fertil Steril 1983;39:44.
25. Rotheram EA, Schick SJ. Nonclostridial anaerobic bacteria in septic abortion. Am J Med 1969;46:80.
26. Shapiro M, Munoz A, Tager IB, et al. Risk factors for infection at the operative site after abdominal or vaginal hysterectomy. N Engl J Med 1982;307:1661.
27. Studdiford WE, Douglas GW. Placental bacteremia: a significant finding in septic abortion accompanied by vascular collapse. Am J Obstet Gynecol 1956;71:842.
28. Sweet RL. Diagnosis and treatment of salpingo-oophoritis Mediguide to Ob/Gyn 1983;2:1.
29. Sweet RL, Schacter J, Robbie MO. Failure of beta-lactam antibiotics to eradicate *Chlamydia trachomatis* in the endometrium despite apparent clinical care of acute salpingitis. JAMA 1983;250:2641.
30. Swenson RM, Michaelson PC, Daly MJ, et al. Anaerobic bacterial infections of the female genital tract. Obstet Gynecol 1973;42:538.
31. Tally FP, Cuchural GJ Jr, Jacobus NV, et al. Nationwide study of the susceptibility of the *Bacteroides fragilis* group in the United States. Antimicrob Agents Chemother 1985;28:675.
32. Tally FP, Cuchural GJ Jr, Jacobus NV, et al. Susceptibility of the *Bacteroides fragilis* in the United States in 1981. Antimicrob Agents Chemother 1983;25:536.
33. Vermeeren J, Telinde R. Intra-abdominal rupture of pelvic absceses. Am J Obstet Gynecol 1954;68:402.
34. Weinstein WM, Onderdonk AB, Bartlett JG, et al. Experimental intra abdominal abscesses in rats: development of an experimental model. Infect Immun 1974;10:1250.
35. Westrom L. Clinical manifestations and diagnosis of pelvic inflammatory disease. J Repro Med 1983;28:703.
36. Westrom L. Incidence, prevalence and trends of pelvic inflammatory disease and its consequences in industrialized countries. Am J Obstet Gynecol 1980;138:880.
37. Westrom L. Effect of acute pelvic inflammatory disease on fertility. Am J Obstet Gynecol 1975;121:707.

INDEX

Page numbers followed by *f* indicate figures; those followed by *t* indicate tabular material.

ISBN 0-397-50735-6

90000

9 780397 507351